THE DISABLED WOMAN'S GUIDE TO PREGNANCY AND BIRTH

THE DISABLED WOMAN'S GUIDE TO PREGNANCY AND BIRTH

JUDITH ROGERS, OTR, ACCE

*D*emos

Demos Medical Publishing, LLC, 386 Park Avenue South, New York, New York 10016

Visit our website at www.demosmedpub.com

The first edition of this book was published in 1991 under the title, Mother-To-Be: A Guide to Pregnancy and Birth for Women with Disabilities, by Judith Rogers and Molleen Matsumura.

The purpose of this book is to provide information to readers; it is meant to be a guide and does not provide medical advice. Always consult your doctor for medical advice.

Library of Congress Cataloging-in-Publication Data

Rogers, Judi.
  The disabled woman's guide to pregnancy and birth / by Judith Rogers.—2nd ed.
      p. cm.
  "First edition of this book was published in 1991 under the title,
Mother-to-be : a guide to pregnancy and birth for women with disabilities, by Judith
Rogers and Molleen Matsumura."
  Includes bibliographical references and index.
  ISBN 1-932603-08-5 (alk. paper)
  1. Pregnancy in women with disabilities—Popular works. 2. Pregnancy—
Complications—Popular works. I. Rogers, Judi. Mother-to-be. II. Matsumura,
Molleen. III. Title.
  RG580.P48R64 2006
  618.2'0087--dc22
                                                              2005007823

ISBN 1-932603-08-5

Made in the United States of America

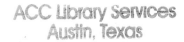

I dedicate this book to the source of its inspiration:
my children, Anya and Ari.
I also want to thank all of the women I interviewed,
who freely gave of their time and of themselves.

"I wanted to have a child so I could be part of the flow of history."

MICHELLE

Contents

Preface   xi

Acknowledgments   xv

1. Meet the Experts: The Experiences of Ninety Women   1

2. Emotional Concerns in Having Children   33

3. The Interaction Between Pregnancy and Disability   41

4. Parenting with a Disability   67

5. Getting Your Health Care Needs Met   83

6. Eating for Two: Nutrition in Pregnancy   115

7. Getting in Shape: Exercises for Pregnancy   131

8. Nine Months of Change: The First Trimester   155

9. Nine Months of Change: The Second Trimester   195

10. Nine Months of Change: The Third Trimester   221

11. The Main Event: Labor and Delivery   257

12. Another Way into the World: Caesarean Section   311

13.   After Delivery: The Postpartum Period   343

Appendix A: Pregnancy Tables for Ninety Women   397

Appendix B: Pregnancy Discomfort Tables   463

Appendix C: Diet Plan and Suggested Food Lists   477

Appendix D: Resource Directory   491

References   503

Index   511

Preface

I HAVE BEEN DISABLED SINCE BIRTH. Being disabled meant being without a role model. There was no person or book I could turn to for information about crucial issues. Most of the writing about disabilities focused on disabled children, and this continues to be true today. Yet, a disabled child grows into a disabled adult with questions of her own. In recent years, there has been greater acceptance of the sexuality of disabled people and more attention has been paid to their needs. The next step has to be validation of the reproductive capacity of disabled women. This validation is especially important now that social services and special adaptive equipment offer new solutions to the problems of pregnancy, labor, delivery, and child-rearing.

When I became pregnant, I again found that there was hardly any literature concerning my particular needs. I searched the abundant material on pregnancy, labor, and delivery, but found little that was relevant to the concerns of the disabled. Most of what was available was limited to single examples in technical journals, personal accounts, and vague generalizations.

At that time I was working at the Center for Independent Living, an organization run for and by disabled people. Finally, I had found role models and peers to share my concerns with, including one co-worker who had been pregnant. At the same time I was receiving calls from other pregnant, disabled women with unanswered questions. I began to see that the best way for women with disabilities to find answers would be to share their experiences. In order to gather as much useful information as possible, I compiled a questionnaire that was based on a series of in-depth conferences with friends and colleagues. I posted notices in pediatric clinics, centers for the disabled, and at disability conferences. Some people heard about the project by word of mouth. Finally, thirty-six women answered the questionnaires in personal interviews. Their responses are at the heart of this book.

While I was conducting the interviews, I supplemented my knowledge about disability by learning more about pregnancy. I trained as a birthing instructor and taught for 4 years. I added to my practical knowledge of pregnancy by questioning my students about their experiences and by attending numerous births. After the interviews of mothers with disabilities were completed, Molleen Matsumura, my co-author on the first edition, and I conducted formal research on pregnancy, disability, and the interaction of pregnancy and disability.

Since the first edition was published in 1991, more has been written on pregnancy and disability. Moreover, working at Through the Looking Glass (TLG) has been invaluable for many reasons. TLG has given me the opportunity to have contact with disabled parents. In addition to doing research and creating adaptive equipment, TLG is the foremost agency in the country conducting research and providing direct services for parents with disabilities. An extensive review of the literature, and interviews with experts in the fields of obstetrics, genetic counseling, physical therapy, nutrition, nursing, psychiatry, neurology, emergency medicine, anesthesiology, and rehabilitation were done for both editions.

All of the women I interviewed were physically disabled. Some of them had a hidden disability, such as thoracic outlet syndrome or fibromyalgia. They represented a true cross section of the community. They were married, divorced, or single mothers; some were full-time homemakers, professionals, white-collar workers, or women needing public assistance; they were lesbian and heterosexual; and there were women of different races and religions. Some of the women who were interviewed for the first edition had given birth 30 years before, but most of the women in this second edition were new mothers at the time the interviews were conducted. Most interviews took place over the telephone. I was careful to include women with a variety of disabilities. The degree of disability varied among those with the same diagnosis. It is interesting that there was more similarity among women with the same degree of disability than among women with the same type of disability.

The most important lesson to be learned from this study is that disabled pregnant women have much the same concerns as all pregnant women. This became even clearer when Molleen, who is able-bodied, kept commenting as she read the material I had gathered, "That's exactly how I felt when I was pregnant!"

Although this book includes much information that will be important to women with disabilities, any pregnant woman may benefit from the problem-solving approaches and specific solutions suggested here. (A personal favorite is sleeping on satin sheets to prevent leg cramps.)

Careful attention has been given to differentiating between the changes and discomforts that are common in pregnancy, and those that are disability-related. In general, disabled women experience many of the same changes as able-bodied women, but they are often unsure whether what they are feeling is disability-related, which can be a source of anxiety.

Health professionals will also find this book valuable because they will learn about the problems their students and patients have been hesitant to express. Some of the information presented here may also suggest new directions for research. Often, simply sharing this book with patients can be helpful.

The opening chapter describes the pregnancies of the women who were interviewed, and underscores how much women with different disabilities have in common. Included are simple explanations of the different types of disability, and descriptions of the physical changes each woman experienced during each of her pregnancies. Finally, it offers the insights the women shared about pregnancy and disability, including their ideas for building cooperation between the pregnant woman and her health care team, and their insistence that a pregnant woman with disabilities be seen primarily as a prospective mother.

Chapters 2 through 4 discuss the many questions that must be answered by a woman who is considering having children. It examines not only the effects on the health of mother and child, but also other practical and emotional concerns, such as "How would I feel about giving birth to a disabled child?" and "How will having children affect my marriage?" The suggested questions that women can ask themselves, their doctors, and their counselors are just as important as medical information. They will enable each woman to make the decisions that are best for her.

Chapter 5 contains advice on how to select a doctor and hospital, what specialists might need to be consulted, and how to assure cooperation and communication among care providers. Again, questions are presented that women can ask in order to make sure their needs are met.

Chapters 6 and 7 focus on prenatal nutrition and exercise and give suggestions on how to maintain health and comfort. The chapter on nutrition explains the role of various nutrients, giving attention to the special concerns of disabled women. Also included is an explanation as to why it is important to gain weight. The chapter on exercise contains exercises that have been adapted for varying levels of disability, so even a woman with limited mobility can maintain flexibility and good circulation.

Chapters 8 through 10 on the three trimesters of pregnancy discuss the physical changes of pregnancy, what to expect during office visits, pregnancy discomforts and ways of coping with them, fetal development, routine and special medical procedures, possible complications, and emotional concerns. These chapters also include a discussion of the special concerns for each trimester. For example, the chapter on the second trimester includes suggestions for choosing a good birthing class. The special concerns of disabled women are addressed throughout the chapters; for example, the different ways some of the interviewees managed to measure their weight, and how to instruct medical office staff in assisting with a transfer from wheelchair to examining table. Again, there are lists of questions that women can ask to help them understand what is happening and get the information they need to choose appropriate medical care.

Chapter 11 describes the course of labor and delivery, ways of coping with the discomforts of labor, and possible complications and how they might be treated. It begins by explaining how to recognize that labor has begun, including a description of the symptoms of labor that might be experienced by women who have reduced sensation. Included are suggestions for relieving muscle spasms and finding alternate positions for giving birth.

Caesarean birth is covered in Chapter 12, and may be reassuring reading for many women with disabilities, who often assume that they will have to give birth surgically. This chapter begins with an explanation of the reasons for caesarean delivery, including a discussion of the concerns of disabled women who are considering this procedure. Next is a description of what happens during caesarean delivery, including what the mother can expect to feel, what happens in the recovery room just after surgery, and recovery and self-care during the weeks following caesarean birth. Special attention is given to the effect of caesarean delivery on mobility and other disability symptoms. The chapter closes with a discussion of vaginal birth after caesarean section, including the comments of two interviewees who gave birth in this way.

The closing chapter describes what women experience during the postpartum period, the 6 weeks after birth during which their bodies return to a pre-pregnant state. It discusses the usual physical changes, variations that may be experienced by women with disabilities, signs and symptoms of infection and other problems, suggestions for self-care, and information about birth control methods. Some of the most important changes at this time are psychological and there is considerable discussion of these issues, including changes in the sexual relationship. This chapter also contains information that will help women decide whether to breast- or bottle-feed their babies, and suggestions for breast care and breast-feeding. It ends with a description of some of TLG's research on equipment, and techniques for making childcare easier for parents with disabilities.

While this book is meant to be a practical guide to pregnancy, the author hopes, most of all, that it will encourage women with disabilities to enjoy their pregnancies. Most of the interviewees were glad they had their children—whether or not they would choose to become pregnant again. Pregnancy is an exciting time. If this book helps you understand the process, if it leads you to try other people's ideas and inspires you to try some of your own, if it can be like a friend who is sharing your excitement—then it is doing what it is meant to do.

Judi Rogers

Acknowledgments

I ACKNOWLEDGE THROUGH THE LOOKING GLASS for providing me with vital experiences and information on parenting, as well as giving me an opportunity to have contact with thirty-four of the ninety women.

I also acknowledge the wonderful support I received from my husband and friends, who were both editors and consultants. Their names are in alphabetical order, because they all made important contributions: Liane Abrams; Barbara Finnin; Pam Inbar-Hansen, MSPT; Johanna Kraemer; Stephanie Miyashiro; Helen Neville; John Neville; Corbett O'Toole; Ken Stanton, RN PhD; and Dr. Michelle Wolfe.

Several other people were also superb consultants: Dr. Selma Calmes; Dr. Graham Creasey; Dr. Pat Dhar; Dr. Eleanor Drey; Elizabeth Gray; George Hage, OT; Dr. Florence Haseltine; Dr. C. Lee; Dr. Judy McKenna McDougal; Dr. Norm Moscow; Dr. Richard Penn; Sid Wolinski and Gabi Marcus from DRA (Disabled Rights Advocates); Dr. Sandy Welner; and Dr. Jennifer Zeidberg. I would like to thank my sister Katherine Rogers for her wonderful drawings.

Thanks to these friends who gave me support: Jackie Brand, Darlene Bubis, Neil Cook, Alicia Conteras, Alexandra Enders, Anya Freedman, Rivka Greenberg, Suzanne Levine, Marcy Mendelson, Lisa Newman, Pam Ormsby, Pam Fadem, Kathy Simpson, and Nicolee Borsen.

Meet the Experts: The Experiences of Ninety Women

THIS BOOK TELLS the stories of ninety women with disabilities who chose to have children and who were willing to share their experiences of pregnancy through the postpartum period. Unlike most women, who experience social and emotional pressure to *have* children, disabled women are under pressure *not* to have children. Yet, disabled women feel the same needs as other women to have children. I support their right to choose motherhood, and offer these primary recommendations:

Take A Positive Approach

The first recommendation concerns the importance of taking a positive approach to the pregnancy of a disabled woman. All of the interviewees encourage other disabled women to have children. For example, in spite of postpartum exacerbations of symptoms related to thoracic outlet syndrome (TOS), Taryn Dion[1] encouraged other women with TOS to become mothers. But she stressed that it is important to get help immediately after birth. Moreover, Taryn Dion thought it was important to have a realistic image of mothering. The interviewees did not deny the potential for problems. Sharon spoke for the whole group when she said, "It may take a toll on your body. You will have to decide if you want to make the sacrifice." As Portia commented, "Pregnancy, labor, and delivery are just the steps you go through to reach the goal of being a parent." Several women felt they had been too fearful and stressed the importance of enjoying pregnancy. Others commented that after they had learned what to expect during a first pregnancy they worried less during subsequent pregnancies.

---

[1] Throughout this book we make reference to the ninety women by pseudonym. They will be individually introduced later in Chapter 1; their detailed pregnancy histories can be found in Appendix A.

In general, the women who were interviewed said they had expected more problems and discomforts than they actually experienced; some even felt better than usual while they were pregnant. The problems that many of these women experienced were not substantially different from those experienced by other women, although mobility impairment was worse for disabled women.

Make Pregnancy the Primary Concern

The second recommendation is that a woman with disabilities be seen primarily as a pregnant woman—both in her own mind and in the mind of her physician.

In their advice to obstetricians, many of the interviewees emphasized their desire to be treated "just like everyone else." For example, Arlene said, "Be open-minded. I am just like everyone else: a woman who is having a baby." Cheryl said, "Treat me like a woman first, and then secondly as a woman with a disability." Much of the advice our interviewees offered to other disabled women centered on ordinary pregnancy concerns: "Try to have your baby vaginally" (Celeste). "Get two people to go in as labor coaches. That way one person can be a back-up" (Marsha). "I found the holistic approach helpful" (Samantha). "Find one nurse who will stay with you. I had my baby that way and I loved it" (Heather).

Yet, some women also expressed the feeling that their pregnancies were different from those experienced by able-bodied women. Some of the advice they offered stressed disability-related concerns: "Consult with specialists other than an obstetrician about the woman's disabilities" (Sylvia). "Hold an in-service training for the obstetrics department and invite some disabled women to come in" (Stacy). "Even if you are only slightly disabled, make sure all the doctors involved know you are disabled" (Priscilla). "Be aware of your limitations and learn about adaptations" (Pam).

Use the Team Approach

The third recommendation is that physicians follow the advice of disabled women and use a team approach to pregnancy and birth.

The pregnant woman, her obstetrician, and the disability specialists should all contribute to planning her care. Cooperation among the obstetrician, disability specialists, and the mother-to-be will ensure the best care. Holly said, "Both of my obstetricians called my neurosurgeon and made sure of what they should be looking for. By the time I got pregnant the second time, I had done a lot of my database work and was quite knowledgeable about pregnancy. I had my own ideas about what to do or not. My doctor was willing to listen to me, even though I'm not an M.D. He was willing to take my suggestions into consideration and consult a high-risk obstetrician. He said to me, 'I'm the expert in delivering babies, but you are the expert on *hydrocephalus* and pregnancy.' He knew I had studied quite a bit about it and he was open to my ideas. The doctor did something I thought was important—he contacted all of his on-call partners (only one worked in his office) and told them the whole story about my hydrocephalus and what to be careful about."

Some of the interviewees suggested additional training for hospital personnel. Many of them had problems with postpartum nursing staff, which seemed to have difficulty imagining a disabled woman taking care of her baby. It is crucial that hospital staff be aware of how they can foster a "can do" attitude. An in-service can potentially help both the mother and hospital staff to become more confident. It is important to remember that supportive staff can help relieve a mother's frustration and help her cope using practical solutions.

Create the Best Possible Outcome

Sensitivity and education are critical in preparing for pregnancy in advance: "Set up a support system before your baby is born" (Clara). "Get a physical exam before you get pregnant" (Hilary). "Have arrangements made before delivery for things like diapers, baby clothes, and furniture. Fill your freezer with enough dinners to last 3 months" (Stephanie). "Don't wait until you're in labor to find out how a medication could affect you" (Priscilla).

Introduction to the Interviewees

The women who were interviewed will be introduced in alphabetical order, according to their disability. The interviews were confidential and, therefore, each woman has been given a pseudonym that has the same initial as her type of disability. For example, Clara has cerebral palsy and Samantha has a spinal cord dysfunction. Because there are many disabilities that begin with the letter "S," they have been subdivided into the following categories: *spinal cord injury, spinal bifida, spinal tumor,* and *sacral agenesis.* All of the interviewees whose pseudonyms begin with "S" are usually affected by numbness and paralysis, as well as urinary tract infections. To avoid confusion in the pseudonym code, the interviewees with short stature are listed under "D" for "dwarfism," even though this is not the politically correct term. Five women were not fully interviewed but a few significant details of their stories have been included.

The tables in Appendix A list the specific physical changes each woman experienced during pregnancy. As a group, they reveal a broad range of possible responses to pregnancy. The tables cannot be used to predict what any one woman will experience, but rather show the kinds of changes an individual woman experienced. The experiences will differ, even for women with the same type of disability. For example, a few women with arthritis experienced an increase in joint pain during pregnancy, although most experienced a decrease. Variations such as these are the subject of continuing research and in the future there may be information that will help women better anticipate what they are likely to experience during pregnancy.

During their interviews, the women were asked to describe the changes they experienced. The tables emphasize discomforts rather than positive changes in order to help women plan for the discomforts of pregnancy. Many of the interviewees commented that they were delighted to find that for once their bodies were working right. They enjoyed looking pregnant, having larger breasts, being able to feel fetal movement, or being able to carry a baby to term.

The Women: Their Pregnancies and their Disabilities

AMNIOTIC BAND SYNDROME

Amniotic band syndrome is a disability that occurs in utero. There is a tear in the amniotic sac and strands of amniotic tissue either wrap around or attach to one or more limbs. These strands act like rubber bands. One or more extremities and/or digits do not develop in some fetuses.

Amanda

Amanda has amniotic band syndrome; her left arm ends at the elbow and her right arm is fused at the elbow. Her right hand has two fingers. Her left leg ends at the knee and her right leg is full length. She wears a prosthesis on her left leg and has arthritis in her left hip. Amanda was born with a type of hip problem that later causes some problems with wearing a leg prosthesis. Amanda primarily used crutches prior to her first pregnancy. She used a wheelchair infrequently prior to the birth of her first child. After the birth of her first child, she found that using a wheelchair to take care of her baby was easier. Amanda sometimes used her crutches after her first child was older. Since her second pregnancy, she has used a manual wheelchair full-time for mobility. She has found that using the chair is easier for both mobility and taking care of children. In retrospect, she said, "I would have been more selective about using crutches if I had known what I know now; for example, three-mile walks on crutches are not a good idea, even if you can physically do it. I never recovered all of the balance and flexibility that I had before my second pregnancy. In fact, I am going to physical therapy to see if I can regain more, as it has not returned on its own."

AMPUTATION

Amputations have many causes, but the most common causes in women of pregnancy age are cancer and traumatic injury.

Amy

Amy was in an accident that not only resulted in a *bilateral lower amputation*, but she also broke her hip, pelvis, sacrum, and wrist. She also had a head injury. One of her legs is amputated above the knee and the other below the knee. She had trouble with transfers and her balance was affected during pregnancy. She had increased phantom and back pain. She experienced headaches and her backache worsened after her pregnancy.

Andrea

Andrea's leg was amputated at the hip because of cancer. She usually uses crutches. She has *carpal tunnel syndrome* affecting both of her hands that started during her first pregnancy. This problem continued long after both of her pregnancies. She has arthritis in her shoulders that started after her second pregnancy. Her balance also got worse during her first pregnancy.

Allison

Allison's leg was amputated below the knee following a car accident. She used a prosthesis for 10 years prior to getting pregnant. She was diagnosed with arthritis in both knees during the second trimester of her first pregnancy. Allison said, "The arthritis in my right knee was the most unbearable part of it. During both pregnancies I experienced dull pain during the night and my right knee locked into position. For example, when I was curled up asleep and tried to shift positions, my knee would be locked and it would be really painful to straighten it out. This problem went away after physical therapy and when I began taking anti-inflammatory drugs after pregnancy. It only happens rarely now." Allison needed a new prosthesis after her second pregnancy. (See "Heather Ann" in Appendix A.)

ARTHROGRYPOSIS

Arthrogryposis is a condition that has different causes and affects the joints to different degrees. At least 30 percent of the cases of arthrogryposis have a genetic origin. The causes of the remaining 70 percent of cases vary greatly. There are two types of arthrogryposis. In *neuropathic* arthrogryposis, nerve function is damaged and, because the nerves cannot stimulate the muscles properly, muscle function is indirectly affected. In *myopathic* arthrogryposis, which is more common, the muscles are directly affected. In either case, arthrogryposis is characterized by multiple muscle contractures that limit movement of the joints. In some individuals, only a few joints are affected. In the most severe cases, nearly every joint is involved, including those of the spine and the jaw. The degree to which the range of motion is limited in the affected joints also varies among individuals. The affected muscles cannot develop normally; instead they atrophy (decreasing in mass and strength).

Arianna

Arianna does not know her type of arthrogryposis, although most of her joints are affected. She had her legs amputated below the knee. Her left hip is fused and she cannot lift her arms over her head.

Arlene

Arlene's myopathic arthrogryposis, which is not hereditary, affects all of her limbs. Her arm and leg muscles have atrophied and she has *lordosis* (swayback). She uses a wheelchair. Her usual disability-related problems include heartburn, poor circulation in the legs, and a persistent *decubitus ulcer* (pressure sore) under her thigh caused by inadequate padding in her wheelchair seating. Arlene had two miscarriages, possibly due to poor circulation. She delivered a child by caesarean section.

CEREBRAL PALSY

Cerebral palsy (CP) is a group of conditions caused by damage to the motor area of the brain. The damage can be prenatal, the result of birth trauma, a syndrome, or damage sustained during childhood. Symptoms vary depending on the site of the injury. From one to four limbs may be affected, trunk and head control may be affected as well. The different types of cerebral palsy are distinguished by the muscle tone and pattern of movement of the affected limb(s). A person may have more than one type of cerebral palsy. The three most common types are:

Spastic cerebral palsy. This condition involves increased muscle tone, which results in the affected limb being stiff. In *spastic diplegic (paraplegia)*, only the legs are involved. The legs are generally adducted (held close together). When the person walks, her legs tend to cross in a manner called "scissors gait." In *spastic hemiplegia*, the leg and arm on one side are involved. The arm is generally held rigidly in a *semiflexed* (bent) position.

Athetoid cerebral palsy. The major characteristics of this condition are involuntary, irregular, slow movements of the affected body part.

Ataxic cerebral palsy. This condition involves a wide-based, unsteady gait and, often, reduced manual dexterity.

Mixed. A person may have a combination of two types (such as spastic and athetoid).

Caitlin

Caitlin has left spastic hemiplegia (one side of her body is affected); although she feels that her right side is affected as well. Caitlin has a *mullerian anomaly* that is rare and happens during fetal development. During normal embryonic development, fusion occurs between the two mullerian ducts to form the vagina, cervix, and uterine body. Although this can result in various abnormalities, it caused Caitlin's uterus to have a unilateral maturation and incomplete development of the ovarian duct on one side. This can also lead to urinary tract problems that are unrelated to cerebral palsy. She has two children.

Carla

Carla learned that she does not have cerebral palsy, but an extremely rare inherited condition known as *familial spastic paresis.* The two conditions have the same signs, and Carla was diagnosed as having cerebral palsy until some of her relatives developed similar signs and the genetic basis of their conditions were identified. Carla commented, "I'm so glad this information will be included in your book so that other people will know they might have an inherited problem." Her walk is similar to those who have spastic diplegia cerebral palsy. She can walk two to five blocks and never used a wheelchair before pregnancy. Her usual disability-related problems include a limited walking range, back problems, difficulty in lifting and carrying, and muscle cramps.

Carla felt that on the whole, her second pregnancy was easier than her first because she had a better idea of what to expect and took a more flexible approach to her problems. She also said, "Taking care of a little kid had gotten me into better shape." Looking back on her pregnancies, Carla commented, "I would have been more comfortable if I had started using a wheelchair in the second trimester."

Carol

Carol has mild diplegic spastic and *ataxic* cerebral palsy. She used a cane to walk after her first pregnancy and during her second pregnancy. Her legs felt "rubbery" after the delivery of her first child which may have been caused by the epidural. This feeling diminished as she gradually stopped breast-feeding.

Celeste

All four of Celeste's limbs are affected with spasticity. Her hand movements are somewhat awkward and she walks with a scissors gait. She used crutches before and during pregnancy, but now she uses a wheelchair. Celeste's usual disability-related symptoms include edema of her ankles and feet, and muscle cramps in her hips.

Charlotte

Charlotte has a combination of athetoid and spastic cerebral palsy on her right side. Her right arm is less affected than her right hand. She often experiences spasms in both her right arm and leg. She used a three-prong cane to help with her balance during pregnancy. Charlotte took baclofen to help control her spasms prior to her pregnancy. After delivery, during which she was given an epidural, she experienced more spasms and tried both Botox® and phenol shots, which helped with her spasms.

Cheryl

All four of Cheryl's limbs are slightly affected; although somewhat more on the left than on the right. Her balance is poor because she has both ataxia and athetosis. Cheryl's usual disability-related problems include tension in her hands and abdominal muscles.

Chloe

Chloe has athetoid cerebral palsy that affects her body in all four of her limbs, trunk, and head. She also has a speech involvement and *scoliosis* (an S-shaped curvature of the spine). Chloe had open-heart surgery in childhood. She stopped being able to roll over during her pregnancy, and her respiration was affected.

Christina

Christina has spastic diplegia and walks without assistive equipment. Her usual disability-related problems are muscle spasms and backaches. She had one miscarriage due to *placenta previa*, which was not caused by her disability.

Clara

Clara has a combination of athetoid and spastic cerebral palsy on her left side. Her left arm is slightly affected and can be used as a helper. She walks with a limp and often twists her left ankle, sometimes falling. Clara's usual disability-related problems include infrequent muscle spasms, edema of her ankles if she walks too far in hot weather, and infrequent backaches.

Corrine

Corrine has spastic cerebral palsy on her left side. Her usual disability-related problems include aching in her upper back and difficulty walking. She has problems walking because it is hard for her to maintain her balance, and she frequently trips and falls. She rides a bicycle rather than walking for long distances.

DEGENERATIVE DISC DISEASE

Degenerative disc disease can happen in any part of the spine. There can be changes in the individual discs that cause pain from a damaged disc. This condition is quite variable in its nature and severity. With age, all people exhibit changes in their discs consistent with degeneration, but not all people develop symptoms (1).

Deirdre

Deirdre had a *laminectomy* and *discectomy* surgery 11 years before her pregnancy at L4-5. Lamenectomy involves the removal of the bony structures on the side of each vertebra. A discectomy is a surgery that removes most of the disc. Deirdre had a discectomy at the L4-5. S1. Her cervical discs were herniated at the levels of 5, 6, and 7 seven years prior to her pregnancy. Her lumbar disc at L3 has also degenerated. Her symptoms include low back pain that affects both her legs and feet. She sometimes has pain running down her leg. Her legs and feet are sometimes numb, and this can affect her balance. She thought that bed rest had contributed to her being out of shape. In the process of rehabilitation, a new problem arose in both feet: *plantar fascitis*, which causes pain in the soles of the feet. Deirdre has upper extremity bilateral repetitive stress injury (RSI), which is shown as *tendonitis*. She experiences it as numbness and pain from her elbows to her fingertips. Her tendonitis can become easily aggravated and quite acute, resulting in her using her arms and hands less. Her shoulders also became deconditioned, as well, because she has limited use of her arms and hands. Deirdre had problems with balance and was immobilized the last 3 weeks of her pregnancy.

DWARFISM

Achondroplasia. Of the estimated two hundred types of dwarfism, *achondroplasia* is by far the most common, accounting for approximately half of all cases of profoundly short stature. The characteristics of achondroplasia are an average-size trunk, short arms and legs, and a slightly enlarged head and prominent forehead. Most people with achondroplasia are born to average-size parents, and they account for somewhere between one in 26,000 and one in 40,000 births. Adults, on average, are four feet tall. Young children with achondroplasia must be examined for such potential problems as *central apnea* (the part of the brain that controls breathing does not start or maintain the breathing process); *obstructive apnea* (an obstruction of the airway such as enlarged tonsils and adenoids); and hydrocephalus.

Darlene

Darlene has achondroplasia dwarfism. She had hip pain prior to getting pregnant, but in spite of her hip pain she was physically active and enjoyed walking prior to pregnancy, during pregnancy, and postpartum. Her hip pain increased during pregnancy, but after the delivery her pain returned to the same level as before her pregnancy.

Diane

Diane also has achondroplasia dwarfism. She has had no back problems. She has four children.

Diastrophic Dysplasia. Diastrophic dysplasia is a relatively uncommon form of dwarfism (about one in 100,000 births). It was first differentiated in 1960. Before then, it had been thought to be a different form of achondroplasia. Diastrophic dysplasia is often characterized by short-limbed dwarfism. In some cases, a person may have *cleft palate*; *clubfeet* (atypical bone formation); *hitchhiker's thumb*; and possibly ears with a cauliflower appearance. Serious orthopedic problems often require numerous surgical procedures. A normal lifespan is expected, but respiratory problems are sometimes present in infancy.

Denise

Denise has diastrophic dwarfism. This type of dwarfism is characterized by bony contractures caused by a decrease of sulfate in the bones, which results in minimal cartilage in the joints. This mainly affects the juncture of the large bone joints, including the *femur* (hip) and *humerus* (shoulder), but she has no contracture of the shoulders. Her right knee is contracted. She has *congenital hip dysplasia* (hip socket is not formed) resulting in her hip being dislocated. Denise had *equinas valgus* (foot that is turned outward) and had surgery to correct her feet so she could walk. After three miscarriages.

Spondyloepiphyseal Dysplasia Congenita (SED). This condition is inherited in an autosomal dominant pattern, which means only one copy of the gene is necessary to have this type of dwarfism. A person with this condition is of short stature (dwarfism). The name of the condition indicates that it affects the bones of the spine (spondylo-) and the ends of bones (epiphyses), and that it is present from birth (congenital). The signs and symptoms of spondyloepiphyseal dysplasia congenita are similar to, but milder than, the related skeletal disorders achondrogenesis, type II and hypochondroplasia.

Dorothy

Dorothy has SED. Her joints get tight and her muscles lack strength. Dorothy said, "My hips were not a problem during or after pregnancy. I had my first hip replacements just a few years before I married, so they were in fine working condition up until 2001." She had some balance and respiration problems in the last month of her pregnancy.

DYSTONIA

Dystonia is defined as "a syndrome of sustained muscle contractions, frequently causing twisting and repetitive movements, or abnormal postures." There are various causes for dystonia, including hormonal abnormalities, brain injury, and genetic factors. Hereditary dystonia first becomes apparent when the affected person is between 5 and 15 years old.

Dawn

Dawn has a type of dystonia (similar to athetoid cerebral palsy) that is caused by damage to the *basal ganglia* in the brain. Her symptoms include involuntary twisting movements of the trunk. All four limbs are involved, and most of the time they are moving. Her speech is also affected. Dawn can walk short distances, but she uses a motorized wheelchair for long distances. Her disability also causes bladder and kidney problems.

FIBROMYALGIA

Fibromyalgia is a chronic condition characterized by fatigue and widespread pain in the muscles, ligaments, and tendons. Previously, this condition was known by other names such as *fibrositis, chronic muscle pain syndrome, psychogenic rheumatism,* and *tension myalgias* (2).

"Fibromyalgia is a noninflammatory syndrome characterized by complaints of widespread musculoskeletal pain for at least 3 months in absence of other conditions to account for the pain. The documentation of discrete tender points on physical examination is essential to making a diagnosis. Fatigue, headaches, and irritable bowel syndrome are other symptoms that are reported. Fibromyalgia is associated with increased psychologic distress" (3).

Felicia

Felicia experienced pain in her shoulders, mid-back, elbows, hands, and knees because of her fibromyalgia. She was especially sensitive to pain and found that she was unable to handle normal amounts of pressure and was unable to have a massage. When Felicia had an exacerbation, her body ached as though she had the flu and she experienced extreme body pain. It took her several days to recover from any physical exertion such as a long hike or a long day at work. Felicia had been asymptomatic prior to getting pregnant. She had been unemployed for several months and, just before getting pregnant, she had started a new, high pressure job. She was working 12 to 14 hours a day, 60 hours a week. Depression is a part of fibromyalgia and she was taking the antidepressant Celexa®, which is not harmful to the fetus. She was told to discontinue it and, as a result, Felicia became severely depressed. (See "Nadine Fiona" in Appendix A.)

Hip Dysplegia

Formerly called *congenital dislocation of the hip*, this type of dysplegia involves a developmental abnormality of the hip that causes instability.

Hannah

Hannah's pelvis is missing a hip socket. She has had bone grafts that failed, resulting in limited mobility. She has arthritis in her hip and spine.

Heather Ann

Heather Ann has *hip dysplasia*, scoliosis, and an amputation. Her *acetabulum* (a cup-shaped cavity in the pelvis that receives the head of the femur) and *femoral head* (the knob at the end of the thigh bone) never developed, so she has no hip joint. Her dysplasia may have caused her scoliosis. Her right leg did not develop normally and was amputated above the knee when she was 14 years old. Although Heather Ann has not been able to find a comfortable prosthesis and uses crutches, she moves quite skillfully. Heather Ann's usual disability-related problems include muscle spasms in the stump, phantom pain when she is tired, and a constant, mild lower back ache.

Congenital Hip Deformity

Hilary

Hilary has *proximal focal femoral deficiency*, a congenital hip deformity in which the femur is short. This condition is caused in utero because of an inability to create bone. The clinical appearance is distinctive, with a very short thigh, flexed abducted and externally rotated hip and often flexion contracture of the knee. There may be associated *fibular hemimelia*. This condition has been classified into four sub-types according to the radiographic appearance (Aitken classification):

- ❖ Type A: Normal acetabulum with located femoral head, subtrochanteric femoral varus with pseudoarthrosis, which usually ossifies by skeletal maturity.
- ❖ Type B: Normal acetabulum and located femoral head. No osseous connection between the femoral head and shaft. The femoral shaft usually lies superior to the acetabulum and has a tufted proximal end.
- ❖ Type C: Dysplastic, flat acetabulum, absent femoral head, short femoral shaft with proximal tuft with no articulation between the femur and acetabulum.
- ❖ Type D: Dysplastic, flat acetabulum, absent femoral head, very short or absent femoral shaft with articulation between the femur and acetabulum.

The characteristics of this syndrome are malformation of the lower spine and short femoral (thigh) bones with missing knee joints. Hilary's uterus is normal size, but it has two chambers. She has difficulty walking and uses artificial legs and *Canadian crutches* (also known as *Lofstran*™ crutches). The artificial legs are similar to stilts because she does not have knees to bend. Moreover, she falls about once a month and has difficulty climbing stairs. Another disability-related problem is stress incontinence. Hilary used a wheelchair when she was pregnant with her second child. She started using the wheelchair full-time when her first baby was a 1½ years old, and she stopped using her artificial legs during the postpartum period.

CONGENITAL HYDROCEPHALUS

Congenital hydrocephalus is a condition in which there is too much cerebral spinal fluid on the baby's brain because the fluid is unable to drain out. In technical terms, there is progressive ventricular enlargement noted either on fetal echo and/or apparent in the first days of life. It can be due to excessive formation of cerebrospinal fluid (CSF) (RARE - choroid plexus tumors), or decreased reabsorption of CSF or obstruction of CSF flow (4). There is obstruction of the normal flow of cerebrospinal fluid because of a blockage in the ventricles in the brain. This problem can be isolated or associated with spina bifida.

Holly

Holly has congenital hydrocephalus without any physical limitations. She has had nine shunt revisions. Her balance was only slightly affected during her first pregnancy, but the shunt had to be replaced 6 weeks after delivery. The probable cause was excess pressure put on the abdomen during the birthing process. Delivery of her first child was difficult because the fetus was large and lying in the posterior position. Her babies all lay on the right side of her uterus, which is near the distal end of her shunt, causing some discomfort. Her shunt tube drains into the peritoneal cavity.

JUVENILE RHEUMATOID ARTHRITIS

Other names for juvenile rheumatoid arthritis (JRA) include Still's disease, juvenile chronic polyarthritis, and chronic childhood arthritis. JRA refers to a group of conditions that all involve inflammation of the joints, similar to adult-onset arthritis. About a quarter of a million children in the United States have JRA; most of them are girls. Joint inflammation in JRA often takes longer to lead to permanent damage than the inflammation of adult arthritis. The systemic symptoms of this condition include eye and skin problems. The exact combination of symptoms depends on the type of JRA an individual has.

Jennifer

Jennifer's joints and skin are affected by JRA. Different joints are affected at different times; every joint is symptomatic at some time. The pain, swelling and limitation of range of motion she experiences are sometimes more severe. In addition, the skin over her whole body usually feels sore and sensitive. Her skin and joint symptoms are worse when she is tired or weak. Jennifer's ability to walk increased dramatically when she was pregnant.

Joan
Joan had bilateral hip replacements at age 13. She uses a motorized wheelchair. Joan's arthritis affects all of her joints. During pregnancy, her arthritis went into remission and she did not feel the sharp grinding pain she usually experienced.

Joy
Joy's joints are affected by JRA, but she walks all the time. She has limited movements in her wrists and one of her shoulders. She has had several joint replacements: her hips 11 years prior to her pregnancy and her knees 7 years prior to her pregnancy. Joy has experienced constant pain in her ankles as well as continued incontinence since her pregnancy.

Julie
Julie's arthritis affects all of her joints. Her usual disability-related problems are difficulty walking and stiffness of the joints. Joint stiffness is especially severe in her ankles. Her disability affects her hands and knees. She usually uses a motorized wheelchair. Despite her joint discomfort, Julie commented that during pregnancy, "I felt better than some of my able-bodied friends did when they were pregnant."

SYSTEMIC LUPUS ERYTHEMATOSUS

Systemic lupus erythematosus (SLE), often referred to simply as *lupus*, is a disease resembling rheumatoid arthritis. It is an *autoimmune disorder*, which means that the immune system attacks other body tissues in a way similar to the way it attacks invading bacteria and viruses. SLE is a systemic disease that affects many organ systems.

Systemic lupus erythematosus causes a variety of symptoms and different combinations of symptoms. The most common problems are pain and swelling in the joints and kidney damage. Other problems include fever, fatigue, weakness, skin rashes, sensitivity to sunlight, headaches, and muscle aches. Seizures, personality changes, or emotional depression may result if the brain is affected. No cure has been found for SLE, but some of the symptoms may be controlled with proper treatment. Many people experience periodic remissions of symptoms.

Laura
Laura's usual problems before pregnancy were aching joints, fatigue, high blood pressure, loss of vision in one eye (probably as a result of high blood pressure) and mental confusion. Laura had numerous problems during and after her pregnancy.

Lea Rae

Lea Rae has both SLE and rheumatoid arthritis. She has arthritis in all of her joints. She has had both hips and a knee replaced. In addition, she needed a hip revision in 1999. Lea Rae was especially tired during her pregnancy.

Leslie

Leslie's SLE was not diagnosed until she had already had one premature baby and one miscarriage. She now realizes that she had experienced SLE symptoms for approximately 13 years before the disease was diagnosed. When working in hot weather that did not affect her co-workers, Leslie experienced severe rashes, vomiting, and hair loss. She had a constantly recurring *streptococcal* infection of the vagina and later realized that the infection kept recurring because her immune system was too weakened by SLE to resist infection. The effects of SLE on her pregnancies led to diagnosis of the disease. Since the time of the diagnosis, Leslie has had continuous problems with psoriasis. Her shoulders, hips, knees, feet, and hands have become arthritic.

MULTIPLE SCLEROSIS

Multiple sclerosis (MS) is an adult onset condition with a variety of symptoms. There are four subtypes. Not only do people have different sets of symptoms, but one person's symptoms will also vary over time. These variations are due to the nature of the condition. In medical terms, the symptoms of MS are caused by *demyelinization* (loss of the *myelin sheath* that surrounds nerves). Myelin sheaths help with nerve conduction of the *axon* at various locations, followed by *glial scar formation* at some sites. Think of your nervous system as a set of telephone wires connecting a central switchboard (your brain) with the various parts of your body. With MS, the insulation of the wires wears away at various points, disrupting communications. If a worn patch is repaired, remission of symptoms will result, but demyelinization (loss of insulation) of a different part of the nerve could cause the same symptom to reappear.

Multiple sclerosis most often first appears in individuals between the ages of 20 and 40 years. The symptoms of MS are so variable and confusing, however, that the disorder may not be diagnosed until years after the first symptoms appear. The cause of MS is not completely understood. It is an autoimmune disorder in which a person's antibodies attack her own body tissues. The cause appears to be a combination of inherited and environmental factors. The reasons that the rate of progression varies among individuals are also not understood. There are medicines to slow the progression and treat the some of the symptoms.

Mandy

Mandy was diagnosed with MS 6 months after the birth of her second child. Her first symptoms were double vision and numbness in her legs. Since diagnosis, Mandy's common symptoms are fatigue, numbness, and depression.

Margie

Margie had been diagnosed with MS before she became pregnant. Her symptoms before pregnancy were weakness in the arm and leg on one side, and occasional bladder problems. Margie commented about her first pregnancy, "I felt great while I was pregnant! I enjoyed feeling so healthy and I had a positive outlook on life."

Marsha

Before her pregnancy, Marsha walked with a limp and used a cane. Many years later, Marsha is still using only a cane.

Mary

Mary tired easily before her pregnancy. She could walk short distances unassisted, but she used a walker for longer distances, especially for getting up and down stairs. Her bladder control was slightly affected. After one miscarriage.

Michelle

Michelle's MS symptoms were mild. The problems that led to her diagnosis were urgency and occasional incontinence, and blurred vision. Later, she had problems with muscle spasms and tired easily.

Mimi

Mimi was taking one of the drugs used to slow the progression of MS prior to pregnancy and "was happy to stop the drug" during pregnancy. She continued to feel well without it postpartum. Mimi walked with a wide gait prior to pregnancy and after delivery. Although she had more numbness on her left side, she felt better without medication. She had a *grand mal* seizure prior to delivery (she is unsure how many day(s) before delivery), but she had no seizure activity for $1\frac{1}{2}$ years after delivery. She felt dizzy and off-balance after her pregnancy. These symptoms could have been due to her seizure medication.

Moira

Moira's main problem is fatigue. She is limited to walking no more than two blocks and uses a power wheelchair for longer distances. Prior to pregnancy she used Canadian (Lofstran™) crutches. Moira has used a cane when visiting friends since her pregnancy. She had *intravenous immunoglobulin* (IVIG) treatment 3 months in a row after giving birth. IVIG is "an immune system booster used to make sure I didn't crash" during the hormone fluctuation from pregnancy to postpartum. Moira is "able to be alert, awake and take care of my child with this treatment and additional medication. I am taking my baby to swimming lessons." She felt better after the pregnancy than she did before as well as during pregnancy, thanks to the IVIG.

Mona

Mona was put on oral baclofen while she was pregnant, but it was not successful and she was switched to tizanidine (Zanaflex®), which reduced her spasticity. Mona said, "I was told that there was no evidence of fetal abnormalities during pregnancy, but that the drug could be passed on in breast milk." In spite of the success of the medication, she had difficulty writing because of tremors in her right hand. In addition, Mona had started to use a walker prior to pregnancy. She had an exacerbation of MS during her first trimester and lost strength in her legs. She also had numbness in her legs. By the end of the first trimester, she had more energy and her walking improved. Mona was encouraged to surgically implant the Baclofen Pump™, an alternative to tizanidine that requires much lower doses. In retrospect, Mona said, "If I could change anything about my baby's birth, I would not have opted for the Baclofen Pump™. I wish I had not tried to breast-feed, but rather stayed on Zanaflex® and spent that time with my son. Also, I was given the choice in the hospital to not breast-feed and stay on the drug, or have the surgery and breast-feed. I let my mother convince me to have the surgery. My doctor left the decision up to me. I was hospitalized after the surgery for 2 weeks without my child and even though I used a breast pump, he basically was fed formula with some breast milk. He was not interested or accustomed to the breast, so after a very short stint of breast milk in bottles I gave up and fed him formula only. I don't know if having two surgeries back to back was right for me, and the pump at that time may have been unnecessary." Mona was prescribed a motorized wheelchair 6 months after her delivery and surgery for the pump. She used it when going outside for both a walk and shopping. Mona found the pump helpful.

Neuromuscular Disorders

"The broad category of *neuromuscular disorders* or diseases covers conditions that involve the weakness or wasting of the body muscles. Some of these conditions are covered by the Muscular Dystrophy Association, but they are not primary diseases of the muscles. These problems may arise in the spinal cord, the peripheral nerves, or the muscle fibers. Some may be hereditary, while others are acquired. Commonly recognized conditions fall into the categories of *myopathies*, which are diseases of the muscle such as *muscular dystrophy*; disorders of the junction where the nerve impulses are transmitted to the muscle such as *myasthenia gravis*; and neuropathies, which are diseases of the peripheral nervous system such as *diabetic neuropathy*" (6).

Charcot-Marie-Tooth

Charcot-Marie-Tooth is an unusual, slowly progressive form of muscular atrophy characterized by weakness and wasting of the feet and leg muscles followed by involvement of the hands.

Naomi

Naomi's doctors are unsure of her diagnosis. The differential diagnosis is between *distal spinal muscular atrophy* and Charcot-Marie-Tooth. She uses leg braces. She used a walker during her first pregnancy and experienced carpal tunnel syndrome during both pregnancies. One of her feet became numb during her first delivery, but the numbness lasted only about 8 weeks. Naomi has since had a second child. She said, "The [second] pregnancy was worse, possibly because I was older. I was tired the whole way through and never really felt great like I had during the second trimester of the first pregnancy. I also got gestational diabetes in the third trimester and had to control my diet. In the second pregnancy the labor and delivery lasted only 1 hour and 15 minutes. Labor was about the same as before, but shorter. I knew the positions that worked for me and it went smoothly. Pushing was only a few minutes, which was a great relief. The first time it was 2 hours. Afterward they gave me Pitocin® for bleeding. Although my uterus was firm, I continued to bleed and got very dizzy. The doctor came back and removed many clots so my uterus could clamp down properly and stop the bleeding. My disability had nothing to do with these problems."

Natalie

Natalie walks with two leg braces. She also has a weak grasp and needs two hands to pick up a glass. She described her hands as being "clawhands." Natalie does not have any sensation in her hands or feet. She had difficulty climbing steps and lifting her legs into the car until 5 months post-delivery.

Nora

Nora uses a wheelchair and cannot use her fingers and toes. She could not transfer after the seventh month of her pregnancy. She felt weaker and had nosebleeds every night. Her physical condition after pregnancy returned to the same as before the pregnancy.

FRIEDREICH'S ATAXIA

Friedreich's ataxia is an inherited, progressive disorder characterized by degeneration of portions of the brain and spinal cord. The disorder progresses slowly, usually causing death by age 30. The earliest manifestation is a wide-based gait—in which the feet slap the ground as they land—and difficulty sensing where the limbs are located in space. Scoliosis and clubfeet are also commonly associated with this disorder.

Noelle

Noelle had walked with the aid of Canadian (Lofstran™) crutches, but she started using a motorized wheelchair a month before she became pregnant. Her other disability-related problems included leg cramps, stress incontinence, back problems caused by scoliosis, and some difficulty breathing. Her ataxia had progressed so much by 4 years after her pregnancy that Noelle could only stand with support for half a minute.

Nikki

Nikki had been walking with a walker but started using a wheelchair during her second pregnancy. She started using a motorized wheelchair in the beginning of her seventh pregnancy. Nikki does not have any difficulty with breathing except during her pregnancies. Her upper extremity ability is slightly affected. Her writing is wiggly now. In addition, reaching is getting hard. She can stand up leaning on the kitchen counter when she is not pregnant. Since her four early miscarriages.

LIMB-GIRDLE DYSTROPHY

Limb-girdle dystrophy is a form of muscular dystrophy. "All limb-girdle muscular dystrophies (LGMD) show a similar distribution of muscle weakness, affecting both upper arms and legs. Frequently, the first reported symptoms will be difficulty climbing stairs, standing from a squatting position, or raising arms above the head" (7).

Nadine Fiona

Nadine Fiona is able to walk, but not up stairs. She has fibromyalgia that went into remission during the second trimester of pregnancy. Her balance got worse during pregnancy. She is also weak in her upper extremities, making it hard to place things in and out of the oven. Her back got weaker and stayed weaker, making it hard to go from sitting to standing. Nadine Fiona also has difficulty straightening up after she bends over at her waist.

Natasha

Natasha has limb-girdle muscular dystrophy and is unable to run. In addition, she has difficulty climbing stairs and bending over. Natasha started having problems getting up from a seated position prior to pregnancy. She has weakness in her arms and as a result she has difficulty lifting things. She has weak upper muscles, biceps, and pectorals. Her upper arm muscles, triceps, and deltoids, are good. Natasha felt stronger during her pregnancy because she was able to maintain a full schedule in spite of being pregnant.

Nicole

Nicole's doctors are unsure of her diagnosis. Nicole was able to walk prior to her pregnancies, but she now uses a wheelchair. She cannot raise her arms over her head. Nicole has a grasp, but it is not strong enough to open tightly closed jars. She did not have any medical problems with any pregnancy except for transfers. Nicole has two children.

Myasthenia Gravis

Myasthenia gravis is an autoimmune disease that affects the transmission of signals from nerve to muscle. The onset is usually in women in their 20s and 30s. Myasthenia occurs when antibodies produced by the body's immune system attack and destroy the acetylcholine receptor located at the muscle-nerve connection. People affected with myasthenia gravis experience weakness that worsens with activity and stress. Myasthenia gravis typically affects facial muscles and other skeletal or voluntary muscles. The eyelid muscles are the most commonly affected, usually causing the eyelids to droop. Sometimes chewing, swallowing, smiling, and talking are also affected.

Nadia

Nadia experienced myasthenia gravis symptoms during the second trimester of her third pregnancy, and could not hold onto a bottle or shampoo her hair. She was diagnosed with myasthenia gravis during the third trimester. Nadia had double vision 6 months after the birth of her child and weakness in her facial muscles as well as her arms and neck muscles. She did not have any problems with her legs until after the diagnosis was made. She was started on steroids the day after the baby was born. Nadia felt weak at the beginning of steroid treatment. She also had a thymectomy a month after her baby was born.

Noreen

Noreen was diagnosed with myasthenia gravis when she was 10 years old. Her disability symptoms vary from day to day, but her eyelids droop most of the time. Many mornings she has a hard time lifting her son.

Spinal Muscular Atrophy

Spinal Muscular Atrophy (SMA) is a type of neuromuscular disorder. It is not one condition, but rather a group of eight similar conditions. All of the different types of SMA are genetically caused, but not all are *familial*, that is, a genetic disorder can result from a new mutation. Spinal muscular atrophies involve degeneration of neurons in the spinal cord, medulla, and midbrain. Dysfunction of these nerves leads to degeneration of the nerves in the muscles that, in turn, leads to muscle atrophy and progressive paralysis. Pulmonary function can also be affected. In some individuals, one set of opposing muscles is weakened more than the opposite set, causing scoliosis. The mode of inheritance, age of onset, severity, and progression of the condition vary among the different types of SMA. Infantile onset is Type 2, which is also known as *Werdnig-Hoffman spinal muscular atrophy (disease)*.

Nancy

Nancy is able to move all parts of her body, although she has little strength in her limbs. She can move her arms more easily than her legs. Her condition has caused scoliosis so severe that her hips are *subluxed* (the heads of her femurs do not rest properly in the sockets). A surgically–implanted Harrington rod helps her maintain an erect posture. Nancy has broken her knees and each of her ankles on various occasions. Her inability to use her lower limbs has also contributed to *osteoporosis* (loss of calcium in the bone), which can lead to easy breaks in the bones.

Nina

Nina is from Sweden and received her medical care there. She is able to move all parts of her body, though she has little strength in her limbs. She can move her arms more easily than her legs. Nina has difficulty getting pregnant because she has irregular menstruation that has nothing to do with SMA.

OSTEOGENESIS IMPERFECTA

Osteogenesis Imperfecta (OI) is an inherited disability that affects *collagen*, a major protein that forms connective tissue in the body. People with OI have less collagen and, therefore, their tissue is weaker than normal, thus causing weak bones. OI is an inherited disability, and a person with this condition has a 50 percent chance of having a baby with OI. There are four different types of OI, which vary in severity and characteristics. Most bone breaks occur before puberty. This is particularly true with Types 1 and 4. Type 1 is the mildest form and most of the fractures occur before puberty. Type 2 is the most severe form and only a few survive. Type 3 is the next most severe type and is associated with respiratory problems, bone deformity, loose joints, poor muscle development, and short stature. Type 4 is between Type 3 and 1 in severity. This type is associated with mild to moderate bone deformity, shorter than average stature, and barrel-shaped rib cage (8).

Olivia

Olivia does not know what type of OI she has. She has had more than 50 broken bones, mostly in the lower extremities. She found that pregnancy was good for her body.

Oprah

Oprah has had 300 to 400 breaks. She has Type 3 osteogenesis imperfecta. She started walking in her teen years and continued to walk throughout both pregnancies. During the third trimester of her first pregnancy, Oprah slipped on wet pavement and fell and broke her hip. She went into labor, but medication delayed labor and delivery by 10 days. Despite breaking her hip, her doctor could not believe how healthy she was. Oprah was also healthy during her second pregnancy. Only one of her children has OI. She has arthritis, 10 years later, and uses a manual wheelchair or crutches, depending on how she feels.

Orielle

Orielle has had around fifty broken bones. She has Type 4 osteogenesis imperfecta of moderate severity, and she uses a wheelchair.

POST-POLIO SYNDROME

Poliomyelitis is a viral illness that affects the *anterior horn cells* in the spinal cord. The anterior horn cell, or motor neuron, is the nerve cell that innervates the skeletal muscle fibers. Post-polio syndrome refers to problems that occur long after the viral infection has ended. When these nerve cells were destroyed, the muscles they served became weakened or paralyzed through lack of information being sent to the muscles, although sensation remains. Later in life, the overuse of the remaining nerve fibers begins to take its toll, and post-polio syndrome develops, often in individuals who had little outward signs of the original disease. Different muscles are affected in different individuals, depending on which nerves were damaged. One person may have difficulty breathing, whereas another may be unable to move her legs.

Although polio has been eradicated in the United States, it has not been in the rest of the world. Therefore, there are a number of women of childbearing age living in other countries—some of whom may have immigrated to the United States—who have post-polio syndrome.

Pam

Pam's arms and hands were weakened by polio; she describes them as "60 percent functional." She can write, cook, and hold a glass of water, but heavy tasks are difficult. Her legs are completely paralyzed and she uses a motorized wheelchair. Pam's abdominal muscles are weak. In order to give her trunk enough support for sitting up, a muscle fascia was transplanted from her right thigh, with one end attached to her ribs and the other to her pelvis. Also, Pam's left shoulder was surgically fused and she has a sway back. Pam had pulmonary function tests before she became pregnant and was assured that she would not have too much difficulty breathing.

Patricia

Patricia's polio affects all four limbs and she has scoliosis. She can walk with the aid of braces and crutches, but usually prefers to use a wheelchair. Her arms are somewhat weak, but she is able to use them to propel a lightweight manual wheelchair. Patricia's comment about her pregnancy was, "I had a better pregnancy than most of my able-bodied friends."

Paula

Paula's arms, legs, abdominal muscles, and back are all affected by post-polio syndrome. Her usual disability-related problems include difficulty in carrying large loads such as grocery bags, tiring easily, hip pain, poor circulation in the legs, and occasional muscle spasms. She walks with Canadian (Lofstran™) crutches. Paula contracted polio during her second pregnancy and the illness caused a miscarriage. She felt that, on the whole, her later, post-polio pregnancies were similar to the first.

Portia

Portia's polio affected her legs, left arm and hand, neck, abdominal and low back muscles, and diaphragm. Her usual disability-related problems include occasional bladder infections, difficulty breathing, and coughing. Portia uses a wheelchair. Because she has had five children, with the last pregnancy occurring several years before her interview, she summarized her pregnancy symptoms as follows:

Portia contracted polio when she was 19 years old. She had her first child 2 years later. Her fifth child was born when she was 34 years old. Anemia was a problem during all her pregnancies. She also had morning sickness with all of her pregnancies and bladder infections during three pregnancies. Pregnancy also exacerbated her disability-related problems with constipation. Portia said that it was easier for her to cough when she was pregnant, explaining, "I didn't need a corset when I was pregnant. The baby did the same job." By the second trimester of each pregnancy, transferring became difficult. Portia was able to adapt, except that by the third trimester using a bathtub was impossible and she avoided going out alone. She said, "I stopped driving when I stopped fitting behind the steering wheel."

Priscilla

Priscilla's polio affected only her right leg. A muscle transplant was performed when she was 9 years old so she would be able to use the leg. When she was eleven, a pin was implanted in her left leg to slow its growth to a rate consistent with that of the right leg. Now, her right leg is somewhat thinner than her left and she walks with a slight limp. Before Priscilla's first pregnancy, her right leg and hip often ached after she carried groceries up a steep hill to her house.

RHEUMATOID ARTHRITIS

There are a number of types of arthritis, all characterized by swelling, pain, and stiffness of the joints. *Rheumatoid arthritis* (RA), which affects about 1 percent of the population, is one of the more common forms of arthritis. People who have rheumatoid arthritis may experience other symptoms, including anemia, eye inflammation, and *pleurisy* (an inflammation of the membrane that surrounds and protects the lungs). Rheumatoid nodules occur in about 20 percent of rheumatoid arthritis patients in areas subject to pressure or trauma (often just under the skin), in the lungs, and in the heart. The causes of rheumatoid arthritis are still not completely understood, but inherited susceptibility, viral infection, and autoimmune response all seem to play roles in this disease. (Autoimmunity is also discussed in the section on systemic lupus erythematosus.)

Rachel

Rachel's rheumatoid arthritis was diagnosed when she was a teenager. One of her shoulder joints was replaced during her late teen years. She has experienced intermittent flare-ups in her hands since her shoulder joint replacement. The aftereffects of the flare-ups have left Rachel with weak hands. She did not have any pain or stiffness in her hands at the time of her first pregnancy. She had an exacerbation when her first child was 2 years old. She "woke up one morning with arthritis affecting every major joint" from her ankles to her neck. Since this flare-up, Rachel has had a hard time getting up from the couch as well as the toilet, getting into and out of the bathtub, walking, straightening her knees, and going up and down stairs. She has difficulty pushing and pulling, and washing her hair. She began her second pregnancy during this flare-up, which has been constant.

Renee

Renee's rheumatoid arthritis was diagnosed when she was 6 months pregnant with her first child. Most of Renee's symptoms were in remission between her first and second pregnancies. A month after the birth of her second child, Renee's feet and hands were constantly painful. The pain and swelling in her hands was so severe that she could use them very little.

Roberta

Roberta's usual disability-related symptoms before her pregnancy included aching and weakness in her hands, aching shoulders and knees, morning stiffness, and susceptibility to bladder infections.

SACRAL AGENESIS

Sacral agenesis is a term applied to a wide range of developmental conditions of the lower portions of the spinal column and pelvis. This term indicates that some portion of the lumbar spine, sacrum, or pelvis is incompletely or incorrectly formed at the time of birth.

Sophia Amelia

Sophia Amelia has sacral agenesis. She has no sacrum or coccyx (located at the end of the spine), and twelve vertebrae in her lower back are missing. Her nerves are composed of clusters of nerve endings, making her hypersensitive in certain places with no sensation in others. She has a dislocated pelvis that is also very small. She has partial arthrogryposis, resulting in skeletal and muscular deformities such as only one bone below the knee, floating kneecaps, and fixed or partially fused joints in her hips, knees, and ankles, with resulting degenerative arthritis. She can only put weight on one leg. When the spinal block for her second child was ineffective, the result was shooting pains in that leg which made it impossible to stand. This caused some difficulty with postpartum recovery and caring for herself and her newborn independently. She has partial arthrogryposis; her feet are fixed and she is unable to flex her feet. She has only one leg bone below her one knee.

Sophia Amelia has a *neurogenic* (spastic) bladder and only one functioning kidney, resulting in frequent kidney and bladder infections. She also has both an artificial bladder and sphincter. Sophia Amelia developed a seizure disorder between her first and second pregnancies. She noticed an increase in seizure activity during her first trimester, which she speculated was due to hormonal changes. She uses a manual wheelchair as well as crutches for short distances. Sophia Amelia used her crutches for a short time during the first trimester. She generally did not use her crutches during her pregnancies, due to changes in her center of gravity that caused problems with balance. She felt more stable using a wheelchair. Sophia Amelia had postoperative complications after both deliveries. Her digestive system had shut down and an NG tube (nasogastric) was inserted. This may have been caused by general anesthesia.

Spina Bifida

Spina bifida is a deformity of the spine that occurs early in embryonic development. There is definitely a genetic component to some cases of spina bifida as well as an interaction between genetic and in-utero environmental factors.

The spinal cord contains a bundle of nerves that is surrounded by a protective covering called the *meningeal membrane*. The spinal cord passes through a column of ring-shaped bones, the vertebrae, which are separated and cushioned by discs of cartilage. The cord occupies the space inside the spinal, or vertebral, column. Spina bifida results from a failure of the canal to close properly. Other problems, such as clubfeet, may be associated with this defect.

There are three types of spina bifida, differentiated by the severity of the defect. The opening does not extend to the surface of the body in *spina bifida occulta* (occulta means "hidden"). The problem is in the vertebrae. Sometimes there are visible changes in the tissues overlying the defect; sometimes it is found by palpation or by X-ray examination. Spina bifida occulta usually occurs in the lower spine and is occasionally accompanied by scoliosis or problems of the feet. Symptoms will depend on the extent of the lesions. It can be very mild, and in some individuals the only symptoms may be backaches. Others may have more severe symptoms such as atrophied leg muscles, bowel and bladder disorders, or sensory loss.

More severe types of spina bifida are *meningocele* and *meningomyocele*. In meningocele, some of the meningeal membrane protrudes through the hole in the vertebra to the surface of the body. In meningomyocele, the nerve roots and spinal cord are attached to the wall of the meningeal sac. As with spinal cord injury, symptoms depend on the location and extent of the lesion.

Sabine

Sabine has the myelomeningocele form of spina bifida (a small protrusion that was not open to the skin of a portion of cord and membranes; a hairy spot designated the site (*hairy nevus*). She also has scoliosis and no sensation in her right foot.

Sabine had surgery to provide bladder control during which the *ureters* (tubes connecting the kidneys to the bladder) were attached to the segments of ileum (last segment of small intestine) so that her urine drains into the ileum and then into a bag attached to the skin rather than the bladder. She had this procedure done many years prior to her first pregnancy and it needed to be redone after her second.

Although Sabine has had *radicular pain* (pain due to disease of the spinal nerve roots) her whole life from unknown causes, she experienced an increase in pain during the fifth month of her first pregnancy. A possible explanation may be that a nerve root was pinched, causing an increase in pain. Her pain started soon after *amniocentesis*. The natural loosening of the joints and the swelling that accompanies pregnancy could have worsened the pain. Moreover, Sabine had surgery to remove her gallstones during this time. This may also have contributed to the radicular pain. Her radicular pain follows the trail of a particular nerve that is being pinched. She had the nerves cut, but this did not stop the pain. Since cutting the nerves was ineffective, Sabine tried medication, which she has found to be effective in controlling her pain.

Sabine's anal sphincter muscle is weak so she takes Lomotil® to keep her bowel movements firm. This required an adjustment in her medication during pregnancy.

Sasha

Sasha had meningocele and two clubfeet. She was able to walk with the aid of Canadian (Lofstran™) crutches. She has used a manual wheelchair more as she has grown older. Her bladder control was poor and she had frequent infections of the bladder and kidneys. Her usual problems included edema and muscle spasms in her legs. Her feet were free of pressure sores only when she was pregnant.

Sherry Adele

Sherry Adele had the myelomeningocele form of spina bifida (an open protrusion of the cord and membranes) at L5-S2, but she has an incomplete lesion. She was born with two clubfeet and some hammertoes. She had one foot amputated and uses a prosthesis. She is able to walk without assistive devices, although both of her legs have diminished sensation. Moreover, she has a spastic neurogenic bowel, and is unable to urinate without using a catheter. She had been doing self-catherization for 10 years prior to her pregnancies. Sherry Adele had many surgeries as a child; some of which may have been experimental. She had surgery to enlarge her urethra then, years later, another surgery to decrease the size of her urethra. Sherry Adele thought that the doctors did not know how to manage her bladder problems. She has had many bladder infections. Her bladder is both hypertonic and hyperactive.

Sienna

Sienna uses both a power and a manual wheelchair and occasionally walks with crutches. She has limited sensation below her waist in both legs and sometimes experiences spasticity in her legs (a condition described by stiff or rigid muscles). Sienna is not aware of any reason why this occurs. She has some sensation in her bladder and a full sensation in her bowels. Sienna does self-catheterization. She gave birth by caesarean section after having three miscarriages.

Sierra

Sierra walks with Canadian (Lofstran™) crutches, but she is unable to bear weight on one of her legs. She has limited sensation below the waist and in both legs. Spasticity in her legs occurs infrequently for no apparent reasons. Her bowel and bladder are not affected. Sierra's child has mild cerebral palsy, cause unknown.

Simi

Simi has the myelomeningocele form of spina bifida (an open protrusion of the cord and membranes at L5-S2). She uses short leg braces and had edema during pregnancy. She also had poor bladder and bowel control. She was constipated during her pregnancy, but has not had any bladder infections since she was 19 years old. Her bladder was numb for a year after the delivery.

Sybil

Sybil has meningocele and arthritis of the spine. The arthritis causes backaches in cold weather. Sybil can walk with crutches, but she has no sensation in her legs. She often gets pressure sores on her legs, and muscle spasms are also a problem. She had a *urostomy*, an operation in which the ureters (the tubes leading from the kidney to the bladder) are detached from the bladder and brought to the surface of the skin. The urine then drains into a collecting bag. Her bowel control is also poor.

SPINAL CORD INJURIES

This type of irreversible damage to the spinal cord typically results from injuries that might be sustained as the result of a driving or diving accident, a gunshot wound, or a fall. The damage can cause loss of movement or loss of sensation, or both.

The spinal cord carries messages between the brain and the rest of the body, in much the same way that a telephone line carries messages between a central switchboard and individual telephones. If a storm occurs, damaging several wires in the cable, not all the houses will lose telephone service, but only those connected to the damaged wires. Similarly, the particular disabilities that a person experiences will depend on which nerves in the spinal cord bundle were damaged. The *level*, or area, of the spinal cord that is damaged—and the extent of that damage—is significant in determining the type of disability. The level of injury is defined by referring to the vertebrae closest to the injury site. Starting from the top, the neck vertebrae are numbered C-1 to C-7; the vertebrae in the upper and mid-back are numbered T-1 to T-12; and the vertebrae in the lower back are numbered L-1 to L-5.

All four limbs will be affected if the spinal cord injury occurs in the neck. This condition is called *quadriplegia*. Injuries closer to the skull cause *high quadriplegia*. Injuries above the C-3 vertebra are almost always fatal due to a loss of innervation to the muscles that control breathing; injuries at C-3 are often fatal; injuries from C-3 to C-5 cause quadriplegia; and people who have spinal cord injury from C-5 to C-7 have some limited hand use. Injury to the thoracic spine level 8 (the part of the spine behind the breastbone) causes paraplegia (affecting the lower limbs) in which trunk control is affected. Injury to the lumbar (low back) spine causes paraplegia. The muscles in the limbs are not the only ones affected. Spinal cord injury affects the abdominal muscles and some of the back muscles. Bowel and bladder control are also affected to varying degrees. Generally people with quadriplegia have difficulty coughing and may have other breathing difficulties.

Women whose injuries are above T-6 (sometimes to T-8) experience *autonomic dysreflexia*, also called *hyperreflexia*. Dysreflexia results from the uncontrolled release of norepinephrine, which causes a rapid rise in blood pressure and a slowing of the heart rate. These symptoms are accompanied by throbbing headache, nausea, anxiety, sweating, and goose bumps below the level of the injury (9).

Sometimes a person may experience nasal stuffiness and changes in heart rhythm. On any one occasion an individual might experience a combination of many possible symptoms. A common term for episodes involving relatively mild symptoms is known as *quad sweats*. Dysreflexia can be stimulated by ordinary events such as bladder fullness or the insertion of a speculum during a pelvic examination. Symptoms may resolve by removal of the stimulus. For example, by emptying the bladder or removing the speculum.

Although most of the interviewees did not feel labor contractions, most were able to feel fetal movement.

Sally

Sally is a quadriplegic whose level of injury is at C-5/6. She has limited use of all her limbs. She can lift her arms and has some use of her hands and wrists. Sally cannot use her fingers but can lift her wrists. She can stand with support by using her spasticity, and she can do a pivot transfer with support. Her spasticity diminished by the second trimester, which prevented her from assisting with transfers. She frequently has bladder infections.

Samantha

Samantha is paraplegic with an injury at T-10/11/12. She was injured after she had already had two children. Her third child was born 10 years after her injury. Her legs are paralyzed and there is some calcification in her hips. She has a *suprapubic catheter*, a catheter that is inserted into the bladder above the pubic bone. Samantha felt that her last pregnancy was much the same as her first two, with the exception of specific disability problems such as trouble transferring. She remarked, "It wasn't as bad as I thought it would be."

Shanna

Shanna has a spinal cord injury at T-11. She had surgery a year before her pregnancy to implant a Neuro-Control™ device to control bladder problems. Soon after the delivery, however, it needed to be removed due to bladder infections. It is unknown why the device was dislodged. (This problem is rare.) Shanna had a second pregnancy without the device and had no bladder infection. She was on bed rest in her third trimester because of early labor pains.

Sharon

Sharon's injury occurred at the T-6 level. Her legs, feet, lower abdominal muscles, and some low back muscles are paralyzed. She had *phlebitis* (inflammation of a vein) in one leg just after she was injured. Another problem is occasional muscle spasms. Because of difficulty with self catheterization during pregnancy, she used an indwelling catheter. After delivery Sharon was unable to resume self catheterization because her bladder had lost elasticity.

Sheila

Sheila is a quadriplegic whose level of injury is at C-5/6. She has limited use of all limbs. She can lift her arms, has some use of her hands, can stand with support, and can do a pivot transfer with support. Her bladder tends to retain urine, but she knows when she has to urinate because she starts to sweat (a dysreflexia symptom). She has problems with dysreflexia and constipation when she is under stress.

Shelby

Shelby is a quadriplegic whose level of injury is at C-7/8. She has use of her arms and good hand grasp. She was able to transfer throughout her pregnancy. She had continual bladder infections. She experienced dysreflexia during her eighth and ninth month of pregnancy.

Signey

Signey had a spinal cord injury when she was 19 years old that resulted in *quadriparesis*, meaning she is not paralyzed and is able to walk. Although she has limited use of her right hand, she can write with it as well as type with one finger. Her fingertips and toes feel somewhat numb. Signey has had bladder control since rehabilitation. She used enemas to manage her bowels prior to pregnancy and through the first trimester.

Sonya

Sonya has a spinal cord injury at C-3/4. She has a Baclofen Pump™ to reduce her spasticity. This device helped reduce her muscle spasms before and after pregnancy, but not during her pregnancy. It might not have worked, because the dosage was not increased even though it is safe to do so. Her paralysis is from the neck down. She does intermittent catheterization. Sonya uses a reclining wheelchair.

Stacy

Stacy's injury was at the C5/6 level. She has some use of her hands. She uses a walker for short distances and a manual wheelchair for long distances. Her usual problems include scoliosis, an inability to sit up without support from a girdle, dysreflexia when she needs to urinate, and occasional light-headedness.

Stephanie

Stephanie has an injury at the T-12 level. She has some sensation in the right hip. She has some internal sensation in her lower abdomen and feels bladder fullness, but needs to use a catheter. She has problems with edema. She sometimes walks with the help of braces and crutches. Stephanie's comment about her pregnancy was, "It didn't seem that different from other people. My cousin has a heart-shaped uterus, too, and she had the same problems as I did."

Sydney

Sydney has a spinal cord injury at T-4/5. She did not feel her baby move unless she had her hands on her belly, which could have been the result of where the placenta was implanted in the uterus. She did feel her baby when he kicked her in the ribs. She had difficulty pushing her wheelchair up an incline while pregnant. She has sensation above the right nipple and below her left nipple. Sydney was able to nurse only from her left breast.

Sylvia

Sylvia is a high quadriplegic, with injury at C-3/4/5. Her whole body is affected from the neck and shoulders down. Her bowels often retain feces, and she has no bladder control. She sometimes has muscle spasms so strong that her body thrashes about. She has occasional episodes of dysreflexia, and often has fainting spells just before menstruating. Sylvia's baby was delivered vaginally using forceps because the baby's shoulder was caught in the birth canal.

SPINAL TUMOR

Spinal cord tumors are abnormal growths of tissue found inside the bony spinal column. *Benign* tumors are non-cancerous, and *malignant* tumors are cancerous. Most primary tumors are caused by out-of-control cell growth. The cause of most primary tumors remains a mystery. They are not contagious and not preventable. Spinal cord tumor symptoms include pain, sensory changes, and motor problems. The three most commonly used treatments are surgery, radiation, and chemotherapy. All of the interviewees had surgery.

Selina Tracy

Selina Tracy had a tumor at the thoracic level (T4) and has been disabled since the age of two. She has full use of her hands and partial use of her trunk. She does intermittent catherization. When she was not pregnant, Selina Tracy only experienced a bladder infection periodically. She uses a manual wheelchair and experiences carpal tunnel. She also has a diagnosis of thoracic outlet syndrome.

Sara

Sara had a spinal tumor removed when she was a child and is now paraplegic. She has some sensation and movement in her left leg but none in her right; she uses crutches. She has never had pressure sores but does have problems with muscle spasms. She has scoliosis and frequent backaches. Her other problems are frequent constipation, susceptibility to bladder infections, and frequent urination.

THORACIC OUTLET SYNDROME

The simple definition of *thoracic outlet syndrome* (TOS) is that this condition includes neurovascular symptoms in the upper extremities due to pressure on the nerves and vessels in the thoracic outlet area. The specific structures compressed are usually the nerves of the *brachial plexus* and occasionally the *subclavian artery* or *subclavian vein*. The symptoms are produced by a positional, intermittent compression. Thoracic outlet syndrome is a group of symptoms arising not only from the upper extremity, but also in the chest, neck, shoulders, and head. The diagnosis is made easier by the physician's awareness and with physical examination using certain criteria, including elevation of the hands, *supraclavicular* tenderness, and weakening of the 4th and 5th fingers (10).

Taryn Dion

Taryn Dion has both TOS and degenerative disc disease. The degenerative disc disease affects her 4th and 5th cervical vertebrae, causing pain in both of her arms, hands, shoulders, chest, upper back, and the lateral vertebral muscles that attach to the ribs and go up the side of the neck (*scalene* muscles). Her pain varies and generally worsens with use. One of the causes is constricted venous return from the arm and hands, which has resulted in a chronic inflammation in all of her upper extremity muscles as well as direct compression of the brachial plexus nerves. She had a breast reduction 15 years prior to her pregnancy.

Tessa

Tessa has TOS *bilaterally* (on both sides) due to constriction under her collarbone. Her first symptoms of TOS started in her 20s. Tessa has 60 percent use of her left arm and 75 percent of her right. She uses her left arm for strength, endurance, and coordination. Although her right side is dominant, she experiences chronic pain in her right shoulder and neck.

Tina

Tina has pain in her upper and lower back, neck, left shoulder, and both arms. The pain in her left hand and left side are worse due to swelling on that side. She also has intermittent numbness in her shoulder. She had a hard labor and was given morphine. The medication altered her perception of pain, which resulted in Tina's clutching the bed bar with her hands. This strenuous activity caused an exacerbation that lasted 6 weeks. Since then, Tina has been in remission with guarded activity.

Closing Comments

Pregnancy is an enterprise of uncertainty and hope, and although no one can guarantee an ideal experience, the most important advice from these women is:

"Enjoy yourself!"

Emotional Concerns in Having Children

MOST OF THE BOOKS that have been written to help people decide whether to become parents fail to address the important concerns of women with disabilities. These books are written with the assumption that most women are under considerable pressure to become mothers, and the authors make a point of reassuring women that the decision *not* to have children is reasonable and acceptable.

The forces of social disapproval and their own fears often work against many disabled women in their decision to have children. Even when they were illegal, abortions were routinely done by American doctors for women with physical disabilities. When Sasha, a woman with spina bifida, was pregnant in the 1960s, she said that she did not seek medical care until her fifth month because she "didn't want a big hassle." Even then, 5 months pregnant, Sasha had to visit four doctors before she found one who would help her. "The others all pressured me to have an abortion." Sasha finished her story by commenting, "I hope some changes have come about and that it is no longer considered a cardinal sin for women with disabilities to have babies." But many disabled women still encounter negative attitudes toward their pregnancies. Sharon, who is paraplegic, says that when she became pregnant in 1979 her gynecologist's first reaction was to ask whether she was going to keep the baby. Such responses are common. Even in the 1990s, women with disabilities faced prejudice based on ignorance. Sabine ran into ignorance from her new doctor, who told her before examining her that she could not carry a child to term. In fact, the doctor was wrong.

Sophia Amelia encountered prejudice early in her first pregnancy when she attempted to sign up for WIC (Women, Infants and Children Supplemental Food Program). She said, "I was told by the technician that she would not file the paperwork until I filed rape charges against the father. She thought there was no way I could have a consensual sexual relationship. I responded with, 'I need to talk with your supervisor'."

Friends, family, and strangers react to a disabled woman's pregnancy in a number of ways, ranging from approval and support to open surprise and even hostility. Whatever the external pressures, women with disabilities often have the same feelings about parenthood as do able-bodied women. They describe the same hopes for building loving families and expressing their creativity by doing a good job of childrearing. Michelle captured this feeling beautifully when she said, "I wanted to have a child so I could be part of the flow of history."

Disabled women's lives are changing. They are claiming a right every woman must have: the right to decide whether and when to become a mother.

For a woman with disabilities, making this decision involves finding answers for many questions: How will pregnancy affect my disability? How will the disability affect the course of pregnancy and the health and development of the baby? How might my disability influence the way I fulfill the emotional and physical tasks of childrearing?

When Holly became pregnant with her first baby, there was almost no information on the subject of pregnancy and maternal hydrocephalus (Holly's diagnosis). She and her husband realized how important it was to find out how others in similar circumstances had fared. Holly used the Internet to find information, and she set up a database with her husband's encouragement.

Tessa's husband wanted a child, but Tessa had a lot of hesitancy because of her disability. Tessa thought that her feelings about her disability affected her feelings about being a mother, so she worked with a therapist on separating her feelings about having a disability and being a mother. Tessa said, "My husband and I did some therapy for 6 months, trying to unravel those issues. We tried to visualize what it would be like to have a child without a disability. It was important because it gave me an idea that I wouldn't mind doing that. I had to think about how I could do parenting safely." Tessa set aside some money to pay for a nanny so she would feel secure that she would not injure herself or the baby.

Rachel decided to conceive a baby while having a flare-up of rheumatoid arthritis. Consequently, she had lots of fears about how she would take care of her new baby, but she still felt it was important to have another child. Some of Rachel's concerns regarding her ability to take care of her baby were addressed by staff at Through the Looking Glass (TLG), a national resource center located in Berkeley, California that specializes in services and adaptive equipment related to parenting with a disability (see Appendix D). This center has had several national grants that have focused on creating adaptive equipment and studying its impact on parenting. The research, the equipment, and answering questions from callers have led to many of the insights that are incorporated in this book.

Sometimes women's feelings or lack of information lead them to make unrealistic assumptions about what will happen to them during pregnancy. One such assumption is, "My pregnancy will be just like my mother's." This was Celeste's belief; she was afraid she would have a stillborn child just as her mother had (Celeste herself had been born prematurely). She should not have assumed that her vomiting in late pregnancy (like her mother) meant she would have a stillborn child. Celeste said, "There isn't any excuse. It was a neurotic fear. My mother was such a dynamic woman and I felt I couldn't do better than she had."

Many of the women interviewed for this book said they were afraid of falling during pregnancy. Ordinarily, they might worry because their disabilities made falling likely or because falls could lessen their mobility. Instead, when they were pregnant, they worried that falling might injure the fetus. Ever since Scarlett O'Hara's tumble down the stairs in the movie *Gone with the Wind*, the idea that falls inevitably cause miscarriages has probably been one of the most common misconceptions about pregnancy in twentieth century America. It is not true, as Celeste discovered when she fell and later said, "It's like landing on a balloon." A variation on this theme was one woman's fear that pressing on her bladder to eliminate urine would cause mental retardation in her child. The fetus is well protected by the amniotic sac and amniotic fluid, the uterine wall, and other structures of the body the majority of the time, and falling or pressing the bladder presents very little danger. Some women did have mobility problems in late pregnancy, and a concern about being injured by falling can be realistic, but a fetus being injured by the pregnant woman falling is rare. This can occur only if the placenta is attached to the front wall of the uterus.

Sometimes feelings will arise that you were unaware of. Heather's answers to the questionnaire exemplify the complex emotions we all experience. In explaining why she decided to have children, Heather said, "I always wanted babies. It never occurred to me I couldn't." Yet, when asked, "What was your reaction to learning you were pregnant?" she replied, "Sheer excitement that I could do it." Clearly, it was difficult for her to recognize her self-doubt. I hope that as you read what other women have to say, you will discover that you are not alone in anything you feel, and perhaps you will make new discoveries about yourself.

One surprising discovery may be that your desire to have a child is more intense than you realized. Some women, not realizing how much they wanted children, had unplanned pregnancies partly because they were unaware of their own feelings. Not only was Julie's pregnancy unplanned, but the timing was unfortunate and she became a single parent in a community that frowned on single motherhood. Later, she commented, "It just happened. Probably subconsciously I was ready for it." Stacy's unplanned pregnancy occurred when she discontinued birth control pills because she thought that "having a lot of X-rays for many years" had made her infertile. One wonders why she took birth control pills for several years then changed her mind. Had she not thought about the X-rays before, or did she, like Julie, unconsciously hope to become pregnant? In either case, the experience shows the importance of carefully exploring your feelings and all of the information available.

The process of self-examination necessitates asking the following questions and exploring these issues:

❖ How does the effect of disability on a woman's self-image influence her decision-making?

❖ Interactions between pregnancy and disability: What are the physical consequences of pregnancy? How will pregnancy affect you? Will your disability affect your ability to give birth to a healthy, full-term baby?

❖ The possibility of having disabled children: What is the possibility that you will have a disabled child? Can genetic counseling help answer this question? What are your feelings about having a disabled child who may or may not have the same disability as you?

❖ Do people with disabilities have unique experiences in their role as parents?

❖ What skills does a good parent need? Are these skills really affected by disability? How do children feel about having disabled parents?

❖ The cost of having a child: How can you plan for the expenses of pregnancy, childbirth, and childrearing?

❖ How will having a child affect your other relationships, particularly your relationship with your husband or partner?

❖ What are some of the advantages and disadvantages of combining a career and family or choosing to be a full-time parent?

Certainly, there is a sense in which any woman considering motherhood feels that her selfhood will be enhanced by having children. She may be seeking self-validation in a broad sense, hoping to join "the flow of history" or to prove her femininity. There may be a more specific motivation such as a desire to "do a better job than my parents did" or to disprove stereotypes about disability.

The unique experiences of women with disabilities lend a special flavor to these concerns. For example, a disabled woman, as she ages, is concerned not only about declining fertility but also about declining physical abilities. She may believe (often correctly) that if she is going to have children, she had better hurry. As Julie examined her unconscious reasons for her unplanned pregnancy, she commented, "The older I get, the more limitation I have to deal with, so having children became more important." Even for women whose disability is not progressive, concerns about aging are strengthened by the knowledge that disability adds to the usual stresses of aging. Whether a woman is eager to have children or nervous about the idea, her feelings may be strengthened by fears of aging. Nicole made a conscious decision to have her third child as a single parent: "I knew what to expect and what my limits were. I made sure I had plenty of help."

Natasha wanted to have her baby "…when I was still capable, because I did not know what to expect with progression of the disability."

Sometimes a love relationship can also change a person's mind about becoming a parent. Amy's amputation was the result of a car accident, and she never expected to get married after the accident. Amy finally realized she could marry when she found the right man: "I realized when we got together that I could be a mom. He built my confidence."

A disabled woman's self-image may have been damaged by negative social attitudes or by the frustrations of physical limitation. The author recalls a painful childhood experience: she was left behind whenever her elementary school had air raid or fire drills.

The principal proudly informed her father that she was being "protected." By excluding her from the fire drills, the principal hoped to protect her from being jostled and knocked down by the other children. Her father insisted that she be included in future fire drills because she needed to know what to do in a real emergency. But, in her mind, the damage had already been done; she felt she was being left behind because children like her were less valuable than others.

Women with disabilities—even more than many able-bodied women—feel a need to prove their femininity, maturity, or worthiness by having children because they know that many people see them as asexual. The wish to prove oneself may have to do with physical self-image or social self-image. For example, Julie "loved being pregnant because for once my body worked right." Arlene said, "Having a baby made me less handicapped because I was able to fulfill one of the female roles in society and I was really rewarded for it." Heather felt that she was "proving I was as independent and as self-reliant as anyone." Noelle "loved being associated with the nondisabled population. It was my only chance," adding that the shared interests and concerns of parenthood offered a basis for friendships with nondisabled people.

You have lots of company if you have these kinds of feelings. But pregnancy and parenthood are full of surprises. The unpleasant surprises can be more unpleasant for people who are unprepared for them, and needless fears can dampen enjoyment of the happy ones. Sasha remembered, "I was afraid. I wish I'd let myself enjoy pregnancy more." The best way to prepare for the surprises is to know the possibilities and to know yourself.

The Interaction Between Pregnancy and Disability

Several of the interviewees feared their disabilities would cause problems in pregnancy or that pregnancy would affect their disabilities. Several thought they would be unable to become pregnant or that the pregnancy would be too difficult. Sonya said, "My husband and I were not sure about having this baby; but now that he is here, we can't even believe we ever had doubts about having him. I feel I have a purpose in life now." Joan "was in shock" when she got pregnant because "for years there was nothing" then "after we started taking ginseng I got pregnant."

Medical professionals had told Sophia Amelia that she could not, or should not, become pregnant. She had a *laparoscopy* performed to confirm whether or not she could become pregnant. (Laparoscopy is a diagnostic procedure that uses a small scope to look inside the abdomen; the procedure includes injecting contrast dye into the fallopian tubes.) She was told that her tubes were completely blocked by scar tissue and she could not become pregnant. She became pregnant soon afterward, but this pregnancy was not planned. She was told that the procedure itself may have cleared scar tissue from the fallopian tubes.

Allison said, "The two things I was most concerned about were weight gain and the fit of the prosthesis. I talked mostly to my certified prosthetist and I was really careful with weight gain."

Celeste was "ecstatic" when she found out she was pregnant; she was also "scared.... I knew it was going to be difficult. My first reaction was: I'll need a caesarean section! I welcomed it." Sasha had thought she could not get pregnant and, "I was afraid I would die in pregnancy or childbirth because of my disability (spina bifida)." Sharon was "shocked, but not really excited. Because of my age and being paraplegic, I didn't know what to expect."

Celeste and Sasha later felt that they had worried more than necessary. Celeste gave birth vaginally and had ordinary pregnancy symptoms such as morning sickness. Sasha said, in looking back at her pregnancy, "I'm sorry I didn't enjoy it more."

Naomi was "deathly afraid" to become pregnant and looked into other options. She went to a muscular dystrophy support group. At that meeting, Naomi was very clear about her fears and found support in deciding not to get pregnant. Once she expressed her fear, however, Naomi rethought her feelings. She and her husband went to a medical library and found one study of seventeen women with spinal muscular atrophy who had become pregnant. She said, "Although it wasn't a large enough number of cases to count for anything, they all had a more severe case than me, and they all did okay. One-third had no residual aftereffects at all; a third had some problems in the pregnancy or delivery with no residual; and a third had some residual that was gone in a year or two. So I said, 'What the heck'."

Most interviewees either experienced remission of symptoms during pregnancy or felt better than usual. Some experienced no change; a very few experienced temporary exacerbations of their disabilities. No one felt that her disability had been permanently worsened or improved, but this is not a guarantee because each person is different. A few of the interviewees wondered aloud in informal conversations a few years after their interviews whether there had, in fact, been lasting effects. It was also possible that aging or continuing disease processes were responsible for the new problems that these women experienced.

Most often, the problems and discomforts that the interviewees described were the same ones that able-bodied women experience such as fatigue or back pain. Although their existing disability symptoms were sometimes exacerbated, a few of the interviewees developed new symptoms and others got relief from their disability symptoms. The symptoms most likely to intensify seem to be those that can also be caused by pregnancy. For example, a majority of pregnant women experience an increased frequency of urination and an increased risk of bladder infection. Therefore, women who are prone to bladder infections may find that they worsen. Back problems and respiratory difficulties may also worsen during late pregnancy. Many pregnant women who use a wheelchair are prone to heartburn. The reason is thought to be the limited amount of room for the baby and the expanding uterus. As the uterus expands, it pushes up on the stomach, causing heartburn. The case of Nikki, who uses a wheelchair and had heartburn during only three out of seven pregnancies, may suggest a different conclusion. One may surmise that the placement of the fetus may be the cause of the heartburn during pregnancy.

The interviews also suggested that often it is the severity of disability, rather than the type, that helps predict the mobility problems that will occur during pregnancy. For example, a woman who is quadriplegic because of cerebral palsy may have more in common with a woman who is quadriplegic due to spinal cord injury than with a woman with milder cerebral palsy.

The next chapter discusses common pregnancy complications as well as those that are known to occur in connection with specific disabilities. This can be the starting point in learning about the possible consequences of pregnancy.

Closing Comments

The next chapter covers a number of factors to aid in decision making, including fertility, pregnancy discomforts, childcare, having more than one child, and the possibility of having a child with a disability. The section on disabled children covers emotional concerns, genetic testing, and immunizations. The information regarding the discomforts of pregnancy is based primarily on published sources.

The Interaction Between Pregnancy and Disability

IT CAN BE DIFFICULT for a pregnant woman to know whether she is experiencing a pregnancy-related problem or a disability-related problem. So, if you are considering pregnancy, it is important to follow Heather's advice: "Try to know your body. Become aware of what is normal for your body so you can decipher what is a pregnancy symptom and what is a disability symptom." Sometimes it may be more important to pay attention to other health conditions that may not be directly related to your disability. For example, if you have a tendency to become constipated, pregnancy could exacerbate this problem. The prenatal vitamins (with or without iron) that are commonly prescribed during pregnancy can also cause constipation.

Common Problems

Specific problems sometimes associated with disability, such as kidney dysfunction, can affect pregnancy and must be evaluated before conception. Other disability symptoms may be worsened by pregnancy. For example, a woman with respiratory problems may have more difficulty breathing during late pregnancy, when pressure from the uterus causes many women to become short of breath; others may go into remission. Some women who have been on medication to control, treat, or reduce disability symptoms may have to stop the medication because of possible harmful effects on the fetus. Therefore, it is important to know the classification of the medication you are taking. It is important to find either alternative medication or alternative treatments if you have to stop a particular medication. Rachel said, "I cleared myself of all medication. I was taking some strong rheumatoid arthritis drugs: methotrexate, Aquanal®, and prednisone. I stopped taking them all about 2 months before we tried to conceive. I started seeing a naturopath. I started changing my diet, which always seems to help a little bit. I also started to get some acupuncture. The acupuncture was amazing. Although it didn't necessarily help my joints, it helped my muscles and my frame of mind."

Olivia said, "I cut my medication in half after I found out I was 3 weeks pregnant."

All medications are classified into the following categories: Class A drugs are safe in pregnancy. Class B is known not to have caused harm in animals but has not yet been studied in humans. Class C is known to cause adverse effects in lab animals. Class D is known to cause fetal harm. Class X is contraindicated.

The medications that are often prescribed to people with disabilities include:

- ❖ Class B: oxybutynin chloride (Diptropan®)
- ❖ Class C: interferon (Avonex®, Rebif®, Betaseron®), tizanidine hydrochloride (Zanaflex®)
- ❖ Class D: carbamazepine (Tegretol®)

You can check the classifications of your medicine(s) in the most recent edition of the *Physicians' Desk Reference*, or you can ask your pharmacist for the package insert.

Women with physical disabilities are likely to have increased mobility problems and fatigue during pregnancy. Most insurance plans allow a person to get one mobility aid once every 5 years and, therefore, it is important to consider your mobility needs before pregnancy. It is also important to consider what your needs might be during pregnancy and the early parenting years. Some women may need two different mobility aids. Some women prefer to walk around the house and use a wheelchair when they are out in the community. Therefore, you may want to purchase the cheaper aid and let the insurance company buy the expensive one. Many women who are able to walk around the house may be unable to walk carrying a baby in their arms. A four-wheeled walker that uses a baby seat attached to the walker's seat was designed by TLG to solve this problem. Since its inception in 1982, TGL has worked with disabled parents, offering both direct services and research. TLG designs accessible baby equipment.

When ordering a power wheelchair, consider the features that you might use while pregnant, even though you do not need them at present. For example, tilt and recline features can help you change position in order to relieve pressure points.

Effects of Specific Disabilities on Pregnancy

LOWER LIMB AMPUTATION

Women who have lower limb amputation may need to modify their prostheses due to problems related to weight gain and edema. Dennis Swigart, former chief of prosthetics at Stanford University, said, "Prostheses with silicone or gel liner and pin-locking suspension are probably the easiest to modify. The number and ply of socks worn between the liner and frame can be adjusted as the volume of the residual limb changes. Also, the liner itself can often be changed from thicker to thinner materials to allow for more comfort. Rigid sockets are more challenging to modify but can be enlarged by grinding down or otherwise opening up the brim. Finally, it is possible to fabricate a temporary socket if the prosthetic limb needs to accommodate large volume changes.

"Women who use belts for suspension of a prosthesis will need to change to a different system, because tight straps across the abdomen are not comfortable during pregnancy. During routine exams, the prosthetist should check for abnormal wear and tear of components and for poor alignment of the prosthesis. Prosthetic feet are rated according to the wearer's weight and activity level. The extra weight during pregnancy can increase the risk of breakdown in the foot. Call your prosthetist immediately if you hear strange noises or the foot feels odd. The knee can become unstable if a woman becomes too sedentary and develops tight muscles, which will require adjustments to the alignment. Adjust your sock plies before skin breakdown. It is also advised to shower at night and wear a shrinker sock to bed in order to maintain a smaller limb volume for putting the prosthesis on comfortably in the morning" (11).

ARTHROGRYPOSIS

The arthrogryposis national Web site did a survey of pregnancy. As with most of the disabilities, there is not a large enough sample to make any recommendations, but here is the information collected. A total of twenty-one responses were received. Of those, seventeen did not know the type of arthrogryposis they had or they did not state it. There were two cases of *distal* arthrogryposis, one *amyoplasia* and one *genetic*. A total of thirty-four children were born to the twenty-one women. Nine mothers had more than one child and twelve had one child. The average age of the interviewees at the birth of their first child was 24 years. Of those who responded, seven were currently in their 20s; ten were in their 30s; one was in her 40s; one was in her 50s; and two were in their 60s. Of the thirty-four births, fifteen were carried to term; seven were not carried to term; and twelve did not state. One of the thirty-four babies died at the age of 7 months of unknown causes. Twenty pregnancies were listed as having no complications. Problems with balance, mobility, or driving were mentioned in nine of the pregnancies. Of those, three women mentioned using a wheelchair during part of their pregnancy. Problems not related to arthrogryposis were mentioned in five pregnancies. These include high blood pressure, morning sickness, and low platelets. Two persons reported back or hip pain.

It is unknown from this data if the interviewees who miscarried were severely affected by having multiple contractures—in other words, did the contractures cause poor circulation and did the poor circulation, in turn, cause an increased risk of miscarriage (12)?

CEREBRAL PALSY

Many women with cerebral palsy experience increased muscle spasms during pregnancy. A small study by Winch and colleagues that analyzed twenty-two women with cerebral palsy found that the rate of caesarean section was about the same as "...from the general population....Nine of the 28 births in our sample were by caesarean section.... All eight of the women who were delivered by caesarean section had lower extremity motor deficit, although some women with contractures delivered vaginally" (13).

DWARFISM

A study in Scandinavia by Kappel and colleagues (14) found that the need for caesareans was three times higher in those with dwarfism than the general public. This study also found higher rates of "intrauterine asphyxia, intrauterine growth retardation, and low *Apgar* scores" in babies of women with dwarfism. The Apgar test is given at the time of delivery; the possible scores range from zero to ten, with ten being the healthiest for a newborn. Having an X-ray prior to pregnancy will help determine the width of the pelvis. A study from India by Desai and colleagues found that many of the fetuses were in the breech position (15). The Indian study found that there was a higher incidence of stillbirth and neonatal death. This study also found increased need for caesarean section. In an article from Canada, Carstoniu and colleagues (16) stated that "the risks of general versus *epidural* anesthesia must be considered for each patient, as the severity of the spinal abnormalities can vary considerable." One may conclude that it is important to follow the growth of the fetus to prevent intrauterine growth, which can result in *intrauterine asphyxia* (the result of any process that deprives the fetus of oxygen).

Diastrophic Dwarfism. Women who have diastrophic dwarfism are at risk for cardiac arrest if the baby shifts against the diaphragm during the third trimester.

HYDROCEPHALUS

Children born with this condition have a shunt inserted to relieve pressure on the brain. There are two different types of shunts, which vary in where the end of the shunt is placed. The *ventriculoatrial* shunt (VA) ends in an *atrium* (one of the chambers of the heart). The end of this type of shunt usually stays open; but, as children grow, the process of growing tends to pull the shunt out-of-place. Therefore, more revisions are required during childhood with the VA shunt, compared with the *ventriculoperitoneal* shunt (VP), which ends in the space inside the abdomen. This type of shunt generally will require fewer revisions during childhood.

According to N. K. Bradley (17), decisions regarding the course of pregnancy with shunts need to consider:

- ❖ The relative value of specific shunt configurations
- ❖ The monitoring of late term headaches and other neurologic symptoms
- ❖ The management of delivery
- ❖ Pregnancy outcomes
- ❖ Unusual complications

According to Farine and colleagues (18), women should be "aware of the potential significance of headaches, drowsiness, irritability, and neurologic signs. Although these signs and symptoms may be nonspecific in pregnancy, they may also imply *shunt occlusion.*"

According to N. K. Bradley (19), "A ventriculoatrial (VA) shunt should be considered the shunt configuration of choice for all young women" who will consider pregnancy. Women who had VP (ventriciloperitoneal) shunt "were not without shunt-related complications."

MULTIPLE SCLEROSIS

Many researchers have written on the issues that must be considered by women with multiple sclerosis who desire to have a baby:

"In women with multiple sclerosis, the rate of relapse declines during pregnancy, particularly in the third trimester, and increases during the first 3 months [postpartum] before returning to the pre-pregnancy rate, as compared with the rate during the year before pregnancy" (20).

"The increased frequency of relapses during the postpartum period can reduce the ability of the mother to provide care for her newborn." (21). This study also found "that epidural analgesic and breast-feeding did not increase the risk of relapse or of worsening disability in the postpartum period."

Dr. Stone of the Edward J. and Louise E. Mellen Center for MS Treatment and Research at the Cleveland Clinic stated in an article in *InsideMS* (22): "If an MS relapse does occur, the use of the steroid *methylprednisolone* is okay, especially after the first trimester. But some neurologists are uncomfortable treating a relapse during pregnancy with steroids."

Dr. Patricia Coyle from State University of New York at Stony Brook "sees nothing to indicate that it is dangerous to use steroids to shorten MS relapses. At one time pediatricians were concerned regarding steroids, but sometimes steroids are in order for a woman who has to deliver early because they help mature a preterm infant's lungs. In other words, while a severe MS relapse during pregnancy is trying for everyone, there are safe and effective treatment options."

"Further studies have concluded that MS has no effect on pregnancy, but female offspring do have a 5 percent risk of developing MS. This is a 50-fold increase over the general population."

Dr. Lael Stone noted, "Most doctors recommend that women discontinue disease-modifying drugs for 1 month, or one cycle, prior to conception. In order to help women, the length of time they need to stop taking disease-modifying drugs is a question of heightened significance to older women, who may need more time to conceive." Dr. Stone recommends using ovulation kits and other non-medical methods to beef up the odds. She observed, "Theoretically, most fertility treatments are safe in MS, but there is virtually no data on this."

MYASTHENIA GRAVIS

In 1998, a study by Batocchi and colleagues (23) was completed that found "pregnancy does not worsen the long-term outcome of myasthenia gravis (MG). The course of disease is highly variable and unpredictable during gestation and can change in subsequent pregnancies." This study examined forty-seven women who had myasthenia gravis and became pregnant after receiving the diagnosis. "During pregnancy, MG relapse occurred in 4 of 23 (17 percent) asymptomatic patients who were on therapy before conception; in patients taking therapy, MG symptoms improved in 12 of 31 pregnancies (39 percent); remained unchanged in 13 (42 percent); and deteriorated in 6 (19 percent). MG symptoms worsened after delivery in 15 of 54 (28 percent) pregnancies. *Anti-acetylcholine receptor antibody* (anti-AchR ab) was positive in 40 of 47 mothers and was assayed in 30 of 55 newborns; 13 were positive; and 5 of 55 (9 percent) showed signs of neonatal MG."

NEUROMUSCULAR DYSFUNCTION

Charcot-Marie-Tooth

There seems to be no evidence of any ill effects of pregnancy on disability. The article that is cited here was based on a case study that stated: "Although respiratory difficulties may be worsened due to the increased respiratory demands of pregnancy.... This is the first report of artificial ventilation in a pregnancy complicated by Charcot-Marie-Tooth disease and illustrates that with careful maintenance of normal ventilation by mechanical assistance, as necessary, a successful outcome may be expected" (24).

In a case study from Israel, the authors wrote that a woman "with juvenile muscular dystrophy including severe scoliosis and severe *kyphoscoliosis* should be advised to avoid pregnancy or consider therapeutic abortion." Although this woman "with juvenile muscular dystrophy" had a difficult pregnancy, her major problem was "severe scoliosis and kyphoscoliosis." The authors also quoted an article that stated: "Cases of severe scoliosis or kyphoscoliosis should be considered high-risk and thus should be carefully monitored for clinical condition, lung function, and blood gases, and managed with hospitalization, respiratory support, intubation, and institution of mechanical ventilation when indicated. This should improve the prognosis of such pregnancies" (25, 26).

Facioscrapulohumeral Muscular Dystrophy

In a study reported in 1997 by Schoneborn and colleagues (27), women with facioscrapulohumeral muscular dystrophy "generally coped well with their muscle disease in pregnancy and after delivery." Three women out of eleven "reported an aggravation of symptoms related to pregnancy. Nonetheless, most patients recovered quickly in the postpartum period."

Friedreich's Ataxia

Respiratory difficulties increase with this condition, and pregnant women may experience frequent periods of shortness of breath. This was the experience of the two interviewees who have Friedreich's ataxia, and while it may indicate a trend, it is not enough of a sample from which to draw a conclusion.

Limb-Girdle Muscular Dystrophy

Schoneborn and colleagues (27) reported, "No deleterious outcome of pregnancy and labor was observed" in a study of twenty-seven women with different myopathies. This group of women had more caesarean sections, however. Moreover, it was noted there was "a significant aggravation of symptoms in gestation with early onset and progressive myopathy than in those with a stable disease course." Five out of the nine women reported a "weight-related worsening of weakness in pregnancy that did not improve after delivery," except for one woman. "All patients had a noticeable worsening of symptoms after delivery and needed a long time to recover postpartum."

In a case study reported in *The Journal of Reproductive Medicine* (28), a woman who had two successful pregnancies did not have any respiratory problems. There was no report of complications during either pregnancy. She delivered both babies vaginally without any complications.

Spinal Muscular Atrophy (SMA)

If lung function is already affected, it is probable that this system will be further distressed during pregnancy. This conclusion was drawn not only from the interview for this book, but also from an article based on two case studies (29). This article also concluded that women with SMA could have a "successful" pregnancy and delivery provided there is "close observation and a careful management planning." It also stated that there was no "obvious deleterious effects of the pregnancy on the progression of the disease."

Osteogenesis Imperfecta

There are four types of *osteogenesis imperfecta* (OI). Type 2 is the most severe form; a few people with this type have lived into early adulthood. Types 1 and 4 are the mildest forms of OI. "Pregnancy does not appear to have a significant adverse effect on the milder forms of OI. Women with OI Types 1 and 4 may experience loose joints, reduced mobility, increased bone pain, and dental problems during pregnancy."

Women with Type 3 have short stature and curvature of the spine. They "may be at risk for medical and obstetrical complications." In women who have severe scoliosis "the likelihood of heart and lung difficulties is increased. As the uterus grows, the shortened distance between the thoracic (rib) cage and the pubic bone can cause discomfort and result in a need for extended bed rest.

"Pregnancy has not been associated with an increase of maternal fractures. However, trauma during pregnancy or obstetrical manipulation at the time of vaginal delivery may result in fractures." Women who have a history of fractures of the pelvis or a contracted pelvis or Type 3 OI should have a caesarean section. "In general, decisions about the best mode of delivery (vaginal versus caesarean section) should be made on an individual basis. There are no definitive research data showing that caesarean delivery is safer than vaginal delivery in women with OI who have normal pelvic dimensions and no other significant complications. A recent study by Cubert (30) found evidence that caesarean delivery did not decrease fracture rates at birth in infants with non-lethal forms of OI, nor did it prolong survival for those with more severe forms. Some physicians believe it is appropriate when planning a mode of delivery to assess the degree of mineralization of the baby's skull. Theoretically, there is an increased risk of central nervous system injury with vaginal delivery when the baby's skull is poorly mineralized. Most caesarean deliveries in a recent study were done for the usual obstetric indications."

Post-Polio Syndrome

The effects of post-polio syndrome on pregnancy depend on an individual's particular symptoms. Women whose mobility is very limited are at risk for developing *deep vein thrombosis* (clots) during pregnancy.

Back deformities resulting from polio might make pregnancy and/or delivery more difficult.

Polio survivors are very sensitive to muscle relaxants because they have fewer neurons to block. "Past reports of not being able to reverse muscle relaxants, most likely due to drug overdose, have contributed to the fear of general anesthesia" (31).

One aspect to consider for women with post-polio syndrome is the effect of pregnancy on breathing. Some post-polio patients—especially those who used an iron lung or other ventilator when they were acutely ill—have poor respiratory reserve. They may even normally use a ventilator at night or during the day. The increasing size of the baby can interfere with marginal ventilation and full-time ventilator support may be needed. Ventilator support should be continued during labor and delivery. As pregnancy proceeds, repeated pulmonary function tests need to be done. A pulmonologist should manage this aspect of care.

Regional anesthesia, which is given near or at the spinal cord, can be used for post-polio patients, especially epidural anesthesia. There can be some technical problems when placing an epidural or spinal if scoliosis is severe, but usually these can be solved. Harrington rods can present a formidable obstacle to epidural or spinal anesthesia, but there are case reports of epidural anesthesia in the presence of Harrington rods. Because of recent information about the effects of local anesthetics on the spinal cord itself, it is probably wise to avoid spinal anesthesia, if possible, and use epidural instead. There is no specific evidence that spinal anesthesia should not be given to post-polio patients. This is a theoretical risk. The risks of all factors for an individual patient should be evaluated and a suitable choice made for that patient. If an epidural is not in place, two other useful techniques may be performed by the obstetrician: paracervical and pudendal blocks. These techniques use a local anesthetic injection around the nerves that carry the pain of labor and delivery. A paracervical block, given through the vagina, anesthetizes the nerves to the opening of the uterus and can be used for labor pain. A pudendal block, also done through the vagina, is used for anesthesia of the perineum (pelvic area). This block is used for the pain of delivery; it is also useful if lacerations occur and repair is needed. Both are useful in relieving pain when an epidural cannot be placed. Other choices for labor pain relief include intravenous narcotics or natural childbirth techniques; however, narcotics can affect the baby and cause a delay in the start of breathing after birth. Natural childbirth techniques need to be learned well before delivery, and classes are available in most parts of the country. A labor coach is also needed and a partner or helper should make a commitment to attend the classes and then help throughout labor (32). (The preceding section was written for this book by Dr. Selma Calmes.)

It is also important that "any blood loss should be promptly replaced" (31).

Rheumatoid Arthritis and Juvenile Rheumatoid Arthritis

"Complete remission of all signs and symptoms leading to no need for medication has been described in about 65 percent of pregnancies that show improvement of disease activity" (33). "Complications during pregnancy are not increased in *ankylosing spondylitis* and fetal outcomes are not compromised" (34). If arthritis has caused hip or spine deformities, delivery may be complicated and caesarean delivery may be necessary.

Nonsteroidal anti-inflammatory drugs (NSAIDs) are generally considered safe in early pregnancy, although studies in animals suggest that they may be associated with infertility related to *blastocyst*. Except for low-dose aspirin, NSAIDs should be discontinued 6 to 8 weeks prior to delivery, in order to avoid both maternal and fetal effects (3).

Gold compounds do not appear to impair fertility or cause neonatal malformations, but most rheumatologists recommend discontinuing these injections.

Scoliosis

The Alfred I. DuPont Institute studied 355 women to determine the impact of scoliosis on pregnancy. Each woman had *idiopathic* (of unknown cause) scoliosis. Of the 355 women, 178 had never been pregnant and 177 had at least one pregnancy. In the women who were observed but not treated, curvature increased more than 10 degrees in 9 percent of the pregnant and 11 percent of the nonpregnant women. In the women whose curvature was treated by surgery, there was almost no curvature progression in either group (pregnant or nonpregnant). Only two women out of sixty-five in the pregnant group had curvature progression of less than 10 degrees in the unfused segment. None of the nonpregnant women had any progression in the unfused segment. It was also found that, in the women who were treated by bracing, there was a greater difference between the pregnant and nonpregnant groups. Among these women curvature increased more than 10 degrees in 11 percent of the pregnant women and only 2 percent in the nonpregnant. The cause for the difference in this group is unknown. An analysis determined that there was a 10 percent higher risk of curvature progression for the thoracic area. Their conclusion was that pregnancy does not increase the risk of curve progression after skeletal maturity (35).

Spina Bifida

The average incidence of spina bifida is one in 1,000 births. Folic acid deficiency is one of the known causes of spina bifida. Prenatal intake of 400 to 800 micrograms of folic acid can prevent up to 70 percent of *neural tube defects*. The neural tube closes completely by day 21 of pregnancy, before most women even know they are pregnant. Therefore, all women of reproductive age should take folic acid regularly *before* they become pregnant. The recurrence risk is plus 5 percent after having one child with spina bifida, and women with spina bifida should take higher doses of folic acid. Spina bifida will not affect the ability to deliver vaginally, but hydrocephalus associated with spina bifida can influence the type of delivery.

Spinal Cord Injuries

Bladder infections are likely to become more frequent. Care should be taken to prevent severe infections, which can cause premature labor. Constipation may also worsen. Pressure from the uterus or impacted fecal matter could worsen breathing difficulties if the diaphragm is paralyzed. Dr. Amie Jackson did a comprehensive study (36) comparing pregnancy with pre-and post-spinal cord injury that indicated an increase in leakage around indwelling catheters and more frequent bladder spasms that expelled the catheter. Other complications, such as morning sickness, anemia, *toxemia*, and vaginal bleeding, did not increase.

Women with injuries at or above the T-6 level (sometimes T-8) have an increased risk autonomic dysreflexia during pregnancy. Autonomic dysreflexia will also occur during labor. Dysreflexia during pregnancy may increase the risk of miscarriage or premature labor.

Systemic Lupus Erythematosus (SLE)
(Commonly referred to as "Lupus")

"Successful pregnancy is now achievable by 85 percent of women with SLE" (37). It is best to wait until one is in remission for 6 months before trying to become pregnant. Some women who have SLE seek the help of a fertility specialist to get pregnant and stay pregnant. Lupus activity during pregnancy has been studied in recent years, and the conclusions reached were that SLE may flare at any time during pregnancy. These flares are usually mild and generally affect the skin and joints. They usually do not affect fetal outcome unless the kidneys are involved. Diagnosis of flares during pregnancy is difficult to determine and should be examined through clinical and laboratory assessment. No evidence supports the belief that steroids prevent flares during pregnancy and prednisone should not be given *prophylactically*. Flares are treated, depending on severity, with nonsteroidal anti-inflammatory drugs such as Plaquenil® or prednisone (38).

"Active renal disease and maternal hypertension are predictors of fetal loss and premature birth, respectively" (39).

Most researchers agree that SLE symptoms can occur during any trimester and postpartum. Control of SLE symptoms in pregnant patients with medications is frequently needed prior to, during, and after pregnancy (40).

"Available data support the use of *hydroxychloroquine* during pregnancy, especially if cessation would risk a flare of disease. This is particularly true for women with SLE, when a flare maybe life-threatening to both the mother and fetus" (3). Most flares are mild and easily treated with small doses of corticosteroids.

Another complication is *pregnancy-induced hypertension*. If you develop this serious condition, you will experience a sudden increase in blood pressure, protein in the urine, or both. Pregnancy-induced hypertension is a serious condition that requires immediate treatment, usually including delivery of the infant.

About 25 percent of lupus pregnancies end in unexpected miscarriages or stillbirths. Another 25 percent may result in premature birth of the infant. Although prematurity presents a danger to the baby, most problems can be successfully treated in a hospital that specializes in caring for premature newborns. About 3 percent of babies born to mothers with lupus will have *neonatal lupus*. This type of lupus consists of a temporary rash and abnormal blood counts. Neonatal lupus usually disappears by the time the infant is 3 to 6 months old and does not recur. About one-half of babies with neonatal lupus are born with a heart condition. This condition is permanent but can be treated with a pacemaker.

Check your health insurance plan. Make sure it covers both your health care needs and those of your baby for any problems that may arise.

Getting Pregnant: Fertility Issues

A home monitoring electronic device called the *Clear Plan Easy Fertility Monitor*™ identifies when a woman is most likely to conceive.

"*Ovulite*™ is a home fertility test that uses a woman's saliva to predict the best time to conceive. The manufacturers claim 98 percent accuracy" (41,42).

One of the new fertility methods involves harvesting multiple ova (eggs) from a potential mother. This procedure requires medication to stimulate ovarian follicle growth. There is a risk that this procedure may increase the chance of blood clots. This is a consideration for women who have limited mobility and may already be at risk for blood clots. A multiple pregnancy is another risk factor. "Pregnancies associated with assisted reproductive technology (ART) and drugs that induce ovulation are more likely to result in multiple births than spontaneously conceived pregnancies in the United States. Triplet and higher-order multiple births are at greater risk than single births to be preterm, low, or very low birth weight, which may result in higher infant morbidity and mortality. This report estimates the connection between these birth outcomes and ART and ovulation-inducing drugs in 1996 and 1997. It also summarizes the trends that indicate ART and the use of ovulation-inducing drugs have increased the ratio of triplet and higher-order multiple births during the 1980s and most of the 1990s (43).

Chelsea, a woman who has triplegic cerebral palsy (three limbs affected, two legs and an arm), decided after her fortieth birthday that it was more important to be a mother than to continue in her long-term relationship without children. She found a supportive infertility doctor and a donor. Chelsea also had the IUI (intrauterine procedure). She did not need any fertility drugs and got pregnant. She paid for the procedure herself.

Diane said, "It took us quite a long time to get pregnant. We were impatient and we did not want to wait any longer, so we talked to a fertility person. I was a little nervous because I wondered what would happen if I had more than twins. I got scared because I knew my body couldn't handle that." The doctors also posed that scenario. Diane said, "I prayed real hard that I would not have more than twins." She had bed rest and delivered two healthy babies.

Although Jackie had juvenile rheumatoid arthritis, she was able to get pregnant twice, but she lost both fetuses. Jackie moved and found a new obstetrician, who found Jackie's inflammatory levels to be mildly elevated. She was put on methotrexate for at least 8 months. During this time, the obstetrician decided to take films of her uterus and ovaries. The test found a fibroid tumor that was acting like an IUD, so that the fetus could not implant into the uterine wall. This illustrates how important it is for the doctor to investigate the more common problems that any woman might have.

Taryn Dion was put on Clomid® for two cycles without a pregnancy. She told her doctor she had noticed she did not have much cervical mucous while taking the drug. Her doctor told her it was possible that the Clomid® was actually blocking her production of estrogen, preventing her from getting pregnant. The doctor advised her to take it for one more cycle "and just before you ovulate, we'll do an ultrasound and measure the thickness of your uterus." Taryn Dion said, "Sure enough, I was just about to ovulate and my uterus wasn't thick enough to support egg implantation. The doctor wasn't sure it was going to work, but she gave me an estrogen patch to put some of the estrogen back into my system. It worked, and that was the month I got pregnant."

Joy tried to get pregnant for 2 years and saw a fertility specialist. She was on fertility drugs for approximately a year and a half. Joy said, "It was finally determined that I probably wouldn't be able to have children unless I had artificial insemination." She and her then husband decided to wait. Joy had experienced a bad flare-up of her arthritis because of the combination of taking fertility drugs and being off her arthritis medication for the past 2 years. She got pregnant with a new partner 7 years later.

Find the Most Current Information

In addition to the information in this book, disabled women who want to get pregnant should look for the most current medical information available, because it changes as new research is done. For example, not very long ago women with MS were told that pregnancy might cause their symptoms to flare up, but more recent studies show that "conception, gestation, and epidural anesthesia will not alter the natural history of their disease" (21). Contact organizations with information about your specific disability, especially if new information might change your course of action.

Your doctor may be able to advise you in more detail about the interaction between pregnancy and your disability, but he may not offer specific advice on your first visit. He may want to review recent research or consult other specialists before making any suggestions. It is usually best to begin by seeing a disability specialist. If you are seeing an obstetrician or family practitioner, you might wish to share the written information you have about your disability. Your doctor may also need to order some diagnostic tests. Blood tests will be done to evaluate kidney function and/or pulmonary function. These tests show whether women with respiratory or kidney difficulties can withstand the additional stress of pregnancy. Hip or spine X-rays or MRIs should be ordered to determine whether spinal anesthesia can be used safely. It is also important to determine whether intubation during anesthesia might be necessary and whether it might injure a woman with arthritis.

Below are several questions you may want to discuss with your doctor:

❖ Will my disability affect the health or development of my baby? For example, "Can my dysreflexia cause premature labor or labor complications that would endanger the baby?"
❖ What problems or pregnancy complications might my disability cause?
❖ How severe could these complications (if any) be? Mildly painful, severely painful, life-threatening? Would they be likely to temporarily or permanently worsen my disability?
❖ Could complications be treated or prevented? For example, autonomic dysreflexia, which causes high to extremely high blood pressure, occurs in people with a high spinal cord injury when pain or discomfort occur, as from an over-full bladder or bladder infection, or skin irritation caused by tight clothing, sunburn, or other irritant, including labor. "Inability to sense these irritants before the autonomic reaction begins is a major cause of dysreflexia" (9). This condition can be life-threatening. "Uncontrolled release of norepinephrine causes a rapid rise in blood pressure and a slowing of the heart rate. These symptoms are usually accompanied by throbbing headache, nausea, anxiety, sweating, and goose bumps below the level of the injury. The elevated blood pressure can rapidly cause loss of consciousness, seizures, cerebral hemorrhage, and death. Dysreflexia can generally be managed with medication. Women who have experienced dysreflexia during labor have successfully given birth with epidural anesthesia."
❖ Do the treatments for complications have any risks or disadvantages? For example, could medicine prescribed for a given problem have unpleasant side effects or be dangerous for the fetus?
❖ What could be the long-term effects of treatment?

❖ Is my disability likely to cause problems during labor or delivery? For example, if you have hip dysplasia, you can discuss whether it is severe enough to necessitate caesarean surgery.

❖ Is there anything that can be done before pregnancy to prevent or minimize problems? For example, you may want to follow an exercise program to strengthen low back muscles before the stress of pregnancy, or change a medication regimen. Tina went to physical therapy for 10 months and worked on both TOS and lower back pain. She said, "We worked on strengthening my core, which includes mostly working on your stomach muscles. Then we looked for gym equipment that is functional in terms of getting you stronger, but not flaring you up."

❖ Are there resources within a prospective clinic or hospital that could be useful during my pregnancy? For example, you may want to consult with a physical or occupational therapist for ideas about taking care of yourself and your child.

Many women said that they had received different advice from different doctors. What then? Chapter 5 examines this question from the viewpoint of women who are pregnant or those who want a child. For them the question is "How will I find the right person to help me carry out my decision?"

It may be that doctors who disagree are both (or all) correct. Perhaps different research has different conclusions, and each doctor is inclined to rely on the research that confirms her own experience. Or a doctor may justifiably believe that a research finding or a method of treatment is too new to be relied upon. To understand differences of opinion, tell your doctor that you have read or heard different advice from different sources and you would like to hear his opinion. Bring any written articles to your doctor(s) and include them in the discussion.

If it seems to you that there really is room for legitimate differences of opinion, rely on the advice that makes the most sense to you and your husband or partner. Or, make your decision on another basis. For example, Michelle had no way of knowing whether pregnancy would end her remission of MS. She decided, "Even if I'd have to be permanently disabled, I'd rather take the consequences than not have the baby." Remember, ultimately you are your own expert.

Additional Concerns

In thinking about the interaction of pregnancy with your disability, you need to be concerned about safety. Another concern is what discomfort or inconvenience may occur. How would you feel about living with certain discomforts? Answering this question is not easy, because no one can predict the severity of discomfort or what discomfort will be experienced, including morning sickness, fatigue, or other problems that can occur with pregnancy. Becoming acquainted with other women's experiences may put the possibilities in perspective. Denise compared her pregnancy with women whose diagnosis is diastrophic dwarfism versus women whose diagnosis is achondroplastic dwarfism. The length of the torsos is different and, therefore, the pregnancies may have different discomforts. Some women compared their pregnancies with those of able-bodied women:

Claudia: "It felt good to be part of the sorority."

Sylvia: "I got jealous of women who had easier pregnancies."

Patricia: "It made me feel good because I had a better pregnancy than they did."

When Naomi compared her pregnancy with those of other women, she found that she experienced no nausea, although she felt worse in other ways because she was quite physically immobilized.

Other women compared the pregnancies they had before the onset of disability with those occurring after onset.

Samantha had two children before her spinal cord injury and one afterward. Samantha said, "I naturally compared. I had a friend who delivered 3 weeks before me, and we compared a lot. This pregnancy was so much like the other two. My second and third were almost the same."

Paula also compared pregnancies before and after polio: "Compared to the first it was different. Physically I was in totally different shape; I wore two leg braces. But I thoroughly enjoyed being pregnant. Not worrying about the baby—that part felt intact—it felt so nice."

Renee had experienced the first, painful onset of rheumatoid arthritis while she was pregnant with her first child. Later, she heard that women sometimes have a remission of symptoms during pregnancy. She was not sure at first that she wanted another pregnancy because she feared that, after she gave birth, the return of her arthritic pain would be unbearable. She eventually decided to have another child.

Sylvia had the most difficult pregnancy, physically, of anyone who was interviewed. She experienced severe muscle spasms, bowel problems, and autonomic dysreflexia. The dysreflexia caused episodes of premature labor and several other problems that were milder but still unpleasant. Not surprisingly, she sometimes wondered, "What the hell am I doing?" Later she said, "I came to the realization that 9 months is a long time. I kept wondering if it was ever going to end."

Even when pregnancy is comfortable and free of problems, it can seem as though it will never end. The mother-to-be can grow tired of carrying the extra weight, waking up several times a night to urinate, and finding comfortable positions for sleeping. But some of the other physical changes that take place may heighten your sense of anticipation. The sight of your growing abdomen is visible proof that something really is happening. The changes in your breasts can be satisfying if you are planning to breast-feed. Probably most exciting is the sensation of fetal movement. In spite of all her problems, Sylvia recalls the joy she felt when her baby moved, "It was great to notice the difference between the baby and her bowels and gas."

Whatever problems or discomforts occur, your way of coping will affect how you feel about your pregnancy. Pam needed bed rest to relieve many discomforts, but it was hard for her to slow down. She wore herself out even more when she resisted the need to rest. Pam commented, "I had learned to manage by pushing myself and ignoring my limitations. It was hard to adjust to being pregnant. I didn't rest as much as I should have because it felt like I was pampering myself."

Indeed, a woman with physical disabilities often has to meet life's obstacles with great stubbornness and a powerful refusal to be held back by her physical limitations. Her experience has taught her not to "pamper" herself. It can be difficult to change these patterns.

Arlene, who usually resented having to rest, thought, "Having a baby was a great reason to rest. I was able to say to myself, 'I'll have more time to read'." Some women tell themselves, "I'm not being lazy when I lie down. I'm working hard at growing a baby."

You may want to consider adoption if you think pregnancy may be too hard on your body and you are open to growing your family in a different way. "Women with significant disabilities who are attempting to adopt need to be prepared to address the wide range of barriers that they might encounter" (44). Yet, there are many adoptive parents with disabilities. Orielle had difficulty adopting 10 years ago, but since the birth of her child she has been able to adopt two children. Orielle credits the American with Disabilities Act (ADA) with creating an environment that supports disabled women's right to options.

Physical Consequences of Childcare

Portia, who has five children, stressed that the problems of pregnancy are temporary. When asked what advice she would give to women considering pregnancy, she replied, in part, "Pregnancy, labor, and delivery are the first steps you go through to reach the goal of being a parent." But afterward, as any mother will tell you, caring for children can be exhausting. Knowing this, Stephanie was pleased and excited to have children, but she was also reluctant because of the physical care of the children. Marsha's doctor did not worry that pregnancy would worsen her MS, but he worried that she would be overly fatigued by caring for a toddler. In fact, Marsha found that toddler care was not too hard for her, but that breast-feeding was exhausting.

Like the difficulties of pregnancy, the body's responses to the physical stresses of childcare are unpredictable. Dr. Amie Jackson, who did a comprehensive study of women with spinal cord injuries, stated that "the abortion frequency was higher in post-injury pregnancies" (36). This may be due to the mothers' concern about being able to physically care for a baby. Results of TLG research found that a majority of women are able to be the primary caretaker if they have the proper equipment, learn baby care techniques, and have adequate support.

Women whose disabilities are worsened by fatigue may want to consider the following issues:

Loss of sleep: Newborns have irregular sleeping patterns and may need middle of the night feedings and comfort. Toddlers and small children wake up with wet diapers, wet beds, nightmares, and illness. You may expect to feel tired and sleepy all the time during early parenting.

Physical stress: Being a playmate in your child's active games or supervising an especially active and curious toddler can be very tiring.

Emotional stress: Sometimes your child will be difficult to live with. The "terrible twos" and the teenage years are the most notoriously difficult stages of development. Some children will be more difficult, especially if your temperaments are not an easy fit. For example, you may prefer to be sedentary but your child is very active.

The physical demands of parenting may be fulfilled, but many of the interviewees did not seek possible solutions. Sara, who felt "overwhelmed" by both of her pregnancies, said, "I was more concerned about birth defects and not so much concerned about the physical aspects of taking care of children." Some people recommend babysitting as a way to learn about caring for a child. This may help you determine what kind of help and adaptive equipment you need.

The Possibility of Having a Disabled Child

One set of questions included in the interviews was, "What were your expectations, fears, and fantasies about the baby? Were they related to your disability? If so, how?" Sara's answer touched on many themes:

"My first thought was the baby could be disabled. I just hoped it would be okay. I didn't know whether my disability was hereditary, but if the child was disabled, I knew I'd be the best person to cope with whatever was there. I had constant fear that the baby would be disabled and I went to the university hospital to make sure it wasn't hereditary. When I found out it wasn't hereditary, I was able to breathe easier."

Naomi pointed out other reasons besides disability that may cause a woman to be concerned about getting pregnant. She said, "My strongest fear might have not been due to my disability. My mother died when I was 12." Naomi's fear was probably increased because she did not want her child to go through the painful abandonment and mourning she went through.

Dorothy pointed out a different opinion held by many in the disability movement: "Many people do not get the humanity wrapped around disability." Dorothy felt that the person with a disability has many other characteristics that make up a person. Some of the problems of being disabled have more to do with how you are viewed than with the disability itself.

I talked to Nora soon after her first child was diagnosed with Charcot-Marie-Tooth. She said, "It was hard to get that diagnosis, but I'm glad I had children. It was one of my biggest desires."

Some of the interviewees had been afraid that their children would be disabled. Several women with spinal cord injuries also worried that their babies would have physical problems. Sometimes it seemed that a woman's own difficulties or discomforts during pregnancy made her more pessimistic. Some women, like Dawn, felt that "my fear was not related to my disability. Every mother goes through that." Sasha's fear was certainly related to her disability, and she was surprised that she could do anything as normal as getting pregnant. She could only imagine that she would have a disabled child.

Some women felt that their concerns about the health of their babies were caused by their feelings about their own disabilities. Several women explained, "Since my body didn't work in other ways, I couldn't help feeling that it wouldn't work when I was pregnant." Celeste doubted she would be able to produce a healthy baby. She had always felt less competent than her able-bodied mother and could not help feeling, "If my mother had a disabled kid like me, I couldn't do any better." Clara's comment was especially illuminating: "I was really excited to have a baby and I did not want my kid to be disabled. Being disabled myself and working with disabled people gave me a fear that physical disabilities are much more common than they really are, and that was scary."

Some of the interviewees reacted to their fear with denial. Celeste was so afraid that her baby would be stillborn that she protected herself "against having any expectations." Others tried to suppress the fear itself. Arlene said she felt some fear but she did not let it rule her. Corinne said of her fear, "I didn't dwell or obsess on it." Tina said, "During my pregnancy I was pretty much in denial until the ninth month when I went to TLG and found out about the adaptations that I would need."

Corinne and Arlene did not dwell on their fears because they had sought information assuring them that their disabilities were not hereditary.

Hilary also consulted a genetic counselor in order to reassure her parents-in-law. Leslie's pregnancies always involved the risk of miscarriage, and she pointed out that sometimes the choice to live with some fear is simply an aspect of trying to have a child. There are really two separate questions to ask about how your disability might affect your fetus:

❖ Will my disability affect fetal development, labor, and delivery?
❖ Can my disability be inherited?

It is important to convey your acceptance of your own disability when you meet with a genetic counselor about the possibility of having a disabled child. Olivia said, "The genetic counselor offered the grim opinion that my baby could already have broken bones, but I held onto the vision of having a healthy baby." Diane said, "I'm pretty healthy and I turned out okay, so we figured why not."

Some women with disabilities might have a greater risk of giving birth prematurely or of having difficult labors that could affect their babies. For example, the high blood pressure of dysreflexia might precipitate premature labor, and premature birth can cause disability.

Another concern may be having a child with a congenital disability. The term *congenital disability* can be confusing. *Congenital* refers to a disability that is present from the time of birth, but although the two words sound familiar, not all congenital problems are genetically caused. Some congenital disabilities are due to problems in the prenatal environment such as certain illnesses in the mother. A well-known example is hearing loss in children whose mothers had *cytomegalovirus* infection during pregnancy. Research into the causes of congenital disability continues and, thus, a genetic counselor can give you the most recent information. Also, ask what immunizations are needed to prevent some disabilities. German measles vaccine, for example, is given in childhood, but to be safe from German measles while pregnant, you need a booster vaccination at least 1 month before you try to get pregnant. Chickenpox is another important vaccine that protects both the mother and the baby (45).

Some congenital disabilities can be inherited and it is important to consult a genetic counselor. Counselors have found that parents often over- or underestimate the likelihood that their disabilities will be inherited. Many genetic counselors do not understand that recommending the abortion of a fetus with the mother's disability is like saying, "YOU should not have been allowed to exist." Some caution should be taken, therefore, in selecting a genetic counselor.

Orielle went to a genetic counselor "because we would receive the best medical care for the baby if the baby had OI (*osteogenesis imperfecta*). We were afraid if the baby had OI it would not be seen on only one ultrasound. They may not do as many ultrasounds as they should to make sure the baby is doing okay." If the baby has OI, it will need special medical care. Although one ultrasound may not pick up OI, it is highly likely that having several ultrasounds will pick it up. She thought that going to a genetic counselor would insure good follow-up during pregnancy.

Some genetic conditions are inherited and a specific gene is passed from generation to generation. This means at least one parent is carrying a specific gene in every cell of his or her body. For example, all the cells of the body contain the gene for eye color. *Tay Sachs* disease and *sickle cell anemia* are examples of inherited disorders. Some other genetic conditions are *not* inherited. That is, the parents do not carry the gene in their bodies; instead, when a sperm or ovum cell was being formed, a change was made in the formation of the genes. Most instances of *Down's syndrome* are examples of this kind of disorder, although some cases of Down's syndrome are familial. A person who has relatives with an inherited disorder, such as Tay Sachs disease (there are five different forms), should absolutely have genetic testing. Someone who has a relative with a disorder such as Down's syndrome may not have a greater than average risk of having a child with this problem. A genetic counselor can advise you about the appropriateness of testing.

Spina bifida is an example of a *multifactorial* condition, one that appears to result from a combination of genetic, non-genetic, and environmental factors. Some families seem to be more susceptible to this condition, although most cases occur in families with no previous history of the problem. It is also known that lack of folic acid is crucial, and someone with spina bifida may need to take more folic acid before becoming pregnant and during pregnancy. Furthermore, there also may be a viral component that interacts with the genetic background of susceptible individuals. Some families have a tendency to be susceptible to ear infections and others to sore throats. *Celiac disease* presents another example of multifactorial illness. Celiac disease is "a lifelong digestive disorder that is found in individuals who are genetically susceptible. It causes damage to the small intestine, which, in turn, interferes with the absorption of nutrients" (46). Celiac disease also may increase the risk of autoimmune diseases.

It is important to remember that new discoveries about the causes of congenital disorders are constantly being made. Hilary received different advice from genetic counselors at different times. Ask your counselor when the research about your disability was conducted and whether any new studies are in progress.

Many genetically caused disorders and the genes responsible for them have not been identified, but literally hundreds of disorders—most of them extremely rare—can be diagnosed, and this number is growing.

A counselor may be able to give you statistical information on the likelihood that your disability can be inherited when prenatal testing is not possible. The genetic counselor will help you assess the likelihood of your child's inheriting your disability according to your age and your family medical history. She will also order blood tests, sonography, analysis of the amniotic fluid (fluid surrounding the fetus), and examination of fetal cells. There are two methods for collecting the cells: *amniocentesis* and *chorionic villus* sampling (see Chapter 8). In both procedures, the fetal cells that have been obtained from within the uterus are analyzed for the presence of genes that cause specific disorders.

In deciding whether to use genetic testing, you need to weigh your desire for information against the possibility a test could cause a miscarriage. Your genetic counselor can provide statistics that will help you compare the risks of having a child with a particular disability versus the risk of the procedure. For example, it is known that the risk of having a child with Down's syndrome is greater for women over the age of 35 than the risk that amniocentesis will cause a miscarriage.

Amanda was advised in her first pregnancy to have amniocentesis because of a low amount of amniotic fluid in the sac. She said, "I chose not to. I felt if there was low amniotic fluid, why were we taking some out? Plus, the doctors stressed that there was a chance of leaking more amniotic fluid after the procedure. I felt there was way too high of a risk for a spontaneous abortion to happen after the procedure."

Felicia was also afraid of a miscarriage and relied on AFP testing. Unfortunately, this test is not completely reliable. The *AFP test* is sometimes called the *MSAFP* or *maternal serum AFP*. Levels of AFP can be checked by drawing a sample of the mother's blood. This test is generally used for detecting neural tube defects, but it can also indicate abdominal wall defects, esophageal and duodenal *atresia*, some renal and urinary tract anomalies, Turner syndrome, some low birth weight fetuses, and placental complications. A low level of AFP could also indicate Down's syndrome (47).

Sophia Amelia had a level two ultrasound during her first trimester, which is more detailed and has better contrast and definition than the typical ultrasound. The technician found "choroid plexus cysts on the brain." A doctor came in to interpret the ultrasound and told Sophia Amelia that "there is a high correlation between choroid plexus cysts and Down's syndrome or trisomy 13 or trisomy 18. Sophia Amelia said, "I was very angry with the doctor for the way he explained the findings to me, especially since he seemed to be fairly young. He told me I could have an amnio done and get the results back 'just in time to terminate the pregnancy.' He explained Down's syndrome as: 'well there's that kid that acts on that TV show (Chris Burke from *Life Goes On*), but most kids with Down's syndrome are severely to profoundly retarded. If you're lucky they can live in a group home and work in a sheltered workshop.' I am glad I have personal knowledge of disability and have friends with Down's syndrome or who have children with Down's syndrome. Many people would have heard such advice from a medical professional and never questioned it. I looked up 'choroid plexus cysts' and learned that they were just deeper than average wrinkles on the brain and 50 percent of the population is found to have them when an autopsy is performed. It has now been removed as one of the indicators of Down's syndrome. I wanted to be happy when my daughter was born, no matter what. I didn't want to go through the shock or adjusting to her having a disability. I wanted to have the appropriate medical staff there when she was born to make sure she would get the best medical treatment possible. Even if my baby had trisomy 13 or 18, which is considered incompatible with life, I wanted this child to born. I wanted this child to be born and live however long it was going to live. The amniocentesis was traumatic, too. I watched them stick the needle in. And on the ultrasound, I watched the baby bat at the needle and [metaphorically] say 'get the hell out of my room!'"

Unlike many of the other interviewees, Tessa wanted amniocentesis and felt that by having a child with a disability she might injure herself further because the disabled child would require more care.

Sabine likes to be prepared with lots of information, so she opted for an amniocentesis, even though she was unsure whether she would have an abortion if the results were problematic. Sabine said, "It was recommended that I get an amniocentesis. I was much more into doing what the doctors said. The doctors thought it would put my mind at ease because I was worried." Also, she had many friends who had opted for this procedure and "it was no big deal." Unfortunately Sabine had a miscarriage at 5 months due to the amniocentesis. The urologist who performed Sabine's reconstruction surgery thought that Betadine® did not kill the germs that were naturally around the *ileostomy*, which produces different flora. He thought the needle introduced germs and the infection caused a miscarriage, but others I consulted (Sandy Welner, M.D., an obstetrician; Dr. Norman Moscow, a radiologist; and Dr. Lee, a urologist) all thought that the germs were killed by the Betadine®. Dr. Lee added that the needle would be far from where the ileostomy bag attaches so it could not have been a factor. Dr. Moscow said, 'This procedure is done by an obstetrician, but I'm unaware of any increased incidence of complication when there is a urinary diversion. This procedure [amniocentesis] comes with a small amount of risk.'"

Taryn Dion was afraid of a miscarriage from amniocentesis and was also afraid of not being able to get pregnant again. She was able to have a *nuchal translucency*, a specialized ultrasound that measures the thickness of the skin on the back of the fetus' neck. The test is performed by either *transabdominal* or *transvaginal* ultrasound scan, and 95 percent of women tested will have a normal result. The test will pick up 80 percent of pregnancies affected by Down's syndrome. The test itself does not carry any risk to the pregnant woman or the baby. If a test is positive (the recalculated risk is greater than 1:300) an invasive test is usually recommended to determine the baby's chromosomal pattern. This may be chorionic villus sampling (CVS)—performed at 11 to 14 weeks—or amniocentesis performed at 16 weeks of gestation. Both amniocentesis and CVS carry a risk of miscarriage of greater than 1 percent (48).

Some genetic counselors believe that, unless a woman plans to terminate a pregnancy if the test results are positive, she should not have genetic testing. They pointed out that the same information will be available when the child is born. This is particularly important for women who have OI. Orielle wanted CVS at 10 weeks to know if her baby had OI so that she and the baby could be monitored more closely. Orielle had ultrasounds every 2 weeks starting at 6 months. Other counselors believe the risk is worthwhile because, if the information is available sooner, parents have more time to adapt emotionally and plan ways to cope with any problems that are diagnosed. A genetic counselor can provide information about agencies to contact for help in the care and education of disabled children.

A genetic counselor can also help you sort out your feelings about the possibility of raising a disabled child. This question was not fully explored in our interviews, partly because none of the women who were interviewed had disabled children, and they focused on pregnancy and birth. Looking back on her pregnancy fears, Margie commented, "I didn't worry as much before my kids were born. Then they were still abstractions. Now that I know them, I worry more about something happening to them."

There are as many different opinions about the possibility of raising a disabled child as there are women who have considered having children. When participants in one survey were asked whether a woman should have an abortion if she knows her child will be disabled, their responses strongly reflected their feelings about themselves. Some women favored abortion, emphasizing the loneliness and unhappiness disability had caused in their own lives. Others rejected abortion, explaining that their lives had been worthwhile. Moreover, they disliked the implication that they should not have been born. Others said that the decision should depend on whether the parents feel able to raise a disabled child. Although some women may be satisfied with their lives, others may not want a child with a disability. Like most parents, Sherry Adele wanted a healthy child. She found that having amniocentesis and knowing her baby had no abnormalities gave her peace of mind.

Oprah had a philosophical point of view: "You take what is given to you and enjoy it."

Your partner's feelings are also important to consider. One of the questions posed was, "Did you have or want amniocentesis? If so, why?" Mimi's answer was, "Yes, because my husband couldn't handle both my disability and a child with chromosomal problems."

When a woman with a disability considers what life might be like for a disabled child, she brings special empathy and insight to the question. Like any other parent, she may have trouble making sure she does not project her own feelings onto the child and assume that the child feels (or would feel) what she feels.

Ask yourself these closely interrelated questions:

❖ How will I feel about my child growing up with the possibility of physical or psychological stigma? Remember Margie, who—when she had a real child in her arms—felt strongly that she did not want the baby to have a disability.

❖ How did you feel about yourself while growing up and how do you feel about yourself now? Many people feel differently about themselves as adults than they did as children. Often they have conquered frustration and loneliness and like themselves much better. Moreover, having yourself as a parental role model could make it easier for your child. If you have friends with disabilities, then those friends will also be role models.

❖ What was it like growing up with a disability? Answering questions two and three can help you imagine how life would be for your child, but this must be balanced by answering question four.

❖ Will my child's life be like mine? Will circumstances be different, making my child's experiences different from mine? Have there been improvements in therapy for my particular disability? Will improved educational opportunities and adaptive devices for children with disabilities make a difference?

❖ Have you compared your childhood experiences with those of other disabled people? Doing so will help you decide which of your experiences and feelings were typical—and, therefore, likely to be shared by your disabled child—and which were unique to you.

❖ How will having a disabled child change my life? How is this different from having an able-bodied child? Would it be possible to provide the extra care a severely disabled child might need?

❖ What will the physical toll on your body be from taking care of a child with a disability? Can you physically continue to transfer your child year after year, as the child gains more weight? If you think you will be unable to transfer your child, how else could it be done?

Other Special Issues

Your thinking will be colored by memories of growing up with your parents. But it would be different for your child with you as the parent. You will bring to the situation different strengths, different weaknesses, and different knowledge. Sasha felt that her parents' overprotectiveness had led to her lack of self-confidence, and she would try to avoid being overprotective herself.

Sara had a special advantage in mind: "I knew I'd be the best person to cope with whatever happened." Most disabled children never hear about successful disabled people; they see no lists of famous disabled Americans to parallel books about famous minority Americans. Often they do not even see disabled adults in everyday life. Some even fantasize about growing into able-bodied adults. But in you and possibly your friends, your child would have a constant example of disabled persons meeting the challenges of adult life.

Although few people with disabilities have felt angry with their parents for bringing them into the world, most are angry at how the world treats them. It is not a surprising reaction in a child, no matter how illogical. They may feel angry, even though their parents did not know they might have disabled children. How would you feel about encountering this anger if you had known you would give birth to a disabled child?

There might be situations in which you feel as though you are reliving your own childhood. For example, on a day your child is particularly frustrated by physical therapy exercises, you might recall the anger and helplessness you felt as a child in a similar situation. Your insight into your child's feelings might enable you to give him understanding and support in dealing with the frustration. You might be able to help the therapist find a more effective way of approaching your child. You might identify with your child's feelings so intensely that it will be difficult to work and communicate with the therapist. Working with educators, therapists, doctors, and possibly social workers, you may frequently find yourself retracing the path of your own childhood. How ready and willing are you to handle these situations?

The Decision to Have More Than One Child

Naomi said, "My reasons had to do mostly with timing. Once the questions about whether I could carry a pregnancy to term without unpleasant effects related to my disability were answered affirmatively with the birth of my firstborn, I wanted to have a second as soon as I thought I could handle being pregnant and still take care of my firstborn. I knew being pregnant would not allow me to carry my son at all, and that I would be quite fatigued most of the time. That meant he had to be old enough to do a lot for himself. But I didn't want to wait too long because of my age. We decided that getting pregnant when my son was around 20 months would be perfect. That would make the kids about two and a half years apart. I wouldn't be really heavy until he was over two. It has worked out quite well—our plan was a good one and the kids are close friends now."

Shanna decided to have a second child before the first child was four because they want to get the diapering over with while they are still used to doing it.

Sophia Amelia said, "I wanted to space the children far enough apart to avoid the financial burden of having two children in full-time daycare at the same time. We wanted our first child to be out of preschool."

Amanda's decision to have a second child "was solely based on the aptitude of my first child. I felt like my oldest child needed to stay by the car door and not run away while I was getting the second one out of the car."

Closing Comments

Having information about the impact of pregnancy on disability is usually not enough for women to make a decision on becoming a parent. Most women want to know what it is like to *be* a parent. They want to understand the different aspects of parenting, including the ability to take care of the baby, the emotional aspects of parenting, child development, and the mother's relationship to her partner, community, and job. The next chapter will explore these issues.

Parenting with a Disability

IS IT POSSIBLE FOR parents with disabilities to be happy, effective parents? The answer is "YES!" (49). Although all the interview questions discussed in the first edition of this book were about pregnancy and childbirth, several women commented on their positive experiences as mothers. None of them felt that her physical disability had detracted from her psychological ability to mother her children. Some of the interviewees, however, had a mixture of fear and anticipation of motherhood. Stacy remembered, "I was acting confident outwardly, but inside I was apprehensive." If you have never had children and you watch the mother of a young baby, it is easy to wonder, "How does she change a diaper so fast when the baby squirms like that?" TLG has developed ways to reduce the level of squirming such as creating a toy mobile to entertain the baby during diaper changing.

Stacy also said, "You work out the fears about nursing, dressing, carrying, and changing." Sasha, who had always had a close relationship with her teenage daughter, said, "Love makes up for what you can't do." Arlene observed, "It takes more than the ability to change diapers to be a mother. I knew I could love and sing to my child."

Disabled women are not alone in wondering how difficult parenthood will be. Many pregnant women find that their joy is mixed with fears of inadequacy. They may have nightmares about failing as mothers. One of the author's nondisabled students told her, "In one of my dreams, I suddenly realized I hadn't fed my baby for days." Another dreamed that she had left her baby someplace and could not remember where. A third woman said, "My fear was what would happen if the baby needed me in the night and I couldn't go to him?" The third woman was the only one who had a disability.

Although physical limitations pose some difficulties, they are not necessarily insurmountable. One study of one hundred "handicapped homemakers" asked: "What do you consider your most difficult problem in caring for your children?" Very few women reported problems for most of the tasks listed (50). For example, only seven women reported difficulty with bathing children and only two felt inadequate in emergencies. The most difficult physical tasks were those involving lifting and carrying (thirteen women). The most frequent problem reported by only twenty-nine women was discipline—a classic problem for all parents with young children. It would not be surprising if 29 percent of an able-bodied group also reported difficulties in disciplining their young children!

It has been the experience at TLG that some of the physical aspects of early parenting can be difficult for some parents without specialized equipment. The research done at TLG found that transitional tasks, such as moving the baby from one surface to another, holding, carrying and moving the baby, and positional changes, are the essential movements involved in baby care, including repositioning the baby for burping or moving a child from the diapering surface to the highchair. These tasks pose the biggest barrier. It was determined that these tasks can be the most difficult aspect of care for parents with disabilities and may impede the parent's ability to do most baby care tasks. The majority of parents with physical disabilities find holding, transferring, and carrying and moving to be the biggest barriers. It is important to note that many of these barriers have been decreased or eliminated with the equipment created by TLG. There are also learnable techniques available to help with baby care tasks. Some of these techniques are used in conjunction with equipment or alone.

Many childcare tasks may be simplified by planning and preparation before childbirth. For example, bathing and dressing children can be made easier with adaptive equipment and adapted clothing. Not only is adaptive equipment for the disabled *useful*, but it can make infant care *easier*. For example, some women put their babies in a commonly available safety harness and use the straps for lifting them. Others mentioned that they preferred feeding tables to highchairs because the tables were more stable. Since 1991, there have been changes in the equipment that is available, and parents with physical disabilities can purchase commercially available equipment. Moreover, the newer baby care equipment is often easily adapted to the needs of a mother with a disability.

The Role of the Occupational Therapist

An occupational therapist can be a valuable resource in planning for future baby care. She can help you:

- ❖ Identify the commercially available equipment that works
- ❖ Locate adaptive baby care equipment and clothing
- ❖ Learn baby care techniques as well as help with other baby care activities

An occupational therapist can also be helpful in planning how to childproof your home. In a childproofed home, medicines, sharp objects, electrical outlets, and other sources of danger are blocked or moved out of the reach of the crawling or climbing infant or toddler. One problem is that childproofing can make the home parent-proof as well. TLG has developed a lock, however, that stops children but is still workable for most parents with a disability. Your best plan may be to find and evaluate safety strategies and equipment before you need them.

You may feel uncomfortable with the idea of working with an occupational therapist. Some occupational therapists have found that women who were recently disabled are more willing to listen to their suggestions for work simplification than those who have been disabled for a longer time. The author, who has been disabled from birth and is herself an occupational therapist, knows both sides of the story. She knows from her own experience that a disabled woman is more familiar than anyone else with her own strengths, limitations, and adaptations. She also recalls that not all suggestions from occupational therapists have been helpful. Yet, her training and work have taught her that an occupational therapist's knowledge, experience, practical training, and contact with other clients may have given her new ideas her clients have not already thought of. It is important to talk to an occupational therapist early in your pregnancy because some pieces of adaptive equipment can take time to make. Moreover, an occupational therapist can help you plan ahead for upcoming developmental changes. The suggestions of a therapist or an experienced parent may be especially helpful during the first few months after childbirth because these months are often a time of tension and exhaustion.

Arranging for Help

Another step in your decision-making and planning process should be to find out what help is available to you in caring for your child. Some women, including some of the mothers who were interviewed, feel that parenting is a way to prove you are self-reliant. In reality, no parent works alone; we all rely on help from daycare centers, babysitters, friends, and schools. The availability of help makes a critical difference for women who may need assistants to help them care for their babies. In these situations, a woman with a disability may feel indebted to the attendant. Although in one case a mother was afraid to criticize her assistant for fear that the assistant would quit, many other disabled mothers have been able to work as a team with assistants in order to make baby care successful. It is legally difficult in many states to have the state pay for a personal care assistant to help with baby care activities, but this is changing. In recent years, some states have changed their policies on paying for personal care assistance for the baby. Some questions to consider are:

❖ Who will be available to help? Obvious possibilities are your partner, babysitters, paid attendants or household help, roommates, relatives from either side of the family, and friends. Many women are surprised when people are willing to help—if they are asked. You may be giving someone a valuable gift of time with an infant. Asking for help can reduce childcare costs.

❖ How much help can you realistically expect? Stephanie said she "got reassurances from both families," but they were not always able to keep their promises. Having a strategy for getting the most important tasks done and being able to wait on the optional ones is very helpful. For example, if a regular routine is to diaper, change, feed, and bathe the baby, perhaps just the diapering and feeding are essential. Obviously, it is also helpful if you have back-up in case your assistant does not show up.

❖ What kind of help would you prefer? You might want or need help with jobs such as bathing the baby, or you might want help with housekeeping chores so you can devote more time and energy to your child. To be of the most help, assistants need to be told clearly just what you expect of them. Sometimes it is all too easy for the helper to slip from helping into taking over. Pam said that, at times, there were problems because her child was confused about who was really in charge. She had to work with her attendants to clarify that they were *only helping* her with the job of parenting. Your baby will see you as the primary caregiver if you are the one who feeds and soothes her from the beginning. Feeding and soothing are important because they allow you to make eye contact, verbal contact, and body contact with the baby. These activities are essential in promoting bonding and attachment between the mother and the child.

The Emotional Aspects of Parenting

Even as mothers talk about the physical challenges of caring for their children, they often mention the emotional aspects of parenting. Children need much more than physical care. If an infant has all of his physical needs met but is not given enough emotional contact, he may not thrive physically. As a child outgrows the need for physical care, he still needs a relationship with his parent(s).

People are often surprised to learn what the real demands on them will be. Arlene, commented, "I never would have guessed that helping with homework and class projects would make me feel like I was going to school all over again."

The next section discusses three sets of factors that influence the kind of relationship you can have with your child: your contribution to the relationship, the child's contribution to the relationship, and the influence of other people in your family and community. In discussing these concerns, I refer frequently to interviews with Jane Carpenter Bittle, who kindly shared the results of her research regarding the feelings of disabled parents about parenthood and their relationships with their children (51).

The Parents' Contribution

When thinking about what you will bring to a relationship with a child, it helps to ask yourself what personal qualities you will bring to the relationship and what expectations you have. Joan gave a beautiful answer to this question when she said, "My daughter will grow up with a broader mind and without the stereotypes that many children grow up with. She will be more opened-minded from the get-go."

It is important to remember that *all* parents bring different strengths and weaknesses to parenting. Ask yourself what your strong points are. Perhaps you have a wonderful sense of humor. In fact, many experienced parents say a sense of humor is vital. Some children with a disabled parent were asked what strengths they got from having a disabled parent and the responses included perseverance and ingenuity. Make a list of the benefits a child might receive from being raised by you.

Some women feel that their disabilities are a source of emotional strength. When Sharon described her feelings about starting a family, she said, "I knew I could deal with the challenge both mentally and physically because I had been able to adjust to becoming disabled. It makes you know you can do it."

In light of Bittle's finding that, "The largest contributing factor to feeling competent as parents is a basic sense of self-esteem," it is important to discuss some of the fears and self-doubts parents have expressed. For example, one of our interviewees said, "I wanted to bond with the baby right away so he wouldn't be afraid of my hands, so he could get used to me." Her remark is doubly significant. First, she had not yet learned what is important to a baby; a newborn infant does not notice the mother's hand very much, at first. It concentrates on the simple features of human faces. It will be years before the child differentiates its mother from others in the environment. Second, and also important, a mother who feels that her appearance is frightening may be less spontaneous with her child.

Even people whose self-acceptance is strong may meet new challenges when they adopt a new role by becoming parents. The parents who participated in a national survey funded in 1997 by the National Institute on Disability and Rehabilitation Research, which was conducted by Through the Looking Glass and Berkeley Planning Associates, found that "33 percent of the respondents had been discriminated against." The survey found that the "top three areas that challenged parents with disabilities were employment, recreation, and transportation/community access" (52).

Sometimes parents have to make hard choices. One of the mothers Jane Bittle interviewed felt embarrassed when she took her children to a public swimming pool because she is an amputee.

Parent-child relationships have ups and downs just like other emotional relationships. Although some of the parents expressed sadness about particular problems, they felt very good about raising their children. All the parents Jane Bittle interviewed felt that their communication with their children was better than average. It is not unusual for *all* parents to feel they are somehow failing their children; yet, at other times, they may think they are doing better than others.

The ideal mother is viewed as being *all-accepting* in our culture. She is not supposed to care whether her child is practical or intellectual, quiet or outgoing, or calm or excitable, but to give unconditional love "no matter what." Expecting mothers to live up to this ideal is as unrealistic as expecting a shy teenager to be a cheerleader. Sometimes our children do things or exhibit characteristics we dislike and we have to find a comfortable balance.

Another common ideal is the mother who automatically loves her child deeply and ecstatically from the moment of birth. Yet, many women are like Michelle, who said, "It took a while to have maternal feelings; I wasn't sure I had any." Like any other relationship, a parent's relationship with a new baby has highs and lows. Some days seem like an endless, boring round of feeding, burping, and changing diapers; other days are remembered for special moments such as the first time the baby turns towards his mother's voice or watches her face while nursing. One day, the mother realizes that for some time now she has loved her baby and formed a special bond with that tiny, unique person.

Finally, examine your expectations. The hopes and fears the interviewees expressed about themselves as mothers were based on specific beliefs about what their children would be like. Corinne, who said, "I worried about not being able to participate in activities like roller-skating," believed children expect parents to share in their play. The most important thing your child needs is positive attention. They will remember the positive attention versus the lack of going roller-skating.

The Contributions of Children to Relationships

Children's awareness and feelings about parental disability change as they grow older. Described below are four age groups: infancy, early childhood (1 to 5 years old), school-aged children (5 to 12 years old), and teenagers. Children's adaptability and growth patterns affect what will happen at each age. Life with each age group offers characteristic challenges and rewards.

INFANTS

In the earliest stage of life, the child's most important emotional need is simply to establish a strong bond with the primary caretaker. Infants are completely unaware of disability. They need to feel loved and cared for, and they need continuity. Babies as young as 5 to 6 months old recognize individual adults and may be upset by change. For example, a baby who has a new babysitter may become more irritable for a few weeks until she is accustomed to the change. Your baby will not judge you in any way; all she needs to know is that you will be available on a consistent, daily basis.

You may often be tired until the baby's eating and sleeping patterns settle down. It will sometimes be frustrating to try to understand your baby. For example, is he crying because he is hungry or because he has a wet diaper? It is not a disaster if you are a little slow in responding. A mother can *always* build a foundation of love with her baby, regardless of her disability. A mother can feed the baby with the use of adaptive equipment or with extra assistance. She can use her head for play by leaning her head forward and tickling the baby with her hair, or play peek-a-boo by shaking her hair over her face. A disabled mother may feel frustrated because she needs other people to warm bottles or bring the baby to her, but the baby will not care.

A growing infant's general adaptability can easily include subtle adaptations to maternal disability. Portia said her infants would crawl to her wheelchair and cling to her arm in a manner that allowed her to lift them. She took this behavior for granted until she baby-sat for an able-bodied friend whose baby did not know how to help Portia lift her up into her lap. Another mother commented, "I change my baby's diaper more slowly than other people do, but she's always more patient with me than she is with other people." Research on inborn infant temperament tells us that some babies are innately more adaptable or are less active and, therefore, more patient during diapering. Unfortunately, one cannot guess ahead of time how easy a particular child will be to raise. Children can have different temperaments, even within the same family.

EARLY CHILDHOOD

At the end of the first year, when parents and child have become comfortable and familiar with each other, new challenges arise when children begin to crawl and then walk and climb around the house. Just how challenging the situation will be depends on factors stemming from the child's inborn temperament, including her activity level, curiosity, and adaptability. A child who is innately slow-moving and cautious will be easier to supervise than a bold, independent child who "gets into everything." Many parents notice that some infants are willing to play in a playpen or crib, but others are frustrated by any confinement. Difficulties or conflicts between parent and child may stem only from differences in temperament.

Once children start crawling, safety and control become even more of an issue. The best ways of dealing with a child will change constantly as he develops. Sometimes distraction can be an effective technique for keeping a moving youngster out of mischief. For example, some extra toys in a handy pocket may help. Many children, especially 2-year-olds, require some physical discipline; not necessarily punishment, but simply being picked up and removed from dangerous situations. If you cannot pick up the child, maybe you can make one or more rooms of your home totally child-proof with safety gates and other devices. During a tantrum another technique is for the mother to leave the room. The important element is the separation for time out. A 2-year-old who resists being strapped into a car-seat or moved away from a curb can make a disabled parent painfully aware of her limitations.

Some parents struggle to find a way of allowing their child to move around and yet be able to pull him back from danger. Children's safety straps can be a solution. Although many people have negative feelings concerning the use of security straps, active toddlers are not only safer while outdoors but also more comfortable than in a stroller or being held.

The role of helpers—whether attendants, daycare staff, or other parents—must be to assist the mother in teaching her child to be more and more responsive to verbal commands, rather than responding only to physical discipline. Nursery schools and play groups can provide physical activities and other experiences that a parent cannot. Many children become defiant around the time of their second birthday.

Children who are 2 and 3 years old are increasingly aware of their mother's disabilities, but not in the ways one might expect. They continue to adapt to the limitations of their mothers in certain subtle ways. Clara recalls being unable to lift her small daughter Sarah when she was pregnant with a second child. Once, when Sarah fell on some steps, she picked herself up, walked over to her mother, climbed into her lap, and then began to cry! This is the kind of behavior that gives disabled parents the impression that their children are unusually independent.

Very young children cannot be expected to make concessions to parental limitations if they are involved in a battle of wills. Most children under five or six are simply too young to imagine another person's feelings. A child who hides behind the dresser to avoid a repercussion is not worrying about how his mother feels; rather, he will stay there just because his mother cannot reach him. (Each of Sheila's children used this trick. Her solution was to simply wait them out!)

Children who are 2 to 5 years old seem to think of disability as being similar to any other individual characteristic such as red hair or freckles. If other children ask them what is wrong with their mother, they might answer, "Nothing." When they do make comparisons, it is from a viewpoint that assumes disability is ordinary. A friend of the author, whose father had lost his hands because of a war injury, remembers expecting her little brother's hands to fall off when he grew up.

SCHOOL-AGE CHILDREN

At about the time they start kindergarten (5 years of age), children become much more aware that a disabled parent is different from other adults. Certainly, they encounter much more curiosity (and even teasing) from their peers. Here are two examples of the change in children's awareness of disability. When Clara's daughter was 4 years old, she simply did not think of her mother as different, even when others commented on her mother's disability. Then, at 5 years old, she said, "You can't be my mother because we don't walk the same way!" Clara's son, at age 4, often imitated the speech of a friend who had speech difficulties. After entering kindergarten, he began to claim that he could not understand what his friend said.

Children, by nature, have the ability to tease, and having a disabled parent makes them an easy target. One good comeback your child can use when other children tease her about having a disabled parent is "SO WHAT!"

There are innovative programs in some cities for teaching children about disabilities, including opportunities for children to experience what having a disability is like. Parents whose children are being teased might try to introduce one of these programs to the child's teachers, or they might prefer to approach the children more informally. For example, the mother who told Jane she visited her child's classroom to discuss her deafness. You can also talk to the principal for assistance in bringing in a program.

Parents with physical disabilities are at an advantage because physical discipline is never really recommended. Discipline takes more creativity in the early years. Children become more responsive to punishment, such as withdrawal of special privileges, as they grow older.

Many schools assume parents will help with homework. This can often be a challenge for both able-bodied and disabled parents. Research on inborn temperament indicates that children who become easily frustrated, who are highly active, or who have difficulty adapting to change, often have more difficulty in a standard classroom and the homework it requires. Parents with limited energy will find this situation especially trying, and they may find that they need to try a number of different approaches before settling on one that works—at least for a while. Often teachers can be helpful with enforcing the requirements of homework if it becomes a battleground for you and your child. It might be better to find a tutor than for you to struggle with your child over homework.

TEENAGERS

Rebelliousness is the result of the developmental need for more and more independence as well as the result of inherent differences between teen and parent temperaments. While growing toward independence, it is common for teens to: (1) identify ways they are different from their parents, (2) point out parental weaknesses, and (3) angrily blame their parents for the difficulties they encounter.

Portia's daughter blamed Portia's disability for her own problems, complaining, "Your wheelchair is ruining my life." The same afternoon Portia's able-bodied friend confided, "My daughter tells me her life is ruined because I am overweight."

Teenagers will encounter new victories as they renew their childhood struggle to balance independence and cooperation with impulsiveness and responsibility. One woman Jane Bittle interviewed said, "I had children in order to create the kind of family I didn't have." She was echoing the hope of many people, disabled and able-bodied alike, to create a climate of love and acceptance they may not have experienced as children. This is a reasonable hope, and fulfilling it demands a lot of work. Parents with disabilities share the universal feeling of "giving more than I get." It was the mother of a loving, sensitive teenager who told the author, "You make up for what you can't do with love."

School issues often continue as children become teenagers. The children who learn easily usually continue to do well, and those who struggle will continue to do so unless help is found. The situation can be exacerbated for the parent whose teenager is having problems. Parents may become increasingly invested in their child's schoolwork and good grades during high school, when schoolwork, in many cases, becomes a measure of future success.

All children have difficulties with major changes in their lives, whether those changes are caused by divorce, moving, or disability. Teenagers dealing with a parent's progressive disability can feel alone. Parents may find their child's behavior and/or peer group unacceptable, as teenagers try different identities and behaviors. This will usually pass, although for many parents it does not pass quickly enough.

A national survey of teenagers and their parents with disabilities was done during 2001 and 2002 by TLG, funded by the National Institute on Disability Rehabilitation Research (53).

The teenagers in the survey who had parents with physical disabilities indicated that they felt they had "more awareness of the feelings of others compared to their friends, and that they are also more comfortable around people with disabilities." Moreover they felt that "compared to their friends: (a) they had the same amount of independence, (b) the ability to stand up for themselves, (c) an awareness of what is fair and just, and (d) the ability to solve problems or overcome obstacles."

An overwhelming majority of the teens felt that they could talk to their parents and their friends and siblings about their parent's disability.

The disabled parents, however, still had worries about: (a) being a good parent, (b) their child's grades and school performance, and (c) their child's emotional development. They did not have any worries about losing custody of their teen or of being abused by their teen.

Community Relationships

Parenting changes an adult's relationship with the surrounding community. As they discussed their hopes and fears for motherhood, many interviewees commented that much of their non-parental social life had centered on friendships with other disabled people. Now, as parents, they wanted to enjoy more friendships with nondisabled people, and they looked forward to meeting new friends through their children. Meeting other parents was not seen as a reason for having children, but as a pleasant fringe benefit. Some women also felt that having children would make it easier to be more accepted in their communities.

Parenthood is very demanding. All parents need social support for this role. It can be painful when strangers just stare. Joan said "The hardest thing was the glares," which may make the parent with a disability feel vulnerable to someone calling child protective services.

People often react with surprise when they learn that a disabled person can be a parent. As more people with disabilities become parents, social attitudes will, hopefully, change, and more people will have an expanded image of the disabled. Media rarely portrays disabled people as parents, so it is often difficult for both disabled and nondisabled people to understand and visualize how a person with a physical or sensory disability can raise a child. TLG refers to this as "visual history," the accumulation of mental images of disabled parents involved in baby care activities. It can be an essential element in solving the problems in baby care.

Sometimes the attitude of surprise that a disabled parent encounters is also one of admiration and encouragement. Sometimes it is disapproving, and such negative reactions, besides being unpleasant, can interfere with the parent-child relationship. Several women told Jane Bittle that they were not allowed to care for their babies in the hospital. One woman was told, "Our insurance rates might go up if you dropped the baby and it was injured." A student of the author told her, "They would never leave me alone with my baby to nurse. They said I might drop him. What did they think I was going to do when I got home?" This lack of support and prejudice is especially painful during pregnancy—a sensitive time for all women.

The director of the agency where Carol worked apparently did not like having an employee with a disability. Carol said, "He was worried about liability. He had a fear that I would fall and have a worker's compensation issue. His fear of my falling only increased when I became pregnant. It just came from him and not my co-workers."

Parents of school-aged children may need to make a special effort to accommodate their children's schools. Sometimes parents find these efforts rewarding, as in the case of the woman who made a point of visiting her son's classroom to talk to the children about disability. Others are annoyed, as in the case of the blind mother who had to call a teacher and tell her, "Please phone me when my son acts up in class. When you send a note home, he simply doesn't read it to me!" Many parents mention the problems created by lack of physical access to schools. For example, many schools have ramps to building entrances, but there is no way for parents to visit second-floor classrooms. Possibly school staff expects the child—who might be an elementary age student—to be the sign language interpreter for a deaf parent.

Some of the older parents who were interviewed commented, "Peoples' discomfort was there all the time. Now that I'm older and more self-confident, I feel I could have handled it differently and reached out more."

Financial Considerations

It is impossible to estimate of the cost of having a child, because these costs will vary by region, but it is possible for you to give some thought as to how you might be affected financially by having a child.

In 2001, the book *Baby Bargain Secrets* by Denise and Alan Fields (54) estimated the approximate cost of diapers for 1 year to be $600; food with formula $900; miscellaneous $500; and baby clothes $500. (It is unknown if gifts and hand-me-downs were factored in.)

It is important to examine your health insurance policy to see if it includes maternity coverage. Many people who do not have pregnancy coverage may want to delay pregnancy. Often, medical benefits will not pay maternity benefits until 1 year after the policy was started. It may be necessary to find out what the costs are and start saving to pay your own expenses. In *Baby Bargain Secrets*, it was estimated that a vaginal birth would cost $6,400 and a caesarean section $11,000.

Your disability health care specialist might be able to advise you about the type of treatments or medications that are typical for a woman with your disability.

If you are employed, it is important to consider the income you will lose if you stop working or miss work to keep medical appointments or care for sick children. In *Baby*

Bargain Secrets, it was estimated that childcare cost $3,000 to 10,000 per year for family daycare, and center care $3,000. The availability of scholarships in the Berkeley, California area for preschool or daycare for mothers with a disability was investigated, and there are none. If you have a child with a disability, however, it may be easier to find available scholarships. If you continue working, you may need to explore such arrangements as job-sharing and part-time work and plan for a reduced income. For many people, the loss of employer-paid health benefits is as great a problem as the loss of wages.

Women who will need help with the physical care of their children must investigate the cost of additional attendant care. If you receive government benefits, such as SSI or SSDI, ask your social worker to explain the regulations to you. In most states, no additional attendant care is funded unless the child is disabled. It may be possible to make adjustments using increases in other benefits, such as rent allowance, but careful planning is needed.

Many people with disabilities have limited incomes and must manage their budgets carefully. Yet, parents often have to meet unexpected expenses such as costs for extracurricular activities and dental care. Even the cost of clothing can be a problem when your child grows faster than your budget.

Many parents who have a disability have been able to find solutions, although it can be difficult. Still, some of the additional expenses associated with having a child are temporary. For example, expenses will be reduced when your child is toilet-trained. If you start a college fund, your teenager can contribute to it as well. You may be able to plan a long-term budget by planning for different expenses at each stage of your child's life and for possible changes in your earning power.

Motherhood and Other Relationships

The arrival of children appears to have a similar impact on a couple in which one partner is disabled to the impact it has on a couple in which both partners are able-bodied. The women interviewed for this book repeatedly raised the same issues that appear in the work of family researchers on nondisabled families. For example, most commented that their marital relationships began to change as soon as they knew motherhood was upon them. The same has been found to be true for all new parents. Some women, like Mary, found that the prospect of having a child increased intimacy with her partner: "I felt more fulfilled as a woman—prouder, and it made it easier for us to come together."

Naomi said, "My husband was absolutely wonderful. He did the chores that I couldn't do any more; he vacuumed. Vacuuming was a problem because the vibration from the vacuum cleaner affected my carpal tunnel problem. There was a time when his job got very stressful and we fought and hashed it out. We redid the chores. We made a whole list of the chores and that helped us figure it out. It got a whole lot better."

Other women, like Dawn, grew more distant from their husbands: "I was more involved in being pregnant than in my relationship with my husband." Again, these types of changes are common occurrences. Arlene said, "Any problems with a relationship are going to be compounded with the birth of a child." Others agreed that the areas that were usually a source of tension became even more sensitive. For example, couples who had difficulty communicating about their sexual relationship experienced more difficulty when stress and fatigue were increased. The most frequently mentioned sources of tension were finances and sexual relationships. The jealousy of partners or fathers seemed to increase when the mothers were absorbed in their new babies. Some women had difficulty in accepting more help than usual. Margie remarked, "I think the difficulty with our relationship is that I react to my multiple sclerosis by feeling and acting dependent. I'm not sure that pregnancy itself was stressful." The positive changes the interviewees mentioned most frequently were increased intimacy with their partners or husbands, pleasure in receiving more care and attention than usual, and shared delight in the new baby.

For some women, the birth of a child was a motivation to change or end an unsatisfactory relationship. Sybil said, "My husband was drinking all the time, and I thought my child deserved better." For others, the changes associated with pregnancy were an opportunity for re-evaluation and growth. These women stressed the importance of frequent and honest communication. Sylvia said, "We were at each other's throats a lot of the time, and we became aware of how important it is to be open in a relationship."

Four women reported that their partners or husbands had not wanted children; all of them experienced considerable strain on their relationships, and two of the four eventually divorced. Sasha said, "Communications broke down totally and there was a switch in the relationship. He became unsupportive and negative." She valued her relationship with her daughter, however, and felt that she had made the right choice. Carla simply said, "Having children was not healthy for the relationship." These statements contrast strongly with those of women whose husbands also wanted children. Heather recalled, "It was like we were pregnant together. We were ecstatic. He spent his time waiting to feel the baby kick." Christina, who had not been married long when she became pregnant, said that during her pregnancy she and her husband "learned to work as a team." The experiences of these women suggest the importance of support from your partner or husband and other family members in the decision-making process.

Another important issue that arises during pregnancy is the mother's need for support. All pregnant women need emotional support, and those who can rely on the help and approval of friends and family tend to be most satisfied with their pregnancies. This issue has special significance for women with disabilities for two reasons.

First, many women have strong emotional conflicts regarding their need to depend on others for help. Others find that conflicts are reduced when they are pregnant. It is important for some women to know that all pregnant women need extra help and attention. Christina explained, "I was always so independent that when he took charge it lessened the clash. My needing help was good for both of us, and it was nice to see how supportive he was."

Secondly, partners and husbands really do assume new burdens when they are needed to help with infant care. When some women discussed how their relationships were affected by pregnancy, they responded in terms of the stress created by such practical problems. Celeste, for example, remarked that, "My housework was not as effective, and my husband had to take time off work to drive me back and forth to the doctor." Pam, whose husband left her when their child was 18 months old, felt that her pregnancy had disrupted the delicate balance they had created to cope with her disability, commenting, "I was so sick, much sicker than most pregnant women, and it and was so much harder for me to get around; it just put too much pressure on him."

Arlene and Renee each made a point of scheduling additional attendant care to ease the burden of their husbands. Pam speculated that her marriage might have survived if she had created a stronger support network. Unfortunately, many public and private agencies will not pay for additional attendant care, assuming that the partner or husband will act as an unpaid attendant. It may be necessary to ask for help from others, if only to give your partner an occasional break. This is not always pleasant for some women, especially if they must turn to their own parents, who may be anxious about the pregnancy. Discussing solutions to these problems before they occur can help considerably. Roberta felt that making careful plans before her child's birth minimized the stresses of the postpartum period, for both herself and her husband.

Another stressful circumstance is when a mother feels helpless. Renee said that even though her husband did not have extra work, "He felt pressured because there was little he could do when I was in pain, and he worried." Undoubtedly, your relationship will undergo some strains that you cannot control or predict, but the experiences of these women demonstrate the importance of cooperation and good communication. As Stephanie said, "Our relationship got even better because we shared something so important."

Combining Career and Family

The issue of combining career and family is often discussed in extreme "all or nothing" terms. Meaning that a woman either stays home until her youngest child is at least 10 years old or goes back to work full-time when her baby is 6 weeks old. In reality, women may be able to work out a variety of ways to combine work and motherhood. For example, a teacher or professor might time her pregnancy to coincide with her sabbatical year. Some types of employment are inflexible, however, and the mother really must make a decision about changing or interrupting her career.

These issues can be more troublesome for women with disabilities because their choices may be more restricted. Besides facing barriers to employment, they must also deal with bias against their disability. A woman with disabilities is likely to have more difficulty adapting her work schedule. Sometimes she must give up a good job and she may not find another one easily. Also, women who have interrupted or given up their careers may sometimes resent their children.

It is important to assess what the demands will be on your time if you want to continue your career. Not everyone is as fortunate as Julie, who said, "I got a tremendous amount of support from my family to make it possible. Plus, I worked for a good firm that was very flexible and supportive. If I needed to take time off for a pediatrician's appointment, it was okay." It might be necessary to make some compromises. For example, while your child is small, you might have to choose to work where there is a flexible schedule but less interesting work.

Meanwhile, there will be varying demands on your free time. Julie said that working was actually easier when her child was younger because, "He would be happy to see me and then go to bed. I had more time to relax. When he got older, he started needing help with his homework. Now I have less time for myself."

Although it is true that (as the bumper sticker says), "Every mother is a working mother," it is also true that an employed mother feels as if she comes home to a second job. The more susceptible to fatigue the mother is, the more essential it is to have help. Couples in which both parents are employed will find that sharing chores can be a major issue in their relationships. It is valuable to discuss these concerns as part of the decision-making process. Ask yourselves: what chores are we willing to do? Can we learn to accept each other's ways of doing things and not criticize our different methods? What is certain is that with careful forethought, you can have something better than the myth of "having it all."

Closing Comments

Disabled mothers believe that a pregnant woman with disabilities should be seen primarily as a pregnant woman. Disability is not necessarily the most important concern for a woman who is deciding whether to have children.

The questions explored in these first four chapters need to be considered by all potential mothers, whether or not they have disabilities. All women need to decide whether they can afford to have children. It is also important to learn what affect pregnancy will have on your health.

Both nondisabled and disabled women express that having children proves that their bodies "work right." Although the values of our society are changing, we still live in a world in which a woman's worth is frequently measured by the old yardsticks of beauty and fertility.

Although disproving some stereotypes about disability can be a pleasant fringe benefit of the decision to become pregnant, what is important for any woman is to make the choice that contributes most to her health and happiness.

Getting Your Health Care Needs Met

NEW QUESTIONS ARISE once the decision to have a child is made: How do I find a doctor? How do I interview a doctor? How do I assess how knowledgeable a doctor is about disability? This chapter answers these questions and addresses the related concerns of deciding where to deliver, consulting with specialists, and—most importantly—assuring that all of your health care needs are met.

Selecting an Obstetrician

Early prenatal care is important and women should begin to search for an obstetrician (OB) as soon as possible. It is ideal to start the search before getting pregnant.

Mimi switched doctors because she felt that her first doctor did not listen or respond to her concerns.

Selina's said, "When I go see a doctor for the first time I ask, 'Where did you go to medical school? Have you ever had a patient like me? Have you ever delivered a paraplegic mother? What complications might I expect?' I interviewed three physicians before I decided. The first two told me I would be automatically scheduled for a caesarean section but they couldn't give me a medical reason. The doctor I chose told me he had assisted with a paraplegic delivery when he did his internship.

"The doctor who delivered my other children is a doctor who likes to do research. He pulled out medical journals and had papers. He was my gynecologist for 6 years before I got pregnant. He sent me to a high-risk obstetrician but I did not like him at all. They made me feel like a laboratory rat. They made me feel like a case study not a human. I went back to my doctor and asked him not to ever send me there again and he said he wouldn't. He gave photocopies of my paperwork to all the nurses. In fact, it was funny, because when I went into labor, the nurses were afraid to touch me for fear of autonomic dysreflexia. When they called the doctor and he asked how far I was dilated, they told him they would not check me and that he had to be there at the onset of labor."

You may be able to put the important changes into motion that are necessary to address your needs by finding a doctor early. For example, the doctor may need to have an accessible exam table. The proper table can reduce the risk of injury, not only to you, but also to the doctor and office staff.

A precedent has been set that may help you get appropriate health care. The Disability Rights Advocates, based in Oakland, California, sued the nation's largest nonprofit health care maintenance organization (HMO), Kaiser Permanente, for discrimination against disabled patients by not providing them with full access to medical care. Kaiser agreed in April 2001 to revamp all of its California health centers and its policies in order to ensure that people with disabilities have access to a full range of health care. This agreement settled the first class-action lawsuit of its kind (55).

It may take some time to find a doctor who has a positive attitude toward your pregnancy. You are likely to meet with a wide variety of reactions from medical personnel. Some of the interviewees met doctors whose first reaction was to advise an abortion (in one case, the woman was 5 months pregnant). Other doctors were doubtful or cautious, but still supportive. During Sabine's first visit to a doctor to explore pregnancy, Sabine said, "The doctor didn't even exam me after I told her I had spina bifida. She said that I shouldn't have children. When I asked her why, her response was that I would not be able to carry a child. I left her office and sat in my car and cried."

The doctor also told Sabine she had a cyst on her ovaries, but Sabine was able to pay for a second opinion. Not only did the second doctor not find a cyst, but he was also very supportive. The second doctor told Sabine, "You can have a baby and I'll help you. All you need is to have someone be your cheerleader."

Meeting with a doctor early in your pregnancy can help avoid future problems. Amy's doctor often explored potential problems with her. Amy said, "It was good to hear him thinking ahead." Darlene said, "My obstetrician was willing to do research and find out more. She was straightforward about it, instead of thinking of me as someone special."

Many of the interviewees had obstetricians who were enthusiastic and welcomed the challenge, as did Portia's doctor. Portia said, "The doctor was happy when I came in. It broke up the boredom of his day."

A woman's body changes drastically during pregnancy. A team approach can assess these changes and provide better care if they get to know you early in your pregnancy or even before you are pregnant. Very few obstetricians have had the opportunity to work with disabled women. Give the doctor time to learn what is normal for you and how your disability may affect your pregnancy.

Health problems that are not necessarily related to your disability may need early attention. Correction of anemia and updating rubella vaccinations, for example, are best taken care of before pregnancy. Medications that must be avoided during pregnancy can be reconsidered and possibly changed before conception.

How to Find an Obstetrician

One of the ways to locate an obstetrician is to call any facility where you have received rehabilitation. Another is to ask for a referral from the doctor who is the most familiar with your medical history. Ask your doctor to call the obstetrician for you in order to provide an introduction and set the stage for future cooperation. You can also ask others in the disability community, an obstetric nurse, or friends. Asking friends can be complicated because not all doctors are signed up with the same insurance company and your needs may be different from those of your friends.

Natasha said, "If I could do it over again, I'd probably look for a doctor who works with disabled people." Because of her OB's lack of familiarity with her disability, he was unable to give her solutions to her problems. Mona had a referral from her neurologist and felt she got good care. Moira also had a referral from her neurologist. She said, "The obstetrician I was referred to was full, but when I told the receptionist that I was referred by my neurologist, she made me an appointment. The obstetrician was phenomenal. She specializes in high-risk pregnancies and told me, 'You're not really high-risk. From everything I know about MS and pregnancy, it is really not that much different from other women's pregnancies. The only thing that is going to change is after you have the baby there is a good chance you will have an exacerbation. It could be really bad, but it might not be. Regardless, you are not going to have a problem during your pregnancy. You'll feel so much better that you'll want to be pregnant forever.' She said this at the first appointment. She also planned weeks ahead of time to get the IVIG (intravenous immunoglobulin)."

Denise received care from an HMO for her first pregnancy; her obstetrician was assigned by the HMO. She believed that the assigned physician's lack of knowledge was the major factor in her losing her first child. Regarding her second pregnancy she said, "I explored different options within the same HMO. I found out about the doctor's experience with delivering dwarf babies and babies of dwarfs, and also their background. This helped me determine the right doctor for my child, because I did not want to make the same mistake again." You can do this even in an HMO, but it will take some time.

Orielle used a Preferred Provider Organization (PPO) instead of an HMO. A PPO is a prepaid insurance plan that may be more expensive, but it may give you a wider selection of doctors to choose from.

Hannah was concerned about being able to deliver vaginally, and asked about options such as using a birthing stool. Hannah said, "The doctor wouldn't answer any of my questions. She said my questions would be handled at the time of labor." Hannah said, "I should have insisted on a new OB, and I should have also asked the labor and delivery nurses for their opinions. Nurses are knowledgeable and they would have answered my questions."

Charlotte called four or five doctors from the *Yellow Pages*. "They said I was too high-risk. I think they were scared because of their malpractice insurance. There is a group associated with the hospitals in town that handles high-risk pregnancies and they can't deny you."

Charlotte is affected by cerebral palsy in the exact same way as Clara, yet Clara was not sent to a high-risk obstetrician. It seems some obstetricians equate any physical disability with high-risk, yet for some disabilities there is no reason for high-risk status. Just because your body does not appear to work correctly on the outside does not mean it does not work fine on the inside.

Evaluating a Doctor

It may be difficult to judge a physician's ability if you are not trained in medicine. Asking for referrals from people you trust can help in evaluating a doctor's ability and practice. The impressions of a doctor's patients and colleagues can also help in assessing her skills and in determining what your priorities are. For example, one doctor might have the best surgical skills, whereas another might have the best ability to help a woman relax during a difficult labor. Friends may even report very different experiences with the same doctor. "I always appreciated the way she took time to answer my questions," said one woman; another reports, "It seemed like she tried to rush me through labor faster than my body could handle it." You may feel more comfortable relying on the experience and intuition of an older doctor, or you may believe a younger one will be more up-to-date. The choice of a doctor is a personal one. As Portia pointed out, there is no single list of requirements for everyone. Instead, you need to identify your own needs. Make a list of your priorities and use it.

Sophia Amelia—who moved back to her hometown during the second trimester of her first pregnancy—wanted to have as her obstetrician the first gynecologist who had treated her as a teenager. He had treated her with respect and assumed she would have a normal sex drive. His office did not take Medicaid insurance, but Sophia Amelia was able to talk with him directly. He remembered her and was willing to take her on as a patient.

You may request that your first visit to a new doctor be for consultation only and delay a physical examination until you are sure which doctor you will choose. Try to bring the baby's father or an advocate along for most of your appointments so you will have someone to share your impressions with and help you make sure all of your questions are answered. Make a list of your questions before your appointments to help you make sure that you do not forget anything important.

Ask questions about the cost of treatment no matter what health plan you belong to. Moreover, you need to find out specifically what types of services are provided.

Reasonable Accommodations: At the Doctor's Office

Title II of the Americans with Disabilities Act (ADA) covers the area of reasonable accommodations.

If you normally use a wheelchair, you already know you should ask whether the doctor's office and the bathrooms are wheelchair accessible. Women who do not need any special accommodations when they are not pregnant may find that they need grab bars in the bathroom when they *are* pregnant. Sherry Adele did not have a problem with giving a urine sample, but she did have a problem getting up from the toilet. Her doctor's office did not have grab bars. It is important to be aware that you have a right to reasonable accommodations in other areas such as having an accessible exam table. (The Welner accessible exam table has been designed especially for disabled patients.) You should also be weighed on a scale that is accessible (see Appendix D). Tell the doctor that he may be eligible for a tax credit if he buys an accessible exam table, if his practice is for-profit.

Sometimes the doctor will want to refer you to a high-risk obstetrician (*perinatologist*), but sometimes this may not be medically appropriate. Just because you have mobility problems does not mean that your pregnancy will cause medical problems to you or the baby. Some women's disabilities do interact with other body systems, however, and may necessitate seeing a perinatologist.

Interviewing A Doctor

When you meet a doctor for the first time, ask yourself, "Am I comfortable with this person?" You are beginning a 9-month relationship—you may see the doctor at least once a week during the last few weeks of your pregnancy. Try to choose someone who is respectful, takes the time to answer your questions, and answers them willingly! Sometimes it may be helpful to tape the interview or have someone take notes. Joan went to a clinic because she thought she was pregnant. She met the doctor on call. She had a good experience and reports, "The doctor was genuinely happy for me."

When a woman with a disability asks her doctor for an opinion as to whether she can carry a baby to term and be physically well, the doctor may not have the medical knowledge necessary to predict what might happen. She may feel legally vulnerable in trying to make predictions. She *might* be able to offer possibilities or probabilities.

Natasha said, "I was too shy to ask questions about whether they had experience with my disability. I now think it is important to ask questions and it is worth taking the time." Sometimes the questions may have to be more probing in nature. Dorothy did not find out her doctor's true feelings about disability until she was carrying a disabled child.

Natalie found one doctor who examined her and thought it was medically necessary to do a caesarean section. Her mother encouraged her to see a new woman OB. This new obstetrician was friendly, personable, and down-to-earth. The new doctor thought a vaginal birth, which was Natalie's preference, would be medically safe.

You will learn more about the doctor's philosophy by asking open-ended questions. For example, you may feel strongly that you want a vaginal birth. If you begin by saying something like, "I think you should know I really don't want a caesarean." you are effectively closing off discussion. It is more useful to ask something such as, "What do you think about my ability to deliver vaginally?" or even, "Do you think I could?" This way, you will learn how the doctor feels about the subject, while leaving room for further discussion. If she tells you, "I don't think you can deliver vaginally" (for whatever reason), you have the opening to say, "I'm really hoping to have a vaginal birth." In some cases, it might be important to ask yourself why you think a vaginal birth is the most important and do some research on the different ways of giving birth.

Felicia was dissatisfied with her doctors. She made a list of questions that she would ask a prospective doctor in the future:

❖ What kind of answering system do you have? "The practice I used really did not have a system. Calls were never picked up by an answering service or machine when the lines were busy. I actually spent days trying to get through. This happened when I trying to learn how much Zoloft® (an antidepressant) I could take. I was finally able to leave a message for my doctor in his in-box. But he was on vacation and no one called me for several days. I finally got through again and told them I didn't care who called me back, just have someone call me. I finally got a response."

❖ How do they get charts from one office to the other if they have offices in two separate locations? "When I went to one location, they would not have my chart or would have lost my lab slips. Finally they said, 'Oh we really don't like patients going between offices. It's too difficult for us.' This was originally why I chose this practice, because it had two locations."

❖ Is it possible to have continual care from the same doctor? "If you are in a group practice, I would like to see you as my primary care doctor. If there is a partner, then I would expect her to read my chart before I'm seen so I will not be starting from scratch each time I see a new doctor."

❖ How will you handle the pain of labor? "I expressed my anxiety about this on day one, but my concern was ignored during my labor and delivery. I wish I had seen the anesthesiologist in advance so we could have made a plan that I could have taken to the hospital."

Sydney chose a doctor that was covered through her insurance plan. She said, "I went and spoke to her before I became pregnant. I came armed with articles and talked about my personal needs. Although she did not have personal experience with disabled mothers, she was willing to learn and work with me."

Sierra went to Planned Parenthood for her medical care when she was 5 weeks pregnant. Sierra felt that her doctor was aware of her special needs. Her doctor discussed with her ways to deliver vaginally, including having extra support for one of her legs, which could not be placed in a stirrup.

Arianna was new to the area when she discovered she was pregnant. She was limited in her choice in a doctor because the only mode of transportation she used was her motorized wheelchair. Arianna switched doctors because the first one was not supportive. Unfortunately, neither doctor took the time to learn about her disability.

Sabine switched doctors for her second pregnancy, going to doctors who were also researchers. She felt they knew how to think and were more informed about women with disabilities. She said, "I liked my doctor because she did not look at the surface of what was happening; she looked beyond that."

Amanda needed to switch doctors early in her first pregnancy. Her OB/GYN dropped her because of misinformation about women with disabilities. This was fortunate for Amanda, because her new obstetrician "was amazingly knowledgeable about it." This obstetrician was able to give Amanda a lot of information about her disability that Amanda had been unaware of.

Noreen felt that her doctors were not sufficiently knowledgeable or willing to research myasthenia gravis. She thought their lack of knowledge affected her care because they were not well versed in treatment options or the risks to her unborn son. Noreen felt stuck because they were providers from her HMO. You can appeal to your HMO to pay for a qualified specialist outside the HMO if you believe your HMO doctors are not sufficiently knowledgeable. First, call member services and ask for a list of the obstetricians in your plan. You can then call those OBs to inquire as to their experience. The HMO will not refer you out if they feel they have a suitable obstetrician in the plan.

The HMO is required to give to you the necessary medical care. It is important to know that this process can be long and arduous. You may be able to appeal on an urgent basis if you are already pregnant. You will need to prove that the providers in the HMO do not have the particular knowledge and skills necessary for your care, but that another provider outside the HMO has the information and skills you need.

Sometimes it may be impossible to change providers, either because your location may limit your choice of obstetricians or because you may feel too overwhelmed to fight for a change in doctors. It is important for your doctor to get a formal consultation from an expert in the field if he lacks crucial information. It was discovered during the interviews that some of the interviewees' doctors made assumptions that were incorrect. In some cases, they were incorrect about the patient's particular medical equipment (Baclofen Pump™ or NDI™ urinary system), although the correct information is available through the companies that make these devices. Some doctors may have inaccurate information. Therefore, make sure your doctor checks with the particular company that manufactures any hardware you use.

Questions to Ask the Doctor

The following questions are phrased in such a way that the doctor's answers will give you information about her knowledge and attitudes, as well as what you might expect during pregnancy:

What are the pros and cons of pregnancy for me?

You need to hear both the positive and negative opinions of your doctor.

Denise's first obstetrician came across as non-informed. She said, "He treated me like an average person having an average baby." She consulted a second obstetrician, who "told me the risks as well as being encouraging. He was very attentive about telling me about what to watch out for."

If the doctor seems opposed to your pregnancy, ask why. The doctor may point out risks that deserve your serious consideration. Then again, you may think her concerns do not really apply to you. Disability specialists may be skeptical about pregnancy. Rachel encountered this attitude; she said, "My rheumatologist discouraged me from getting pregnant. He based this on how difficult it would be for me to care for two kids. He was still willing to treat me, but I started seeing a new rheumatologist." Rachel's obstetrician was supportive. "He thought it was our choice. He thought it was a good choice if that was what we wanted. He said to me, 'People with disabilities and people who are born with disabilities have children every day, and it doesn't stop them from being good parents. You shouldn't worry about your rheumatoid arthritis and whether or not you would be a good mom.' I was really encouraged by that. We both did some research. He talked with my current rheumatologist to find out how long I had to wait for my arthritis medication to be out of my system before trying to conceive. We waited $2\frac{1}{2}$ months before trying, and then it took 6 months before we got pregnant."

The first doctor Marsha talked with immediately asked if she wanted an abortion, stating that it would be too exhausting for a woman with MS to care for a toddler. Marsha decided to continue the pregnancy, and she later found that caring for an infant was much more wearing than caring for a toddler. In any case, whatever the risks of pregnancy, the decision is yours and you need a doctor who will be truly supportive. A referral to an occupational therapist and a physical therapist, as well as consulting with staff at TLG can help you with some of the obstacles you may face in finding a doctor (see Appendix D).

WHAT DO YOU KNOW ABOUT MY DISABILITY? HOW MUCH EXPERIENCE HAVE YOU HAD WORKING WITH DISABLED WOMEN? HAVE YOU TREATED OTHER WOMEN WITH MY SPECIFIC DISABILITY?

All of the interviewees stated that it was important to be aware of the doctor's experience with disability. Dorothy felt that she was given the same treatment as the other disabled patients who had been treated there, although they had different disabilities than she did. She felt that her doctor may have not been knowledgeable about her specific needs.

Many women also felt that it is not so important for your doctor to have special knowledge about your disability, as long as she is willing to work with you, learn about your needs, and adapt to them. Arlene said, "Even though a doctor doesn't have experience, an open mind is most important."

Roberta felt that her treatment had been adversely affected by her doctor's lack of experience. Her doctor was supportive, but she said she could not talk openly with him because she felt that he did not know what to expect. She added, "I had a team, and I wasn't comfortable unless my obstetrician consulted my rheumatologist." Her primary care physician had referred Roberta to the OB. The two doctors conferred frequently, and she felt that these conferences filled any gaps in the OB's knowledge about her disability.

Joan's doctors did not know if she could deliver vaginally, and she was referred back to her orthopedist to see if her prosthetic hips could handle the vaginal birth. Joan was also followed by a perinatologist every 2 months, "Just for a follow-up to see how my pelvis was doing."

Naomi interviewed her doctor and decided to stay with him because of his response to finding out about her disability and her fears. The doctor told Naomi, "I don't know anything about it; let's get you hooked up with a specialist; let's find out about it. I'm calling this person. I'm looking in the medical journals.'" Naomi said, "He took the bull by the horns. He was unbelievable. He got my records. He read the articles I brought in. The best thing he said was, 'I don't know, but I'm going to find out.'"

Diane suggests that the referring doctor should tell the obstetrician about your disability so they can make the appropriate accommodations "and so they won't be totally shocked."

An article published in *InsideMS* suggests, "You might start looking for an obstetrician with your neurologist. Ask them to e-mail or speak to each other" (22).

Moira's neurologist read about intravenous immunoglobulin treatment, talked with colleagues, and did research on treatment after delivery.

Nadia's disability was not diagnosed until her eighth month of pregnancy. She still needed to be in charge because she needed to that feel she was safe and that her doctors were coordinating with each other. Nadia said, "It was quite confusing. They weren't quite conferring. They had differing ideas about hospital schedules and how to coordinate everything. There was a lot of miscommunication between the neurologist, the perinatologist, and the hospital, and I had to be the one who got them all to communicate because they weren't communicating very well. I called the neurologist and drew out what his plan was and then I asked the perinatologist for his plan. When the plans contradicted, I had to get them to come up with a plan that was coordinated. I'm glad I realized they were contradicting each other."

Natasha said, "I had my neurologist write a letter to my obstetrician telling them I have muscular dystrophy and this is what it is like."

An article in *The Archives of Physical Medicine Rehabilitation* talks about the team approach. "Pregnancy in a woman with SMA (spinal muscular atrophy) requires a team approach, with physiatrist, pulmonary, and perinatology specialists involved early in the course" (29).

Another article also finds that the team approach results in good outcomes. "Our data on maternal morbidity, both in terms of lupus complications and non-rheumatic obstetric complications, dictate that every mother with lupus should be seen by a high-risk obstetrician throughout pregnancy and should see a rheumatologist at least once a month" (56).

Sophia Amelia's urologist was a part of the caesarean section team "because the obstetrician wasn't going to touch anything without the urologist there. The obstetrician didn't want to mess up anything that was done in my prior urologic surgery."

How will you work with my primary doctor?

During your first talk with your obstetrician, make sure that she agrees to confer with your primary doctor. Most physicians are willing to work with the specialists who are the most knowledgeable about your disability. Disability specialists who write about pregnancy emphasize the importance of the team approach to prenatal care.

Of the women who were interviewed, the ones who were the happiest with their prenatal care were the women whose OBs had conferred with the referring primary doctors who were treating them for their disabilities. The following are examples of three situations in which teamwork was helpful:

- ❖ Roberta felt that her obstetrician minimized her disability at first. She described his initial attitude toward her arthritis as being limited to "take aspirin and the pain will go away." She said that his conference with her rheumatologist, however, made him more aware of how her disability specifically affected her pregnancy.
- ❖ Elinor knew she might need a caesarean section. She told her doctor that she was worried about having spinal anesthesia because she had previously had lower back surgery. Her doctor offered to use general anesthesia. She was unhappy about this alternative because she wanted very much to be conscious when her child was born. The solution to the dilemma was a telephone call to her neuro-surgeon, who assured her that spinal anesthesia would be no problem.
- ❖ Patricia's doctor was doubtful that a woman with post-polio syndrome could with-stand the physical stresses of pregnancy. Nevertheless, he conferred with her pri-mary doctor and read more about her disability, which enabled him to narrow his concern to specific problem areas and perform the appropriate diagnostic tests.

Be sure to follow up after asking your obstetrician to confer with your primary care doctor. Michelle remarked that her obstetrician agreed to confer with her regular physician but did not do so. On your second visit, ask whether your obstetrician has met with your regular physician or spoken with him by telephone. Do not worry about being perceived as nagging. Your doctor needs to know that this issue is important to you. Have a deadline in mind. One reason you found a doctor early was to give yourself time to make a change if necessary. If your deadline has passed and you do not want to change obstetricians, ask your regular doctor to make the first contact.

Who should I call if I experience unusual symptoms and do not know whether they are related to pregnancy or disability?

It can be difficult to know whether worrisome symptoms are caused by pregnancy or disability, or by another condition not related to pregnancy or disability. Your HMO will assign your obstetrician to be your primary care physician for the remainder of your pregnancy if you request it. This allows one doctor to coordinate your care as well as referring you to a disability specialist as needed. Beth had kidney stones, which eventually caused premature labor. Her response to the earliest symptoms was to assume that they were caused by disability. She was referred to her obstetrician when she called her disability specialist. Cheryl attributed a normal pregnancy symptom to her disability, until her obstetrician reassured her that the muscle spasms in her lower abdomen were a reaction to stretching caused by uterine growth.

HOW WILL LABOR AND DELIVERY BE AFFECTED BY MY DISABILITY?

Make sure to ask for explanations about anything you do not understand. Your doctor's reply to this question may include positive solutions to special problems. For example, Julie's doctor said they would use a birthing stool, rather than a bed, to give her more hip abduction (so she could move her legs farther apart).

Amy had been in a car accident that affected her pelvis. She had a team meeting with an orthopedist and an obstetrician, who looked at the possible problems and solutions that could arise during pregnancy and birth with a pelvis that had been broken.

DO YOU THINK I WILL NEED CAESAREAN DELIVERY? WHY? WOULD YOU SET A DATE OR WAIT FOR LABOR TO BEGIN SPONTANEOUSLY?

Again, your doctor may not be able to answer this question until your pregnancy has progressed further. For example, you may have *fetopelvic* disproportion (the baby's head is bigger than the pelvic opening). Be sure your disability specialist is consulted if you feel that the doctor's opinion reflects incomplete or inaccurate knowledge about your disability.

There may be other areas in which the doctor may make incorrect assumptions. Many people assume that weak muscles (such as from muscular dystrophy) or a total lack of muscle strength (from spinal cord injury) means that a woman may not be able to push during delivery. It is important to note that the uterus is innervated by the autonomic nervous system, not the voluntary (somatic) nervous system. Conscious pushing on the mother's part is not necessary to deliver a baby! Delivery may be difficult due to a uterus that becomes overly tired due to a long labor. The uterus will work regardless of disability in the same way that the heart works.

CAN YOU GIVE ME A REFERRAL FOR GENETIC COUNSELING?

Your doctor may be the best person to help you find out where to obtain genetic counseling. Darlene was referred to genetic counseling because the doctors assumed she and her husband had the same form of dwarfism and that they would be concerned about having a baby with dwarfism. Moreover, they felt the doctor did not know there are different forms of dwarfism and two different forms will not produce a baby who has dwarfism.

Many women who have an inherited disability may encounter a doctor who has his own agenda. This can translate into having numerous genetic tests, so before you see a doctor for the first time, write down the questions you want to ask. Start with, "I have some questions to ask." You can refuse any or all genetic testing. A discussion with a genetic counselor will highlight the pros and cons of having genetic testing.

Most likely, not all of your questions will be answered during your first consultation. Certainly more questions are bound to come up in the course of your pregnancy, but by the end of your first visit, you should know who in the office or clinic will be available to answer your future questions. A nurse, nutritionist, health educator, or a combination of these may be responsible for providing information about what to expect and how to care for yourself.

During Sabine's second pregnancy, she was advised to have a test called a *triple screen*. This is a blood test that screens for Down's syndrome, spina bifida, and trisomy 18. The doctor told her the results were positive, but offered no further explanation. Sabine was skeptical and checked on the information. She said, "I looked it up and read about this test and what my scores meant. Because of my age—and age is always factored in—it is impossible to get a negative score."

When Liane Abrams, a genetic counselor, was asked about the triple screening test, she said, "If the woman has a *screen positive*, it merely means she has increased risk for whatever she is screen positive for. An ultrasound will be offered if she is referred for genetic counseling. Often amniocentesis is also offered if her due date does not change. She may be screen positive because of wrong dates, twins, or some other reason."

The Physical Examination

Asking questions is not the only way to evaluate a doctor. Notice how she behaves when examining you. Does she make an effort to let you know what is happening by making reassuring comments, such as, "Now I'm going to insert the speculum" or "You'll feel a slight pressure now"? Does she give you time to relax? The doctor's behavior during an examination is a good indicator of whether you will be treated with sensitivity and consideration during childbirth. Notice, also, what questions the doctor asks you. Does she ask specific, relevant questions about your level of sensation, your mobility and flexibility, or the physical positions that are the most comfortable for you during the examination?

Fertility Considerations

Some women have difficulty in becoming pregnant and they may blame their disability when the disability is not the actual cause for their inability to become pregnant. Simi's periods were very irregular. She was also told that she had flaccid muscles. Sperm always find their way to an ovum without help from contracting muscles. It would seem that the relevant obstacle to Simi's getting pregnant could have been her irregular periods. Equally important was her husband's own fertility problem, which was repaired by surgery.

Connie has diplegic cerebral palsy (affecting both legs), and was unable to have sexual intercourse because her vagina was too tight to allow penetration. She and her husband tried all the possible positions for sexual intercourse without success. They also tried dilators without success. The doctor then ordered larger sizes of dilators. They opted for artificial insemination in the end, because they did not want to wait. They were able to get it covered by health insurance because of "female infertility." The insurance code for this problem is listed in the *ICD 9 Codebook* and your doctor can bill for this procedure. The doctor used an intrauterine procedure. Connie said that the first time the procedure was done it was very painful. "My vagina is very tight and inserting the speculum caused a lot of pain. Plus, my doctor said that my cervix is also tight and tender, so inserting the sperm also made it awful. The second time I found the procedure less painful." Connie later called TLG to say that the insemination procedure did not work and she was going to have surgery on her hip abductors because they were the cause of her inability to have vaginal intercourse. She has since called back with the information that she became pregnant the old-fashioned way.

Andrea also needed artificial insemination because of her husband's disability. She said, "I only ovulated every other month, so they put me on a very low dose of a fertility drug so I would ovulate every month. It took 2 months before I got pregnant the first time; for my second pregnancy it took only once." The insurance paid their share of everything. She also said, "I did not face any prejudice."

Although Orielle was not able to adopt, she was able to get the needed medical intervention in order to conceive. She was prescribed Clomid® (clomiphene citrate) and had artificial insemination in order to conceive.

Although Andrea, Connie, and Chelsea did not experience discrimination when getting fertility intervention, some women might and it is important to know what is covered in your medical plan. "If your medical plan has provisions for fertility intervention, then you should not be discriminated against in being able to participate in the fertility program" (55).

The Doctor's Partners

It is important to meet your doctor's partners and the physician on call. Schedule one of your regular office visits with your doctor's partner(s) as early as possible. You cannot predict which doctor will deliver your baby because you cannot predict when labor will start. Childbirth is likely to be a more satisfying experience if there are some familiar faces among the people helping you. Also, you need the opportunity to make sure that the other doctors who may care for you fully understand and support any plans you have made with your own doctor. You cannot assume that all partners in a practice will take the same approach. Sybil had a doctor who was highly supportive, but it was her doctor's partner who attended the birth. This partner was horrified that a woman with spina bifida was having a child and pressured Sybil and her husband into signing forms permitting him to sterilize her during caesarean delivery. Although this happened many years ago and is illegal, this can still happen. Michelle, on the other hand, found her doctor's partner to be even more helpful than her regular obstetrician and more careful in taking her disability into account. If you have strong disagreements with one of your doctor's partners, bring up the problem with your own doctor. He can help you resolve the problem or arrange for another doctor to attend your delivery if he is not available. Make sure your feelings are known if you find that you cannot work with a partner. Clara was uncomfortable in telling her obstetrician that she was uncomfortable with the possibility of having a certain doctor in his practice perform her delivery. She had her husband talk with her obstetrician. Clara received an absolute guarantee that she would not have that particular doctor during her delivery.

When Holly became pregnant with her second child, her obstetrician recognized Holly as being an expert in hydrocephalus. She had set up a database to collect information on hydrocephalus and pregnancy. Holly had switched obstetricians between her first and second pregnancies. She said, "My new obstetrician did something very important the moment he found out I was pregnant with my second child; he called his on-call partners in and had a meeting about me. He told them what they needed to be aware of and gave them some understanding of hydrocephalus."

If you and your doctor make special plans for your care, make sure they are written in your record, and be sure to bring your own photocopy of these plans to your labor and delivery because this may be the only copy available at the hospital. It is equally important to have a guarantee that all of your doctor's partners will be notified and agree to follow these plans. When you meet with your doctor's associates, tell them, "I'm sure you've noticed in my chart that Dr. "X" and I have discussed ... (a particular aspect of your care). I'd like to go over these plans with you." These precautions may help you avoid a disappointment like Hilary's, who had planned very carefully for her caesarean delivery. She hoped she could have regional anesthesia, and so she took the required class and found a position in which she could receive the spinal injection. Hilary met with an anesthesiologist who was willing to give her husband the required permission to be at the birth, but when her labor started, both her obstetrician and the anesthesiologist were away. The only available anesthesiologist would not allow her husband in the operating room, and the obstetrician could not, or would not, call for a different anesthesiologist. Hilary's disappointment was deepened because her disability prevented her from receiving regional anesthesia. She had planned on trying hypnosis, but it did not work for her and she had to have a general anesthetic. When Hilary was asked, "Did you have an unplanned caesarean section?" She answered, "Yes," because nothing happened according to plan. To the question, "How did you cope?" she answered, "I cried."

Hospitals

It is important to call your local hospitals so you can learn about their policies and how they apply to you. Some hospitals may make an exception to a policy if you give them an important reason. Disabled Rights Advocates wrote in *Through the Maze* regarding hospital stays related to childbirth: "Health plans generally cannot limit coverage for hospital stays for childbirth to less than 48 hours following a vaginal delivery or 96 hours following a caesarean section. You and your doctor may decide that you want to leave earlier, but you cannot be pressured to do so. This protection comes from the Newborns' and Mothers' Health Protection Act (for group plans, including self-funded plans) and state law (for individual plans and non-self-funded group plans)." (57)

The hospital would not let Arianna's husband video the birth because she did not want an epidural. Arianna said, "I didn't find out until a week before the C-section that my husband wouldn't be allowed in, and by that time I had already bought a camcorder so I could record the birth." You must get permission from your doctor and the hospital before you can take a camera into the delivery room. Be sure to bring your copy of any written consent forms when you go to the hospital to have your baby.

Rachel liked her first obstetrician, but she switched doctors because she did not like the hospital that the doctor was associated with.

Sienna said, "Although my doctor understood my disability and the special needs related to my disability, it would have been more helpful to have an environment with nurses and other medical care providers who had some understanding or knowledge of access, assistance, and general disability." You may want to ask your doctor to set up an in-service consultation in order for the labor and delivery staff to learn about your special needs. This may help prevent the problems Sienna and others have faced.

Many people with disabilities have experienced past traumas that are associated with hospitals. Simi said, "To me, walking into the hospital means losing all control over who touches you and what they do. Hospitals are filled with pain and misery for me."

One way to be in control and not feel victimized is by negotiating with the hospital and doctors to get them to meet as many of your needs as possible.

Reasonable Accommodations: At the Hospital

Some women may need a raised toilet seat and/or a shower chair during labor. Simi said, "The maternity ward was not set up for anybody in a wheelchair." Simi was lucky to be in a hospital with a rehabilitation unit, because the hospital staff was able to find a shower chair. Unfortunately, she had to wait, which was difficult because "after sweating for 24 hours and being covered in blood all anybody wants is to take a shower."

Most hospital beds are higher than home beds, and getting in and out of bed was too difficult for her to accomplish without proper equipment.

Charlene had a problem transferring into the hospital bed because the bed was too high. Because she could not do the transfer, she needed to keep her catheter in longer and could not take a shower. She wanted to be able to urinate and shower whenever she needed. Get an early consult with a physical therapist to help find a possible solution if you know that transferring from a high bed will be difficult.

Amanda felt that the hospital staff was not prepared and that her doctor should have oriented them to her needs in advance. She wrote a letter to the hospital before her second labor, telling them that she needed an accessible bathroom as well as what she would need during labor. She said, "We sent three letters before it was all said and done because we were ignored. We ended up having to file a Department of Justice complaint. I still had to stay in the labor and delivery room for my entire stay because they did not have an OB/GYN recovery room that was accessible." (Unfortunately, it can take years to get state approval to change anything structurally in a hospital.)

Calling risk management can be helpful if the hospital is not cooperative in making reasonable accommodations to your medical needs.

Questions to Ask About Hospital Services

Hospitals differ in the services they offer and in some of their rules. The following questions can be asked in order to determine if the hospital will be able to meet your needs:

WHAT BIRTH-RELATED SERVICES DO YOU OFFER?

A hospital may offer a number of birth-related services, including classes about birth in general and the hospital's own procedures; classes about caesarean birth; classes about preparing for childbirth; prenatal exercise classes; classes for other children who will be present at the birth; referrals to classes given outside the hospital and other information sources; nutrition counseling; and referrals.

WILL A REGISTERED NURSE BE IN ATTENDANCE AT ALL TIMES?

The position statement of the Association of Women's Health Obstetric and Neonatal Nurses, the professional organization for nursing support of women giving birth, maintains that continual, available labor support by a professional registered nurse is a critical component in achieving improved birth outcomes.

With the advent of managed care, some hospitals do not keep to this standard. You might want to bring an additional coach with you to attend your labor and delivery in case hospital staff members become busy with other patients. Clara's husband had to hold her leg because her leg went into spasm during labor; this prevented him from coaching her and they needed another coach. Make sure the hospital will make an exception in the event you need extra help for an essential medical reason. Again, make sure to bring your own written copy of the consent form.

HOW LONG DO WOMEN STAY IN THE HOSPITAL AFTER A NORMAL DELIVERY?

Some delivery units have an early release program that allows mothers to go home within 12 hours after giving birth. Such a program should also provide for a home visit by a nurse on the third day after the birth.

WILL THE BABY BE ABLE TO STAY WITH ME AFTER THE BIRTH?

In some hospitals, the baby is taken to the nursery immediately after birth to have its health evaluated and/or be cared for until the mother is moved to her room. When the baby is born at night, sometimes it is kept in the nursery until morning.

DOES THE HOSPITAL ALLOW ROOMING-IN?

This means that the baby stays with the mother in her room, rather than in the nursery. Some mothers prefer that the baby be cared for in the nursery because they need to rest. Others want to keep the baby near them at all times. Rooming-in is much more convenient if you are breast-feeding. Hospital policies about rooming-in vary; it may be allowed around the clock, daytime only, or may require your doctor's consent. Find out your hospital's specific policies. Find out if the nursery is wheelchair accessible if the hospital does not offer rooming-in.

Many women who are wheelchair users find the nursery and the baby's bassinet inaccessible. These women have to rely on the postpartum nurse to bring them the baby. They have generally found themselves continually waiting for their baby.

Natalie said, "Unless my mom or husband was there, the baby mostly stayed in the nursery. I could not get out of bed to take care of him. I had to call for a nurse to come and get him." Natalie said, "I could not hang onto the glass bottles." When one nurse found out that Natalie had not fed the baby in the hospital, she questioned Natalie's competency. This nurse called in Natalie's pediatrician, who would not release Natalie and her baby from the hospital until she fed him in the hospital. Her husband came in and fought for her rights. It is important that your obstetrician leave orders to have the nurses feed the baby *and* make sure the hospital staff understands why those orders are left. In the alternative, Natalie could have brought in bottles that she was able to use so early bonding could take place and she could show hospital staff that she could care for her baby. Natalie needed to use bottles that were plastic *and* had a narrower base. Make sure your pediatrician understands your special needs and agrees to assist in filling them—in writing—long before the birth of your baby.

If you are willing to pay for a private room, in some hospitals your partner may be able to spend the night with you, or the hospital may provide a private room because of the legal requirement of reasonable accommodations. Simi needed a private room because it was difficult to move around with a wheelchair in a regular room with two beds. Also, it was impossible to close the bathroom door because it was not wheelchair accessible.

IS THE HOSPITAL FLEXIBLE ABOUT THE FEEDING SCHEDULE IF I BREAST-FEED?

Find out whether babies are brought to mothers on demand (for example, when they cry from hunger) or according to a set schedule. If a schedule is used, find out if the schedule allows the nurses to meet the needs of newborns at least every 2 hours.

DO NURSES HELP MOTHERS LEARN TO BREAST-FEED?

You might want to ask friends who have given birth in the hospital what they experienced. You can also talk with nurses. Beth recalls that she was never left to breast-feed in privacy. She could not understand why an attendant was necessary when she knew she would be alone with the baby at home. This policy is in place because the hospital is legally responsible and is liable if anything happens to the mother or baby, so there may not be any opportunity to be alone with your baby. It is important to ask for help from an occupational therapist, or call TLG or a breast-feeding consultant if you are having difficulty.

DOES THE HOSPITAL PERMIT SIBLINGS TO VISIT? CAN MY OTHER CHILD (OR CHILDREN) BE PRESENT DURING THE BIRTH?

Some hospitals allow siblings to watch the birth. The usual requirements include the following: the child must be above a certain age; an adult must be present to care for the child; and the child must take a special class about what they will see during the birth. You may want to consider how your child might react to seeing you in pain.

DOES THE HOSPITAL REQUIRE FETAL MONITORING?

Fetal monitoring equipment can be uncomfortable or interfere with mobility, and you may wish to refuse it until it is clearly necessary to evaluate the well-being of the fetus.

DOES THE HOSPITAL REQUIRE THE USE OF AN INTRAVENOUS NEEDLE (IV)?

This question is not as simple as it seems. An IV is a hollow needle that is inserted into a vein to deliver fluids and medications, and to take blood for tests. You may need assurance that an IV will be used only when specific needs arise and not as a matter of routine. If you have the use of only one hand—and that would be the hand in which the IV would be inserted—you would lose much of your ability to move freely during labor. (The use of IVs and fetal monitors is discussed in more detail in Chapter 9.) It is also possible to have a saline lock in place without the IV fluid. This is a small plug in the vein that can be used if necessary.

CAN MY PARTNER AND/OR ANYONE ELSE BE PRESENT IF I HAVE A CAESAREAN SECTION?

The hospital may want you to meet certain conditions in order to allow the father to be present such as taking a class or obtaining consent from the obstetrician. The same applies to anyone else who might come with you. The hospital will likely limit the number of people who can be present.

How much will it cost?

Check on the difference in the financial implications of each option. One program might be completely covered by your insurance, but another one might involve additional charges. Be sure to ask specific questions about any charges that might be associated with your access needs. Someone in the financial office will tell you what the basic charges are and what you might be charged for additional procedures. Remember, you have rights under the Americans with Disabilities Act (ADA). For example, all of the rooms should be wheelchair accessible, not just the rooms in the more expensive section. You should not be charged extra for an ADA accommodation. Will you be charged for additional staff to help you or will this covered by your insurance or the birthing center? You may need to have specific discussions with the medical staff *and* with the financial staff.

Taking a tour of the birthing programs at the hospitals in your area is the best way to know what option is best for you. There is no standardized system for labor and delivery units across the United States. Each hospital has its own arrangement. Some hospitals have labor, delivery, and recovery in different rooms. Other hospitals let you stay in the same room that you labored in. It is important to see whether each hospital room you may be put in is accessible.

You should have an opportunity to meet the staff that works in the labor and delivery unit. Moreover, you should have an opportunity to discuss any special needs you think the staff should know about you before you arrive at the hospital for labor and delivery.

You can take a tour of the delivery rooms, alternative birth center (if any), and nursery. You will be able to see for yourself what the facilities are like, including whether the nursery is accessible to wheelchairs; whether any of the delivery rooms have birthing chairs; and whether there is a shower in the alternative birth room.

There may be a freestanding birth center in your city. This type of center is physically separate from any hospital and is exclusively a childbirth facility. It should have the same professional staff as a hospital and the necessary equipment for normal birth and minor emergencies. It should also be near a regular hospital delivery unit in case the mother needs to be transferred.

Home Birth

A number of women who are non-disabled, and one spinal-cord-injured woman who was interviewed for this book, have had good experiences with home birth. Many women who have higher-than-average risk factors, such as multiple birth pregnancy (such as twins), high blood pressure, or certain disabilities (such as spinal injury T6 and above), will require the facilities that only a hospital can provide. Although home birth can be a good choice, it is a choice that demands very careful consideration. It is important to find out if you are at high risk for complications.

First, think over your reasons for considering home birth. Some common reasons for choosing home birth include:

❖ The desire to keep the family together to ensure that the partner and/or siblings will not be excluded from the birth, and that the mother and infant will not be separated afterward

❖ The desire to maintain control of the birth process and avoid unpleasant hospital routines

❖ The conviction that childbirth is a safe, natural process and medical intervention is best avoided

❖ The wish to have a midwife as the birth attendant (many people feel that a midwife is most likely to give more sensitive, personalized care)

❖ The desire to avoid the expense of a hospital birth (normal uncomplicated home birth, whether attended by a physician or a midwife, is certainly less expensive than a hospital birth)

Make sure your midwife understands your special needs. It is also important that your midwife is formally associated with an obstetrician.

Whatever your reason for considering home birth, understanding exactly what you want will help you decide if home birth is really best for you.

The concerns mentioned here are the same ones that motivate the consumer demands that have caused changes in many hospitals all over the country. Many of the procedures that used to be routine are now done less frequently. You can infer from our list of suggested questions for hospitals that it is possible to have a satisfying childbirth experience in a hospital setting. You can ask these questions and find out whether a local hospital has the features that satisfy the goals you wish to achieve.

Certainly it is true that pregnancy and childbirth are natural processes, and a woman should not be treated as though her pregnancy is an illness. It is also important to remember that *natural* does not automatically mean *uncomplicated*. Another natural process is fever, which is the body's defense against invading germs. Most fevers harmlessly run their course, but sometimes it is essential to treat the underlying illness with antibiotics. Similarly, pregnancy usually poses no threats and the associated physical changes serve useful purposes, but occasionally there are serious complications.

The question to ask, then, is how safe is childbirth for you? If you are considering home birth, you need to begin by getting a medical opinion about your general health and the risks posed by your disability. You may want to delay discussing home birth with your doctor if you think this information will affect her evaluation of your general health. Once your general health has been assessed, you can explain that you are considering home birth and ask what she thinks the advantages and disadvantages might be. Remember, the course of a pregnancy can be unpredictable. One woman's physician was willing, at first, to attend a birth in her home, but he advised her to give birth in the hospital when her blood pressure became too high. Many changes can occur during 9 months and the decision to give birth at home is always somewhat tentative.

The decision of where to give birth involves both practical and personal considerations. Think about your goals. Investigate the potentials of both hospital and home birth, and compare the advantages and disadvantages of each. The more information you have, the clearer your answer will be.

WILL HOME BIRTH BE CONVENIENT FOR ME, CONSIDERING MY DISABILITY?

You might need assistance with changing positions during labor. Hospital staff should be available. Would there be people available to help you at home at any hour? Would a birthing chair or other equipment at the hospital make labor significantly easier for you?

One possibility is using a doctor and midwife team. Ask how they would share the task of caring for you. One common pattern is for the midwife to come to the mother's home when labor begins and call the doctor when labor is well advanced and/or if problems arise.

MIDWIVES

Tina preferred a midwife. She asked her gynecologist about a referral to a midwife, but her gynecologist did not work with a midwife. Tina was referred to a midwife in another medical practice "but she did not take my insurance." Tina said, "A lot of insurance does not cover midwives." Finally, Tina found a midwife who worked in the same office and billed through a doctor, so Tina was able to use her. "I wanted her to deliver the baby, not some third-party doctor or midwife. I asked her how many deliveries she had been present for." Another option is to talk to several mothers who have worked with the midwife. Find out how flexible she is about working with your disability, just as you would with a doctor. Discuss how to differentiate between normal pregnancy symptoms, signs of a problem pregnancy, and warning signs that your disability is causing problems.

PREPARING FOR EMERGENCIES

Ask the people who will attend your birth what emergency equipment they usually bring. Does it include oxygen, intravenous equipment, and saline solutions? Two dangerous complications of childbirth (again, excluding disability-related complications) are blood loss in the mother and oxygen deprivation in the infant. If you will not have emergency equipment, find out if it is available from paramedic or ambulance services. Find out *exactly* what emergency services are available in your community. A public librarian can help you locate such services, or you can contact the fire department, because many paramedic units are attached to city fire departments.

HOW FAR ARE YOU FROM THE HOSPITAL?

The distance between your home and the hospital is an important factor. An emergency physician said that severe blood loss should be treated within 30 minutes. He pointed out that part of this time might be spent waiting for an ambulance to arrive, transferring the pregnant woman to the ambulance, and driving to the hospital. The farther you are from the hospital, the greater the risks are due to loss of blood. He added that saline solutions can be injected after arrival at the hospital, but it takes time for blood typing before transfusions can be given. He suggested the precaution of going to the hospital early in labor for blood testing, and then returning home to give birth, or you can have blood typing done anytime prior to labor.

Other Medical Professionals

Your obstetrician may not be the only specialist you need to consult. In some situations, you may want to get a second opinion—which is your right—about a particular aspect of your care. You may want to have a vaginal delivery after a previous caesarean section, and you want more than one recommendation. Use any of the methods suggested for selecting your obstetrician if you are uncomfortable asking for this referral. Another source of information is the National Second Opinion Hotline.

Obstetric Anesthesia For Disabled Women

An anesthesiologist is a physician who specializes in administering anesthetics, pain and related medication, and monitoring the patient's response to these medications, usually during surgery.

The individual medical situation of any patient coming for anesthesia for any surgical or obstetric procedure should be carefully evaluated beforehand. Planning for anesthesia is based on the patient's medical condition and the technical requirements of the surgical or obstetric procedure. This pre-procedure planning is especially essential for disabled women who will be coming to the hospital for a delivery or other obstetric procedure.

The woman's past experiences with anesthesia should be discussed prior to delivery. Any unpleasant experiences from the past can generate great fear as delivery approaches. This situation should be discussed proactively with an anesthesiologist. Sometimes it is prudent to talk with a general anesthesiologist rather than an OB anesthesiologist, because they are more familiar with doing epidurals on an atypical body.

An anesthesiologist should be consulted as delivery approaches, and a physical exam should be done of the lower back (to evaluate for possible technical problems with regional anesthesia) and mouth, neck, and teeth (to evaluate for possible airway problems). It is not always easy to see an anesthesiologist before delivery, especially given the nationwide shortage of anesthesiologists. This shortage results in long hours in the operating room and little time for other patient-related activities. If a patient has a definite medical or other possibly anesthesia-related problem that is known before delivery, it is best to consult with a hospital that offers perinatal services. This type of hospital is experienced in handling obstetric patients and babies who might have problems, and usually can also provide a pre-delivery anesthesia evaluation. The obstetrician would request this. Because no one knows when a particular patient will deliver, the anesthesiologist consulted in advance may not be available for the actual delivery, even though the patient has already been evaluated and an appropriate plan has been made. The information about the patient and the plan should be available for other staff in the department.

Each type of obstetric anesthesia has possible drawbacks. By discussing the patient's needs with both the obstetrician and the anesthesiologist, and by being at an institution that has an established perinatal unit, disabled women can have the best obstetric outcome possible (32).

It is a good idea to have an appointment with an anesthesiologist, whether or not you are planning to give birth by caesarean section. It is now common for many women to have an epidural during labor for pain control. Felicia needed anesthesia because her fibromyalgia caused a low pain threshold. She filled out an anesthesiology intake form. She said, "I answered all the questions and I put fibromyalgia down as a complication. The anesthesiologist asked 'how does it manifest for you?' I told him about my sensitivity to pain. The labor and delivery nurse were insensitive to my needs and ignored what I had to say."

One of the reasons Darlene chose a scheduled caesarean was to make sure she would have the anesthesiologist she interviewed in advance attend her delivery. Darlene said, "I wanted to have an epidural so I could be awake during the C-section. I heard from another small person that most small women need a general. I did not hear this from the medical community. I also think it's important for physically small women to do their own research on anesthesia."

Sienna said, "If I could do it over again, I would request an anesthesiologist who was experienced, or at least had some interaction with women with disabilities. I would also meet him prior to delivery." Sometimes pain medications are used during vaginal birth, as well, and the anesthesiologist can explain why anesthesia might be used and the effects of various medications, in order to determine which procedures are most appropriate for you.

As mentioned previously, some hospitals require permission from the anesthesiologist for the partner to be present during surgery. Our consultant commented, "I could not agree more with the concept of talking ahead of time to one or more members of the anesthesia department before labor."

Naomi's obstetrician set up an appointment between her and the anesthesiologist. Naomi had found information that an epidural might cause the progression of her specific disability, and so they decided that if she needed a caesarean, a general anesthesia would be used.

The consultant went on to say that most hospitals routinely allow the partner to be present during caesareans sections performed under regional anesthesia, adding that anesthesiologists sometimes do not want to be distracted by a partner's presence while they are actually administering anesthesia, but they would be comfortable allowing the partner in the delivery room during the baby's birth.

Orielle used the same anesthesiologist for her caesarean section that she had used for other surgeries. She said, "I handpicked my anesthesiologist." If you do not have a relationship with an anesthesiologist, it is better to have your doctor make the referral.

Deirdre wanted to have the option of pain management; she wanted an epidural if she found labor too painful. Her doctors (the obstetrician and anesthesiologist) were at a different health care facility from her spine doctor. The obstetrician refused. Deirdre said, "They were unwilling to do an epidural on me because of my spinal history. I talked to my spine doctor, who said, 'they should be able to go up a level or below from where the surgery was and the scar tissue is'. I brought all my records and films into the anesthesiologist, whom I was referred to from my spine doctor. I left those items with him. The anesthesiologist then said, 'no problem.' I made him put it in the notes. I also had short and long labor plans for my friends to help me with. I made sure this was on file and included the physician's names I had spoken with, as well as their phone numbers and beeper numbers. Make a list of all your doctors' names, numbers, and critical information, including what you and they have agreed to such as the types of preferred medications and anesthesia. Keep this list with you so you can show it to each medical professional."

As Sally learned, having information on a file is not enough. She said, "We had our doctors' numbers available, but the replacement doctors wanted to do their own thing." The pregnant woman should have a copy of the plan in her own hands, as well as in the medical file. The woman should have the knowledgeable doctors' phone numbers in hand in case there are any concerns that an alternate staff person is not following the plan.

An MRI may be used if you do not have any X-rays. It is unknown whether MRI is a safe procedure during pregnancy, but the anesthesiologist may want to use an MRI so it can be determined if a regional anesthesia (spinal or epidural) is workable.

You or your physician(s) may need to give the anesthesiologist information beyond what is usually required. Be sure to ask the anesthesiologist to contact the doctor most knowledgeable about your disability. Heather's experience will give you an idea of the kind of advance planning you can do with your anesthesiologist.

Heather was instructed to lie flat on her back after she was given anesthesia, but she is very uncomfortable lying on her back without a pillow because she has congenital hip dysplasia and scoliosis. She had to put up an argument to get a pillow because the doctor had given firm instructions that she should lie flat. She could have arranged during a meeting with the anesthesiologist ahead of time for permission to use a pillow or lie on her side, because many hospitals allow patients to do this after receiving spinal anesthesia.

The anesthesiologist may also need time to schedule diagnostic tests to help determine the choice of anesthetic. For example, women who have myasthenia gravis may need thyroid function tests and an *electrocardiogram* (a test of heart function), or the anesthesiologist may want to do some research on a drug or a procedure that is contraindicated with a particular disability. Diane is a good example of this. "It is common for dwarfs to have unusual discs; they are closer together." Having the discs closer together may make the administration of regional anesthesia difficult.

The information required for a caesarean should be reviewed in case emergency surgery is needed, even if a caesarean section is not planned. Noelle, who has Friedreich's ataxia, had an unplanned caesarean birth and general anesthesia was used because it was unknown whether spinal anesthesia would be safe for her. She was very disappointed that she was not conscious when her baby was born. If Noelle had consulted with an anesthesiologist ahead of time, he may have had time to investigate the options. Noelle would have known what to expect; she could have done her own research if he still found that general anesthesia might be necessary; or he could have consulted with her neurologist.

If you have spinal cord dysfunction or a neurologic disability (such as cerebral palsy) or neuromuscular disability, the anesthesiologist will need to examine you in order to determine the muscle tone and reflexes below the level of the lesion. This information can be useful in monitoring your recovery if you need regional anesthesia for control of dysreflexia or for surgery.

You may have other kinds of questions for which you want answers as well. For example, you might be afraid of having headaches for several days after spinal anesthesia. Some of what you hear and read about the experiences of other people may not apply to you. You may hear about a person who has a rare allergic reaction to medication, and you might be afraid that this can happen to you. Therefore, you may want to ask the anesthesiologist how likely it is that you will experience this or any other problem.

Get the information before you visit the anesthesiologist that can help you pinpoint your questions. Even if you had a previous caesarean section before having subsequent caesarean sections, make sure that each anesthesiologist has read the information in your chart. Diane had a regional anesthesia for each of her caesareans. She said that in the first two caesareans she found the administration of medication easier. Diane laid on her side in the fetal position. During her third delivery, the new anesthesiologist had her sit and bend over. Diane found this position to be difficult because it was hard to breathe. You can get information from written sources, hospital classes about caesarean births, childbirth educators, or C-SEC, a support group for caesarean parents.

Discuss the following questions with your anesthesiologist:

❖ Have you given anesthesia to other women with my type of disability?
❖ Do you feel comfortable giving me this type of anesthesia?
❖ What are the advantages of each method of anesthesia?
❖ What are the risks of each method for me and for the baby?
❖ What can I expect to experience with each type of anesthesia?
❖ What are the possible side effects?

Your contractions and the sensations you experience will be affected differently by different anesthetics. For example, people who have spinal anesthesia often notice that they cannot feel themselves breathing. This experience can be frightening until someone reassures them that this lack of sensation is to be expected.

DO YOU RECOMMEND A PARTICULAR TYPE OF ANESTHESIA? WHAT CIRCUMSTANCES, IF ANY, WOULD CHANGE YOUR RECOMMENDATION?

You might also want to ask the anesthesiologist to explain the basis for any recommendations. If there is any question about what anesthesia would be appropriate for you, the anesthesiologist could refer you to a specialist; you could also consult with the doctor who has treated you for your disability.

Tell the anesthesiologist if you strongly prefer one type of anesthesia, and if he recommends against it, ask any questions that help you understand why. If the anesthesiologist's recommendations are based on disability concerns, a consultation with your disability specialist may be helpful. Ask the anesthesiologist these questions:

❖ What information will you insert into my medical record?
❖ What instructions will the staff will be given when I am admitted to the hospital?
❖ What might be done differently by another doctor if you are not available when I give birth?
❖ Would you be willing to give me a copy of the information?

Hilary was disappointed because the anesthesiologist she interviewed in advance of labor was willing to let her husband attend the birth, but the one who actually attended the birth was not. Your preferred anesthesiologist may be willing to insert information into your record that will explain any special arrangements. Make sure the correct information regarding anesthesia is noted in your chart, ask for your own copy, and be sure to take it with you to the hospital.

The Perinatologist

A *perinatologist* is an obstetrician who specializes in high-risk pregnancy. After obstetrical training, the perinatologist spends 2 years gaining supervised experience in treating the complications of pregnancy. Some of the more common complications are placenta previa, multiple pregnancies, diabetes (diabetes may be pre-existing or the type that appears in pregnancy), high blood pressure, or a history of miscarriages or premature labor during previous pregnancies. A perinatologist treated some of the interviewees. Most of the interviewees who had sought one on their own found that this effort had been unnecessary because the perinatologist discovered that their disabilities did not put them in a high-risk category. On the other hand, you may want to choose a perinatologist. One woman changed obstetricians because the first one she saw seemed to be a bit uncomfortable with her plans to become pregnant. She had heard great things about the perinatologist and made an initial visit. She changed doctors because she liked the perinatologist so much, not because she actually needs a perinatologist.

Amanda had moved to a new area, and for her second pregnancy she chose a doctor who had been a perinatologist but dropped the specialty. He saw Amanda and her pregnancy as a "walk in the park."

It is not necessary to consult a perinatologist unless there is reason to suspect you have a specific complication of pregnancy. If complications develop in the course of your pregnancy, however, your obstetrician might refer you to a perinatologist or a hospital high-risk center. In some situations, a perinatologist might become your primary doctor, in others she will act as a consultant. Sylvia felt that her perinatologist provided technical expertise, but did not offer the kind of empathy and reassurance her obstetrician provided. As a result, Sylvia considered her obstetrician to be her primary doctor.

Although a perinatologist has been trained in the complications of pregnancy, she will still need to obtain additional information about the interaction of disability and pregnancy. Most physicians receive very little training and education in physical disabilities. It is important to have the perinatologist get a consult with a disabilities specialist. Carol's story illustrates this point:

"I was referred to a perinatologist when I was hospitalized because my liver enzymes had become twice that of normal due to preeclampsia. A lot of the problems arose when my regular doctor went away for the weekend. He is a good advocate, but it's hard to advocate when you're away. The biggest issue for the perinatologist was that the hyperflexity of my legs was interpreted as a sign that my brain was swelling due to preeclampsia. My son was delivered sooner than necessary due to this misconception. My regular doctor said, 'we could have waited longer.' I think they need a doctor who knows about CP to consult with the perinatologist and explain what is normal for the mom's condition and how not to aggravate the tone or spasticity (such as when my water was broken for my son's birth)."

The biggest issue for the perinatologist was when the deep tendon reflex test of Carol's legs showed that she had hyperreflexia. This can be a sign that the brain is swelling due to preeclampsia, but it is also common in cerebral palsy. A doctor needs to be able to distinguish between these two conditions, or between preeclampsia and other physical disabilities.

Genetic Counselors

A genetic counselor can help you determine how likely it is that your child will have a disability. They can also help you explore your feelings about the possibility of having a disabled child. You can ask your doctor for a referral for genetic counseling or you can call any March of Dimes agency for information. If you seek genetic counseling, you may also be working with a team composed of doctors and/or ultrasound technicians who perform diagnostic tests; laboratory personnel who grow and analyze the fetal cells; and the genetic counselor. You may wish to meet with a genetic counselor to discuss your options before conceiving. There may be some testing available prior to the pregnancy to determine your risks for various disabilities. There may also be new information on testing for genetic problems that is more advanced than at the time of your disability diagnosis. In addition, you can review all of the options available so you have time to consider them prior to your pregnancy.

The genetic counselor can explain the appropriate tests, possibly in consultation with your obstetrician or family doctor. Later, the genetic counselor will explain your test results and provide other information. An important part of the counselor's role is to give you emotional support as you absorb the information you are given and help you try to reach any necessary decisions. The genetic counselor will rarely interject his own opinion because it is his job to assist you only with the decision-making process. You may encounter a genetic counselor who exhibits his own prejudice, however.

Simi went to talk to a counselor. Simi said, "The counselor couldn't imagine how anybody in a wheelchair could possibly have a child." The counselor even had the audacity to tell Simi to get a foster kid for a little while "so I could get over it; so I could figure out I really can't handle this."

Be sure to discuss the counselor's report with your physician. Discussing this information with two advisers can help you to be sure that you understand your test results correctly.

Many genetic counselors stress the importance of working with an established genetic counseling center. They point out that the procedures for obtaining fetal cells can be done by many doctors, but that the crucial step is the culturing and analysis of the cells in a reliable laboratory. The following are some questions you might want to ask when considering a particular genetic counseling center:

ARE THE COUNSELORS BOARD-CERTIFIED OR ELIGIBLE FOR BOARD CERTIFICATION? DOES THE CENTER OFFER HIGH-RESOLUTION ULTRASOUND AND CHORIONIC VILLUS SAMPLING, AS WELL AS AMNIOCENTESIS?

As the term suggests, high-resolution ultrasound provides more detailed images. Chorionic villus sampling (CVS) is not as widely available as amniocentesis, but it is worth knowing whether the test is available. It is important to know the pros and cons of each procedure. There is a 1 in 100 chance for miscarriage with CVS, which is performed before the second trimester (10 to 12 weeks). Amniocentesis is performed in the second trimester (15 to 16 weeks); its risk of miscarriage is one in 300. Not only does amniocentesis identify the same genetic issues as CVS, but it also identifies neural tube issues. Having an abortion late in pregnancy can be more emotional for some women because you may be more bonded to the fetus. In addition, by the second trimester, many friends and family are aware of the pregnancy. Your pregnancy is more public and this makes you more vulnerable to outside pressures.

HOW LONG HAVE THEY BEEN PERFORMING THESE TESTS? HOW MANY HAVE THEY DONE?

If you have a choice between centers, you may prefer the one that is more established. What is most important is that the staff is experienced.

WILL THE MEDICAL GENETICIST BE AVAILABLE TO HELP EXPLAIN RESULTS IF THE TEST RESULTS ARE UNCERTAIN OR DIFFICULT TO INTERPRET?

The geneticist specializes in the field of genetics. Most likely she will work with the counselor in explaining test results to you.

HOW MUCH EXPERIENCE DOES THE CENTER HAVE WITH THE PARTICULAR CONDITION YOU ARE CONCERNED ABOUT?

There may be a staff member who is highly experienced in analyzing the ultrasound images for specific conditions.

WHO WILL PERFORM THE DIAGNOSTIC TEST? HOW MUCH EXPERIENCE DO THEY HAVE?

The procedure may be performed by a resident under the supervision of another physician more experienced in the procedure if the center is attached to a medical school or a teaching hospital. Some women might want to request that the procedure be done by a more experienced staff member.

Get the Support You Need

You may have many unpleasant and even quite painful memories about your medical care, especially if you have had your disability since childhood. Long, anxious waits in crowded waiting rooms; hurried nurses; receptionists who ignored you; painful surgeries and lonely nights in hospital beds; embarrassing examinations by strangers; years of unanswered questions—these may be your memories. If you add to these memories the vulnerability felt by any pregnant woman, you may feel very unenthusiastic about the idea of facing a new round of doctors, hospitals, tests, and examinations.

Whatever medical attention you need, your providers should be working for you, not on you. You need support in coping with your fears as well as support for your desire to create and care for a new human being. Your tools for getting what you need are threefold:

- ❖ Your ability to communicate and plan ahead
- ❖ A treatment plan clearly agreed upon by you and your obstetrician and other doctors, when indicated
- ❖ The assistance of an advocate

When a patient advocate at a university obstetrics clinic was asked what the most important advice she had to offer was, her answer was one word: *Communicate!* The author recalls an incident related to her by Sharon, who had visited that very clinic. Sharon was assisted in getting ready for an examination and then left alone for a long time in the examining room. The wait was not merely annoying, but infuriating to Sharon, who is paraplegic and could not shift position or get off the examining table. She made a point of telling all concerned that she must never be left alone like that again. The advocate remembered appreciating Sharon's willingness to talk about her needs and agreed that this incident was a perfect example of the kind of situation in which communication is all-important.

You may be one of the first patients with your disability in the obstetrics clinic or maternity ward. You will not only get what you need by communicating your problems and needs, but you will also help smooth the path for other disabled pregnant women. There is increasing professional recognition that patients are often the most knowledgeable about their disabilities. They will welcome the information you give them if you make comments such as, "Please let me know and help me if the doctor is going to be delayed. Remember, I'm stuck up here on this examining table," or, "May I have a pillow? With my scoliosis, I'll need it in order to lay the way you want me to." Misunderstandings can happen very easily. When Stacy gave birth, she had not yet made it clear that she had some pain sensation even though she was quadriplegic. It hurt when the obstetrician began to stitch Stacy's episiotomy without anesthesia! It is often helpful to have your patient advocate with you as much as possible when you have a medical appointment.

Find out who is the best person to contact for each problem or question. A nurse or health educator may be able to answer most of your general questions about pregnancy; the doctor will help you with medical decisions. If your doctor refers you to a specialist, ask whether the specialist or your own doctor will explain your test results. Many large clinics have patient advocates who are responsible for helping you make sure your needs are met.

Advance planning can prevent much confusion and frustration. Obstetricians' schedules can be very erratic. Appointments are often delayed when a doctor is detained at the hospital. It is a good idea to call ahead before leaving home and ask whether to come at the appointed time or later. Do not schedule appointments too closely together. If you must travel far, plan ahead for delays and consider whether you will need to change your transportation plans or bring along a project to work on while you wait.

Bring along a pencil and paper, or even a tape recorder if you know you will be covering a lot of information during an appointment. Keep a written list of your questions to ensure that you cover them all. It can be difficult to search your mind for one last question when your appointment started 20 minutes late. Give the doctor a copy of your list of questions at the start of the visit.

Keep copies of any forms you fill out. Bring copies of medical questionnaires with you when you go to the hospital. Information can be misfiled even in the best-run hospital. You will not want to answer questions about your medical history between labor contractions!

Advance planning is a process that you should share with your obstetrician. You and your doctor will develop a more or less detailed plan of action for your childbirth as the months go by and you discuss a variety of concerns. The important features of your treatment plan should be in written form and signed and dated by your doctor. You should have a copy to bring with you to the hospital. This plan should include your doctor's instructions to the hospital staff for your care after you are admitted to the hospital. Some aspects of the plan may be specifically related to your disability. For example, a common hospital policy is that nothing should be taken by mouth once labor is confirmed, but you may be taking medications that should not be interrupted. Your doctor can give instructions for you to continue your medications or for you to be given medications by injection.

Other aspects of your treatment plan may deal with issues that would concern any pregnant woman. For example, your doctor may agree that your baby can be given to you to hold and nurse right after the birth, rather than being sent straight to the nursery.

Perhaps not all of your treatment plan will be listed in your signed copy. It depends on what is comfortable for you and your doctor. In addition, some aspects of the plan might change with changing circumstances. For example, you will not be able to hold the baby right away if your baby's breathing is irregular or if the pulse is abnormal, even if that was the original plan. Some aspects of your treatment plan serve as guidelines for what you may reasonably expect rather than as unalterable procedures.

At times you will want to share the task of assuring that your needs are met. The person you share this with is your advocate. The advocate may be your husband, a friend, or a health professional. The health professional should be someone with whom you are already comfortable and familiar. Your advocate should be someone who is comfortable helping you in the following ways:

- ❖ He may accompany you on some or all of your doctor visits. Many of us are uncomfortable asking questions or expressing our concerns. An articulate forthright advocate can help you express yourself. Your advocate may also help you remember your doctor's explanations and instructions more clearly.
- ❖ An advocate may collect written information about your disability for others involved with your care.
- ❖ He may accompany you on a hospital tour, help you formulate the questions to consider, and work with nursing staff to create special provisions for your care.
- ❖ Having an advocate is also helpful when you are in labor. His role will not be the same as in other situations, so you may decide to choose a different person for this role. The role of the advocate (or coach) during labor will be covered in more detail in Chapter 11.

You and your advocate should discuss in advance how you will work together. It should be understood that you are in charge, but you also want assistance in communicating your needs. You and your advocate can help other people realize that you are competent. For example, answer for yourself if someone asks your advocate a question they should have asked you.

Getting Preauthorization

Deirdre needed preauthorization from her insurance carrier for physical and occupational therapy, but she was too tired to be persistent in getting the preauthorization. This is the time to ask your patient advocate for help. Your doctor or the staff at your doctor's office should also help you get preauthorizations. They know how to maneuver their way through the insurance system. A good doctor should also be your advocate.

Planning Ahead for Mobility Equipment

Plan ahead for the type of equipment or equipment features you may need because mobility is affected by the second trimester. For example, a reclining and tilt wheelchair could help relieve heartburn and gastro-esophageal reflux. It can take at least a month for an insurance approval. The DME (durable medical equipment) provider may not be able to rent a reclining and tilt wheelchair. Therefore, going to the supplier may prove to be helpful.

Closing Comments

This chapter has discussed a number of issues pertinent to medical care, and provided questions that you can ask yourself and medical professionals. Answering these questions should help with all aspects of finding a doctor who is knowledgeable, who is willing to work in a team with you and your other physicians, and with whom you feel comfortable. Each woman needs to explore all of the options available in order to decide how to meet her own specific needs.

Eating for Two: Nutrition in Pregnancy

THE OLD SAYING, "A pregnant woman is eating for two," used to mean that a mother-to-be should eat an amount of food that would be enough for two people, but it has been criticized for sounding too much like an excuse for *over*-eating. Eating well is important for you and your baby, but a pregnant woman should not simply increase the amount of food she eats. She must make a point of choosing foods that will supply the additional protein, vitamins, and minerals she needs. One key way to ensure a good diet is to eat 6 to 8 ounces of protein-rich food every day, with an increase in vitamin and mineral consumption ranging from 15 to 100 percent. Each nutrient plays a role in fetal development and has value for pregnant women.

This chapter explains the basic nutritional requirements and includes a discussion of the special concerns of women with disabilities, including special diets, weight gain and its effects on mobility, and avoiding constipation. The chapter outlines the nutrients that are required for a balanced diet, as well as ways to ensure that a vegetarian diet is adequate for pregnancy.

Special Concerns of Women with Disabilities

Women with disabilities have essentially the same nutritional needs as other pregnant women, although there are a few minor differences. These differences are related to the effects of special diets and weight gain.

Some disabled women try special diets in an attempt to alleviate the symptoms of disability. Many of these special diets are controversial. A pregnant woman and a developing fetus have very specific nutritional needs, and unusual diets can be inadequate or even harmful. Michelle was thinking about trying a special diet to see if it would improve her MS symptoms, but she told us: "My doctor's nutritionist told me I was taking too much vitamin A for the baby." Michelle added that the nutritionist's advice made a significant difference in what she ate: "I would have tried another MS diet I'd heard about, but I found out my baby needs specific vitamins."

If your doctor has told you to modify your diet in a way that is related to your disability, it is important to ask him if you should change your diet again when you become pregnant, or even before you get pregnant. Women who use medications regularly will need to ask their doctors whether to change medications. For example, a pregnant woman needs extra calcium, but calcium interferes with the absorption of most medicines, some antibiotics, and iron.

One interviewee saw a biochemist 2 months before her baby was born because she wanted help with her muscular dystrophy. She said, "He gave me a strict diet to follow in addition to taking five different vitamins a day. After 2 weeks of this regimen, I felt hungry all the time. Plus, I did not think pregnancy was a good time to start a new diet. I was also worried that my baby was not getting all the nutrition he needed." Pregnant women are advised to inform their obstetrician regarding any recommendations made by the doctor who regularly treats their disability symptoms.

You may need to ask for a referral to occupational therapy if preparing food is difficult for you. Mona said, "I needed help learning to work in the kitchen because of my tremors." She was eating frozen dinners because it was hard for her to cook. In occupational therapy you can learn how to work in the kitchen.

The best plan for a pregnant disabled woman is to follow the nutritional guidelines given below. Any modifications to diet should be discussed with a nutritionist or obstetrician.

WEIGHT GAIN

Pregnant women with disabilities may be concerned with the recommendation to increase calorie intake during pregnancy because it can exacerbate the problems caused by disability. Many of the interviewees experienced difficulties with mobility and transfers because the weight gained during pregnancy is not distributed evenly over the body. Balance became more difficult for several women. Others found that the joints that were painful with weight-bearing became further stressed during pregnancy. The increasing fatigue and clumsiness that all women begin to experience in the second trimester was of greater concern for many disabled women. Several of the interviewees needed to start using canes or wheelchairs; others found that they simply could not accomplish their normal daily activities because they needed to slow down. If weight gain is significant, the loss of mobility may be even greater. Carla pointed out: "I gained 50 pounds the first time I was pregnant. It caused a lot of back problems and my range of motion was less. The next time, I was much more nutrition-conscious. I only gained 30 pounds, and I had a much easier time."

Weight gain can increase the risk of pressure sores during pregnancy. This was not a problem for the women who were interviewed, as explained below.

Some disabled women try to avoid loss of mobility by keeping their weight down. Pam, for example, was careful to keep her weight gain to 15 pounds. Minimizing weight gain can be a sensible strategy, but this should be discussed with a doctor. Pam's restricted diet may have contributed to her fatigue.

The need to maintain mobility is a strong motivation to keep weight down, but it is important for women with disabilities to understand why they need to gain at least 24 pounds while they are pregnant. Most of the weight increase represents the growth of the mother's "products of pregnancy," as shown in Table 6-1.

The weight gain representing fetal growth is very important. It could be tempting to take the same approach as Patricia, who told us: "I actually lost weight at one point because I was afraid the baby would be too big to go through my pelvis." There was a time when women were often advised to keep their weight down in the hope that having smaller babies would make childbirth easier. More recent studies have shown this approach to be highly inadvisable. Birth weight is a major indicator of an infant's health. Babies with low weight (less than 5.5 pounds) are more vulnerable to illness and a number of neurologic and learning problems.

If your pre-pregnancy weight is average, the recommended weight gain is between 25 and 35 pounds. Women who are underweight at the beginning of pregnancy are advised to gain from 28 to 36 pounds. The recommended weight gain for women who are overweight when they become pregnant is 15 to 25 pounds. The recommended

TABLE 6-1
PRODUCTS OF PREGNANCY

Products	Weight Increase (lbs)
Baby[a]	7.5
Placenta	1.0
Amniotic fluid	2.0
Uterine tissue	2.0
Increased blood supply	4.0
Breast growth[b]	3.0
Maternal reserves[c]	4.0–8.0
Total	24.0–28.0

[a] This represents average birth weight of infants.

[b] It should be remembered that even if a woman does not intend to breast-feed, her breasts will grow, and she needs to eat accordingly.

[c] Reserves are a small amount of fat tissue needed to support the fetal growth spurt in late pregnancy, provide the mother with energy during labor, and provide energy during early lactation.

weight gain is 35 to 45 pounds if you are having twins. It may be necessary to modify the usual weight gain guidelines when considering whether a woman with disabilities is underweight, normal weight, or overweight. For example, a woman who has lost muscle mass from atrophy and is underweight, according to the charts, may be at a normal weight in all other respects. Thus, a woman who appears to be underweight might actually not be, and she could suffer increased mobility problems—while deriving no benefit—from too great an increase in weight.

The pattern of weight gain is as important as the amount of weight gained. A healthy pattern is usually 4 to 6 pounds by the end of the first trimester, and roughly one pound per week for the remainder of the pregnancy. A sudden increase in weight can be edema caused by preeclampsia, a dangerous condition. Weight gain may be low during the first month or two of pregnancy as a result of the loss of appetite, but a pregnant woman does not need to worry if she eats nutritious foods and begins to gain weight normally by the end of the first trimester. (If her appetite is poor, she may want to ask her doctor to prescribe a prenatal vitamin.) The slight increase in calories recommended in Table 6-2 (an additional 100 calories per day in the first trimester, and 300 calories per day in the second and third trimesters), will support the slow, steady weight increase that is normal in healthy pregnancies.

"When you are pregnant, your blood volume increases by 50 percent; your baby is immersed in one quart of amniotic fluid; and tissue fluid volume increases by 2 to 3 quarts. You need to drink at least two quarts of liquid a day (64 oz) to meet these extra fluid needs" (58).

Vitamins and Minerals

Some of the vitamins and minerals that are important to health are not well enough understood to warrant special recommendations for pregnant women. Even a very small increase of some minerals may actually be toxic, and pregnant women are usually advised not to take supplements in amounts exceeding those recommended for all adults. Two important nutrients not mentioned in Table 6-2 are water and sodium, which is found in table salt. These are discussed in the following section.

Nutritional Requirements

Calories

Both the pregnant woman and the fetus are growing new tissue, and energy is required to support this growth. Many studies have shown that growth of the fetus and the placenta are impaired when a pregnant woman restricts her intake of calories.

Calories are a measure of the energy supplied by foods. In addition to eating enough to meet her energy requirements, a pregnant woman also needs to assure "protein sparing." If her diet does not include enough calories, her body will start breaking down

TABLE 6-2
DAILY NUTRITIONAL NEEDS DURING PREGNANCY

Nutrient	Nonpregnancy Need	Pregnancy Need
Calories	2,100 (approximate) (may be adjusted for age, height)	2,400 (approximate) (36–40 Cal/2.2 lbs body weight)
Protein	44 g	74–100 g
Vitamins		
Vitamin A		
(Do not take in supplement form)		4,000 IU
Vitamins B		
Folic Acid	400 mcg	800 mcg
Niacin	13 mg	15 mg
Riboflavin	1.2 mg	1.5 mg
Thiamine	1.1 mg	1.5 mg
B6	2.0 mg	2.6 mg
B12	3.0 mcg	4.0 mcg
Vitamin C	60 mg	80 mg
Vitamin D	200–400 IU	400–600 IU
Vitamin E	8 mg	10 mg
Minerals		
Calcium	800 mg	1,200 mg
Phosphorus	800 mg	200 mg
Iron	15 mg from food,	15 mg from food, plus 30–60 mg supplement
Iodine	150 mcg	175 mcg
Magnesium	300 mg	450 mg
Zinc	15 mg	20 mg

proteins to provide the necessary energy. Pregnant women cannot afford to let this happen because protein is needed for building the tissues.

By simply eating more foods that are rich in the recommended nutrients it is easy to add the necessary 300 calories per day. For example, if a woman who does not ordinarily drink milk simply adds a quart of fortified skim milk to her daily diet, this will supply all the calcium she needs, significant amounts of vitamins and protein, and 360 calories. A chicken thigh adds 237 calories, most of the minimum additional protein (29.1 g), and a third of the riboflavin requirement (0.48 mg). A 6-oz serving of cooked red beans, at 236 calories, provides significant amounts of iron and calcium, and almost 15 g of protein.

FLUIDS

The body contains a large amount of water, and a pregnant woman needs to drink enough water to support her own growth and the growth of the fetus. Drinking enough water also helps to prevent the dry, itchy skin that bothers many pregnant women. Pregnant women urinate more frequently, and need more water for the health of their kidneys and urinary system. Drinking enough water helps prevent urinary infections and heartburn, and may also prevent or relieve constipation by keeping the stools soft.

Women who have disabilities that make them susceptible to bladder infections have even more reason to drink plenty of water. Sylvia recalled, "I drank two or three times as much as usual, and I didn't have any problems with bladder infections." Women who are unable to exercise might already have problems with constipation, which could become worse during pregnancy. They, too, need to be careful to drink plenty of water.

How much is enough? The equivalent of eight 8-oz glasses of water daily is sufficient for most women. This might seem like a lot at first, but it helps to remember that you are not restricted to drinking only plain water. Milk, fruit juice, broth, and coffee substitutes all provide water. You should also have at least three glasses of milk daily if you are not milk-sensitive (lactose intolerant).

PROTEINS

Proteins are the essential building blocks of the body. Pregnant women need 75 to 100 g of protein daily for fetal growth, as well as the growth of the maternal tissues. Protein is in found meat, eggs, dairy products, and vegetable foods such as peas and dried beans. It is important to have at least three servings of protein a day. There is evidence indicating that pregnant women should avoid fish "because freshwater and ocean predator fish may contain large amounts of mercury." The Food and Drug Administration (FDA) warns against king mackerel, swordfish, certain tuna, and tilefish, which may be high in mercury. "Developing fetuses and young children are thought to be disproportionately affected by mercury exposure, because the presence of mercury affects both general development and, in particular, the brain maturation of fetuses and children. Therefore, minimizing mercury exposure is essential for optimal child health" (59).

A study at the University of Connecticut showed that mothers with high intakes of the omega-3 fatty acid docosahexaenoic (DHA) during the third trimester reported that their newborns had more consistent sleep patterns, compared with other newborns. DHA seems to help reduce depression in mothers and lower the risk of heart disease in babies. The best sources are supplements and fish (59).

Many disabled women have an additional reason to make sure they eat enough protein-rich foods: prevention of pressure sores. Disabled women are often warned that increased weight may put them at increased risk for pressure sores when they are pregnant. This risk can be reduced by eating a balanced diet that includes enough protein to keep the skin in good condition.

MINERALS

Sodium

One important function of sodium is maintenance of the body's fluid balance. It was once thought that excess sodium contributed to edema and toxemia, which is why many of us have heard our mothers mention that they were on salt-restricted diets while they were pregnant. An interviewee said, "I watched my salt intake to reduce swelling. I also read that watermelon was a diuretic, so I ate a lot of watermelon."

More recent studies have shown that some increased sodium retention and moderate edema are normal responses to the increase in blood volume and the hormonal changes associated with pregnancy. Researchers have observed *hyponatremia* (low blood sodium) in the infants of mothers who were on severely salt-restricted diets while they were pregnant. Thus, your physician will not necessarily recommend that you restrict salt. Sodium is abundant in many foods, and using table salt for seasoning will help women get the 1 to 3 g of salt they need daily. Reading a few food labels will show how easy it is to find salt in food. Women who crave salt—perhaps because they avoided salt before pregnancy—can satisfy their craving by occasionally using salt on healthy foods. A doctor should be consulted if the craving continues, however. Iodized salt is also a good source of dietary iodine.

Iodine

Iodine is a constituent of an important hormone, *thyroxine*, which is necessary for energy and mental stability. Iodine is also needed for normal fetal growth. Lack of iodine in the maternal diet will make the mother sick. Iodine deficiency is also a factor in cretinism, a birth defect characterized by growth retardation, mental retardation, and a number of physical abnormalities. Excess iodine also causes birth defects. Iodine-related birth defects in humans are caused by the medications for bronchitis and asthma, which contain iodine, not excess dietary sodium. Seafoods are rich in this mineral, but the most reliable way to get iodine is to use iodized table salt.

Calcium and Phosphorus

Women who do not bear weight are prone to thinning bones, and taking 1,500 mg of calcium with 800 units of vitamin D per day can help reduce the risk of osteoporosis. Disabled women should check with their doctors as to whether this amount of calcium is safe for their kidneys. It should be safe, even for those who have kidney stones. This amount of calcium can cause constipation. Take calcium and iron 4 hours apart, because calcium interferes with the absorption of iron. If this is too difficult, take iron with calcium, rather than not take iron at all. It is best to take calcium throughout the day, but if that is not possible, taking it once a day is better than not taking it at all. Calcium plays many important roles in the functioning of the body, but the main reason for eating more calcium-rich foods during pregnancy is to provide enough calcium for fetal development of teeth and bones. Early in pregnancy, hormonal changes cause a woman's body to retain more calcium than usual. In this way, her body builds a reserve supply of calcium that can be used when the fetal skeleton mineralizes in the third trimester. Thus, even though the fetus does not absorb much calcium until late in the pregnancy, the mother should eat plenty of calcium from the beginning. Other calcium-rich foods are listed in Appendix C for women who cannot tolerate milk products.

Calcium combines with phosphorus to make *hydroxy-apatite*, the crystal that hardens bones and teeth. Phosphorus is so common in food that nutritionists do not make special recommendations concerning phosphorus-rich foods.

Studies have shown that babies of mothers who did not get enough calcium have lower bone densities than those born to well-nourished mothers. It has been theorized that severe calcium deficiencies, especially over several pregnancies, may also cause loss of calcium from the mother's bones, but not all studies support this theory.

Although the research is not conclusive, there is some evidence that the calf-muscle cramps that bother many pregnant women may be relieved by calcium supplements. Women who are bothered by leg cramps can ask their doctors if calcium supplements are recommended. If a woman's disability already makes her susceptible to muscle spasms (as in cerebral palsy), then during pregnancy she may experience much stronger and more painful leg cramps than other women. Clara's cramps were so intense that only a strong person could flex her foot enough to ease the spasm. Clara said, "I was having lots of problems with leg cramps, and when I started taking calcium pills, the cramps got better." Carol began taking 1,300 mg of calcium in supplement form per day instead of drinking milk, and she noticed a decrease in leg cramps.

Iron

Iron is part of the hemoglobin that is found in red blood cells. Hemoglobin carries oxygen throughout the body. A pregnant woman needs iron for the red cells in her increased blood supply, and the fetus needs iron for making hemoglobin. "All pregnant polio survivors should be on a supplemental iron, as well as regular recommended supplements, throughout pregnancy and immediately postpartum period to maintain hemoglobin and tissue oxygenation to normal levels" (60).

Anemia can be caused by a lack of sufficient iron, vitamin B_{12}, B_6, or folate, resulting in exhaustion and stress. In addition, an anemic woman is less able to tolerate blood loss during delivery. Some women take iron supplements to treat the more common form of anemia. Hannah said, "I was anemic even though I was taking prenatal vitamins, so the doctor added an iron supplement."

Joy said, "I had nutritional concerns because of rheumatoid arthritis. I'm concerned that I'm deficient in iron and things like that to begin with. I knew with the rheumatoid that my body would go through the nutrients faster or wouldn't utilize them the way that it should. I was extremely concerned." Joy not only took prenatal vitamins, but also drank Ensure™ to make certain of good nutrition.

It is also possible for women who are not anemic to be iron-deficient. In this case, they have enough hemoglobin, but their iron reserves are low.

During early pregnancy, the fetus of an anemic mother usually obtains enough iron for its developing blood supply, but the fetus may not build up a sufficient reserve of iron. A premature baby of an anemic mother is also likely to be anemic. These infants may have low iron reserves, and will have a greater tendency to develop anemia during their first year of life. The hemoglobin levels in full-term infants will probably be unaffected unless the mother's iron deficiency is severe.

Iron is the only nutrient listed in Table 6-2 for which a supplement is recommended. Nonpregnant women can easily get enough iron from foods, but pregnant women cannot get enough without consuming a large number of calories. Anemia occurs in one-third to one-half of the pregnant women who do not use supplements. Women with rheumatoid arthritis are often anemic, but iron supplements will not improve the anemia associated with arthritis. Women with arthritis-associated anemia, who also develop pregnancy-related anemia, can minimize this problem by taking iron supplements on a regular basis.

For most pregnant women, the iron included in a prenatal vitamin is sufficient to prevent anemia if the label states that it contains 30 to 60 mg of elemental iron. Women who are not anemic need to avoid taking excess iron, because too much iron can interfere with the absorption of other nutrients.

Unfortunately, iron tablets can cause stomach upset, constipation, or diarrhea in many women. Some doctors recommend that women who are not anemic should wait until they are 20 to 24 weeks pregnant before taking iron tablets. Indigestion is usually not as much of a problem for the mother by that time, and the fetus is just beginning to build up its iron reserves. Taking iron tablets with meals or at bedtime helps many women avoid indigestion. Exercise, fluids, and high-fiber foods, such as kidney beans, garbanzo beans, dates, dried fruit or prune juice, can help with constipation. Laxatives should not be used, except for products that add bulk, such as Metamucil™. Women who have ongoing indigestion or constipation should tell their doctors. Different types of iron supplements are available, and the doctor may suggest a change.

Many women, whose disabilities make it difficult to exercise, have problems with constipation. They may find that their usual problems get worse when they are pregnant and might be tempted to avoid taking iron supplements because they are afraid of making their constipation worse. In this case, injectable forms of iron may work.

Magnesium and Zinc

Although zinc and magnesium are known to have important roles in metabolism, their functions in pregnancy are not fully understood. The need for magnesium seems to increase with pregnancy, and magnesium deficiency is linked to preeclampsia. Dr. Michael T. Murray recommends 350 to 500 mg of magnesium per day (61).

Zinc deficiency is clearly associated with birth defects in animals, and there is evidence that the same is true for humans. Therefore, pregnant women who are taking vitamin and mineral supplements should take a supplement containing zinc.

VITAMINS

Vitamins A, C, and E

Each of these three vitamins has several functions. One important function is that they contribute to maintaining the integrity of some tissues. There is strong evidence that too little or too much vitamin A can cause birth defects. Therefore, vitamin A supplements must be avoided during pregnancy. A study published in the *New England Journal of Medicine* stated that doses larger than 10,000 I.U. should be avoided during the first 2 months of pregnancy (62).

Vitamin C is necessary for the maintenance of connective tissue such as cartilage.

Vitamin E protects the membranes of the individual cells and helps maximize the absorption of vitamin A in the intestines.

These vitamins are usually well supplied in food, so it is rare to find women with deficiencies. In some studies, women with comparatively low blood levels of vitamin C were found to have a higher incidence of premature births; other studies contradict those findings. On the other hand, when a woman takes large amounts of vitamin C during pregnancy, her fetus may become so dependent on the vitamin that after birth it develops scurvy, a deficiency disease. Research has shown that "women with low vitamin C intake (<10th percentile), both before conception and during the second trimester, had quadruple the risk for preterm membrane rupture than did women with intake at or above that percentile during both periods" (63).

The maximum recommended dosage of vitamin C while pregnant is 500 mg. Sally took 10,000 mg of vitamin C and she did not have a reoccurrence of a kidney infection. She can only speculate that taking vitamin C helped her urinary system. Sally also said, "I used it to change the acidity of my urine."

B Vitamins

Thiamine (B_1), riboflavin (B_2), and niacin are important in energy production. Severe deficiencies of thiamine can cause babies to be born with deficiency disease. Deficiencies of thiamine and riboflavin have been associated with extreme vomiting in early pregnancy.

Folic acid, vitamin B_6, and vitamin B_{12} are needed in a number of chemical processes; they also increase energy. Folic acid and vitamin B_{12} are especially important in cell division. Vitamin B_6 is necessary for the building of proteins, sometimes independently and sometimes in combination with niacin. There is evidence that B_6 helps reduce nausea and vomiting for some women during pregnancy. It is a first-line treatment that some doctors use for morning sickness. (Additional information on the control of morning sickness can be found in Chapter 8.) Do not take more than 100 milligrams of B_6 per day.

Folic acid is necessary for the synthesis of hemoglobin, and lack of folic acid causes one type of anemia. Folic acid taken before and during early pregnancy has been determined to reduce neural tube defects by 48 to 80 percent.

In rare instances, a woman may experience agitation and/or insomnia from folic acid supplementation. Sherry Adele said, "The news came out after my first pregnancy about folic acid being helpful prior to conception, so my OB/GYN actually put me on a pregnancy dose of folic acid prior to conceiving my second child." The Spina Bifida Association of America recommends that women who are at risk for having a baby with a neural tube defect should get a prescription for 4,000 mcg of folic acid, 1 to 3 months prior to getting pregnant. This amount of folic acid will reduce the risk of neural tube defects by 75 percent. It is important to note that you may get side effects from taking large doses of folic acid, including insomnia and/or heart palpitations. Still, it is clearly important to eat enough foods rich in these vitamins because they are necessary for the growth that occurs during pregnancy.

Vitamin D

This vitamin is necessary for the absorption of calcium and the proper calcification of the teeth and bones. It is important to have 800 units of vitamin D daily so that calcium supplements can be completely absorbed. Vitamin D deficiency is associated with malformed teeth and bones, and other problems in newborns. Pregnant women must obtain enough vitamin D from diet and exposure to sunlight in order for the fetus to get enough, although it is not yet understood how an excess of vitamin D might affect the fetus.

FINDING THE RIGHT BALANCE

Even a well-balanced diet may not meet all of the nutritional requirements of pregnancy, and supplementation may be necessary. Vitamin and mineral supplements must be used with care because excesses of some nutrients are toxic. In addition, vitamins and minerals that work together, such as calcium, phosphorus, and vitamin D or vitamin B_6 and niacin, must be present in the correct proportions.

Vegetarian Diets

Vegetarians might need to change their eating habits when they become pregnant. The main challenge is to get enough protein from a vegetarian diet. Five of the women interviewed for this book are vegetarians, but they all ate meat while they were pregnant. Sharon said that talking to a nutritionist influenced her decision to change her diet. Both Naomi and Sylvia craved meat. Sylvia said, "I went from being a vegetarian to eating everything. I craved salty meat. After the baby was born, I became a vegetarian again; I didn't even want meat. But I just couldn't do it while I was pregnant." A strict vegetarian diet is almost certain to be deficient in B_{12}, L-carnitine, calcium, and iron.

TABLE 6.3
COMPLETE VEGETABLE PROTEIN COMBINATIONS

Beans	+	Milk products
Beans	+	Cornmeal or tortillas
Beans	+	Rice
Milk	+	Rice, wheat, or potato
Wheat	+	Beans
Wheat	+	Peanuts
Wheat	+	Milk
Peanuts	+	Milk
Rice	+	Sesame (including tahini, or sesame butter)
Rice	+	Soy products

These combinations are found in many familiar foods, especially if you enjoy ethnic foods. Many of these ingredients are also among the calcium-rich foods. Sample meals might include the following: a peanut butter sandwich with whole-grain bread and a glass of milk; scalloped potatoes; burritos made with corn tortillas and cheese; pita bread with falafel and tahini sauce; rice pudding; red beans and rice; and bean soup with whole-grain biscuits or cornbread.

Women who eat fish and/or milk and eggs can easily get all of the protein they need. Those who avoid all animal products will have more difficulty getting enough protein. Pregnant women can use the protein combinations listed in Table 6-3 to be sure that they are eating complete proteins.

Proteins are chains of different types of amino acids. Humans need eight different amino acids. A protein chain containing each of the eight essential amino acids is a complete protein; a chain containing only some of the eight is an incomplete protein. Animal proteins are complete, but vegetable proteins are incomplete. By combining foods from the vegetable protein, bread and cereal, and milk product food groups (see Appendix C) vegetarians can improve the quality of the protein in their diet. Some combinations are better than others. For example, beans and cornmeal are a better combination than beans and peanuts. Combining grain and beans, as in a bean burrito, or by eating bean soup with bread, provides complete protein. Table 6-3 presents some particularly nutritious protein combinations. Women should eat nine or more servings of bread, cereals, and grains; at least four of the 4-oz servings should be whole grain.

Vegetarian diets also tend to be low in calories, and it is important to eat enough so that the protein in the diet is spared for building new tissue. Sometimes vegetarians need to make a point of eating energy-dense foods. For example, substituting dried fruit for fresh fruit, or a serving of cheese for a serving of milk, will add calories without making one feel too full.

A pregnant woman needs seven or more 4-oz servings daily of fruit or vegetables that are rich in vitamins C and A. It is also important to note that the only safe way to get enough vitamin A is by eating fruits or vegetables high in vitamin A. (As previously stated, vitamin A supplements may cause birth defects.)

Iron is also difficult to obtain in a vegetarian diet, so vegetarians will need to take iron supplements.

Strict vegetarian diets also tend to be low in calcium and vitamin B_{12}, and supplements are often recommended. Nutritional yeast and some fortified soy products contain vitamin B_{12}, but women who dislike these foods should consider taking supplements. One thousand mcg of B_{12} in the morning is a good minimum starting dose. Increase the dose by 1,000 mcg once a month, but lower the dose to 250 mcg if you experience insomnia. Then, gradually increase it by 250 mcg once a month.

A woman who is on a strict vegetarian diet should consult a nutritionist because it can be difficult to get good prenatal nutrition from such a diet.

Allergies and Cravings

Like vegetarians, women with milk allergies can find nondairy sources of calcium on the list of calcium-rich foods in Appendix C. They might also consider using calcium supplements. Generally, allergies should not pose a problem because most nutrients are contained in a variety of foods. For example, a woman with citrus allergies can get plenty of vitamin C from other fruits and vegetables such as cantaloupe and broccoli. The lists in Appendix C should make it easy for you to find acceptable sources of the recommended nutrients.

Individual food cravings can be dealt with in different ways, depending on what is craved. Craving a certain food is not necessarily your body telling you what you need. For example, some women experience *pica*, which can be a significant sign of iron deficiency. Pica is the strong desire to eat non-foods such as ice, paint chips, or clay. Women with pica should have their doctor check for underlying problems. Food cravings can be reasonably indulged if eating the desired foods does not diminish the appetite for nutritious foods. A craving for fresh fruit will not hurt anybody, and neither will an occasional scoop of ice cream.

What to Avoid or Limit

SMOKING

Babies born to smokers tend to be smaller and have more health problems than those born to nonsmokers. Smoking harms the fetus both directly and indirectly. When the mother smokes, nicotine and other toxins enter her bloodstream and cross the placenta to the fetus. The blood vessels constrict when a mother smokes, and the change in blood flow reduces the amount of oxygen and nutrients available to the fetus. Over time, there is possible damage to the placenta, which may interfere with nourishment of the fetus.

Furthermore, smokers are more likely to suffer complications of pregnancy, including placenta previa, premature rupture of membranes, and placental detachment—all of which are dangerous to both mother and fetus.

It is never too late to stop smoking! Women who stop smoking during pregnancy are less likely to have placental problems than those who continue to smoke. Women who are unable to stop smoking should be aware that nicotine enters breast milk. Babies who have allergies or asthma are affected by second-hand smoke.

The effect is proportional: one pack of twenty cigarettes per day has a huge effect compared with smoking just one cigarette. Some women would not dream of smoking tobacco during pregnancy, but think that smoking marijuana is safe, even though it may not be. Studies suggest that maternal exposure to marijuana leads to behavioral changes in animal and human newborns, as well as physical changes in animals. Smoking marijuana can also interfere with milk production.

ALCOHOL

Heavy drinking leads, at worst, to *fetal alcohol syndrome* (FAS) in which the newborn has growth retardation, mental retardation, and certain typical physical deformities. Many infants who do not have full-blown FAS may have other severe health problems, including some of the symptoms of FAS and alcohol addiction at birth.

There is evidence that smaller amounts of alcohol may cause more subtle changes, especially behavioral and emotional changes. The effects of moderate drinking are difficult to assess for three reasons:

1. Different studies have used different definitions of "moderate" drinking.
2. Mental and behavioral functioning, which are not always easy to assess, have been studied in different ways and at different times. For example, it can be difficult to determine whether a newborn who is not very responsive has been affected by prenatal drinking or by the anesthetics used during childbirth.
3. Studies cannot take into account the possible differences in fetal susceptibility to alcohol.

According to the available evidence, it is clear that even moderate drinking is risky. Health professionals advise pregnant women to stop drinking alcohol altogether.

CAFFEINE

Studies of the effect of caffeine on the fetus have had variable results. In animal studies, huge amounts of caffeine (the equivalent of 12 to 40 cups of coffee a day in humans) were required to cause birth defects. Some studies suggest a relationship between heavy coffee drinking and lowered birth weight. Other studies have shown that large amounts of caffeine should be avoided, but there is no risk from the consumption of decaffeinated coffee. In addition, moderate caffeine consumption during pregnancy does not appear to meaningfully influence fetal growth.

MEDICATIONS

Sometimes nonprescription medications can be as dangerous as prescription medication. There is even a case on record of a baby born with fetal alcohol syndrome because the cough syrup the mother used during pregnancy contained alcohol. (Not all brands of cough syrup contain alcohol.) Therefore, pregnant women are advised to always check with their doctors before taking any nonprescription medications.

Sometimes people wonder whether they can save money by substituting a less expensive medication for the one that has been prescribed. When a pharmacist asks if you would prefer a *generic* medicine, he is referring to a less expensive medicine that is made from the same or similar chemical compounds as the one prescribed, but that is manufactured by a company other than the manufacturer of the brand name version of the same drug. Keep in mind that many patients report to their doctors that some generic substitutes seem less effective. Inform your doctor if you are considering a generic medicine. Possibly you and your doctor will decide that you should try both forms of the medication in order to see if there are different results. If you want brand name medications, you need to request them at the time the doctor writes the prescription.

The same principles that apply to nonprescription medications also apply to herbal teas and/or alternative remedies, as they may also have harmful side effects.

"EMPTY CALORIE" FOODS

Empty calorie foods do not provide significant amounts of the necessary vitamins, minerals, and protein, but they do provide extra calories from fat and sugar. Examples of empty calorie foods include soft drinks (which may also contain caffeine or excess phosphorus), chips, most crackers (read package ingredients), candy, cookies, and cakes. Even fruit pies have excessive fat in the crust. Ice milk, frozen yogurt, and "light" ice creams are preferable to regular ice cream, but they still have plenty of sugar. Snack meats and soft cheeses have too much fat in comparison to protein, and often contain too much salt as well.

Besides lacking nutrition, these types of foods can make a woman feel full and unable to eat the foods she really needs. Let empty calorie foods be occasional treats.

Closing Comments

Eating a balanced diet during pregnancy is an opportunity to improve your eating habits for life. It contributes to your health and comfort during pregnancy. For many women, the greatest benefit of eating a balanced diet is the knowledge that they are doing all they can to assure the health of their babies.

Getting in Shape: Exercises for Pregnancy

THIS CHAPTER PRESENTS exercises for women who have a variety of disabilities and differing functional abilities. There really is something for everyone! The exercises begin with variations in which a partner or attendant assists with the exercise, and then become increasingly challenging.

Exercise creates a general sense of well-being. Signe went back to a type of physical therapy known as the *Feldenkreis* method prior to getting pregnant. She said, "I went with the intent of getting myself in shape so I would be ready for pregnancy." She said, "I gained an awareness of how I stand and do things, as well as a sense of well-being."

Oprah enjoyed walking, but her doctors expected that by the time she was 3 months pregnant, she would be on bed rest or using a wheelchair full-time. Oprah said, "I walked throughout my pregnancy, and only gained 15 pounds. The constant exercise was better than sitting around and doing nothing."

Amanda compared her two pregnancies; during one she was active and during the other she was sedentary. She did a lot of walking on crutches as well as general stretching during her first pregnancy. Amanda started to exercise during her second pregnancy, but she was so tired during the second trimester that she did not continue. She was still able to do some stretching. Amanda was asked if she noticed a difference between her two pregnancies, and she said, "My stamina was not as good the second time."

Shanna was sorry she stopped lifting weights while she was pregnant. She felt it might have helped her feel better during her pregnancy and after delivery.

Sienna felt that sticking with an exercise regime would have increased her circulation and helped her control her diabetes.

Exercise enabled Deirdre to stop taking most of her pain medication. She said, "By exercising and keeping the endorphins going, I was able to gradually lower the dose of my medication. I was able to use the mental focusing that I learned from pain management and mindfulness meditation."

Olivia said, "I exercised prior to becoming pregnant, and also the entire time I was pregnant. I was stretching, walking, and swimming. I did not gain much weight, which was essential to my condition. If you have OI (osteogenesis imperfecta), you can become very clumsy and fall if you become too heavy. I was worried about the possibility of falling, and I also had a phobia about wheelchairs. I had this vision of walking around being able to handle it. The pregnancy gave me more energy and made me feel better."

Studies have shown that the blood contains more *endorphins* after exercise. Endorphins are natural chemicals produced by the body that are associated with feelings of pleasure and happiness.

Exercise during pregnancy is important for a number of reasons:

❖ Exercise helps maintain strength and flexibility, and the ability to perform such daily activities as transferring.

❖ Exercise can preserve and even increase muscle strength, as well as help maintain endurance for some women.

❖ Exercise can help a woman feel more comfortable walking and standing as her weight increases, and prepare her for the physical exertion of giving birth.

❖ Exercise helps the circulatory system function well, enabling it to handle the increased blood volume of pregnancy.

❖ Pregnancy hormones loosen the ligaments, so it is important to strengthen the back and abdominal muscles in order to keep the pelvic joints stable.

❖ Exercise can keep all of the joints flexible. Oprah felt that walking helped her the most because it kept her active. She said, "The more you sit still, the more you are prone to having breaks."

❖ The appropriate exercises can prevent or reduce many of the discomforts of pregnancy, including muscle spasms in the calves, back pain, groin pain, shortness of breath, constipation, and, for women with edema, tingling and numbness in the arms. Felicia said, "The only time I didn't have back pain was when I was in the pool and an hour or so afterwards."

❖ Women with pelvic and abdominal muscles that have been strengthened by exercise during pregnancy are likely to recover more quickly after childbirth. Strengthening exercises can be good preparation for the physical demands of childcare.

❖ Exercise can help maintain a normal level of functioning during pregnancy and the postpartum period.

It is important to do more than one type of exercise. Stretching exercises alone cannot maintain strength. They can actually reduce flexibility of the joints. A balanced exercise program includes four types of exercise:

❖ General conditioning or endurance exercise
❖ Strengthening exercise

❖ Relaxation exercise
❖ Flexibility exercise

Often a single flexibility exercise may be described as either a stretching exercise or a range-of-motion exercise. A stretching exercise is a movement that lengthens muscle fibers; a range-of-motion exercise is a movement that enhances the range of motion of a joint. For example, some range-of-motion exercises enable the elbow to bend and straighten as fully as possible. Relaxation exercises ease or prevent muscle pain and improve circulation because blood flows better in relaxed muscles. Carol said, "Hydrotherapy helped me ambulate to the best of my ability. I would get range of motion in the pool. It kept me limber. The hydrotherapy helped reduce my spasticity." Salina Tracy said, "Swimming really makes a big difference in keeping down spasms, whether you're pregnant or not."

Stretching exercises that relieve specific discomforts of pregnancy are located in one section of this chapter. Other stretching exercises can be found in the section titled "Relaxation Exercises." All of the exercises can help a woman prepare for the relaxation techniques used during childbirth. Salina Tracy said, "I went through physical therapy to learn how to do my own stretches. I would put my leg up on a chair. I also liked the butterfly stretch."

It is important for each woman to be kind to her body. Some prefer gentle exercise; others prefer to exercise until they sweat. A woman will be happier and perform better if she incorporates exercise into her pregnancy, no matter what form of exercise she chooses.

Active and assisted range-of-motion exercises are both beneficial. *Active* exercise refers to exercise a woman performs independently. *Assisted* exercise refers to exercise in which another person moves her body. Since no stretching exercise is active in the sense of requiring voluntary contraction of the affected muscles, these exercises are described as *assisted* or *unassisted*.

Exercises for pregnant women follow certain safety guidelines. Exercise patterns that are safe and appropriate for nonpregnant women might not be equally safe for women who are undergoing the changes of pregnancy. Many of these changes continue to affect women for several weeks after birth, so they must continue to modify their exercise during this period. It is also important to remember that the fetus is affected by changes in the mother's body. Both the American College of Obstetricians and Gynecologists (ACOG) and the American Physical Therapy Association have offered recommendations for appropriate exercise during pregnancy. These recommendations are designed to assure the safety of the pregnant woman and the fetus.

A number of physiologic changes affect the kinds of exercises women can do during and after pregnancy:

❖ Joints are more vulnerable to injury because of hormonal effects on connective tissue.

❖ The growth of the uterus and breasts changes the body's center of gravity and increases strain on the lower back and hip joints.

❖ The increase in blood volume affects heart function, so pregnant women must exercise less vigorously. Sedentary women and women with anemia must be even more careful not to stress their hearts.

❖ Late in pregnancy, as uterine growth presses upward, the space available to the lungs is reduced. Pregnant women are able to breathe in enough oxygen at rest and during mild exercise, but cannot breathe as efficiently during prolonged, intense exercise.

❖ Pregnant women become dehydrated more easily.

❖ The basal body temperature is higher during pregnancy. This temperature increase, coupled with the temperature increase that occurs during prolonged, heavy exercise, may be cause for concern because fetal development is affected by temperature changes.

❖ Blood sugar levels tend to be lower when women are pregnant, and overly strenuous exercise can lower blood sugar even more.

❖ The fetal heart rate is affected by maternal exercise, and it seems wise to avoid prolonged exercise sessions.

Because of these normal changes, all healthy, pregnant women need to follow the exercise guidelines listed in Tables 7-1 and 7-2.

Specific health problems or complications of pregnancy may also make it necessary for a woman to avoid exercise. Women who have one or more of the health problems listed in Table 7-3 should *always* avoid strenuous exercise.

Women who have one or more of the health problems listed in Table 7-4 should be evaluated by their physicians and/or physical therapists. They may be advised to limit exercise or to avoid certain types of exercises.

Women with disabilities may be advised to modify their exercise program for specific reasons. For example, a woman with MS, who must be especially careful to avoid fatigue, may be advised to shorten her periods of intense exercise. In some cases, exercises appropriate for those with a disability may have to be avoided because of pregnancy considerations. Leslie was advised to do range-of-motion exercises, but even these mild exercises stimulated uterine contractions. Leslie had to discontinue exercising because she was already at risk for premature labor.

Besides having some concerns about safety, women with disabilities sometimes have other reasons to feel skeptical about the value of exercise. When Nancy's doctor suggested that she see a physical therapist, she felt it would be "more of a hassle than it was worth." She did not see a physical therapist, and she does not regret her decision, because "I just had too many negative experiences when I was a child, and trying to exercise just reminds me of all the things I can't do." The author remembers thinking as a child that exercise would make her able-bodied. When she did not become able-bodied, she decided that exercise was useless. It took her time to learn that exercise can help a person make the most of her abilities. In her work as an occupational therapist, the

TABLE 7-1

SAFETY GUIDELINES FOR EXERCISE DURING PREGNANCY AND THE
POSTPARTUM PERIOD

Pregnancy and Postpartum

- Women who are not used to exercising should begin slowly, and gradually increase exercise intensity.
- If a woman experiences any unusual symptoms, she should stop exercising and contact her physician.
- Exercise regularly (three times a week), rather than intermittently. [a]
- To avoid raising body core temperature, do not exercise in hot, humid weather, or when sick with fever.
- Exercise on a firm, but not hard surface such as a carpeted floor. Avoid bouncy, jerky motions or rapid swinging movements.
- Avoid exercises that strain the pelvic floor or the abdominal muscles.
- Avoid extreme bending or stretching of joints. If soreness or discomfort lasts more than 60 minutes after exercising, the stretch was too much.
- Warm up before vigorous exercise with activities such as slow walking. After exercising, cool down with gentle stretching.
- Check heart rate during exercise. Do not exceed recommended limits (Table 7-2).
- Always rise from the floor slowly and exercise the legs briefly after rising to avoid sudden blood pressure changes.
- Avoid dehydration; drink plenty of water before and after exercising. Stop to rest during exercise if necessary.
- Women at risk for, or who have had, a caesarean section can have appropriate exercises prescribed (see Chapter 11).
- Exercises using a knee-to-chest position are inappropriate postpartum.

Pregnancy Only

- Check heart rate during exercise. Heart rate should *not* go higher than 140 beats per minute.
- Strenuous exercise should not last longer than 15 minutes.
- Avoid prolonged exercise while lying on the back after the fourth month. If a woman lies on her back too long, the weight of the uterus on major blood vessels will interfere with circulation.
- Avoid the *Valsava maneuver* (holding the breath and pushing as if defecating). Instead, breathe rhythmically during exercise.
- Maternal temperature should not rise higher than 38°C (100.4° F) while exercising.

Cautionary Symptoms: When a woman experiences any of the following signs or symptoms, she should stop exercising and contact her physician: pain, bleeding, dizziness, faintness, shortness of breath, rapid heart rate or palpitations, back pain, pubic pain, or increased difficulty walking.

[a] If a pregnant woman must exercise less frequently, do not try to compensate by exercising strenuously and risking muscle strain.

TABLE 7-2
RECOMMENDED MAXIMUM HEART RATES DURING EXERCISE

Age	Beats per Minute
Pregnant (all ages)	140
Postpartum (20 years)	150
25	146
30	142
35	138
40	135
45	131

This table offers general guidelines. Some women may be advised to exercise less strenuously. For example, a woman who is not used to vigorous exercise might be advised to keep her heart rate lower than suggested here.

author has seen that, over time, exercise increases a person's capacity to meet the demands of daily living. It is especially valuable for coping with the increased physical stresses of pregnancy. Most disabled women have not seen other people who move the way they do exercising. This can make it more difficult for disabled women to think about exercise in a positive way.

Through the Looking Glass conducted a study of the impact of managed care on the delivery of health care to disabled pregnant women. One of the women interviewed in that study experienced a broken leg after delivery which was probably caused by prolonged bed rest during her pregnancy. She did not receive any assisted range-of-motion exercise during her pregnancy-related bed rest, although she needed to rest in order to reduce her spasticity because she has cerebral palsy (65). Other interviewees also wanted or needed a referral to physical therapy.

TABLE 7-3
CONTRAINDICATIONS FOR STRENUOUS EXERCISE

- Diagnosis of multiple gestations (twins)
- Diagnosis of heart disease
- Incompetent cervix
- Dilated cervix
- Vaginal bleeding or diagnosis of placenta previa
- Ruptured membranes
- Episodes of premature labor, or high risk of premature labor
- Conditions exacerbated by stress or fatigue, such as myasthenia gravis or multiple sclerosis, unless under medical advice

TABLE 7-4
CONDITIONS REQUIRING RESTRICTIONS ON EXERCISE

- Hypertension (high blood pressure), anemia, or other blood disorders
- Thyroid disease
- Diabetes
- Cardiac arrhythmia or palpitations (irregular heartbeats)
- History of precipitate labor
- History of intrauterine growth retardation (fetus too small)
- Extreme underweight or overweight
- History of bleeding during pregnancy
- Breech presentation
- Extremely sedentary lifestyle (women who do not get much exercise should not suddenly start exercising vigorously)
- Toxemia or preeclampsia
- Diastasis recti (separation of abdominal muscles)
- Uterine contractions lasting several hours after exercising
- Phlebitis (inflammation of the veins)
- Systemic infection
- Backache, headache, pain radiating to the legs, pubic pain, or other pain after exercising
- Fatigue

Mona asked for a referral to physical therapy to help with her tremors and balance. Sonya was also referred to physical therapy to help reduce the shoulder pain caused by the enlargement of her breasts, which had been caused by pregnancy. Allison had pain in her knee from arthritis, and she was sent for physical therapy during her second pregnancy to strengthen the muscles around her knee. Allison said, "The physical therapist helped me, and exercising became a part of my daily life."

The interviewees who did some sort of exercise, active or passive, felt less tired from their daily activities and were generally more comfortable. Exercising does not have to be a formal routine. Carla said that "running after a toddler" was enough to make her feel stronger and healthier during her second pregnancy. It is beneficial to have range-of-motion exercise on a regular basis. Sheila had passive range-of-motion exercise during her first pregnancy, but not her second. It was during the second pregnancy that she had problems with muscle spasms. When she compared her pregnancies, Sheila wished she had gone to physical therapy for range-of-motion exercise the second time. Sonya had range-of-motion exercise every day, which reduced her spasms for an hour. There are other ways to do range-of-motion exercises. Michelle had problems with muscle spasms during only one week of her pregnancy. She said, "I was expecting a lot of muscle spasms, but I didn't get any because of my yoga classes."

Michelle and Priscilla all said that the stretching exercises they did in yoga class helped them feel even better. They felt their mobility and general sense of well-being improved. Mona said, "I've never been to a yoga class; but I watched a program on PBS. I practiced one position called 'down dog' that was useful in stabilizing my center of gravity. It stretched out and stabilized my lower back. I wish I had taken the time to learn more and put my personal issues on the back burner."

If you take yoga classes, it could be useful if your teacher is familiar with pregnancy and disability. Some of the interviewees experienced other benefits from yoga. They had less muscle pain. Tessa felt that a prenatal yoga class could work for women who have thoracic outlet syndrome if they use an exercise ball to support their torso. Renee found that doing hand exercises reduced her pain. She said, "It's a good idea to keep active because it usually keeps the pain down. Looking back, I'd exercise more." Denise needed to stretch because of her bony contractures. She said, "The soft tissues have a tendency to tighten up if I don't move. I did morning stretching. I needed to stretch my hips and my knees, and usually a hot shower loosened me up."

The exercises described in this chapter were chosen because they are useful for pregnant women. Most of them are commonly taught to all pregnant women. Some are modified pregnancy exercises, which makes them easier for women with disabilities. Some of the exercises were originally designed for people with disabilities, and are included here because they are particularly useful for pregnant disabled women.

Some of the exercises are particularly useful for disabled women who use certain mobility aids (manual chair, crutches or canes(s)) because repetitive stress injury can be caused by using one of these aids. Judi decided to add exercises for shoulder pain and carpal tunnel to her routine because a wheelchair may become ill-fitted during pregnancy.

Think of this chapter as a set of flexible guidelines, not as the last word. Women with specific problems, such as high blood pressure, blood disorders, or multiple pregnancies, may be advised to avoid vigorous exercise. Certain exercises will work better than others for some women. It may not be feasible to follow each detail of the instructions. Many women will have to modify the exercises according to their abilities. For example, when the author does curl-ups with her hands at the back of her neck, she cannot keep both elbows back, but she still benefits from the exercise.

It is important to follow the instructions for coordinating the breath with exercise. Any exercise can be modified to give each muscle group the appropriate exercise if necessary. A doctor or physical therapist can be consulted for assistance in creating an exercise program that works best.

The guidelines in Table 7-1 state that women who are more than 4 months pregnant should avoid lying on their backs for long periods of time. Some of the suggested exercises require lying on the back briefly, however. These are valuable exercises, and it would be worthwhile to ask whether your physician approves of your lying down just long enough to do them. If any exercise learned from this book, in a prenatal exercise class, or in a childbirth preparation class feels too difficult or uncomfortable, stop the exercise and talk it over with your doctor or physical therapist.

Remember to drink plenty of water and empty your bladder before exercising, and never hold your breath while exercising. If a pregnant woman experiences any of the warning signs listed at the end of Table 7-1, she should stop exercising immediately and contact a doctor. But, generally, exercise should contribute to well-being.

Conditioning Exercises

GENERAL CONDITIONING

Swimming and walking are good general conditioning exercises. They promote cardiopulmonary function and increase muscle tone. Swing the arms vigorously when walking in order to exercise the upper body as well as the legs and hips. "Aquatic therapy is one of the best forms of exercises for polio survivors" (60).

Conditioning exercises can be adapted to many disabilities, and to the changes of pregnancy. Swimming can be a good way to exercise and stretch the muscles if it becomes difficult to move around during late pregnancy. Amy was able to swim during her first two trimesters and found that it relieved her backache. She said, "Swimming helped strengthen my arms." Nora said, "The physical therapist said that swimming was the best exercise for me because I couldn't walk or ride a bike. The water was about 92 degrees, so it felt real good on my muscles and bones." Swimming is also valuable for women who suffer joint pain during weight-bearing exercises. Carol found that swimming helped lower her blood pressure. She said, "My blood pressure was taken before and after swimming and they found it had dropped 20 points."

Deirdre liked walking so much that she volunteered to walk dogs for people who had AIDS. She said, "I asked for the smallest, dingiest dog they had. I helped with some puppies and one Yorkshire terrier. It pushed me to get out on a schedule, even when I really didn't feel up to it."

Women with good upper body functioning have several ways of exercising. Stacy exercised by doing laps on an indoor track in a manual wheelchair. Women who decide to start using a wheelchair during pregnancy can try doing what some women do all the time: use the chair for going long distances, but maintain strength and flexibility by continuing to walk short distances. It takes a while to get used to each new piece of equipment and see how it impacts your body. Increase your use of wheelchairs and crutches slowly, so as not to cause shoulder and wrist problems.

Women who are able to exercise vigorously enough to increase their heart rates should talk to their doctors about safety guidelines.

EXERCISES TO STRENGTHEN ABDOMINAL AND LOWER BACK MUSCLES

The abdominal (stomach) and back muscles work together to support the spine and pelvis. The back muscles alone cannot support the pelvis adequately, so it is always important to keep the abdominal muscles as strong as possible. Abdominal exercise is even more important during pregnancy for two reasons:

❖ As the uterus grows, the forward shift of weight stresses the lower back. The lower back tends to become sore and painful unless the abdominal muscles are strong enough to help support the increased weight.

❖ Even strong abdominal muscles are stretched during late pregnancy. After birth, these muscles are significantly weakened. Muscles that were well exercised before birth will recover more quickly.

Pelvic Tilts

The pelvic tilt is a commonly prescribed exercise that stretches the lower back muscles. It strengthens the abdominal muscles and reduces the excessive swayback (*lordosis*) so common in pregnancy. The pelvic tilt is one of the pregnancy exercises specifically recommended by ACOG. They can be done on the hands and knees, lying down, standing, or seated. Pelvic tilts can also be done in other positions, because getting onto the hands and knees is awkward for many disabled women.

In an *assisted pelvic tilt* adaptation, the woman lies on her back on a bed or table at the assistant's waist level, with her knees bent or supported by pillows, and her head supported. Her assistant gently lifts and lowers her hips, rocking them in a way that will flatten the back against the bed or table. The tilt will not be at the correct angle if the assistant's hands are not properly placed. Figure 7-1 shows the best position for this exercise. The back should be as flat as possible for 5 seconds. The woman should exhale while her hips are being lowered.

In the *active seated pelvic tilt*, the woman hooks her arms around the sides of a straight-backed chair, as if to join her hands behind her lower back. Alternatively, she can hook her arms back over the top of the chair. Then, she presses her lower back against the back of the chair, feeling the abdominal muscles tighten. For some people, it may be easier to grip the back of the chair seat while doing this exercise.

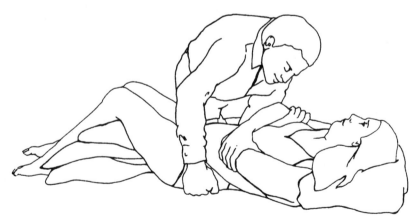

FIGURE 7-1   Assisted pelvic tilt.

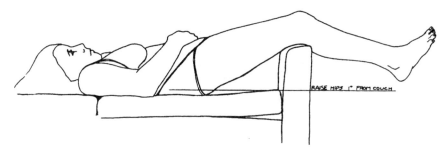

RAISE HIPS 1" FROM COUCH.

FIGURE 7-2 Pelvic tilt on couch.

Use the floor or a firm bed to do an *active supine pelvic* tilt (lying on your back). Rest the feet flat on the floor about 18 inches from the hips (shins almost vertical). Let the arms lie relaxed beside the body. Press the lower back flat against the floor. Rock the hips upward slightly, gradually increasing the lift as the muscles grow stronger. Squeeze the buttocks together and tighten the abdominal muscles while lifting. Increase the amount of lift as strength increases. Alternatively, lie on a couch, knees resting on the armrest. It may be necessary to use an assistant to help get into this position. Press down with the knees, squeeze the buttocks, and tighten the abdominal muscles to flatten the back. Hold this position with the back flat for about 5 seconds, and then breathe out slowly while releasing (Figure 7-2). Rest and repeat. This exercise can be done with the knees supported by pillows rather than an armrest. Keep in mind that the armrest will be stable, whereas the pillows may slip.

For a more challenging exercise that is closely related to the pelvic tilt, try *bridging*, an exercise wherein the knees are unsupported. The lift is continued until the body is held in a straight line from the shoulders to the knees. Hold this position as long as it is comfortable. Then, breathe out slowly while gradually rolling back down. At the end, the hips are once again resting on the floor. This variation is the most effective when the buttocks are squeezed and tightened during the lift.

At any point, but especially when it is no longer appropriate to lie on the back, a *standing pelvic tilt* may be substituted. Stand with the feet apart (at shoulder width), knees slightly bent. Contract the buttocks and abdominal muscles so that the pelvis is rolled upward. Stand with the back lightly touching the wall at the beginning of this exercise in order to feel the lower back flatten against the wall.

Curl-ups

Curl-ups are especially good for strengthening the upper abdominal muscles located just below the ribs. More tightening can be felt in these muscles than in the other abdominal muscles when these exercises are done properly.

For an *assisted curl-up*, the woman lies on the floor, knees bent or supported by pillows, and feet flat on the floor. Her assistant lifts her head until her chin is touching her chest and then raises her shoulders slightly (Figure 7-3).

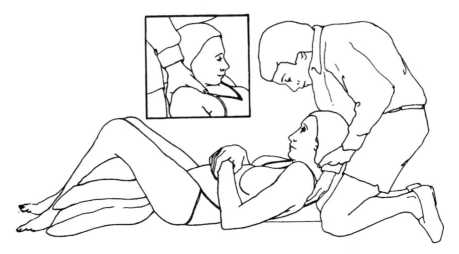

FIGURE 7-3   Assisted curl-up.

To do an *active curl-up*, lie down in the same position that would be used for the assisted curl-up. The hands can be clasped behind the neck, with the elbows held back (upper arms parallel with tops of shoulders), or the forearms can be lightly crossed on the chest. In the easiest curl-up, just the head is lifted from the floor or bed, with the chin touching the chest. As strength increases, it may be possible to lift the shoulders away from the floor. It is important not to use the hands to pull the neck upward if this exercise is done with the hands clasped behind the neck. The abdominal muscles should be doing the work. Only curl up until the shoulder blades are off the floor (Figure 7-4).

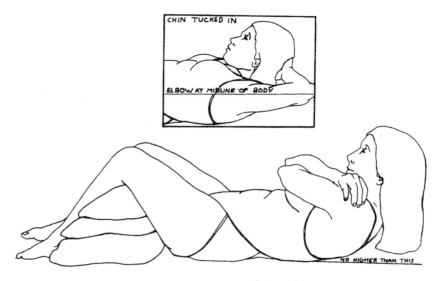

FIGURE 7-4   Correct full curl-up.

Lifting to full sitting position can injure the lower back, and it might injure the abdominal muscles in pregnant women. It is helpful to begin by taking a deep breath, then breathing out slowly while curling up.

Women who do not have leg spasticity can make curl-ups more effective by pressing their feet against a vertical surface such as a wall or the footboard of a bed.

Leg Lifts

Leg lifts are especially good for the lower abdominal muscles (below the navel). More tightening can be felt in these muscles when the exercise is done properly. Leg lifts may cause low back pain when not done properly. It is important to hold a pelvic tilt position while doing leg lifts. One way to accomplish this is to place a rolled towel or firm cushion under the lower back. Straight leg lifts should be discontinued after the fifth month of pregnancy. As the growing uterus increasingly separates the abdominal muscles, they do less and less of the work in this exercise, and the lower back could be strained.

For *assisted leg lifts*, a woman can recline in her wheelchair, or lie on her back and have someone else raise and lower her legs.

In another type of *assisted seated leg lift*, the woman can act as her own assistant. She places a loop made of rope, webbing, or a folded towel around her foot. Then, sitting on a bed or a firm surface with her back supported, she grasps one end of the loop, and swings her legs onto the bed or a nearby piece of furniture. The loop should be long enough to permit her to lean comfortably against the back support as she lifts her leg. Remember to do the pelvic tilt first.

For more challenging *active leg lifts*, sit supported in bed, legs outstretched, and slowly raise and lower the legs. Alternatively, sit on a chair, raise the legs onto a footstool, relax, return the feet to the floor, relax, and repeat. Although this exercise is more effective when the legs are kept straight, doing it with knees bent can still be useful.

There are two more types of advanced leg lifts. Only one leg is outstretched in the easier variation and, in the other, the knee is bent, with the foot resting on a footstool or placed flat on the floor. The straight leg is slowly raised and lowered, and then the exercise is repeated on the other side. Done this way, the exercise is somewhat less effective than the more advanced variation, but it is safer. More repetitions make the exercise more beneficial.

For the most advanced leg lifts, lie flat on the floor or a reasonably firm surface, with the arms resting at the sides. Exercise one leg at a time. The resting leg may be bent or straight. Raise the other leg slowly, keeping it straight, then slowly lower it. Breathe out while lowering the leg. During this exercise, the pelvis should be tilted to keep the back from arching upwards, because the lower back can be strained if arched. For some women, it is helpful to support the lower back by putting the hands under the hips (palms to the floor). This tilts the hips slightly, making the pelvic tilt easier. Others may wish to support the back by placing a small, rolled towel or a foam pad under the small of the back.

Deep Breathing

These exercises are useful for women who are quadriplegic, or who have weak abdominal muscles. Breathing involves the abdominal muscles. Variations on normal breathing—such as grunting, coughing, laughing, talking in a deep voice, or special deep breathing—will exercise the abdominal muscles. Any woman can check the effectiveness of these exercises by resting her hand on her stomach and feeling for tightening, or asking someone else to check for her.

Rapid, deep breathing can make a person hyperventilate and feel dizzy. If this happens, lie down and breathe normally, and the dizziness will go away. Remember to breathe slowly and do not push while holding your breath! Do not hold your breath longer than 10 to 15 seconds.

An easy, basic deep breathing exercise consists of taking a deep breath, then slowly blowing out until there is no air left. Rest before repeating. This exercise can be done in any position, and it is good practice for the slow, deep breathing needed early in labor.

For a slightly more difficult exercise, simply hold the breath for about 10 seconds, breathe out, rest for 23 seconds, and repeat. To make the exercise easier, rest longer between deep breaths, or hold the breath for a shorter amount of time. Start with as many repetitions as are comfortable, in order to avoid tiring the abdominal muscles, and then slowly increase the number.

Laughing is a wonderful abdominal exercise. Find out what will make you laugh. Get silly with friends or children, listen to a favorite comedy tape, or get someone to lightly tickle your ear lobe or neck. Just remember to stop short of getting dizzy or tiring the abdominal muscles.

For another simple exercise, take a deep breath and slowly repeat "ha, ha, ha, ha..." or "oh, oh, oh, oh...." Rest a few minutes and repeat.

"PC" Muscle Strengthening

These exercises are specifically recommended by ACOG. They are often called *Kegel exercises*, after a researcher who emphasized the importance of strengthening the muscles of the pelvic floor. The figure-eight-shaped muscle surrounding the vagina and urethra in front, and the anus in back, is called the *pubococcygeal* muscle, or *PC*. If possible, *every* woman should exercise the PC muscle regularly before, during, and forever after pregnancy. This exercise is for life.

The ability to hold urine is not only a matter of bladder control; it is a matter of PC muscle control. During pregnancy, bladder volume decreases as the uterus grows and presses on the bladder. A pregnant woman has to go to the bathroom more often, and waiting becomes more difficult. She may have problems with *stress incontinence* (leaking when sneezing or coughing). At the same time, hormonal changes contribute to relaxation of the pelvic muscles. A strong PC muscle will help prevent urinary problems during pregnancy, the postpartum period, and throughout life.

The vaginal muscles will be stretched during childbirth, and they will recover more quickly if they have been exercised and strengthened beforehand. Some older women may need surgery for a *prolapsed uterus*, which is a condition wherein the uterus drops down into the vagina. Exercising the PC muscle may help prevent this problem. Women who have done these exercises know how to relax the vagina during childbirth.

The easiest way to learn the PC exercise is to simply stop and start the flow of urine repeatedly, which will alternately contract and relax the PC muscle. Do this exercise while urinating until it feels familiar. *Once learned, do not do this exercise while urinating.* Too much stopping and starting might prevent the bladder from being completely emptied. This exercise can also be done anywhere, anytime, standing or sitting, waiting in line at the bank, or waiting for a traffic signal to change. Begin by doing the exercise at least ten times a day, and work up to twenty-five times a day over a period of a few weeks. It is not necessary to do twenty-five repetitions all at once; five at one time and ten at another is just as beneficial.

Next, make the exercise a little more difficult. Relax the flow slowly while urinating, allowing only a few drops to escape, and then immediately contract again. For variation, imagine that the vagina is an elevator and tighten from the bottom up, stopping at the "first floor," the "second floor," and on up to the "tenth floor." Next, relax from the top down, stopping at each floor. Continue all the way to "the basement," pushing outward a bit.

Some women enjoy tightening the PC muscle during intercourse. Just tighten the muscles against your partner's penis, and hold for a count of five, or longer. Your partner can tell you whether the PC muscle stays strong. This exercise will add to the pleasure of lovemaking.

Stretching Exercises

Stretching exercises should be done immediately after strengthening exercises. Muscle fibers shorten during strengthening exercise, and need to be stretched to prevent cramping. Clara swam once or twice a week, but she did not take time for stretching exercises. As a result, she experienced severe leg cramps, also known as "Charley horses."

Stretching exercises are easier to do after conditioning and strengthening exercises, because warm muscles stretch more readily. Evening is a good time to do stretching exercises, especially leg stretches. Muscle spasms are most likely to occur during sleep; stretching at bedtime can help prevent them. If you do not exercise before stretching, relax your muscles by taking a warm bath or shower, or by applying localized heat.

It is very important to do stretching exercises *regularly*. If your daily routine changes, find a new time to stretch. It only takes a few days for muscles to become tight.

It is also important not to bounce while doing stretching exercises. Bouncing alternately shortens and lengthens the muscles, which makes stretches less effective and can even cause injury. The best way to maximize a stretch is to hold it as long as it is comfortable; usually a slight increase in stretch is felt at the end of the hold. If you exercise regularly, the amount of stretch and the length of time the stretch can be held will gradually increase until a given stretch can be held for up to 30 seconds. Remember, the maximum amount of stretch for pregnant women will be less than that for nonpregnant women. Breathing out during a stretch is also helpful. Start breathing out slowly just before beginning the stretch. The number of repetitions can be increased gradually. It is better not to do too many repetitions at first. Six repetitions, for a total of 3 minutes stretching, is a reasonable goal.

LOW BACK STRETCHES

The same pelvic tilt exercises that strengthen the abdominal muscles also stretch the low back muscles. By helping to maintain good posture, this exercise helps to alleviate the backaches that are so common in late pregnancy.

SEATED TRUNK FLEXION

Sit with the feet flat on the floor or supported. Grip the back of the chair at the level of the buttocks, then lean forward, resting the upper body on the thighs. Slowly curl upwards, straightening first the lower back, then the middle back, and then the upper back.

CALF STRETCHES

Assisted Calf Stretch

Sit with the legs outstretched for an *assisted calf stretch*. The assistant rests the heel of one foot in his cupped hand, grasp the ball of the foot in the other hand, and bends the whole foot toward the knee, keeping the leg straight. The exercise is then repeated on the other side (Figure 7-5). The woman can also loop a towel around the bottom of the foot and pull the ends to assist in the stretch.

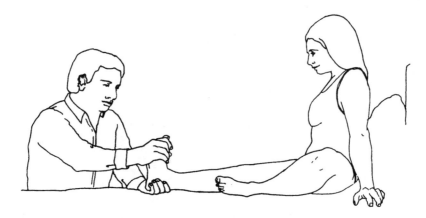

FIGURE 7-5   Assisted calf stretch

Seated Calf Stretch

Unassisted calf stretches can be done standing or seated. One type of seated calf stretch is for women who are able to sit with their legs outstretched; another is for those who need to keep their legs bent. To do the first exercise, sit with the legs stretched forward, heels supported on the floor, feet at right angles to shins, and toes pointing outward. (The foot is dorsiflexed and everted.) Sitting in this position, bend forward at the hips as if to rest the upper body on the thighs. A stretch should be felt in the calves, and may be felt at the back of the thighs. If the stretch is felt more strongly in the thighs than in the calves, modify the starting position by sitting on a higher chair or placing pillows on the seat of the chair. The idea is to lower the foot with respect to the hip, while keeping the knee straight.

If the seated calf stretch cannot be done with the leg outstretched—because the foot cannot be bent with the toes facing upwards—this position can be done with the foot supported against a large book or block, with the heel resting on the floor.

Standing Calf Stretch

For the *standing calf stretch*, start in a modified lunge position facing a wall, just close enough to lean forward slightly and rest the forearms on the wall. If your balance is good and your wrist joints are not painful, rest your palms on the wall with your arms stretched straight forward. Place one leg forward, slightly bent at the knee; the other will be straight back, with the whole foot contacting the floor. Lean against the wall to do the stretch. Bring the hips toward the wall, allowing the front leg to bend more. Keep the back leg straight, and feel the stretch in the calf muscle (Figure 7-6). Repeat the stretch a few times on each side.

INNER THIGH STRETCHES

The inner sides of the thighs, just where the thighs join the body, also become vulnerable to muscle spasms as the increasing weight of the fetus and uterus put more pressure on the area. Many disabled women experience muscle tightness in this area. These exercises can help prepare a woman for childbirth, because she will need to spread her legs as widely as possible during birth. If any of these exercises cause hip pain, they should be discontinued *immediately*, and not be started again until a doctor or physical therapist is consulted.

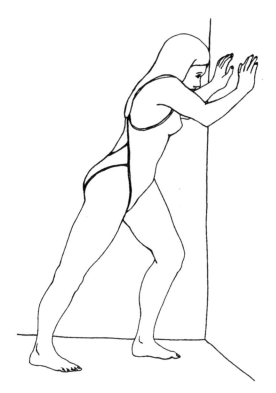

FIGURE 7-6 Standing calf stretch.

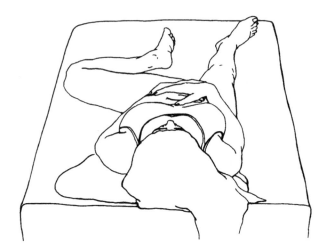

FIGURE 7-7: Inner thigh stretch.

These exercises can be done with or without assistance. To do the first inner thigh stretch, sit with the outer side of the ankle resting on a low stool, with the knee bent and pointing outward. For an *assisted inner thigh stretch* variation, an assistant can lift the foot onto the stool. At first, simply rest in this position for as long as it remains comfortable. As the stretch becomes more comfortable, try putting on shoes, and then tying them while seated in the stretch position. Leaning forward will increase the stretch. Putting on shoes while sitting in the stretch position will make this exercise very easy to work into a daily routine. This is a very gentle stretch. To increase the stretch, put both feet on the stool at once, with the soles of the feet facing each other.

Resting the ankle on the opposite knee while putting on and tying shoes can give a more challenging stretch. It can also be done without shoes. Gradually increase the amount of time the stretch is held, up to about 30 seconds, but *never strain*. Again, if this stretch causes hip pain, *stop immediately*. Another challenging stretch involves taking the position shown in Figure 7-7 and gently pressing the bent knee against the mattress.

For a practical, effective stretch, sit up in bed, with the back supported if necessary. Sit with legs straight and spread as wide apart as possible. Keep the ankles relaxed, and be sure not to point the toes, because pointing can cause spasm of the calf muscles. Lean forward between the legs for a comfortable stretch. For an *assisted inner thigh stretch*, an assistant can push the legs apart by placing her hands on the inner thighs, just above the knees, and/or sit between the pregnant woman's legs.

UPPER BODY STRETCHES

Many people experience repetitive stress injuries. Disabled people are not an exception. Repetitive stress may be due to computer use, an ill-fitting wheelchair or use of crutches or canes. Some pregnant women, regardless of being disabled, are at risk for carpal tunnel problems. Therefore, it is important to reduce the risk of repetitive injury by stretching your neck, arm, and wrist muscles.

These exercises stretch the *intercostal* muscles, which are located between the ribs. A "stitch in the side" is usually a spasm of the intercostals. Stretching these muscles helps prevent muscle spasms, eases the discomfort of increasing pressure on the ribs during late pregnancy, and sometimes relieves heartburn. These exercises also stretch the arm muscles. They can also help with tingling and numbness in the hands.

For an *assisted intercostal stretch*, a woman can sit while an assistant lifts her arm straight up (Figure 7-8). Then, with one hand on the wrist and the other hand on the upper arm, the assistant gently pulls upward slightly, just enough to stretch the intercostal muscles. The stretch will be greater if the woman is leaning toward the side opposite the lifted arm.

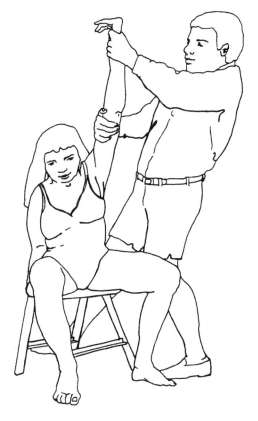

FIGURE 7-8   Intercostal stretch.

The intercostal muscles can also be stretched while lying on the back. Start with the arms at the sides, keeping them straight; slowly sweep the arms across the bed in a half circle, finishing with the arms stretched over the head (the upper arms will be next to the ears). In this position, stretch a little further by stretching the fingers. An assistant moves the woman's arms in the assisted intercostal stretch variation. For the last bit of stretch, the assistant has one hand on the forearm and the other hand on the upper arm in order to make sure the intercostal area is stretched, not the wrists or elbows.

The next exercise is an *unassisted intercostal stretch* for women who have a spinal cord injury, and women who have difficulty raising their arms or cannot keep their arms raised overhead. This exercise stretches both the arm muscles and the intercostal muscles. To do this exercise, a woman grasps an overhead trapeze or strap and allows herself to sag or hang a bit, so that her ribs are stretched upwards. Women who cannot grip a trapeze could ask their doctors or therapists about hooking their wrists over the trapeze. This variation should not be tried without the approval of a doctor or therapist, because this type of pressure on the wrists might be a problem.

For a more challenging stretch, the woman sits up with her back against the wall. She begins by lifting her arms up and out to the side, elbows straight, palms facing outward or upward, and fingers outstretched. Moving slowly and gradually, she raises her arms higher and higher, and "walks" her arms up the wall. When her arms are stretched over her head, her intercostal muscles will also be well stretched.

Upper Limb Stretches

For the *unassisted stretch*, stand or sit straight with the arm outstretched to the side. Place the palm flat on a wall with the fingers pointing upward. As the arm bends at the elbow, bend the head toward the opposite shoulders of the outstretched arm. Next, straighten the elbow and hold for 5 seconds. Repeat on the opposite side. If this stretch causes pain that lasts after the stretch is released, STOP and consult a physical or occupational therapist.

For an *assisted stretch*, have an assistant hold the arm at the wrist and elbow, and stretch the arm straight out at shoulder height, with the fingers pointed towards the ceiling and palm facing out. The assistant should bend and straighten the arm. While the arm is being bent, the head should be tilted towards the opposite shoulder. Next, the assistant should straighten the elbow and hold for 5 seconds. Repeat using the opposite arm.

Wrist Exercises

Wrist Extension Bilateral

For an *unassisted stretch*, put the palms together, and bend the wrist toward the left side, and then the right side. Bend until the stretch is felt, and hold for 5 seconds.

For an *assisted stretch*, the assistant interlaces his fingers with the woman's fingers, and holds her hand so that the wrist is at 45-degree angle. Next, the assistant should push on the upper part of the palm near the knuckles so that the wrist goes back.

Wrist Flexion

For an *unassisted stretch*, hold the arm out in front of the body with the elbow straight and palm down. Bend the wrist down using the other hand and hold for 5 seconds.

For an *assisted stretch*, have an assistant hold the arm at the wrist and elbow, with the elbow straight, palm down. Next, the assistant should bend the hand toward the woman and hold for 5 seconds.

Relaxation Exercises

Relaxation exercises encourage good circulation and a general sense of well-being. Many of the techniques taught in birthing classes will be easier to learn if other relaxation exercises have been previously practiced on a regular basis. The relaxation exercises we suggest below are for areas of the body that were not included in the section on stretching exercises.

FEET

Aching feet are more likely to be a problem as pregnancy continues. Extra weight puts more of a load on the feet, and increased blood volume often leads to swollen feet. Taking time for a good foot massage can make the feet more comfortable and contributes to a general sense of relaxation.

Some people like to combine a foot massage with an inner thigh stretch by sitting with one ankle resting on the opposite knee or thigh and massaging their own feet. Have someone else give the massage if this position is not comfortable. Begin by gently and briskly patting the whole surface of the foot with both hands. Next, grasp each toe, one at a time, and gently pull. Finally, gently rub the ball and arch of the foot.

Women who cannot bend to reach their feet can place a tennis ball on the floor and rub one foot at a time on the ball, slightly rolling the ball with the sole of the foot. Women with leg spasticity need to do this gently to avoid causing muscle spasms. This exercise can also be done using a larger ball.

BUTTOCKS

The extra weight of pregnancy can cause tension and discomfort in the muscles of the buttocks when the woman is seated. Rocking from side to side can release some of this tension. For some women, it might be easier to press their hands on the arms of a chair and bounce up and down slightly. Shifting the weight in this way can also help prevent pressure sores.

There is an increased risk of pressure sores during pregnancy, and women who cannot exercise may need to change position more frequently, either by transferring between wheelchair and bed more often, or by getting help to change position.

NECK

For many people, the neck muscles are the most likely to become tense in response to stress, and relaxing these muscles contributes greatly to a general sense of relaxation. Relaxation exercises can help prevent neck pain and prevent headaches.

Chin Tucks. One of the best exercises for relaxing the neck is the chin tuck (*dorsal glide*). To do this exercise, look straight ahead, and tuck the chin in slightly to make a double chin. Hold about 2 seconds, relax, and repeat about ten times. During this exercise, the back of the neck will seem to tighten like a rubber band. This exercise should be discontinued if it causes pain or tingling in the arms, or pain in the shoulder blades or shoulders.

Head rolls are also relaxing. First, drop the chin to the chest, breathe deeply, and relax. Slowly roll the head to the right, and then reverse direction, rolling toward the center and all the way to the left. Return to center, breathe deeply once or twice, and then repeat the head roll in the reverse direction. Repeat three or four times in each direction. This exercise will be even more relaxing if you breathe out slowly while rolling the head. Try pausing

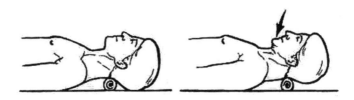

1. Lie on back with 2-3 inch towel roll at base of skull
2. Tuck chin so that you feel a stretch in the back of your neck
   and the base of your skull
3. Hold _____ seconds
4. _____ repetitions, _____ times a day
Goal_____

FIGURE 7-9   Suboccipital release.

before changing the direction of the roll if this exercise makes you dizzy. Do not bend the neck backwards without the advice of a doctor or physical therapist.

The *neck side bending* exercise is designed for stretching the neck muscles in order to reduce repetitive stress. It can be done sitting as well as standing. Looking straight ahead, bring the ear toward the shoulder. Make sure that the arm opposite from the bend is hanging down and the shoulder is down. Hold the head in that position for at least 5 seconds. Then bend the head toward the other shoulder.

For the *neck stretch (suboccipital release)*, the man or woman lies on her back with a 2- to 3-inch rolled towel at the base of her skull. Tuck the chin until the stretch is felt in the back of the neck (Figure 7-9).

Neck and Shoulder Massage. Neck and shoulder massage is also very helpful. Begin the massage gently, kneading more firmly only at the woman's request.

Exercise to Relieve Constipation

Conditioning exercises such as walking and swimming help prevent constipation, but there is also an exercise specifically designed for relieving constipation.

Sit on the toilet with your legs stretched out in front of the body. Imagine a line coming down from the ceiling through the center of the toilet. Slowly circle the body around the imaginary line. If it is difficult to hold your legs out, rest them on a chair or footstool. If balance is a problem, hold onto the grab bars or the sides of the toilet seat and, if necessary, modify the circling motion by rocking slightly from side to side, or back and forth. Women should not do this exercise if they have hemorrhoids.

Closing Comments

These exercises do not have to be strenuous or painful, and they are effective when a woman exercises to the extent that is comfortable for her. It takes time to see the benefits of exercise. Many women must wait as long as 6 to 8 weeks for noticeable results. But the results are very worthwhile: prevention or reduction of discomforts such as back pain and muscle spasms, increased endurance, and better general health. The interviewees made the strongest recommendation for exercise during pregnancy when they said, "I should have done more."

Nine Months of Change:
The First Trimester

Pregnancy is divided into three trimesters, each lasting approximately 3 months. The next three chapters discuss the following topics as they apply to each trimester: normal physical changes; common pregnancy symptoms; typical discomforts and ways of coping with them; medical care, including office visits and diagnostic tests; fetal development; possible complications; emotional concerns; special concerns for each trimester (for example, how to choose a birthing class during the second trimester); and the special concerns of women with disabilities.

Some of the common discomforts and disability problems associated with pregnancy are listed in Tables B-1 through B-6 in Appendix B. Table B-1 shows how many of the interviewees experienced these problems, and communicates a sense of what pregnancy can be like during each trimester, including the different symptoms that might appear, intensify, or disappear. Tables B-2 through Table B-6 illustrate the same discomforts as Table B-1, but they are organized into disability categories with only five women (or more) with similar disabilities. Table B-1 indicates whether there is a tendency towards a pregnancy discomfort, and provides a general sense of the experience of pregnancy. It does not include all possible symptoms, however, and should not be taken as a definitive guide. Some common pregnancy symptoms were under-reported, possibly because the interviews often focused on disability. For example, some women who mentioned feeling tired or faint may have been anemic without knowing it. Others may have simply forgotten some of their symptoms. Clara, for example, who remarked during a casual conversation that took place after her interview, "I forgot to mention that with one of my kids my nose was stuffy most of the time." Minor symptoms may have been forgotten because others were more important or memorable. When Celeste was asked what symptoms she experienced, she replied, "I was so afraid I'd have a disabled child, I blocked everything else."

Being disabled appears to affect the perception of pregnancy symptoms. For example, most women who have spinal cord injuries might not be aware of vaginal infection because they cannot feel genital irritation. Sometimes a woman cannot be sure whether she is experiencing a symptom of pregnancy or of disability. Jennifer described the swelling of her feet as a pregnancy symptom, but commented that the sensation resembled arthritic pain. Any woman who is experiencing an unpleasant or confusing symptom should not hesitate to discuss her concerns with her doctor. A sign is anything that a doctor, nurse, or physician's assistant can see, feel, hear, or smell. A symptom is what you feel. For example, a headache is a symptom. Swollen feet are both a symptom and a sign.

Initial Signs and Symptoms of Pregnancy

Many of the interviewees did not recognize the initial signs of pregnancy until their husbands or friends suggested the possibility. This was not limited to women who did not believe they could become pregnant. Although the common symptoms of early pregnancy may have other causes, a woman who experiences one or more of the following should consider the possibility that she is pregnant:

AMENORRHEA (ABSENCE OF MENSTRUATION)

This symptom is not always noticed immediately. Jennifer, who had been taking fertility medications, said, "I was paying attention to every sign, so I was particularly aware of my periods." But Patricia was caught by surprise. She explained, "I wasn't using any birth control, and I was telling a friend of mine about some of my sexual relationships when she said, 'If you go on like that you could get pregnant.' When she said that, I suddenly realized I *was* pregnant—I had already missed one period."

REDUCED MENSTRUATION

This may also be a sign of pregnancy. Women who experience a light flow at the time they are expecting to menstruate, and even some women who have stopped menstruating, may not realize they are pregnant until other symptoms occur.

NAUSEA

Morning sickness is the second most common symptom of early pregnancy. Sheila commented, "It wasn't until I got sick to my stomach that I started looking for my period, and I realized I was late and I was pregnant." Many women think at first that they really are sick. Julie said, "It didn't occur to me that I was pregnant. I told a friend of mine that I got sick at the same time every day, and then felt fine for the rest of the day. I couldn't believe it when she said I might be pregnant, but she badgered me into getting a pregnancy test." While some women feel nausea at the same time every day (not necessarily the morning!), others become sensitive to particular sights or smells. They may even dislike the smells of foods they normally enjoy. Celeste recalled, "I was watching the movie

Vertigo, and when I saw one particular scene, I started feeling sick and the feeling just wouldn't go away. Then I knew I was pregnant again." Tina said, "Smells that I am normally sensitive to really began to affect me. It happened right away and got worse in the second trimester. I traveled to Italy in the fourth and fifth months and smells made me sick all the time."

BREAST CHANGES

Some women notice changes in the appearance of their breasts. The nipples and areolas darken and take on a bumpy appearance during pregnancy, and the veins become more prominent. Others notice swelling, tingling, or soreness. Fay remarked, "I was sure I was pregnant, even before I took the test because my breasts hurt."

INCREASE IN BASAL TEMPERATURE

The basal temperature is the resting temperature of the body. It should be measured with a special thermometer before getting out of bed in the morning. Basal temperature varies during the menstrual cycle, but it rises in a different pattern when a woman becomes pregnant. Clara said, "We wanted to have a baby, so we were keeping track of my temperature. My husband knew I was pregnant when he took my temperature and it went up and didn't go down again. It might have been only a half a degree."

All of these early pregnancy symptoms, as well as other symptoms such as urinary frequency or fatigue, are easily confused with other conditions. Stacy said, "I thought I was sick until my husband commented, 'Your breasts are looking bigger. Maybe you're pregnant.'" Nikki said, "I would get very tired and fall asleep anywhere, but I didn't know I was pregnant until I got sick."

Even a physical examination can be misleading. The most reliable sign that a woman is pregnant is a positive pregnancy test. Sophia Amelia had a severe urinary tract infection, which made it hard to confirm her pregnancy.

Pregnancy Tests

Pregnancy tests detect the presence of a pregnancy hormone, human chorionic gonadotropin (HCG), in the urine or blood. Many women use home pregnancy tests for common reasons: they want to be sure they are pregnant before calling the doctor; they want privacy; or they want to avoid the inconvenience of going to a laboratory or clinic. A home pregnancy test may not be worth the extra expense, however. Your doctor will include a pregnancy test in your physical examination that will be covered by your medical insurance, whereas a home test will not be covered. Laboratory and office pregnancy tests also measure the presence or absence of HCG in urine. Blood tests are used only when there is a need to measure the quantity of HCG.

Home tests require only a small amount of urine, and some are 99 percent accurate. Women who have indwelling catheters can use the home test with a sample of urine taken from the leg bag. Women whose hand control is poor may not be able to use home tests without the help of an assistant, because a sample of urine must be poured into a small vial up to a measuring line, and some test ingredients must be measured with a dropper.

Office Visits

MEDICAL HISTORY

The first office visit for pregnancy is usually the longest, because your doctor needs to ask a number of questions about your medical history and perform a thorough examination. The medical history will cover four areas: personal medical history, family medical history, gynecological history, and social history. In a busy office, you may be asked to complete a questionnaire, or a nurse or medical assistant may interview you. The doctor will review this information and ask you to explain any unusual answers. You will also be able to ask questions about your concerns.

Personal Medical History

Discussion of your personal medical history is very important. Although it can be helpful for you to have copies of your medical records sent to your obstetrician, there is no substitute for a discussion of your past experiences. The doctor may need to ask some questions to gain a clearer understanding of what has happened in the past. Sometimes it might be beneficial to have her talk with your other doctors to have a better understanding of your medical issues.

It is clear from the literature that women with disabilities benefit from the team approach, including communication between all of her doctors via letters, telephone calls, or even conference calls. Given the pressures of managed care, written communication will help, unless the situation is complicated. For example, if your disability has caused you to have a predisposition to urinary problems, your urologist will know what antibiotics work for you, and your obstetrician will know more about how urinary tract infections can affect the fetus.

Family Medical History

A discussion of your family medical history will alert the doctor to the possibility that you may have certain medical problems. For example, if your mother has diabetes, or had diabetes of pregnancy, you might be more susceptible to this problem, and your doctor will want to make sure you know the warning signs.

Gynecological History

The gynecological history includes a discussion of your menstrual experiences, past pregnancies, past pelvic or genital infections, surgery, and other conditions.

Social History

Discuss your past and current life circumstances, including your marital, emotional, and economic situation, with your doctor. She can care for you better if she knows whether you have the help you need for pregnancy and childcare, whether you have other children to care for, and so forth. It is important to discuss these issues thoroughly and honestly, because many disabilities are exacerbated by stress.

MEDICAL ISSUES FOR DISABLED WOMEN

Disabled women will need to discuss a number of special issues with their obstetricians. As you discuss these questions, you and your obstetrician can decide which questions should be answered by her and which by your disability specialist.

Current Status of Your Disability

At your first and all subsequent visits to your obstetrician, you will need to discuss the current status of your disability. The problems you discuss will depend on your particular disability. Most women need to discuss how pregnancy affects their mobility and daily functioning. Dennis Swigart, who was the Chief of Prosthetics at Stanford University, stated, "Any amputee who is pregnant should at least notify her prosthetist during the first trimester. Good communication with your prosthetist at this time is the key" (11).

Women who experience autonomic dysreflexia need to discuss this problem thoroughly with their doctors, including a description of the circumstances that stimulate dysreflexia, so that their care can be planned accordingly.

Bladder and Kidney Problems

Many different disabilities can make a woman susceptible to urinary tract infections. Both myasthenia gravis and systemic lupus erythematosus can be exacerbated by such infections. Preventing infection depends on the appropriate use of medication, good hygiene, and good bladder drainage. It is important to do everything you can to prevent bladder infection. This includes making sure you completely empty your bladder periodically throughout the day. It is important to discuss all of these issues with your doctor. Many women with spinal cord dysfunction have long-term problems with urinary tract infections. Some of the interviewees wanted to stop their antibiotics. Sheila said, "During my first pregnancy, my doctor and I agreed to try stopping my antibiotics, but I had to start them again when I got a bladder infection. With my second, I just kept on taking antibiotics, and it went better." Sharon and Sybil also developed bladder infections when they tried discontinuing antibiotics.

Sienna took antibiotics during her first trimester, but she said, "I agreed with the doctor to stop taking medication because it was not crucial, and I was psychologically uncomfortable being on antibiotics." Sienna also said, "My doctor and I both thought I could control the infections by increasing the amount of fluids I took in." Sienna controlled her bladder infections by drinking more water. Some women may be more comfortable taking antibiotics. If you need to take medication in order to feel comfortable, make sure it is safe. Your doctor may decide to substitute a medication that is known to be safer during pregnancy. There are several medications that are class A and B. This means that they are safe during pregnancy. Medications classified C and higher, however, may be harmful to the fetus.

Sally's doctor chose to treat her bladder infections during pregnancy. She said, "We chose to treat my bladder infections because I was pregnant. I have bladder infections regularly when I'm not pregnant, but I don't always treat them." The risks of side effects are sometimes smaller than the risks of leaving a condition untreated. For example, the possible side effects of a particular antibiotic may be less worrisome than the risk that a severe urinary infection may lead to premature labor or injury to the mother or fetus.

Pregnancy increases susceptibility to urinary infection, and it is important to ask what symptoms merit a call to your doctor's office. The late Dr. Sandy Welner believed that being on antibiotics could prevent kidney problems (67). Women with spinal cord injuries can reduce the incidence of dysreflexia by keeping bladder infections at a minimum.

Women with spinal cord injuries can use the NDI Medical system for bladder control. "The NDI Medical bladder system is a surgically implanted device similar to a pacemaker, which can be used by people with a spinal cord injury to empty their bladder or urinate on demand. This device sends electrical signals through electrodes to the nerves to the bladder that lead to the bladder and bowel. It usually empties the bladder fairly thoroughly and therefore reduces urinary infection. Some women have used this device successfully to empty their bladder during pregnancy" (68).

It has been documented by the staff associated with NDI that five women had this device during and after successful pregnancies. One of those women had two successful pregnancies. Although Shanna used the device successfully during her first pregnancy, she did experience problems post-delivery that were caused by an unknowledgeable emergency room doctor. The device needed to be removed because of the doctor's lack of knowledge. Shanna decided to wait and have the control device reinstalled after her second pregnancy. Even without the device, Shanna did not have any bladder infection during her second pregnancy.

Breathing Problems

Women with a number of disabling conditions, including myasthenia gravis, post-polio syndrome, high spinal cord injuries, dwarfisms, and kyphoscoliosis (scoliosis of the upper spine), may have respiratory difficulties during pregnancy. Upward pressure from the growing uterus can cause exacerbation. The placement of the placenta in the uterus can also be a cause, as well as sitting most of the time. The seated position puts extra strain on the respiratory system, because in this position the baby pushes up against the diaphragm.

Breathing problems may first become noticeable at the end of the first trimester, when the uterus begins to rise into the abdominal cavity. Women with these problems must be careful to avoid respiratory infections, and call the doctor as soon as they notice symptoms, so that a slight infection does not become dangerous. It is probably best to have lung function checked periodically, because having a high thoracic or cervical spinal cord injury affects breathing. This can be done with a simple breathing test called a *vital capacity measurement*, which can be done quickly and easily in the doctor's office.

Breathing difficulties can be hazardous not only for the mother, but also for the fetus, which depends on the mother for oxygen. You and your doctor need to discuss whether respiratory testing is necessary, and what treatment will be required if problems arise. One possible solution is a mechanical device called the Advanced Respirator™, which can help improve respiration. This device was invented in Canada and is used for a variety of disabilities. The Advanced Respirator™ is a vest that is attached to a generator, which inflates and deflates the vest, thus compressing and expanding the chest wall.

For some women, particularly those with high spinal cord injuries, another cause of breathing problems can be pressure from the large intestine if it becomes impacted with fecal matter. This should be treated immediately.

Pressure Sores

Women who have occasional problems with pressure sores should tell their doctors. The increased weight of pregnancy, and pregnancy-associated anemia, sometimes put women with a spinal cord injury at an increased risk for pressure sores. Treatment plans can be developed to try to prevent this problem. For example, the doctor may order tests for anemia more frequently.

It is important to perform twice daily skin checks, eat a healthy diet, drink a healthy amount of water, and shift your weight every 15 to 20 minutes. A few of the interviewees experienced pressure sores that were caused by a body part continually rubbing against an unpadded surface. Shelby got too big for her wheelchair, but the sores quickly healed. Changing your weight-bearing positions from sitting to lying down may help prevent pressure sores.

Other Disability Issues

The interviewees with spina bifida were all put on folic acid because the neural tube closes completely by day 21 of pregnancy, which is before most women even know they are pregnant. The Center for Disease Control estimates that a large number of neural tube birth defects could be prevented every year if women took 400 mcg of folic acid per day before pregnancy and early in pregnancy (69). Many doctors prescribe a prenatal multivitamin in addition to folic acid. Folic acid can cause insomnia and/or agitation in rare cases.

Some women are troubled by constipation caused by iron supplements. If constipation has been a problem for you, your doctor can prescribe stool softeners, which are often prescribed for pregnant women. Constipation can be a problem for women with a spinal cord injury. After a spinal cord injury, it takes longer for the intestinal muscles to push the stool through the intestines and colon, putting the woman at greater risk for constipation. Moreover, constipation can cause dysreflexia in women with injuries at T6 or above (see Chapters 6 and 7 for suggestions on how to prevent constipation). Sydney said, "I haven't used suppositories since about 3 years after my injury. I find that simple digital stimulation works for me. When I have to go to the bathroom, the back of my arms tingle, so I know it is time. I usually go every couple of days. I've never really had the need for stool softeners, even during pregnancy."

MEDICATIONS

A review of your medications is a crucial part of your examination. Your doctor needs complete, accurate information about your medication schedule. In order to be sure you give him the correct information, you should:

(a) have your medical records sent to your obstetrician before your appointment;

(b) arrange for your all of your specialists to send a formal letter to your obstetrician discussing your medications; and

(c) bring all your medications to your first visit—in the original containers with the prescription labels attached—with your typed or clearly printed notes stating the time of day each medicine is taken and any side effects. Your obstetrician and disability specialists should confer about your medications if necessary. Roberta told us, "My obstetrician would order my lab tests, and my rheumatologist would tell him how to adjust my medication. It worked out fine." If your physicians need to confer about a particular medication, or if your dosage needs to be adjusted according to laboratory test results, make sure you ask whether to continue the medication in the meantime. Also ask who should be contacted and which doctor you should call and when. Sometimes you will be asked to contact a nurse, nurse practitioner, or physician's assistant. These specially trained people can usually tell you what the doctor wants you to do.

One possibility is that your doctor will ask you to substitute a medication that is known to be safer during pregnancy for one you took before pregnancy. For example, Stephanie regularly took an antibiotic to prevent bladder infection, but when she became pregnant, she was prescribed a different antibiotic that was safer for the fetus.

Not all medications have the same effects. Some are chemically changed by the placenta before they reach the fetus, others are not. Sometimes only small amounts of a medication the mother is taking will reach the fetus, while others reach the same concentration in the fetal blood as in the maternal blood. Many medications have been studied in order to understand their effects during pregnancy. It is often possible to treat the mother with a medication that is known to have no effect on the fetus. Some medications might need to be stopped, therefore, but others might need to be changed. Mona's neurologist changed her medication for spasticity because her original medication can cause fetal abnormalities.

Women who take medications such as Betaseron® or Avonox® to decrease their multiple sclerosis activity need to stop taking them while they are pregnant. Mimi was very happy to stop taking Betaseron® because she did not have to receive the painful injections every other day. Moira stopped taking Betaseron® 3 months before she got pregnant, but she kept taking her other medications until she became pregnant (Prozac® (antidepressant), Oxycontin® (pain medication), Neurontin® (pain medication), and

Oxybutynin (bladder medication)). Moira said, "I felt so great while I was pregnant." She found it a little bit more difficult to get around and her balance was a little off when she got off the Betaseron®.

Sabine had her pain medication, which was also an antidepressant, and her other medication lowered. She said, "I stayed on the lowest dose that would control the pain." Her doctor was up on the research and had her stop taking aspirin. Some antidepressants are considered safe during pregnancy.

Joy stopped all her medications when she found out she was pregnant. She was taking Embrel® for her arthritis, and Doxycycline®, an antibiotic. Joy did not have any reaction to stopping her medications. She said, "I went into remission almost immediately."

Although women are usually advised to avoid prescription medications during pregnancy, there are important exceptions to this rule. Reducing or discontinuing medication can be life-threatening for some women. Women with disabilities need to discuss all medication changes with their doctors in order to carefully weigh the possible risks and benefits of each medication. Noreen's perinatologist told her to take as much of her myasthenia gravis medication as she needed. Noreen saw no negative effects. She said, "It kept me breathing."

Felicia's obstetrician told her to stop taking Celexa® (an antidepressant) in her second month of pregnancy, "because it doesn't have a clear green light during pregnancy." Felicia experienced a severe depression as a result, and had to start taking Zoloft® in her sixth month. She was not seeing a psychiatrist. Her medication had been first prescribed by her rheumatologist, who diagnosed fibromyalgia. Felicia could have avoided depression if her obstetrician had consulted with a psychiatrist or checked on-line regarding this medication, because the available information shows that Celexa® can be safely taken during pregnancy. Furthermore, depression in pregnant woman can be harmful to the fetus.

Medications used to treat some symptoms may cause other symptoms. For example, drugs for treating preeclampsia or premature labor can increase the muscle weakness of myasthenia gravis. Medications used to suppress the symptoms of systemic lupus erythematosus, thereby averting miscarriage, may increase susceptibility to infection. According to Dr. Dhar, a rheumatologist, "Drugs such as aspirin and blood thinners, which are used to treat coagulation problems, can result in miscarriage. They can also cause excess bleeding in lupus patients. Corticosteroids are relatively safe to use in lupus patients, but the side effects include increased water retention, weight gain/edema, hypertension, and diabetes. These are all problems that can occur in non-lupus pregnancies, but they are exacerbated by the addition of corticosteroid medications." The mother, her obstetrician, and her disability specialist can discuss all these considerations. Information about the safety and effectiveness of various medications and combinations of medications are continuously changing, and the recommendations of your doctors may change from one pregnancy to the next.

Deirdre said, "I was very impressed with my HMO's advice line. They have a geneticist available by telephone who will research the effects of any medication on the fetus, both prescribed and nonprescription. They will also type out the results and mail them to you."

Sophia Amelia read the handout that accompanied the antibiotics for her urinary tract infection. Her urologist had prescribed them without consulting her obstetrician. She asked her urologist to change her antibiotic after she read the precautions.

Ask your doctor to explain what side effects you should look for, and whether the dosage of your medication will need to be adjusted. You should be aware of any special instructions for taking medication. For example, taking medication with meals can lessen indigestion.

Some of the interviewees commented on what happened to them when their medications were altered. Cheryl actually felt better when she stopped taking tranquilizers. She said, "I noticed I didn't need them. I found I had an inner sense of peace." Michelle had difficulty sleeping when she discontinued taking tranquilizers. Carol's doctor, who is also a licensed pharmacist, said she could continue taking Valium® when necessary. Carol later found out that taking Valium® close to delivery could cause her newborn baby to have problems with temperature regulation.

Sara said, "I did okay when I lowered my dose, but when I stopped altogether, I felt very tense and got more muscle spasms. Staying on a small dose worked best."

Roberta did not notice any change after discontinuing some of her medications before pregnancy. She did not say how long before pregnancy she stopped taking these medications. It is possible that she did not feel any change because pregnancy caused a remission of her symptoms.

It is also possible that the medications she continued taking during pregnancy provided adequate relief of her symptoms. Laura said, "I had to start my cortisone again because my lupus flared when I was $5\frac{1}{2}$ months pregnant." Leslie pointed out, "I didn't get prednisone till my third pregnancy and that went much better than the first two." Prednisone is crucial for women with systemic lupus erythematosus, but it might not be as important for women with other disabilities. Rachel was prescribed prednisone on a regular basis, but she took it only when she really needed to move. Rachel said, "It doesn't help me enough to make me want to take it every single day." When discussing medications with your doctor, be sure to also mention any nonprescription drugs you take.

All women are well advised to stop smoking, drinking, and taking drugs before pregnancy. Although Hannah was addicted to cigarettes, she was able to quit smoking early in her first pregnancy. She thought that quitting might have triggered her depression. She incorrectly believed that cigarettes contain antidepressant qualities. Arianna said, "The day I found out I was pregnant was the day I quit smoking." Sometimes your doctor can help you to stop with prescription medication, or perhaps a non-smoking group or hypnosis can help.

Any medications you take can affect your baby. Stopping as early as possible is the best protection for your baby. Sometimes the doctor can change medication. Deirdre was taken off Motrin® and put on Tylenol with Codeine®. She took it rarely, and then only a quarter of the pills, because "it would allow my muscles to get back on track and for me to become more independent more quickly."

If your medications for back or joint pain have been stopped because you are pregnant, you may want to ask your doctor to recommend occupational or physical therapy to help alleviate symptoms.

PHYSICAL EXAMINATION

The first examination includes a general evaluation, including the heart, lungs, etc., and some tests that will not be repeated until the final weeks of pregnancy. The pelvic examination usually will usually not be repeated until the final weeks of pregnancy. Other aspects of the examination are repeated at every visit, including measurement of temperature, blood pressure, pulse, weight, and urinalysis. (Note most offices do not have an accessible scale.)

Routine Examination

During a routine examination temperature, blood pressure, urine test, and weight will be taken. Temperature is taken because elevated temperature is often the first sign of infection. High blood pressure is a health problem that requires careful attention. Increases in blood pressure may be a sign of pregnancy complications and/or exacerbation of disability. A sudden increase or decrease of weight is also significant. Urine is tested for the presence of infectious bacteria, sugar (a sign of diabetes of pregnancy), and protein (a sign of pregnancy complications and/or exacerbation of disability).

Blood Tests

Several blood tests are done at the first visit. The blood type is determined, so that the doctor knows whether maternal and fetal blood might be incompatible. Blood tests also record the mother's blood type, in case she needs a transfusion. It is important to determine the Rh type (positive or negative), because untreated Rh incompatibilities can lead to fetal illness or disability, miscarriage, and premature labor.

The level of antibodies to rubella (German measles) is determined by a blood test. If the antibody level is low, the mother will not be vaccinated until *after* she has had her baby, because rubella vaccination during pregnancy is risky for the fetus. A woman should be tested for rubella *before* pregnancy and vaccinated if she is not already immune.

A VDRL or RPR test is used to diagnose syphilis, other venereal diseases, or hepatitis B (women who have systemic lupus erythematosus may react with a false positive).

A complete blood count (CBC) can reveal the presence of systemic infection or anemia. The CBC may be repeated at later visits.

If you or any of your sex partners has ever used illegal, injectable drugs, consider having an HIV-antibody test. This test can tell you whether you have a risk of developing AIDS, or transmitting the HIV virus to your fetus. Your doctor can advise you about confidentiality (keeping test results secret), understanding test results, and AIDS prevention and treatment. Proper treatment may prevent transmitting HIV to the fetus or embryo.

A blood test to determine thyroid function should be performed. *The New England Journal of Medicine* reported a study that showed babies born to mothers who do not produce enough thyroid hormone are prone to short attention spans and slightly lower IQs than other babies (70). There are many symptoms indicating low thyroid function, including anger, depression, agitation, low energy, constipation, weight gain, and migraine and other headaches. Low thyroid can run in families.

It is important is to have routine thyroid level checks throughout the three trimesters and postpartum. A test for thyroid stimulating hormone (TSH) is usually considered the most reliable blood test. The level of TSH goes up when the quantity of circulating thyroid hormone goes down. Many doctors will not prescribe thyroid hormones until the TSH is up to 10. Many people develop severe symptoms of low thyroid (hypothyroid), even with a TSH of 5 or 6. The reference range varies between 0.4 and 4.4, depending on the laboratory performing the test. Some use the 0.4 to 5.5, or 0.4 to 6.6 micro international units per milliliter (micro I.U. per ml.). You need to know the exact number of your TSH. If you have symptoms of low thyroid, you may have to interview several doctors to find one who will treat your low thyroid condition completely. Some psychiatrists are experts at treating hypothyroidism because it often includes psychological symptoms.

You may feel better if you take thyroid hormone. Usually the dose is increased slowly because the body takes about 6 weeks to adjust to a new dose of medication. Many people do not feel better until the TSH is lowered to 5 or 6. Other people do not feel better until the TSH is lowered to between 0.5 and 3. You should increase the dose slowly until you feel better, *not* until the blood test reaches a preset number. Your dose may need further adjustment.

THE PELVIC EXAMINATION

The pelvic examination serves a number of purposes. The appearance of the vagina and cervix can show signs of infection. At the first visit, the examination usually includes a Pap smear and cultures for gonorrhea and chlamydia. These are sexually transmitted diseases, and a baby who is exposed to herpes or gonorrhea in the vagina during birth may contract the infection and be blinded as a result. Examining the appearance of the cervix and the size of the uterus will help to confirm pregnancy, and determine how advanced the pregnancy is. The size of the uterus will help the doctor estimate the size of the fetus and the probable date of conception. During a bi-manual exam, which is an examination of the vagina and anus, the doctor can assess whether the size and shape of the pelvic opening, and the mobility of the coccyx (tailbone) are adequate for the birth process. Pelvic exams are usually not repeated until the last 4 weeks of pregnancy.

The pelvic examination alone may not provide enough information to determine how advanced the pregnancy is. When Pam's doctor examined her, the height of the fundus (top of the uterus) suggested that she had been pregnant longer than the time indicated by the date of her last menstruation. This discrepancy occurred because Pam's lordosis (excessive curvature of the spine) affected the angle of her uterus. The due date is not an exact prediction, but rather an estimate that can be incorrect if the woman does not have a 28-day menstrual cycle; she had a light flow after becoming pregnant; or she does not know the date of her last menstrual period. There are individual variations in the length of gestation. The estimated due date sometimes seems almost mythical. As a woman nears the end of pregnancy, often she can hardly wait for the due date, and she worries if it passes without the birth of the baby. It may be better to add a week to your doctor's estimate.

Transferring Issues

Transferring onto the exam table can present its own difficulties. Most offices do not have an accessible exam table, and many women have to ask for assistance.

Hilary said, "After my doctor lifted me onto the examining table, he decided to order one that had a hydraulic lift." Using the widest table available may help if the table's height is not adjustable. Removing the paper covering makes it less likely that you will slip or slid, but this method is far less sanitary. If you get on and off the table by yourself, make sure someone is there to put your crutches or sliding board out of the way, but within easy reach when you are ready to leave.

Although medical office staff in some states are required to help with transfers, it may be preferable to call ahead. In addition, women who need help transferring onto the exam table may prefer bringing their own assistants. Sylvia explained, "It's easier to go with your attendant, because they know the routine and you don't have to go through a long explanation." Portia, Pam, and Stephanie had their husbands help them.

In some cases, your attendant can show the office staff how to help you so they will be able to work with you at later visits if you need help. Olivia said, "The doctor's office staff helped me by just being there. They asked me what I needed, and their attitude was absolutely wonderful. There was a time when I would go to the doctor's office feeling depressed, but then they would tell me what a beautiful baby I was carrying."

Others find their own adaptations for transfers. Dorothy found that using a step stool was helpful in transferring onto a regular exam table. She also said she needed to ask for the step stool. Although Diane used a step stool, the office staff had to give her a boost. Darlene's obstetrician examined her on the floor. Rachel found that the best way for her to transfer was to back up against the exam table, and use her backside to inch up onto the table. Moira used her cane to balance herself and transfer onto the exam table.

You can encourage your doctor to purchase an accessible exam table if you do not want to struggle with transfers. Tell him that by purchasing an accessible exam table he can get tax credits.

Dr. Sandy Welner designed an accessible exam table that changes heights *and* positions (see Appendix D). This type of accessible exam table makes transferring easier. It also makes the exam itself more comfortable. Until accessible exam tables are the norm, however, some women will need to ask for help with transfers during office visits.

If you must tell your doctor or a member of his staff how to assist you with transferring, clarify the following points:

❖ Make sure you are not transferred onto the examining table until someone is able to remain in the examining room with you. It is often routine to have a patient wait in the examining room for anywhere from a few minutes to an hour, while the doctor finishes with another patient. Explain in advance that you can wait in an office chair or your wheelchair, but you must *not* be left alone on the examining table.

❖ The examining room and other equipment must be readied for you in advance. For example, somebody may need to move furniture aside so your wheelchair can be brought close to the table. Explain how to set the brake on your wheelchair, turn off the motor on an electric wheelchair, and move armrests and footrests out of the way. If adaptive devices such as leg braces must be removed, explain how they should be removed and set aside. Make sure jewelry, loose clothing, and tubing are not in the way.

❖ Have the examining table adjusted to the appropriate height, if possible.

❖ Any of the common transferring methods described below can be used, depending on individual preference. If you have developed a special method of transferring, these descriptions can help you decide how to explain your own method. You should consider getting a referral to physical therapy in order to determine the best way to transfer, because your center of gravity will have changed with your advancing pregnancy. Describe the entire transferring procedure in advance. It is better to have more than one assistant available, but if you have only one, discuss what to do if she drops you. It may be safest to simply to lower you to the floor, and then get help. Have your assistant practice lifting you over your wheelchair, and then lowering you into the chair. Remind your assistants to protect themselves by keeping their backs straight, bending their knees, and lifting with their legs.

Pivot Transfer: The table should be low enough for you to sit on for a pivot transfer. For this type of transfer, your assistant should stand in front of you, take your knees between his knees, grasp you around the back and under the armpits, and then raise you to a standing position. Next, he should pivot you onto the table. The assistant can help you lie down, once you are seated on the examining table. When returning to your wheelchair, have the table readjusted to a position that allows you to place your feet firmly on the floor before you are brought to a standing position.

Cradle Transfer: The cradle transfer is done with one or two assistants. The examining table should be at about the waist height of the assistants. If there is one assistant, she should squat beside you, and put one arm behind your knees and the other arm around your back and under your armpits. Next, she should stand and carry you to the table. Alternatively, two assistants can grasp each other's arms behind your back and under your knees, and carry you to the table. They must be careful to coordinate their movements.

Other Two-Person Transfers: Two other types of two-person transfers can be used to lift a woman in a sitting position over the arms of her wheelchair and onto the table. With these methods, the taller, stronger assistant should lift your upper body. The assistants must be careful to work together. In the first method, you should cross your arms across your chest. One assistant starts by kneeling behind you and reaching around you, putting his elbows under your armpits and grasping your opposite wrists (right hand on your left wrist). The other assistant should support you under the knees, and they should lift together. If you cannot cross your arms, the assistant standing behind you should put her hands together, or grasp her own wrists, so that she will not drop you.

Some aspects of the physical examination may pose problems for women with disabilities, but there are possible solutions for each problem.

During the Examination

A woman may have trouble getting on the examining table or finding a comfortable position. Muscle spasms, incontinence, or dysreflexia may occur during the examination. Many women with disabilities are unable to assume the usual position for a pelvic examination. A number of modifications are possible. Some women are more comfortable with obstetric stirrups that support their knees rather than their feet. Jennifer was able to stay in position for a short time by resting her heel in the stirrup, rather than the sole of her foot. Celeste had her husband hold up her legs. Amy had her legs held by the nurses.

Sienna's doctor allowed her to keep her shoes on during the exam because she had difficulty taking her shoes on and off, and her shoes helped keep her feet in the stirrups. Sydney thought it was important to have padded stirrups.

Sophia Amelia was unable to use the stirrups, so she rested her legs on her doctor's shoulders. She would sometimes have the doctor's assistant hold onto her legs, or she would hold one and an assistant would hold the other. Sometimes Sally would lie in her reclining wheelchair while the doctor examined her. This is a poor substitute to being examined on the table. Heather Ann needed a nurse to hold her stump up during the pelvic exam.

You may need some assistance in finding a comfortably balanced position once you are on the table. If you have a catheter in place, it does not need to be removed for the examination, but someone should make sure that the tubing is not caught or kinked. During transfer, the leg bag must *always* be 1 to 2 full feet below your bladder. Otherwise, the urine can easily drain back into your bladder.

If a woman must catheterize herself to urinate, or manually stimulate her bowel movements, the pelvic examination can cause her bowels or bladder to empty. This is less likely to happen if she empties her bladder and bowels before her appointment. It is also helpful to empty any leg bag before an examination.

Sometimes the touch of the speculum, or a slightly awkward position, will stimulate muscle spasms in the limbs or abdomen. An assistant should gently support the area that is in spasm. The examination can continue after the spasm resolves.

The internal pressure of a pelvic examination can occasionally cause dysreflexia. Your doctor will perform the examination during the first visit, but at later visits assistants may examine you. They should do so only when a physician is available on short notice, and should know that you must not be left alone if symptoms occur. Many physicians have found that applying an anesthetic jelly to the vagina and rectum before they begin will prevent this reaction. Cold objects touching the legs or feet can also cause dysreflexia, so it can be helpful for you to wear thick, warm stockings, or have towels placed on the table and stirrups. If you experience symptoms of dysreflexia, the stimulus must be found and removed; for example, the speculum must be removed, or a kinked catheter straightened. Bringing you to a sitting position may reduce your blood pressure if it becomes elevated during an exam. If your blood pressure does not drop, or symptoms such as a throbbing headache or stuffy nose become severe, the doctor should be called immediately to decide whether you need medication. Another examination can be scheduled for a later time.

SPECIAL DIAGNOSTIC TESTS

At the first office visit, samples of blood and urine will be taken for routine testing. These same samples may be used for the special diagnostic tests that are needed by women with disabilities. Ask the doctor what tests you will need, how test results will influence your care, and when test results will be available. Some of the tests that may be requested include:

Kidney Malfunction Tests
Women who have kidney malfunction for any reason need to be tested.

Maternal Alpha Fetoprotein (AFP)
This is an antibody screening test for fetal abnormalities. Other tests will be done if results indicate possible problems. Alpha fetoprotein is a chemical that is secreted by the fetus, and some of it enters the maternal bloodstream. The AFP level in the mother's blood may be tested any time between weeks 15 and 20 of pregnancy. It is recommended, however, that the test be done before the eighteenth week, because if the mother needs to consider terminating an abnormal pregnancy, an earlier screening test will allow time for further testing before she must make a decision. The length of pregnancy must be determined before the screening is done, so that test results can be interpreted correctly. The age of the mother also needs to be factored in. During Holly's second pregnancy, her AFP test result was abnormal. She had always worried about pass-

ing her condition on to her children, because women with congenital hydrocephalus have a 1 to 2 percent chance of passing it on to their babies. Holly was surprised when the results came back at the low end of the reference range. (A high result indicates a neural tube defect such as spina bifida).

The APF test is not nearly as accurate for assessing chromosomal disorders, but a low result can mean the presence of a chromosomal disorder. Simi was 32 when she became pregnant. Her blood test results for AFP came back elevated, indicating a possible neural tube defect, so her doctor recommended amniocentesis. A low level may indicate Down's syndrome.

Systemic Lupus Erythematosus

Women who have systemic lupus erythematosus need to have blood tests for the presence of SS-A and SS-B antibodies. These antibodies indicate there is an increased risk that the fetus will be born with heart damage. Other diagnostic tests will be needed later in pregnancy. The presence of lupus anticoagulant and antiocardiolipin antibodies is associated with an increased risk of miscarriage caused by blood clots in the placenta. If these antibodies are present, appropriate medication will be prescribed, which can greatly improve the outcome of systemic lupus erythematosus pregnancies.

Muscle Strength and Lung Function Tests

These tests may be ordered for women who have myasthenia gravis. Since medication dosage needs continuing adjustment as weight and blood volume change during pregnancy, these tests may be repeated.

Blood Samples

Having a blood sample taken in the doctor's office or at the laboratory can be difficult for many women who may have spasticity, involuntary movement, or other problems. There are only a few ways to draw blood from Amanda, "I have no veins left that are worth a hoot because of all the surgeries I had as a child. The only easy, safe way is in the neck, or a femoral stick. With my first child, we did one femoral stick to get the whole smattering done. We did everything through finger sticks with the second. I was impressed that my doctor let me do it this way. He felt comfortable if I was willing to get stuck until I couldn't stand it anymore."

If you have one "good" arm, decide in advance whether you would prefer to have blood drawn from that arm or the opposite arm. Some women prefer to have blood drawn from the good arm because it is more difficult to draw blood from the affected arm, and the technician may need to try more than once. Some prefer to have blood drawn from the affected arm because they do not want a sore spot in the good arm. Tell the technician about any methods that have been helpful in the past, or if you have a preference. You may try leaving your arm hanging in a downward position for 5 minutes. Then, ask the technician to put the tourniquet on *before* raising your arm. This method leaves the vein more engorged and much easier to find.

URINE SAMPLES

Giving a urine sample in the office can present difficulties. Some women are not comfortable using a catheter in the restroom at the doctor's office, and prefer to bring a sample to the office in a clean jar. Shanna's, Sonya's, and Nicole's doctors had them bring in urine samples. Shanna said, "I would take several sterile cups to use at home." Amanda's doctor put the toilet pan in the toilet to collect urine because Amanda could not hold a cup to collect the urine.

WEIGHING IN

Being weighed is difficult for many women with disabilities. Arianna got weighed only a couple of times. Most women were assisted by their partners. The partner stepped on the scale first and had his weight measured, and then took his partner in his arms to re-weigh. The woman's weight is determined by taking the total number and subtracting the partner's weight. This may not have been the best procedure for Pam, who tried to avoid gaining weight so her husband would not injure his back while lifting her. Sophia Amelia's doctor weighed her in the same way. There is a type of scale available that allows a person to transfer into a seat attached to the scale. The armrest can be raised for horizontal transfers. Sally's husband transferred her to a sit-down scale during her first pregnancy. Several women solved the problem by weighing themselves on special scales and reporting their weight to their doctors. Sylvia and Sara used a freight scale at a nearby hospital; Stephanie used a laundry scale; and Samantha used a special scale at the nursing home where she worked. Sydney found a nursing home near her house and asked them if she could use their scale before she went to her doctor's appointments. One woman laughed when she said, "I even thought about trying a veterinary scale." She used an industrial laundry scale during her second pregnancy. Selina said, "With my first baby, I was small enough to sit on my scale, but with my second they used a wheelchair scale at the hospital where I later delivered.

The Detecto™ is a scale that works with a chair (see Appendix D). The Sammons Preston Catalog has several versions, including a scale that allows a wheelchair to be driven onto it.

HEART RATE

The doctor or his assistant will listen to the baby's heartbeat every time you go to the office for a visit, starting when you are 11 to 12 weeks pregnant, and record it in your prenatal record. The first time a heartbeat can be heard on a sonogram is at 5 to 6 weeks of pregnancy. At 12 to 13 weeks of pregnancy, a simple device called a *Doppler*™ magnifies the baby's heartbeat so that it can be heard. The Doppler™ is placed on your stomach over the uterus, and the angle of it is changed until the heartbeat is found. If your doctor has a Doppler™ with a microphone built into it, you will also be able to hear your baby's heartbeat at every visit. The usual heart rate at 12 to 13 weeks is about 160 beats per minute. The heart rate slows to 120 to 140 beats per minute as the fetus grows.

CONCLUDING THE OFFICE VISIT

After the examination, you and your doctor can discuss any remaining questions about your pregnancy. He will advise you about nutrition and other aspects of your care. Many women begin discussing their concerns about what will happen during labor, a discussion that will continue during later visits. Office visits normally take place once a month during the first trimester.

OTHER DIAGNOSTIC TESTS

Two other tests that may be done outside your doctor's office are *sonography* (often called *ultrasound*) and chorionic villus sampling (CVS).

Sonography

Sonography may be done at any time during pregnancy for a variety of reasons. During the first trimester, a sonogram may be used to determine the gestational age of the fetus; to verify that the pregnancy is in the uterus if symptoms of extrauterine pregnancy occur; locate the fetus for chorionic villus sampling; or detect Down's syndrome.

Sonography resembles sonar, the method used on submarines to navigate and locate objects under water. High-frequency sound waves bounce off the fetus, and a transducer sends the resulting image to a screen without causing any damage to mother or fetus.

The woman lies on her back during the procedure. A special gel that improves the transmission of the sonogram is applied to her abdomen. The gel feels cool and slippery, and helps the transducer glide more easily. If this test is conducted during early pregnancy, the woman will be instructed to drink several glasses of water just before the examination in order to fill the bladder. The filled bladder is more easily distinguished from other organs, and lifts the uterus so that it can be examined more easily. Filling the bladder in this way obviously poses a problem for women who use indwelling catheters, and those who experience dysreflexia when their bladders are full. They will need special instructions from their doctors. Other women should be aware that the examination may become uncomfortable. Even the light pressure of the transducer can be unpleasant because the urine is held in during the procedure. If a woman has good control but becomes uncomfortable, she may be allowed to partially empty her bladder.

Nuchal translucency (NT) is a term used to describe a *sonolucent* area in the *nuchal region* (back of the neck) of the fetus, typically observed in the first trimester. Nuchal translucency screening provides a couple with an individual, specific risk for having a child with Down's syndrome, trisomy 13, and trisomy 18. Increased NT refers to a NT measurement of greater than 3 mm. This does not mean your baby has a chromosome abnormality, but it does mean that the baby has an increased risk for some disorders and birth defects (71). This test is performed by either transabdominal or transvaginal ultrasound scan. Of the women tested, 95 percent will have a normal result. The test will pick up 80 percent of the pregnancies affected by Down's syndrome. The test itself does not carry any risk to the mother or the baby. If a test is positive, meaning the recalculated risk is greater than 1:300, further testing is usually recommended to determine the baby's chromosomal pattern.

Women who have systemic lupus erythematosus are likely to be scheduled for sonography at the time of their first prenatal visit. It is important to determine gestational age accurately because their babies are at increased risk for both preterm birth and growth retardation. Using this test, a baby who is simply small will not be considered premature.

Chorionic Villus Sampling (CVS)

This method of genetic testing was developed more recently than amniocentesis. Although it is no longer considered experimental, it still is not as widely available as amniocentesis (see Chapter 9 for further information on amniocentesis). Some women prefer CVS over amniocentesis because the procedure can be done earlier in pregnancy and test results are available much sooner. If the mother decides to terminate her pregnancy, she can do so earlier, when it may be safer and less stressful emotionally. When a woman is deciding whether to use CVS, her doctor or genetic counselor will discuss the advantages and disadvantages, including the risks of infection or miscarriage.

Early in pregnancy, the embryo is surrounded by a sac called the *chorionic membrane,* which will develop into the placenta. This membrane is covered with small projections called *villi.* Some of the villi are removed through a thin tube that is introduced into the uterus through the cervix (transcervical CVS). Sometimes the procedure is done using an abdominal puncture (transabdominal), although this method is more complex than transcervical CVS. A sonogram is used in CVS to locate the embryo. A small amount of local anesthetic will be injected to prevent discomfort if the transabdominal procedure is used. The genetic material in the villi is then analyzed for abnormalities.

Physical Changes

The most commonly noticed changes are described below. A number of complex hormonal changes take place during pregnancy, and the level of each hormone rises and falls in a characteristic pattern. Some changes in the levels of hormones in the blood or urine can be measured for diagnostic purposes.

Changes in hormones and other physical changes are not always directly perceptible to the pregnant woman. For example, a woman may not be aware that there is a change in the way her body uses insulin; she simply knows she feels hungrier.

BLOOD VOLUME

The blood volume begins to increase during the first trimester in order to support the growing fetus, placenta, and uterus, and to create a reserve in case the mother loses blood during delivery. Sometimes the volume increases so quickly that the amount of hemoglobin (iron-containing protein) seems relatively lower; this type of mild anemia is not unusual.

UTERUS, CERVIX, AND VAGINA

The uterus and vagina begin to change, even in the first trimester. The nonpregnant uterus is a pear-shaped organ, with the "neck" of the pear, the cervix, extending into the vagina. The uterus does not simply stretch during pregnancy; the muscle tissue in the walls grows as well. Some enlargement can be found during pelvic examination by the fifth week. The uterus is spherical in shape by the twelfth week.

The cervix, the area where the cervix joins the uterus, and the muscles in the vaginal walls become softer and looser. These changes begin the process that will allow the tissues to stretch enough for the birth of the baby. Some couples may notice a change in the vagina during intercourse.

The uterine muscles begin to contract slowly and irregularly in order to prepare the uterus for the eventual childbirth. These early contractions are too slight to be noticeable to the mother, but her doctor may be able to feel them during a pelvic examination.

The lining of the vagina thickens and the woman may notice a thick white discharge. This discharge is normal, but it differs in texture, color, and odor from the discharges commonly caused by infection (see Chapter 10 for a discussion of *vaginitis*).

BODY TEMPERATURE

The increase in temperature that follows conception stabilizes for the remainder of pregnancy. Some women enjoy feeling warmer; others may be uncomfortable.

BREASTS

Several changes in the breasts occur during the first trimester. Many women notice soreness, tenderness, or a tingling sensation during the first few weeks. Breast size increases noticeably during the second month, and the veins become more visible and appear as a network of blue and pink lines. The nipple and surrounding area (*areola*) may darken, and the nipple begins to enlarge. The little bumps on the areola (*Montgomery's glands*) also enlarge.

The Discomforts of Pregancy

Pregnancy affects all of the bodily systems, including the digestive, urinary, and muscular systems. The discomforts of early pregnancy often seem to be the most dramatic. Laura spoke for many women when she said, "The first trimester was the worst of all."

Nausea and Change in Appetite

Perhaps the most common pregnancy discomfort is morning sickness. From about the sixth week of pregnancy, approximately one-third of all pregnant women experience only a slight loss of appetite. Other women become extremely nauseated or even suffer from vomiting. Symptoms usually improve or disappear by about the fourth month. It is not possible to predict who will be troubled by morning sickness. Some women are bothered during every pregnancy; others are bothered only during some of their pregnancies. Nicole was sick all the way through her first pregnancy, and needed to be hospitalized in order to receive intravenous therapy. She experienced only a small amount of nausea during her subsequent pregnancies.

Nausea occurs at the same time of day for many pregnant women, but not necessarily during the morning. Julie said, "It was like clockwork. It happened at the same time every morning." Pam said, "The awful feeling happened every day in the late afternoon." Nausea can also happen at any time in response to tastes, sights, or smells. Corrine said, "The smell of coffee made me sick."

The causes of morning sickness are not completely understood. Some doctors suggest that human chorionic gonadotropin somehow causes it, because morning sickness is most likely to occur when levels of this hormone are high. Nadine Fiona's morning sickness was so bad during the first 4 months that she actually lost 4 to 5 pounds. She said, "I would get most of my calories in the morning from fruit and vegetables because I knew at night I would be sick."

Negative or ambivalent feelings about pregnancy may contribute to nausea, but it is unlikely that they are the sole cause of nausea. Sasha had no problems with morning sickness, although the anxiety of her family made it difficult for her to enjoy her pregnancy. Sheila had morning sickness during both pregnancies, but she only felt ambivalent about the second one because her husband was unsure whether he wanted another child.

A number of remedies have been tried to relieve nausea and vomiting, but no single solution works for all women. Experiment with the suggestions in this chapter and do what works best for you. Although Holly had nausea with all three of her pregnancies, she vomited only once during her first and second pregnancies, and never with the third. Holly said, "I hate to throw up. It's a psychological thing, because every time I vomited as a child, my parents would rush me to the neurosurgeon. In fact, if I get any stomach ailment, I hardly ever vomit."

There have been many studies about the impact of vitamins and other supplements on pregnancy. A double-blind study showed that 30 mg of vitamin B_6 is considered to be a useful treatment for morning sickness. Dr. Michael T. Murray (61) recommends that it may be successful to take a combination of 250 mg of vitamin B_6 with ginger root powder four times a day. Some of the interviewees did not find ginger helpful. Check with your doctor as to the length of time and the amount of B_6 that should be taken.

Holly tried ginger root in both pill form and ginger snaps, but they were only slightly helpful. Nadia also tried ginger, and found it did not relieve her nausea. Rachel said, "I found that true ginger ale with real ginger in it seemed to help a little bit. I got it at the health food store. Occasionally toast would also help." Laura said her nausea was horrible, and she ate popcorn and sipped ginger ale for relief. Sienna found that the vibrations produced by deep humming helped reduce her nausea.

Sophia Amelia said, "I knew what to expect during my second pregnancy. I took much better care of myself. I learned the trick of always keeping something in my stomach, and also eating crackers before I even lifted my head off the pillow. I took my prenatal vitamins at night."

Eat a few dry, low-fat crackers, such as soda crackers or matzoh, when you are likely to feel sick. Some women, including Christine and Clara, kept crackers by the bed and ate a few before rising. Dawn was helped by beginning her meals with a few crackers.

Eat yogurt, cottage cheese, or milk in small portions. Try not to become too hungry or too full. Eat small, frequent snacks, not full meals. Make sure each meal or snack includes a high-protein food, which will satisfy hunger longer than sugar or starch.

You can also try sipping carbonated water or hot mint tea. Another option is to drink ginger or cinnamon tea 2 or 3 times a day, or lick a lemon. Amy tried ginger and ginseng teas, and found them to be useful. Ginger tea helped soothe Joy's nausea.

Some women prefer a combination of remedies. Michelle's afternoon nausea was relieved by dry toast and mint tea. Drink between meals in order to get adequate fluids without feeling too full. Notice the foods that make you feel worse and avoid them. Leslie said, "I stayed away from greasy food, otherwise I would get sick."

Sometimes taking a nap or becoming involved in an absorbing activity can help with nausea. Pam said, "I tried to occupy myself, but sometimes I needed the medication."

There are also many remedies that have not been proven by any medical studies to be safe or effective. Nikki had morning sickness all day, every day, for 4 months during all seven of her pregnancies. During her seventh pregnancy, she rubbed an essential oil called Di-Tone™ on her ear lobes twice a day (72). This reduced her morning sickness by 90 percent. Nikki thought her success was because the ear has many acupressure points. Ellie had terrible nausea, but her doctor was not comfortable with her using Di-Tone™ because he did not know if it was safe. He prescribed Zofran®, an anti-nausea medication, instead. This medication is generally used in treating cancer; it has not been proven to be safe for pregnancy.

Seabands™ are wristbands that stimulate acupressure points in order to relieve nausea. Orielle and Sophia Amelia found the wristband to be helpful, but Amy and Joy did not find them to be helpful. A study done at the University of Rochester in New York found that it can make a difference if a person expects the remedy to help.

Ordinary morning sickness is not dangerous. Some women, however, develop a condition called *hyperemesis gravidarum*, which means literally "too much vomiting during pregnancy." You may become malnourished and/or dehydrated and need hospitalization if excessive vomiting continues. It is important for your doctor or midwife to watch and correct for dehydration and electrolyte deficiencies, or inappropriate levels of blood electrolytes. Typically, this relates to abnormal level of sodium, potassium, or chloride in the bloodstream (73).

Joan threw up everything, including water, and she lost a lot of weight. She said, "I couldn't eat for 2 weeks. When I couldn't take it anymore, I went to the emergency room. They put me on IV fluids and gave me an anti-nausea shot. It eased my nausea enough so that I could start eating, but I still felt queasy and was sensitive to smells."

Urinating less than usual, or not at all, can be a noticeable sign of dehydration. Other signs can be found on examination by a physician or midwife. It is unwise to allow such severe problems to develop. If you experience frequent vomiting, consult your doctor about the advisability of medication, because it can be very helpful for some women. Sylvia commented, "When I started medication, it helped me gain weight." Natalie did not vomit, but her nausea stopped her from eating, so her doctor prescribed an anti-nausea medication. Natalie quit taking it because it "knocked me out!"

Nausea creates special problems for women with disabilities. It can be dangerous for women with myasthenia gravis, who can become seriously weakened if vomiting interferes with absorption of their medications. Contact the doctor immediately if this happens, and discuss using injectable medicines or anal suppositories. Women with other disabilities may have trouble keeping oral medicine down. They may also need the dosage of their medicine changed after weight loss or gain.

Some women have difficulty reaching the bathroom quickly when they feel nauseated. Some may not be able to bend over to clean up vomit. Some of the interviewees thought it was fortunate that they had nausea at the same time every day because they were able to schedule attendant care accordingly. Others made sure to keep a bowl for throwing up within easy reach.

The fetus is not harmed by mild morning sickness. Taking prenatal vitamins helps assure that the mother and fetus have sufficient vitamins and minerals. Sydney had difficulty swallowing prenatal vitamins. Her doctor told her to take Flintstone® children's chewable vitamins with calcium and iron. Ask your doctor how many tablets per day you need if you prefer chewable vitamins.

Some women have an increased appetite in early pregnancy. Jennifer remarked, "I ate constantly. I was impressed at how much I could eat." Clara said, "I usually don't eat breakfast, but when I was pregnant it felt as if someone else inside of me made me eat." Both women said they felt as though they would develop nausea if they did not eat.

Other women start craving unusual foods—the "pickles and ice cream" syndrome. Food cravings are harmless as long as they do not interfere with eating a sensible diet. Cravings for non-foods such as ice or chalk may be a sign of illness, including iron deficiency, and should be reported to your doctor.

Fatigue and Faintness

Feeling flushed, faint, or dizzy is common in early pregnancy, but the degree of tiredness varies widely. Many people believe that fatigue occurs because extra energy is required for growth of the fetus and placenta, and maternal tissues. That cannot be the only reason, however, because even more growth occurs during the second trimester, when many women feel more energetic.

Many women do not feel equally tired in every pregnancy. Others may not experience fatigue at all. Mimi said, "I think I was already tired because of MS, but I learned how to handle it. I have stools around the house because standing in one place gets me really tired." Moira said, "I could feel the difference between MS fatigue and pregnancy fatigue. With MS fatigue you sleep, and when you wake up you do not feel rested, but when I was pregnant, I took naps and felt rested."

Other women may find it difficult to distinguish between pregnancy-associated fatigue and the exacerbation of multiple sclerosis or myasthenia gravis.

Some women with MS recognize their fatigue as multiple sclerosis exacerbation. Michelle said that she experienced an exacerbation of MS in her first trimester. She said, "I was really tired in the first and third trimesters. I felt so tired that I stayed in bed most of the time." Mary said, "Increased tiredness was my main problem."

Multiple sclerosis and myasthenia gravis can be worsened by fatigue and stress. Women with these disabilities must be very careful to get adequate rest, and to report their symptoms to their doctors in case an adjustment of their medication or other treatment is needed. A corticosteroid may occasionally be given if the woman has a disability-related exacerbation (74).

Women with other disabilities can also have varying degrees of fatigue. Carla commented, "It was easier the second time. I was in better shape from running after my first child, and I had a better idea of how my body works."

Rachel said, "I am very tired and I have a 3-year-old, as well as a flare-up, and things are very difficult." She needed a different coping technique when she was pregnant with her second child. She said, "I am able to handle it because I'm very fortunate to have a supportive husband who has a flexible schedule. I also handle it differently, in that things that mattered to me before don't matter to me now. For example, if the dishes don't get done, they don't get done. I'm not going to fret about it because I can't afford the energy to do that now. I do what I can, when I feel I have the energy to do it, and that has freed both my mind and my body." Allison had a helpful husband and went to bed early.

Depression can contribute to fatigue. Sheila remarked, "I think I was more tired the second time because I was having relationship problems and I was depressed."

Sometimes fatigue is a symptom of health problems such as anemia or infection. These problems can be diagnosed during regular office visits, and treated if necessary. Naomi needed the dose of her thyroid medication raised. She thought that low thyroid played a part in her being so tired. She was tired "the whole way through" her second pregnancy. It is important to call your doctor if you feel extreme fatigue between office visits.

Women are given prenatal vitamins containing iron to prevent or alleviate anemia, but many women are tempted to stop taking them when they cause constipation or indigestion. Instead, they should discuss the problem with their doctors, and use the suggestions for avoiding constipation given in Chapters 6 and 7. Sophia Amelia said, "When I got really constipated, they told me to take a break and stop taking the vitamins temporarily."

Even when fatigue is not associated with other problems, many women are simply upset at being unable to accomplish as much as usual. Nora said, "It was hard for me to do anything. I would lie down, but I'd feel fidgety because I had things I wanted to do."

Some disabled women may be upset because they have been taught to be tough. Pam said, "When I needed to rest, it felt like I was pampering myself." A useful solution to fatigue and feeling faint is to rest as much as possible. Elevating your feet to improve circulation may also be helpful.

Felicia said, "I slept in my car at lunch time. Sometimes I would sleep in my car after work for half an hour before I would attempt to drive home." Priscilla said, "It was upsetting. I was used to having so much energy. I read an article about the effects of pregnancy hormones, and that helped me get over my frustration about not keeping up with the demands on my time."

Moira rested two or three times a day during her entire pregnancy. She said, "Sometimes I would have to force myself to lie down, or I would read. I would do deep breathing or meditate to make sure I was calm and healthy."

Oprah thought that listening to her body was important. She said, "If I pushed myself, I would have broken something." Sally took catnaps to handle her tiredness. It is important to try to arrange times for resting or napping. Paula said, "I would collapse on the couch whenever my children were napping or busy playing." Sonya said, "Prior to pregnancy, I would take an hour nap. When I was pregnant, I would take a 2 to 3 hour nap in the afternoon." Sonya could not sleep in her chair and arranged for attendants to transfer her into bed. Andrea's solution was to nap during her lunch break. Corrine said, "I felt more tired with my second pregnancy, so I took a nap whenever my first child was sleeping." Heather Ann "kept to a regime. I just stopped what I was doing and watched TV. I made sure I kept my leg up."

Some women have difficulty getting into bed or arranging cushions to support their feet. It is hard for some women to rest if they do not have additional attendant care. Some women adapt by using reclining chairs or reclining wheelchairs. Recliners that raise the feet as well as recline are useful for some women, but having a recliner wheelchair can be difficult or impossible to maneuver if the house is small. At first, Nancy managed by carrying a pillow with her. Several times a day she would place the pillow in front of her and lean up against a piece of furniture to rest. She said, "I eventually realized I would just have to spend more time in bed. I found things I could do in bed and stayed there 12 hours a day." Having your feet raised can help with both tiredness and faintness.

Feeling faint is more common during the second trimester, but Stephanie felt faint during the first. She noticed that she was especially likely to feel faint after meals and after her bowel movement, which occurred every third day. She found that when she became faint after bowel movements, it was best to remain seated and put her feet up on the bathtub bench. She added, "I made sure I carried smelling salts with me. One time when I was out with my husband and I got dizzy, I had him lay me down right there on the ground." It is wise to stop and rest if you become dizzy, because you may fall and possibly cause an injury. Alter your schedule accordingly if you become faint at predictable times.

Several women emphasized that finding ways to reduce housework and other responsibilities is just as important as finding time to rest. Margie said, "I worked only part-time." Patricia said, "I didn't go to work, and cut down on my social life for the first 2 months." Paula cut back all of her responsibilities. Naomi said, "I quit my demanding job."

Women who cannot afford extra help must find other solutions. Sometimes a partner can take over some tasks, but that approach may cause other problems. Stephanie's and Cheryl's husbands did not mind doing more chores, but Pam's husband felt so burdened that he left her when their child was 18 months old. Portia rented out a spare room in exchange for housework. Some women simply eliminate non-essential chores. Heather Ann said matter-of-factly, "My house wasn't as clean as it had been before I was pregnant."

URINARY PROBLEMS

Some increase in urinary frequency is normal throughout pregnancy. The increased volume of body fluids and the pressure of the growing uterus on the bladder contribute to the frequent urge to urinate. Some women find that the pressure is relieved later in pregnancy, as the uterus grows upward out of the pelvis. Some of the interviewees were not troubled by frequency or incontinence. Other women had more severe problems. Mary and Marsha both stopped wearing underwear so they "wouldn't waste any time." Other women suggested staying close to a bathroom, or wearing absorbent underwear.

Urinary tract infections are more serious. Women whose disabilities increase their susceptibility to bladder or kidney infections are even more susceptible during pregnancy. Some of the symptoms of kidney infection are chills, fever, and blood in the urine. Sometimes blood in the urine may be caused by local irritation. This symptom should always be reported to your doctor.

Women who are pregnant must be alert for early symptoms of infection, because severe infection may exacerbate the disability or cause preterm labor. Increased frequency of urination is only one symptom of bladder infection. Other symptoms include pain or burning before or after urination, or feeling the urge to urinate but only passing a few drops.

"During pregnancy, women who intermittently catheterize may want to use a sterile technique as a way of preventing infection. If a urinary tract infection is suspected, aggressive treatment must be instituted. This is especially true for women with spina bifida and spinal cord injuries, who may have a high incidence of *pyelonephritis* (kidney infection). Other complications have been reported" (75).

Women who have neurologic disabilities seem to have a higher incidence of kidney stones. Ultrasound can help evaluate this problem. One way to reduce this risk is by drinking more fluids, as well as maintaining the pH of the urine by taking adequate vitamin C and drinking cranberry juice.

Sophia Amelia said, "They put me on antibiotics for bladder infections, and they would change them if they became ineffective. They would prescribe the antibiotics according to the side effects for each trimester."

Several of the interviewees tried drinking large quantities of water to prevent or combat infections. Sylvia said, "I was getting a lot of quad sweats. This is a sign of dysreflexia; sweating is *above* the level of the spinal injury secondary to vasodilatation. I drank lots of water to replace the fluids I had lost. I must have been drinking two or three times as much as normal. Maybe that's why I never got a bladder infection, even though I usually get one."

Sheila and Samantha reported that increasing fluids was not as effective as taking antibiotics. Adequate fluids can sometimes help prevent infection, and may increase comfort during a bladder infection. Contact your doctor as soon as symptoms develop, and take medication as prescribed. Moira drank five to six glasses of water a day. She had only one bladder infection, and was put on antibiotics. Treating infections early is important, because during pregnancy, the *ureters* (tubes leading from kidneys to bladder) are dilated, making it easier for a bladder infection to spread upward to the kidneys. The interviewees rarely had a kidney infection.

One possible way to limit bladder infections was suggested by someone who has had a spinal cord injury for $17\frac{1}{2}$ years. This method is for people who do intermittent catheterization. He had a reflexic bladder and experienced urinary leakage until he began coating his bladder with the antispasmodic Ditropan®. He catheterizes himself 4 to 6 times a day. After dissolving the Ditropan® in tap water in a 2-oz, catheter-tipped syringe, he catheterizes himself and injects the Ditropan® into his bladder. Then he pulls out the catheter, leaving the Ditropan® in until the next cathing. He said, "I never experience leakage now, and as an extra bonus, I haven't had a bowel accident in many years." He has experienced very few bladder infections in the last 12 years (about once every 2 years). Dr. Graham Creasey, a noted urologist, confirmed the use of Ditropan®.

"Regarding Ditropan® and the bladder: this is something that people do, and some doctors recommend it, although Ditropan® is not supplied in a liquid form, so it has to be dissolved. I would suggest that it is better to dissolve it in sterile water rather than tap water. The main effect is to reduce bladder spasms and leakage. Some people may also find that when they have fewer bladder spasms they have fewer infections" (68).

On the other hand, in a study of 28 pregnant women with cerebral palsy by Winch and colleagues (13), only three of the women had a history of pyelonephritis, and only one had it during pregnancy. Bladder infections in women with certain disabilities occur at the same rate as those without disabilities. Only two of the interviewees with cerebral palsy had bladder infections during pregnancy. Moreover, none of the interviewees with neuromuscular disability had urinary problems.

ABDOMINAL MUSCLE STRETCHING OR CRAMPING

As the abdominal muscles are stretched by the growing uterus, some women experience a stretching sensation or muscle cramps. Sometimes the cramps can be relieved by stretching. Massage or firm pressure on the cramped muscles might also help. These sensations usually do not last long, and as Carla said, "I just lived with it." Cheryl remarked, "I knew it was the uterus expanding, but I still felt maybe my cerebral palsy added to it" (see section on ectopic pregnancy).

LEG MUSCLE CRAMPS AND BACK PAIN

Some women whose disability involves back pain or muscle spasms may experience exacerbations as early as the first trimester. However these problems are more likely to occur during the second and third trimesters.

Two women with spinal muscular atrophy who were presented in a case study by Carter and Bonckat (29) had musculoskeletal problems: either costochondritis (inflammation of the joints between the rib and sternum) or low back pain. These problems were treated with physical measures, including heat and ice, a transcutaneous electrical stimulation (TNS) unit, and wheelchair modification. Another treatment was modification of the wheelchair. A change was made for positioning, and a lumbar support was added.

Prior to pregnancy, Sonya's Baclofen Pump™ controlled her spasticity, but the medication did not control her spasticity during her pregnancy. The pump is surgically placed, usually just under the skin of the abdomen. Medication is dispensed inthrathecally, which means directly into the cerebrospinal fluid. It does not cross the blood brain barrier, and it does not circulate to the rest of the body. Only tiny doses are required to be effective; side effects are minimal; and a neurologist can adjust the dosage non-surgically (76).

Sonya's doctor did not increase her medication during her pregnancy, although it is unclear why. The author called Medtronics, the manufacturer of the pump, to find out more information. She was referred to Dr. Richard Penn, a neurosurgeon with the University of Chicago, because he has experience with ITB Therapy (Baclofen pump™) for adults, including pregnant women with spinal cord injury. According to Dr. Penn, "There is no contraindication to increasing the amount of baclofen in order to decrease the spasticity during pregnancy, because the medication never gets to the embryo." Some women may not want to use medication, but some may have a strong reaction without meds.

Shelby experienced severe spasticity. She was thrown out of her manual chair during one incident, and so she put anti-tippers on her wheelchair.

CONSTIPATION

Constipation refers to hard, dry stools and difficult bowel movements involving strain, discomfort, or infrequent movements. Constipation is a common problem during pregnancy for most women, disabled or not, due to the increased hormones of pregnancy, the uterus putting pressure on the rectum, and the decrease of motility of the intestines. Some women experience constipation as early as the first trimester, but the problem is much more common in the third trimester. Simi drank prune juice the whole time she was pregnant. Sophia Amelia handled her constipation by eating cherries and the stool softener Colace®. In this case, the brand name seemed to be far more effective than the generic.

HEADACHES

You are more likely to get a headache during the first trimester. If you have headaches, it may be worthwhile to visit an optometrist and find out whether you need glasses or a change in your prescription. Headaches can also be caused by sinus congestion. There is often no obvious cause, and the problem disappears spontaneously by mid-pregnancy.

Try the following suggestions instead of using nonprescription medications for headaches:

- ❖ Get more rest.
- ❖ Drink plenty of fluids. During the first trimester of her first pregnancy, Sophia Amelia went to the emergency room, where she received IV fluids for a severe, prolonged migraine. She also was prescribed Tylenol 3 with Codeine®, but she could not keep it down. Shanna experienced migraines and drank chamomile and green teas, which helped some. Amy tried to tough it out.
- ❖ Learn relaxation techniques. Allison worked with her midwives on relaxation techniques, which helped alleviate her migraines. Neck relaxation exercises help prevent the muscle tension that can cause headaches. Find a place to relax and rest when a headache occurs. Use heat or massage to relax tense neck muscles; some women prefer scalp massages.
- ❖ Avoid noise and bright lights.
- ❖ Try covering your eyes with a cold compress.
- ❖ Try alternating hot and cold compressions if your sinuses are congested.

Call your doctor if your headaches are persistent or severe, or if they are accompanied by swelling of your face or hands, blurred vision, or double vision, as these conditions can be dangerous.

NOSEBLEEDS

Nora stated, "Right after I got pregnant I would wake up with red blood on my pillow." She also said, "I wasn't concerned, because nosebleeds are listed in the pregnancy books as being common during pregnancy." They are caused by an increase in the hormones progesterone and estrogen, and the fragility of the capillaries.

SKIN AND HAIR

Sharon commented, "My hair and skin were never better." The hair of pregnant women seems healthier and thicker during pregnancy because it grows faster and stops falling out. Both Naomi and Joan said their skin and hair were better than ever when they were pregnant.

There is much individual variation in skin changes. The skin of some women becomes dry and itchy, even painfully so. Women with this condition will be more comfortable if they wash with mild soaps, or no soap, and moisten their skin with unscented lotion. Others find their skin is oilier. Dawn recalled, "I started breaking out. It was like being a teenager again. My skin was oilier and my hair grew more." Sally had acne on her back with her first child and on her face with her second.

A woman's abdominal skin is marked with a very faint vertical line from the navel to the pubic hair. During pregnancy, this line grows darker on women with lighter skin. Some women experience *chloasma*, a condition in which patches of skin on the face and neck grow darker, especially on the forehead, nose, and cheeks. Some women develop *telangiectasias*, red, spidery markings on their skin, especially the limbs. Some of these color changes are reversed after pregnancy. Chloasma is enhanced by sunlight, and using a sunscreen lotion outdoors may keep it from becoming more noticeable.

Women who are at risk for pressure sores may be at further risk during pregnancy because of the added weight of pregnancy. The anemia associated with pregnancy can also worsen pressure sores. If pressure sores become infected, the infection can become systemic. Only a few of the women who were interviewed for this book had problems with pressure sores. Shelby got a pressure sore from rubbing against the side of her wheelchair after she gained 40 pounds during her pregnancy. Her skin improved in other ways, however. Shelby's sides got skinned, but they healed easily.

Several women noted that their skin had never been healthier than when they were pregnant. Sasha said, "It was the first time in my life that the sore on my foot healed." Sherry Adele said, "I had no problem during pregnancy with my prosthesis. The skin around my stump improved." Sabine said, "I was worried about skin ulcers, but I never got any." Amanda had a crack in a bone from falling, and thought her bone healed faster than usual. She said, "It usually took 6 to 8 weeks to heal. But when I was pregnant, I could touch my stump against things without pain after only 3 weeks." Sylvia said, "When my skin got red over the pressure points, I started using a special pillow, and that kept it from getting worse." Good care and nutrition can also prevent and heal pressure sores.

Interaction Between Pregnancy and Disability

Some of the changes related to disability, such as increased incontinence, are not so obviously related to the changes of pregnancy. Some remissions and exacerbations of disability can be related to hormonal changes. The nature of these relationships is still being studied.

Although rheumatoid arthritis often improves during pregnancy, sometimes it grows unpredictably worse. In some cases, arthritic symptoms first appear during pregnancy. Joan said, "I went right into remission. That was one of the first clues that I was pregnant. I had no pain." Amanda's chronic hip pains from arthritis went away. She said, "It was the most fabulous time in my life." This was not the case during her second pregnancy. Jennifer's joint pain improved starting in the first trimester, but her skin sensitivity worsened in late pregnancy. Roberta's arthritic pain did not improve until the second trimester. Renée's arthritic pain first appeared early in her first pregnancy, and gradually grew worse as her pregnancy continued. "About 75 percent of rheumatoid arthritis patients improve during pregnancy" (77).

Nadine Fiona's fibromyalgia got worse. She said, "I was in constant pain. It was horrendous." This was during her first trimester. Other types of disability are also prone to exacerbation.

The type and degree of exacerbation also varies among women who have systemic lupus erythematosus. For example, Laura had increased joint pain. She said, "Each morning when I woke up, different joints ached." Leslie's joint pain went away, and her psoriasis improved when she was pregnant.

Leslie's temperature fluctuated between 96 and 101°F throughout her first two pregnancies. This lasted until she was given medication in her third pregnancy. The average temperature when taken under the tongue is 98.6°F, but this can vary from person to person.

Although exacerbation of the symptoms of multiple sclerosis is not expected to worsen during pregnancy, some women have had exacerbation. Marsha, for example, had difficulty gripping small objects. She could not write, hold things, or use a can opener.

Some women with high spinal cord injuries may have more frequent episodes of dysreflexia. It is not clear why, but one possibility is that the bladder and bowel are more quickly filled as the uterus enlarges.

Another woman experienced stabbing pain caused by her shunt because both the baby and the shunt were lying low in her abdomen.

Complications

CHOREA GRAVIDARUM

Chorea gravidarum means "the dance of pregnancy." This condition is rare. Women who have systemic lupus erythematosus are more susceptible to this disorder, which is characterized by repetitive involuntary movements. There are medications for this condition, but there have been few opportunities to study the effects of these drugs on fetuses.

ECTOPIC PREGNANCY

This unusual complication occurs when the fertilized ovum implants anywhere other than the lining of the uterine cavity. This usually occurs in one of the *fallopian tubes* (tubes leading from the ovaries to the uterus), but not always. Although it is frequently used, the term *tubal pregnancy* is incomplete, because some ectopic pregnancies occur elsewhere.

A tubal ectopic pregnancy can occur when an obstruction, such as adhesions caused by past pelvic infections, or a tumor, interferes with the passage of the ovum into the uterus. This is a dangerous complication because of the risk that the pregnancy will rupture the fallopian tube, causing potentially fatal bleeding. The usual treatment is surgical removal of the fetus. The signs and symptoms of ectopic pregnancy may also be caused by other conditions. For example, abdominal pain and tenderness might also be caused by localized infection. Abdominal pain may be the first presentation in serious complications. Appendicitis should be suspected in any woman having abdominal pain. Appendicitis can be confused with other more common problems in pregnancy that cause abdominal pain, including ectopic pregnancy, *abruptio placentae*, twisted ovarian cysts, and pyelonephritis (78).

Blood tests and sonograms are used for diagnosis. The signs and symptoms vary for ectopic pregnancies, and any of the following might indicate ectopic pregnancy, justifying an immediate call to your doctor:

❖ Bleeding or spotting following a missed period or confirmation of pregnancy
❖ Severe cramping pain and tenderness in the lower abdomen, sometimes one-sided
❖ Nausea and vomiting
❖ Sharp shoulder pain
❖ Sudden dizziness, weakness, or fainting, possibly accompanied by clammy skin and/or a fast, weak pulse

MISCARRIAGE AND THREATENED MISCARRIAGE

Miscarriage is a common term for spontaneous abortion of a fetus that is too immature to survive after birth. After about the twenty-second week of pregnancy, the fetus has some chance of surviving. Birth after the twenty-second week, and before the thirty-seventh week, is considered preterm or premature birth. *Threatened miscarriage* refers to the presence of signs or symptoms of impending miscarriage.

Miscarriages occur for a variety of reasons, including fetal death, Rh incompatibility, placental abnormalities, hormonal insufficiencies, fibroid tumors, and infection. In some cases, the cause is unknown. It is highly likely that Felicia had a miscarriage. She said, "The doctors believed that I miscarried one of my twins. At 5 weeks, my hormone levels dropped, and the doctors expected me to miscarry. I bled heavily for several days. When I went in for a D and C (dilation and curettage), the doctors found a heartbeat, much to their surprise. They said, 'So you still have a baby.'"

It is *extremely rare* for falls or accidents to cause a miscarriage. Many disabled women worry about falling, but the uterine wall and amniotic fluid cushion most blows. Ninety percent of miscarriages occur in the first trimester, usually before 8 weeks. Some women blame their disabilities. A few disabilities can put women at risk for miscarriages. They can also occur if the placenta is implanted in the front wall of the uterus. Some of the interviewees fell during pregnancy, but only Carla had a miscarriage after an incident she correctly described as "a freak accident." Her abdomen was struck by the handle of a baby carriage in just such a manner that the fetus was injured. She realized the circumstances were very unusual, and commented, "I didn't feel guilty. Somehow I didn't feel like I wanted to punish myself."

Often the only possible treatment during the first trimester for threatened miscarriage is total bed rest. Many women feel frustrated and discouraged when they are forced to neglect their responsibilities in order to rest. It may be heartening to know that rest was effective for Sara, who said, "I had some spotting during my second pregnancy. I was told to rest for several days, and I didn't have any problems after that."

At week 13, Natalie woke up to spotting. She said, "It was awful. I did not expect to see bright red blood. The emergency room doctor said not to worry because there wasn't any cramping. I went to see my regular doctor the next day, and he heard the baby's heartbeat. The blood went from bright red to brown, and then it stopped." Resting does not guarantee a good outcome, but it offers the best chance to avoid a miscarriage. Laura explained, "I knew that I only had a 50 percent chance of a successful pregnancy, so I took it one day at a time. I listened to my body and didn't push myself."

Women who have systemic lupus erythematosus are at increased risk for miscarriage because they may have antibodies that cause formation of blood clots in the placenta and eventual placental rejection. Appropriate medications can be prescribed if a threatened miscarriage is related to the complications of systemic lupus erythematosus. Studies suggest that medical treatment of systemic lupus erythematosus has improved the rate of successful pregnancies. Leslie's experience is an example. Her longest lasting pregnancy was her third, during which she received medication. Her miscarriage of one twin in the first trimester was due to cervical incompetence, meaning her cervix was too weak to hold the fetus in. The second twin was born prematurely and died.

Often sonography is necessary to evaluate a threatened miscarriage. When Cheryl experienced spotting after her pregnancy was confirmed, a sonogram showed that her fetus was of normal size and activity. Then it was determined that the problem was localized bleeding in the cervix. Christina's experience was different, "I wasn't even sure I was pregnant. I thought I might be having either a period or a miscarriage. I went to the doctor, who confirmed that I was pregnant. An ultrasound was done when I kept on bleeding heavily. It showed I had placenta previa; my placenta was lower than the fetus, possibly covering my cervix. They said there was a chance it would improve as the baby grew." Christina was able to give birth vaginally.

The symptoms that indicate a possible miscarriage require urgent medical attention, including:

❖ Bleeding with lower abdominal cramps or pain
❖ Pain that is severe or lasts more than a day, even without bleeding
❖ Heavy bleeding or light staining lasting more than 3 days

Women who experience these symptoms should call their doctors immediately, before blood loss reaches a dangerous level.

Other symptoms also represent an emergency. If a woman experiences these symptoms and her doctor is unavailable, she should leave a message at the doctor's office and go to a hospital emergency room:

❖ Bleeding and/or cramping in a woman who has had previous miscarriages
❖ Unbearable pain
❖ Bleeding heavily enough to soak several pads in an hour
❖ Passage of clots or grayish material. (Your doctor might instruct you to bring this material to the hospital in a clean container).

If a miscarriage does occur, a D and C may be necessary. During this procedure, the cervix is dilated and instruments are inserted to remove the materials of pregnancy from the uterus. This procedure prevents infection, and the possibility of bleeding caused by tissues retained in an incomplete miscarriage.

Perhaps the most difficult problem any woman can face is a miscarriage. It is important that a woman who has had a miscarriage not minimize her feelings. She needs to know that it is common for women in her position to feel just as much grief as women who suffer late pregnancy losses. She needs to allow herself time to grieve rather than telling herself (or letting other people tell her) that "it was only a miscarriage," and that she can "try again soon." It is appropriate and important to join a support group for parents who have had similar experiences, or to seek counseling. It is also important for her to take care of herself physically. The blood loss and other changes associated with a miscarriage are stressful on the body. Adequate rest, nutrition, and medical care are important and necessary for a full recovery. Physical recovery can contribute to a good emotional recovery. Remember that sleeplessness and loss of appetite can be manifestations of depression. These problems can be worked on with professional help, if necessary, so that recovery is possible. This way, the miscarriage will have less of a negative effect on you and the people you are close to.

Arlene's comments reflect many of the feelings women express after some time has passed. "When I had those miscarriages, I knew it wasn't meant to be. I think now that my daughter has been born, I pushed the other two aside. I have learned to be philosophical because of my background of being disabled and a research example."

If a woman feels emotionally ready to try again, she should first discuss it with her doctor to make certain she is physically ready. At the same time, she can discuss any questions she has about the possibility of preventing another miscarriage.

THROMBOPHLEBITIS

Thrombophlebitis is an inflammation of a vein. When inflammation occurs, blood clots (thrombi) may form. *Deep vein phlebitis* is potentially dangerous because of the risk that clots will break loose and be carried to the lungs (thromboembolism). Superficial vein phlebitis is less likely to be dangerous.

During pregnancy, the risk of thrombophlebitis in the leg or pelvic veins increases. Women who have post-polio syndrome or spinal cord injuries are already at increased risk, and must be especially watchful for symptoms during pregnancy. Symptoms may include local pain, tenderness, or swelling. Sometimes the whole limb swells. Women with reduced sensation need to watch closely for visible swelling.

Rest, elevation, elastic support of the limb, and mild pain relievers may be sufficient treatment if the problem is in a superficial vein. Deep vein thrombosis is difficult to diagnose, and special diagnostic procedures and treatment with anticoagulants (medication to prevent further clotting) may be necessary.

Adequate exercise is important for preventing thrombosis, but do not exercise if symptoms occur. Contact your doctor immediately and rest until you receive further instructions.

Only one of the women who were interviewed encountered this problem. Sharon had had phlebitis in one leg prior to pregnancy, and it became swollen again in the third trimester. Sharon was not very concerned. She said, "I was conscious of the problem. I made sure I kept the leg elevated both at work and at home." She chose not to use anticoagulants. Sharon's decision worked for her, but this is not a safe guideline for other women. In each case, the relative risks of treating or not treating are different, and should be carefully discussed by the woman and her physician.

Fetal and Placental Development

The fetus remains very small during the first trimester. It is no larger than a grain of rice by the end of the first month. By the end of the third month, it is about 3 inches long, weighing half an ounce. Most of the organ systems, including the skeleton, heart, liver, etc., begin to develop in the first trimester. The limbs are "buds" in which the fingers and toes have not separated. The reproductive organs have started to form, but it is still difficult to distinguish boys from girls at the end of the third month. The fetus can kick and clench its fists, but the mother cannot feel these movements.

The placenta begins to develop as part of a membrane surrounding the fetus and eventually becomes a large, specialized organ. It attaches firmly to the uterine wall by means of many villi (finger-like projections) that penetrate the wall. Nutrients and oxygen pass from maternal vessels in the uterine wall, through the placental blood barrier, and into fetal vessels in the placental villi. Under ordinary circumstances, the maternal blood and the baby's blood never mix. It is usually dangerous for the infant on the rare occasions when they do mix. In addition, many medicines, street drugs, and alcohol are able to cross the placental barrier, enter the infant's circulation, and cause harm, including potentially severe harm. The umbilical cord contains blood vessels connecting the placental vessels to the fetal heart. Normally, the umbilical vessels close at birth.

Besides being the organ that provides nutrients to the fetus, the placenta is an important source of certain pregnancy hormones.

Emotional Concerns

Women who have just learned that they are pregnant react with a variety of emotions, including shock, delight, amazement, and/or fear. Their emotions are also linked with how their loved ones react. Sophia Amelia had an unusual reaction—she found that her sex drive dramatically increased during the first trimester of her first pregnancy. She said, "I partied my tail off without any drugs or alcohol. Men paid more attention to me than ever before because I had large breasts. I would go out with my friends as the designated driver because I couldn't sleep!"

For some women with disabilities the first reaction is surprise that pregnancy is even possible. Stacy, who had thought she was merely ill, said, "I was shocked and skeptical. I thought all the X-rays had made me sterile." Oprah was also totally surprised. She said, "I figured I couldn't have kids because of OI and all the breaks and surgeries."

Women who have been trying for a long time to get pregnant can experience a dreamlike feeling of unreality. Samantha said, "I was absolutely thrilled. I had wanted it for so long!" Nora said, "*I couldn't believe it!* I had tried everything: infertility treatment, adoption. I wasn't able to adopt because of prejudice. Becoming pregnant was my ultimate dream." Emotions are strong, and women who have wanted to be pregnant speak in glowing terms. Sheila and Priscilla both said they were ecstatic. Sheila said, "I didn't have any fears for myself or about the baby." Paula said, "It was pure joy." Amanda said, "I was afraid during my first pregnancy that I would drop the baby when she was born. It was totally irrational, because I had taken care of plenty of children and I'd never come close to dropping a child. I think I took on this fear because so many people brought it up."

Most of the interviewees had mixed feelings. Noelle described her reaction to her first pregnancy as "a combination of emotions somewhere between panic and exhilaration." Some women's ambivalence had nothing to do with disability. One woman recalled, "I was ecstatic when I found out I was pregnant with my second child, but I also felt some apprehension because my husband and I were having problems with our relationship." Sienna said, "I didn't have a lot of patience or tolerance for the first couple of months. I was irritable and short-tempered, especially with my husband, but thankfully he endured me." On the other hand, Sally thought it helped her relationship, "I think it was positive because we did a lot of research about doing it right. It was well planned and well thought out." Several other women also stated that pregnancy strengthened their relationships.

Other women worried about the effects of pregnancy, delivery, or childcare on their disability. Stephanie said, "I was excited, but at the same time I was reluctant because of all the physical work required in taking care of a child." Both Hannah and Celeste were anxious about the delivery itself. Hannah was worried during her first pregnancy about the effect the delivery would have on her. She did not have this concern with her second pregnancy until a few days before delivery, when she found out how big her baby was. Celeste said, "I was frightened of giving birth, and afraid I might not get a C-section." She gave birth vaginally without any difficulty. Other women, including Carla, Cheryl, and Sara, worried that their children would be born with disabilities. Many aspects of the interaction between pregnancy and disability are discussed in Chapter 3, and women will find many of their questions answered there.

Most women's emotions change over time. A woman who feels pure joy at first may begin to have a few practical worries. A woman who is shocked at first may begin to enjoy being pregnant. Nina tried to get pregnant for 2 years, and was not sure if she could. She hardly believed it when she was finally pregnant. Nina felt conflicted because she had decided to go back to school. She had just won her fight to be trained as a teacher. She said, "It was hard for me to be happy at that time." Celeste recalled, "I was ambivalent at first because my husband wasn't sure he wanted children. But then we went out and shared a milkshake, and we began to giggle, and he said that it was wonderful." Like Celeste, many women find that their feelings are affected by the reactions of others. In the first trimester, a woman has some control over the situation; the only people who know that she is pregnant are the ones she chooses to tell. Their reactions can be very influential.

Most parents are worried about how the pregnancy will affect their daughter. But one of their larger fears is how their daughter will be able to physically take care of the baby. They are also concerned that they will have to take over that responsibility. Amanda's husband was very supportive during her second pregnancy. Even though she had successfully parented her first child, her mother was not supportive during the second pregnancy. Her mother felt that Amanda's plate was full enough.

Andrea's mother had the same attitude. When Andrea was pregnant with her first child, her mother was very concerned about how she was going to get around, and whether she would be able to carry the baby. Her mother relaxed completely after Andrea had her first child because she saw that Andrea could manage with some minor adaptations. Andrea was fortunate that her family was supportive of her leading an independent and productive life.

Nadine Fiona's situation was similar to many women with disabilities. "My mom and my grandparents were mad, even though I was married. They thought it was going to be harmful, and they treated me as if I was an invalid. This was at the beginning. They weren't so worried after they saw that I was doing okay." Women who want support while being pregnant should offer information to their families explaining how women with disabilities can have good pregnancies and can be successful parents. Women who do not get the support they need should seek out support. Nadine Fiona felt alone, until she found support. She said, "I've learned to deal with whatever I have to." Rachel's parents were apprehensive about her ability to handle the experience of childbirth and be a parent. She had a problem birth when her first child was born. Rachel said, "My mother, father, and brother were worried about my ability to care for this baby, but I knew that I would find a way." Sasha said, "I was horrified when I found out I was pregnant because my family was always so fearful for my health. I never enjoyed my pregnancy because they were so worried."

Julie's story was different from Sasha's. She was upset by her unplanned pregnancy, and worried that she could not afford to have a child. She feared that her family would reject her for being a single mother. In addition, she worried that her pregnancy would worsen her disability. She was at work when she found out that her pregnancy test was positive, and she went to the bathroom to be alone. Another worker found Julie crying, and when she poured out her feelings, the co-worker said, "This is such a beautiful miracle for anyone to experience. Forget about anyone thinking badly about you. All that matters is you and the baby." Julie said, "I began to feel hopeful because she was so sympathetic."

Julie's experience confirms many research findings that women feel better about their pregnancies when friends and family are supportive.

Unlike many of the interviewees, Sophia Amelia's first pregnancy ended her relationship with the baby's father. Although the pregnancy ended that relationship, it strengthened her relationship with her parents. Nevertheless, her parents were worried and concerned about how the pregnancy would affect her body. Her relationship with the father was re-established after the birth of her first child, and they married when the child was 2 years old. They now have a second child.

Although Joy's parents were concerned about the health of both Joy and the baby, they were very helpful.

Natasha had been engaged for 2 years when she became pregnant and got married a few months later. Her relationship with her husband was strengthened, even though her parents and in-laws were worried whether Natasha could handle pregnancy and parenting. Natasha was able to get support from her grandmother.

Many women begin to wonder whether their emotions will ever return to normal. The physical and hormonal changes of pregnancy often cause women to overreact to ordinary situations or change moods suddenly. Tessa found herself more irritable. She wished she had known that being irritable in the first trimester was part of the hormonal changes, because then she could have told her husband "I'm really crabby, but it's just an adjustment to pregnancy hormones." Tessa also felt the pregnancy bonded her relationship to her husband, and that they "were in it for the long haul."

Some of the emotional responses women experience are because of physical sensations. For example, frustration at feeling tired all the time. Sylvia said, "My mood would depend on how I was feeling physically. It was depressing when I got sweats or a lot of spasms." Shanna became depressed because she felt more dependent. Noreen also felt depressed, and had to drop out of her last year in college because she was so tired. She went home to live with her mother. She said, "My mother was a big support throughout my pregnancy. I tried to keep busy with reading and watching videos. I was used making the best of my time without having much visible strength because I have myasthenia gravis."

A few of the interviewees specifically mentioned being troubled by emotional extremes; many described strong reactions to particular problems. Arianna's doctors did not know her prior to her pregnancy. She felt it affected her pregnancy. She said, "All of the doctors felt that I wasn't going to be able to carry any baby, and especially twins, long enough for them to survive. They made me feel that if I did make it, it would be a miracle. I *knew* I was going to have a baby. I tried not to let anything they said bother me."

Women find a variety of ways to cope with their emotions. They may distract themselves by getting involved in shopping for the new baby, or calm themselves with special relaxation techniques. It is helpful to compare notes with other pregnant women. Pam did not like having to spend more time resting, but she said, "I have an able-bodied cousin who was pregnant at the same time I was. I told myself, 'If she can lie down, I can lie down.'" Several women made similar comments. A few enjoyed the unusual experience of feeling better than other people. Priscilla's only problem in the first trimester was fatigue. She said, "It helped to compare notes with women who had many more discomforts than I did." Sophia Amelia said, "I thought my pregnancy might be unique, but most of it seemed pretty typical." Sabine also agreed, "I wanted to compare myself with other women in order to have more to understanding of what was normal." Andrea said, "It was wonderful to know that I was feeling the same thing as other women. I got more information from my girlfriends than my doctor." Darlene had similar feelings. She said, "I did not talk to many little people (dwarfs), but I did talk with other women. It felt good to compare my pregnancy with theirs because it made me feel normal. I felt like I fit in with other women, and that I, too, was a woman who could become a mom."

Joy compared her pregnancy to that of her sister and mother. She said, "I compared how I felt and what was going on with me. I wanted to compare my pregnancy to theirs to find out if I was going to end up with the same problems. Joy did not have preeclampsia like both her sister and mom, but she did have nausea.

Closing Comments

When a woman realizes that she is pregnant, she generally experiences a myriad of emotions. These emotions can range from sheer joy to ambivalence and anxiety. During the first trimester, the joy of pregnancy outweighs the discomfort that many women experience during this time. Women look forward to the second trimester because they know they will start to feel better, *and* the baby will start to move.

Nine Months of Change:
The Second Trimester

MOST WOMEN FEEL COMFORTABLE with pregnancy by the beginning of the second trimester. The discomforts of early pregnancy, such as morning sickness, will have begun to abate. The baby will begin to move, and can be visually seen on a sonogram. For many women, the second trimester is a time of great joy.

Office Visits

You will visit your doctor once a month during the second trimester. These visits are usually shorter because the full physical examination is usually not repeated. The visit will include routine measurements of your weight and blood pressure, and a urine test. The level of alpha-fetoprotein level will be measured by a blood test sometime between the fifteenth and twentieth weeks of pregnancy (see "Diagnostic Tests"). Your doctor may order periodic blood sugar tests if you are at risk for developing the diabetes of pregnancy, also known as gestational diabetes. Your risk of developing diabetes is higher if you are obese, you previously gave birth to a large baby, or if you have a family history of diabetes or had gestational diabetes. If an earlier blood test showed you were anemic, your doctor may repeat this test. Some women with disabilities may need repeated blood tests to assess medication levels or kidney function.

The uterus has grown enough by now to make it possible to measure the height of the *fundus* (top of the uterus) at each visit. These measurements help determine the how long you have been pregnant and the growth rate of the baby.

The office visit will include an opportunity for you and your doctor to discuss any physical or emotional changes you are experiencing. Write down your questions before each visit in as much detail as possible. No symptom is too unimportant to mention to your doctor, who can then reassure you, give practical advice, or order diagnostic tests if necessary. For example, tell your doctor if you have been feeling tired, even though it is common for pregnant women to experience fatigue. Your doctor may ask you questions in order to determine whether to test you for anemia, exacerbation of your disability, or thyroid problems. She may also suggest ways you can reduce stress. For example, if you have been experiencing headaches, note whether they are located at the front or back of your head. Is there a constant ache or throbbing? Does the headache occur at a certain time of day? Is it accompanied by other symptoms?

If you are at risk for a premature birth, a hormone injection of 17-alpha-hydroxy progesterone caproate, given between the sixteenth and twentieth weeks of pregnancy can help reduce the risk of premature births (80).

Your doctor will also ask whether you have felt the fetus kicking. At first this sensation is difficult to recognize. You will find descriptions of this amazing experience below in the section on physical changes. Whether you feel your baby kick hard or soft will depend on where the placenta is implanted. Amanda said, "I felt the second baby move less than the first."

Mimi said, "The baby's grandmother saw her move before I even realized it was the baby moving. It didn't feel like the butterflies everyone told me I would feel."

If you have had genetic testing or other special tests, your doctor will explain the results to you during your office visit. Make sure he explains the test results in sufficient detail.

Diagnostic Tests

SONOGRAPHY

Sonography may be used during the second trimester to determine the cause of pain or bleeding, or to arrive at a more accurate assessment of fetal size and age than is possible from external examination alone. If the fetus seems to have stopped moving, or its heartbeat is difficult to detect, sonography can help determine whether there is a problem. It can also be used as an adjunct to amniocentesis. Sonography produces a *sonogram*, an image that looks like a still photograph. "Real-time" ultrasound produces a screen image that shows the fetus in motion.

Sonography can also reveal whether there is a normal amount of amniotic fluid, locate the placenta, and determine whether the fetus is of normal size and activity. Some deformities, including neural tube defects, may be detected during this procedure. Joan was offered amniocentesis because the doctor found an echogenic focus in the baby's heart that showed up as a bright spot on her ultrasound. This type of bright spot can indicate a possible abnormality, Joan's baby showed no abnormalities.

Depending on when the sonogram is taken, and the position of the fetus, it may be possible to see the fetal heartbeat and determine the baby's gender. Twins are often discovered during sonography.

During the second trimester, the uterus is large enough that the mother will not need to intentionally fill her bladder before the procedure. Sonography is often rather routine at this stage of pregnancy. Many parents feel it is an exciting opportunity to see their baby for the first time. Hearing a heartbeat and seeing a picture makes it feel like the baby is "real." In some scrapbooks, "baby's first picture" is a sonogram!

Women who have systemic lupus erythematosus will need sonography monthly, starting at the twentieth week, because of the increased risks of growth retardation and stillbirth. They will need this procedure every 1 to 2 weeks if there is evidence that the fetus has congenital heart block.

FETAL ECHOCARDIOGRAPHY

This procedure uses ultrasound to study the fetal heart. If the fetal heartbeat shows signs of congenital heart block (an infrequent complication of systemic lupus erythematosus), it can be determined whether there are also structural defects in the heart. This procedure is usually done at 20 to 22 weeks of pregnancy.

AMNIOCENTESIS

During this procedure, a very small amount of amniotic fluid is withdrawn from the amniotic sac through the anesthetized abdomen. The doctor will determine the positions of the fetus and placenta by using real-time ultrasound. A sample of amniotic fluid is then taken using a syringe. A local anesthetic is used, and having an amniocentesis is no more uncomfortable than having a blood sample drawn. There is a small (as low as 1 in 300) but real risk, however, that the procedure will cause infection or miscarriage. Therefore, this test is only used for specific important indications. Discuss the risks and benefits thoroughly with your doctor and/or a genetic counselor before you have an amniocentesis. This discussion should include safety and accuracy statistics at the facility where the test will be performed. If you think there may be a high chance of having a child with Down's syndrome, you may want to consider nuchal translucency (see Chapter 8).

The amniotic fluid will be chemically analyzed, and the results should be available within 24 hours. If the maternal alpha-fetoprotein (AFP) test or the family history suggests that the fetus may have a neural tube defect, measuring the amount of AFP in the amniotic fluid can determine whether there is a problem. Having abnormal results caused Holly to debate with her husband whether she should have amniocentesis. She worried about the procedure causing infection of the peritoneal cavity wherein her shunt lies and premature labor. She said, "We finally decided to do it because I did not want to spend the rest of the pregnancy wondering if something was wrong with the baby. Her baby had trisomy 13. This is an extra chromosome on the 13th chromosome pair, but unlike some chromosomal disorders, such as Down's syndrome, trisomy 13 is always fatal. Holly said, "There is no hope for these babies. That is the only reason we terminated the pregnancy. My doctors felt there was a good chance that the baby would die inside me. They worried the baby would turn septic and infect my shunt system."

Sometimes the amniotic fluid is examined for the presence of infectious organisms.

Genetic testing involves obtaining some of the cells that the fetus has shed into the amniotic fluid. These are collected from the amniocentesis sample and cultured until there is enough genetic material for analysis. Results are available approximately 3 weeks after the amniocentesis. Women who are over 35, or who have a family history of genetic disorders, may want to consider genetic testing.

Women who do not want to terminate their pregnancies may also choose genetic testing. One woman said, "Even though I knew I wouldn't abort the baby, I had amniocentesis because of my age. I just wanted to know." Weighing the value of this knowledge against the risk of genetic testing is a very individual decision. Noelle agreed to have an amniocentesis in order to assist with research on her disability (see Chapter 3).

Joan was offered amniocentesis because something suspicious was seen on her ultrasound. She said, "They told me there was a less than 1 percent chance there was anything wrong because all my blood work came back great. They asked me if I wanted amniocentesis to make sure it wasn't some chromosomal dysfunction. I decided that there was more risk in having the amniocentesis than having an abnormality. Plus, if the baby had a disability we would make great parents because we would understand what she was going through."

Some women want to know the sex of the fetus after genetic testing, because knowing the sex helps with preparations such as shopping for clothing and choosing a name. Others enjoy being surprised, and wait until the baby is born to find out whether it is a boy or a girl.

STRESS AND NON-STRESS TESTS

These tests are more commonly used during the third trimester, but may be performed in the second trimester if there are signs of fetal distress or threatened miscarriage. Women who have myasthenia gravis, systemic lupus erythematosus (SLE), or spinal cord injuries are at increased risk for preterm labor, and they may need these tests (see Chapter 10).

ADDITIONAL BLOOD TESTS

Women who have kidney problems will need frequent kidney function tests. "Correct diagnosis of a lupus nephritis flare during pregnancy relies on recognition of signs of disease activity in other typical SLE target organs. For instance, true arthritis, cutaneous vasculitis, mouth ulcers, or lymphadenopathy, coexisting with worsening *proteinuria* (protein in the urine), point to a lupus flare. Rising levels of anti-DNA antibodies and/or active urinary sediment, including hematuria and red, white, or granular cell casts, are also suggestive of SLE. The sensitivity of these laboratory tests is not 100 percent, however, because they are not uniformly positive in every case of lupus nephritis" (81).

Medical Procedure

PLASMAPHERESIS

If symptoms of myasthenia gravis are severe and resistant to medication, *plasmapheresis* may be considered. During this procedure, the mother's blood plasma is replaced by donor plasma. The exchange is made very slowly, so that normal blood pressure can be maintained. During the procedure the mother must lie on her left side, unless her disability forces her to lie on her right side. If she lies on her back, pressure from the uterus might interfere with blood circulation. This procedure is usually not too uncomfortable. You simply have to anticipate spending $1\frac{1}{2}$ to 2 hours lying on your side with an IV needle in your arm.

Physical Changes

As the uterus and fetus continue to grow, and the amount of amniotic fluid increases, the abdomen becomes more rounded. The pregnancy will be obvious by the fourteenth week, and most women will need to start wearing maternity clothes early in the second trimester.

You must not lie flat on your back or sleep on your right side, if possible, because the enlarged uterus will put extra weight on major blood vessels, which can interfere with circulation. The uterus also puts pressure on the vein that brings blood back to the heart. You may also find it difficult to lie on your stomach. Try sleeping with pillows under your knees if you must sleep on your back.

Many of the changes experienced in the first trimester, such as breast growth, increased vaginal discharge, and changes in skin color, continue during the second trimester. Olivia said, "My breasts became really big, and I felt sexy."

Tessa found that having bigger breasts required additional bra support. This additional support usually results in having tighter bra straps, causing the bra straps to pull down on the shoulder muscles and the collarbones (the clavicles), which constricts the nerves even more. Tessa recommends wearing a strapless bra or an exercise bra.

Increased blood flow often makes the genitals appear darker and more swollen. Most women notice that their hair and fingernails grow faster, an interesting coincidence, because the fetal hair also starts growing in the second trimester.

FETAL MOVEMENT

Feeling the baby move is even more exciting than hearing its heartbeat. Christina recalled, "I was in church when I first felt him kick, but I yelled anyway. I couldn't help myself." Cheryl said, "The joy of feeling life inside me made me glad to be a woman." By the end of the second trimester, most women can share their excitement by inviting other people to feel the baby kick.

The fetus starts moving during the second month, but movement is generally felt between 18 and 22 weeks, usually about week 19. A thin woman may feel the baby move earlier than heavier women. Whether you feel your baby's kick as hard or soft will depend on where the placenta is implanted. Amanda said, "I felt the second baby move less than the first."

A woman who has already experienced pregnancy is likely to recognize fetal movement earlier, because the sensation can be difficult to recognize at first. Nadia said, "The kicking of this baby was like the other two."

Sharon explained, "It was muted. It felt more like pressure. Then I would put my hand on my belly and feel the movement." Stacy and Samantha said they saw the movement before they could feel it. Sally said, "It felt like little tickles, or butterflies."

Sydney did not have the internal sensation of her baby kicking, except when he kicked her in her ribs. She said "I kept my hand on my belly so I could feel him kick." The location of the placenta can affect how much movement you feel. If it is at the front of your uterus, it will tend to cushion your baby's movements, which could make it hard to notice the movement (82).

Signey said, "I visually saw them move by the end of the second trimester. I started seeing bumps and movements on my belly. I don't know if I could have felt them moving if I had closed my eyes."

Natalie did not know if her disability was the reason she did not feel the baby kick. She said, "I'm a small person, so he did not have much room to move." She was able to feel the baby kick when the kicks were strong. She said, "The hard kicks would only happen occasionally." Natalie's doctor wanted her husband to feel for the baby's kicks and count them. During her second pregnancy, Natalie said, "I felt strong fetal movement throughout my pregnancy. The baby kicked so hard this time that other people could see my stomach jerk or ripple through my clothes." Sienna said, "The movement felt like a rolling marble."

Noreen had the opposite experience. She thought she felt her baby kick, but the doctors disagreed. They said there was an excess of amniotic fluid, and the baby had contractures. In spite of this, Noreen said, "The thought of my son being born always excited me."

Nikki said, "My kids never kicked hard; maybe they are calmer than other kids."

Many women describe it as a fluttering movement; others compare it to gas pains. Nora, Patricia, and Laura all said, "It felt like the baby had hiccups." Laura added, "Sometimes it felt like a wiggling fish."

Diane said, "The movement felt like bubbles popping." Natasha experienced it as "a muscle twitching, or a muscle spasm that lasted for a few minutes; except I had it in my stomach area."

Other women have found the kicking difficult. Orielle said, "He was pretty active. He was sideways, so he kept kicking my ribs. He would get his little feet under my ribs and push on them. He never broke any of my ribs, but it wasn't very comfortable.

Several of the interviewees remarked that the fetal movement felt the same as it had in pregnancies that occurred before they had become disabled.

The Discomforts of Pregnancy

Most women find the second trimester to be the most comfortable, because they are no longer bothered by the unpleasant symptoms of early pregnancy such as nausea and vomiting. Nadine Fiona said that her fibromyalgia disappeared during the second and third trimesters, and she had "zero pain." Corrine commented, "The second trimester was the only time when I had no problems at all." Most women feel more energetic, but a few are still troubled by fatigue. Naomi was lethargic during her second pregnancy. She said, "I felt spacey a lot of the time. These feelings were probably due to gestational diabetes, although this was not diagnosed until her third trimester. Naomi was able to control the diabetes through diet.

Gestational diabetes is caused by pregnancy, but it has been theorized that women who develop diabetes during pregnancy have a predisposition to type 2 diabetes (adult onset diabetes). Research shows that 50 percent of the women with gestational diabetes will develop type 2 diabetes. Medication is recommended if diet cannot control it.

Some disabled women find that weight gain limits their mobility during the second trimester; others feel great. Christina said, "I felt so good that I went out in my wheelchair and did all kinds of things." Looking pregnant and feeling the baby kick can also be so satisfying that many women are less annoyed by the discomforts they experience.

Dorothy said, "I felt more immobilized. The extra weight was hard to accommodate." Women also need to be aware that weight gain can have other consequences in addition to mobility problems. For example, Shelby said, "When I gained 40 pounds, I did not fit in my wheelchair." When she borrowed a larger size wheelchair, she had problems putting the chair in her car.

Allison's midwives sent her to an orthopedist because of pains in both of her knees. She found it difficult to step up onto curbs and climb stairs. Allison had an X-ray to help diagnose arthritis in her knees. Dennis Swigart has stated, "Concentrate on taking big steps while walking. Look for softer, shock-absorbing surfaces like grass" (11).

Noreen felt very bad during the fourth and fifth months. She said, "The myasthenia symptoms were all exacerbated. I had trouble walking even a few steps. Most of the time I needed help with sitting up and getting up. I had trouble eating and chewing. I had trouble with every activity."

Although Nadia was first aware of symptoms and diagnosed with myasthenia gravis during her second trimester, she may have had some other symptoms in the first trimester. She said, "There was a marked difference between my first two pregnancies and this pregnancy. I had to lie down to rest whenever my kids were lying down. I had to go to bed by 7:30. I had a bad sinus infection during the first two trimesters, which could have contributed to the fatigue."

Sabine had experienced radicular pain (pain at the site of a nerve root or along the path for which a nerve supplies function) all her life, but during her first pregnancy the pain increased. It felt like a spasm. The pain began to increase just prior to her amniocentesis, and continued to increase in intensity soon afterwards. The pain was at the T-6,

T-7, and T-8 levels (the level of the ribs). It was sharp and knife-like, and would set off a spasm. Any kind of clothing could trigger the spasm, and "then an ungodly pain around the stomach." Sabine also had a gallstone attack that could have triggered this problem.

CRAMPS AND MUSCLE SPASMS (CLONUS)

The interviewees did not always differentiate between the two types of muscle spasms, cramping and clonus. Muscle cramps bother all women during pregnancy, but women with disabilities may have more frequent or severe cramps. If they experience clonus or cramps when they are not pregnant, it may become more frequent during pregnancy. These problems usually begin during the second trimester.

Cramps

Cramps are strong, painful, involuntary muscle contractions. The cramped muscle feels like a hard knot. Calf muscle cramps are the most common type of cramps. They usually occur at night. Sometimes a cramp in the calf can be relieved by firmly bending the foot upward. Some women sit on the edge of the bed and press the foot against the floor or wall. Others find the cramp so painful that they wake up their husbands and ask them to grasp the ball of the foot and bend it upwards (see Figure 7-5).

Some cramps can be avoided by taking preventive measures. Pointing the toe downward can cause a cramp, so try moving your foot in an upward direction. Tight bedclothes may cause a woman to point her toe as she sleeps; some women have fewer problems when they stop tucking in the top sheet. Many disabled women prefer satin sheets even when they are not pregnant, because they can move more easily between slippery sheets and have fewer problems with muscle cramps or tension.

Heat relieves soreness after cramps, and seems to prevent further cramping by relaxing the affected muscle. Many women take hot baths, but for some women with disabilities it is difficult to get in and out of the bathtub. Sara pointed out that it can even be difficult to check the water temperature, so she used a heating pad instead, even though she thought a bath might have been more effective. Sybil used massage, liniment, and a hot water bottle. Twenty minutes of heat should be sufficient to promote relaxation and good circulation. Women who have reduced sensation should check frequently for reddening of the skin when using a heating pad or hot water bottle to avoid a burn.

Noelle found that ice packs relieved her muscle cramps. Ice may have worked for her because of her particular disability, but other women may find that the cold makes the cramping worse.

Several of the interviewees discovered that sleeping position affected muscle cramping. Samantha only had cramps at night when she was very tired. She found it helpful to sleep with pillows between her knees, with her legs slightly bent. Sleeping with pillows between the knees also helped Cheryl to prevent groin cramps. Several of the other interviewees avoided thigh cramps by sleeping in this manner.

Amanda also experienced cramping from arthritis. She said, "I curled up when I slept, but when I shifted positions, my knee would be locked and it would be really painful to straighten it out."

Some of the stretching exercises in Chapter 7 can be very effective in preventing muscle cramps. Michelle remarked that she never had cramps until the last week of her pregnancy, when she was too tired to exercise.

Calcium supplements may also prevent cramping. Clara remarked, "I never drink milk, but taking calcium tablets eased the cramping" (see Chapter 4). It is important to consult your doctor before taking calcium supplements. Nikki said, "During my third pregnancy I had muscles spasms at night, so I took extra calcium, which alleviated my muscle spasms. Four hundred to 800 units of vitamin E (D Alpha, not d1 Alpha) may help, as well as B_{12} and iron supplements.

Clonus

Severe muscle spasms are called *clonus*, and they usually include involuntary movements. It is marked by contractions and relaxations of a muscle, occurring in rapid succession (83). Clara remarked that her ordinary calf cramps seemed to stimulate clonus. The spasm often ends more quickly when another person holds and supports the affected limb (Figures 11-1 and 11-2). Women who use anti-spasmodic medications when they are not pregnant should not resume or increase these medications during pregnancy without consulting the doctor about possible risks. Shelby had clonus more frequently during both pregnancies.

Botox® has been used for reducing spasticity. Moser and colleagues (84) have stated that although it was contraindicated for botulinum toxin type-A to be used during pregnancy, there were sixteen women who were given Botox® injections during pregnancy. The women who were given Botox® had *strabismus* (uncontrollable squinting), limb and cervical dystonia, *blepharospasm* (abnormal eyelid closures), and *oromandibular dystonia* (involuntary movement of the mouth). There were ten women who were injected during the first trimester; three women were injected during the second trimester; and two women were injected in the third trimester. In addition, one woman had taken the medication throughout her pregnancy. "There were fourteen full-term normal deliveries, one of which was twins." There were two miscarriages, however. "None of the newborns were floppy or had any problems during the postnatal period." The authors also stated, "Botulinum toxin type-A (Botox®) administered during pregnancy seems to have no adverse effects on the fetus or the mother. It should be given during pregnancy only if clearly needed."

Back Pain

Several physical changes can cause back pain in pregnancy. First, the hormones of pregnancy cause ligaments to relax, and pelvic joints become less stable. This is an advantage during childbirth. Second, the abdominal muscles are stretched and weakened as the uterus grows, and the back muscles must work harder. Third, the weight of the uterus puts additional strain on the muscles in the lower back. Hilary could feel the difference, and commented, "My back wasn't as rigid."

Women who are disabled are often more vulnerable to back pain, and may experience it earlier in pregnancy. Able-bodied women usually have no problems until the third trimester. Paula commented that she had no back problems during her first pregnancy, which occurred before she was disabled, but she did experience back pain in later pregnancies after her abdominal muscles were weakened. Noelle, too, thought that she felt more back pain in her third pregnancy because her abdominal muscles had become weaker. Several women with spinal cord injuries noticed back pain during pregnancy. It is not surprising that their backs were strained, because their abdominal muscles were already weakened by the disability. Possibly the pain was caused by putting additional strain on functioning muscles.

Felicia experienced back problems on and off during her pregnancy. She said, "My ability to walk was limited because I was in so much pain. I lost my ability to do my regular exercise to control my fibromyalgia. I did gentle walking, and then I had to switch to swimming."

Deirdre felt that her back became sore because she was more sedentary, and because she was getting out of bed more often at night. This exacerbation often made it impossible for her to lift her legs. She had to use Thera-Bands™ (exercise bands) to lift up her legs. She experienced major pain in her hips. Adaptive equipment is available to help you lift your legs up. One device lifts the leg at the thigh; the other lifts the leg at the foot. You can get this equipment by contacting an occupational therapist or ordering it from a rehabilitation catalog.

Exercises to stretch the lower back muscles and strengthen the abdominal muscles may reduce back pain. Rest, heat, and massage can also alleviate pain. Sitting in a straight-backed chair may also help. When a woman is not pregnant, sitting upright can make back problems worse by straightening the normal curve of the lower back. Sitting upright can be helpful during pregnancy, however, when the curve is exaggerated.

Women who have difficulty exercising, or who have persistent pain including back pain, should talk to their doctors about getting physical therapy. The physical therapist can help with active or passive exercise, and suggest ways to avoid back strain when performing daily activities, including the best ways to bend and lift.

Mobility Difficulties

Able-bodied women usually find that their mobility is unaffected until the third trimester, when the size of the uterus may affect their sense of balance and cause them to feel clumsier. Some of the interviewees with reduced mobility felt that they had time to adapt. Celeste explained, "Looking back, I see it didn't affect me as badly as I thought, because the body accommodates." Portia remarked, "If I had to go immediately from not being pregnant to being 8 months pregnant, it would have been impossible, but I managed because it was a gradual process." Other women are unable to adapt quickly enough. This can be due to injury. For example, Cheryl had difficulty walking for 6 weeks after she fell and strained some of the muscles in her groin area. Denise started to use her disabled placard so she did not have to walk so far.

Sally's ability to transfer was affected. Prior to pregnancy, Sally was able to use her muscle spasms to help her stand and pivot, but her spasms decreased during pregnancy, making transfers more difficult and dangerous. Sally also found getting repositioned in her chair difficult. She was unable to stay upright and would slide down in the seat.

Rachel had a flare-up prior to getting pregnant with her second child; she had an exacerbation in the second trimester. The flare-up made it difficult for her to move. She said, "The only thing that I can count on that really works for me in terms of keeping moving is my will. I move easer when I *make* myself move." Rachel was unable to bear any weight on her right leg because of pain, which resulted in her walking with a severe limp to protect her right knee. She weighed the pros and cons before deciding to have a procedure on her leg. She was concerned that even local anesthesia might cross over into the placenta. Rachel also worried about permanent damage being done to her joint, so she decided to have a shot of cortisone. Some women whose disability symptoms are mild also experience less difficulty. Margie, for example, said, "I walked the same as I did before, dragging one leg."

Some women begin to have more difficulty transferring or being lifted during the second trimester. Nadine had problems with balance because of her bigger belly. Natasha said, "Getting up from a chair or a couch is another area I normally have difficulty with, but it became more difficult when I was pregnant because my center of gravity was thrown off." There is a cushion available that will help a person stand (see the North Coast Medical Rehabilitation Catalog and the Fred Sammons Catalog in Appendix D). Natasha was also worried about her need to be in a twisted position in order to get up. She was concerned that the pressure on her spine when she got up would put extra pressure on the fetus and placenta. Her worry was needless, however, because babies suffer no ill effects from the extra physical maneuvers required of disabled pregnant women.

Amy had her bed taken off the frame so it would be lower, making an even transfer. Deirdre wished she had a trapeze to lift herself out of bed. An alternative to a trapeze is a transfer handle, which is a device that is mounted onto a metal bed frame (see Appendix D).

Some of the interviewees found their mobility compromised in other areas besides bed transfers. For women with limited upper extremity function, another technique for getting out of bed is to lie on your side, swing your legs out of bed, and then lean on your arms to bring yourself to an upright position.

Being able to transfer in and out of the bathtub affects most women by the second trimester. Most of the interviewees ended up using some form of bathtub seat. Amy said, "I ended up getting an over-the-tub shower bench. Shanna said, "The shower was the most difficult transfer. I did not shower until my husband was home or someone came over. I couldn't carry my legs." Nora transferred into the tub without using a step stool. She would get on a Rubbermaid™ stool in the tub in order to get out. She would first transfer onto the side of the tub and then into her chair. Using a bath chair and a hospital bed can make transferring easier for you or your attendant.

Other types of transfers become difficult as well. Shanna said, "I could transfer into the car, but I could not put my chair in the car." Both Sydney and Sophia Amelia found that they were unable to wheel up an incline. Amy found pushing on the carpet difficult, so she switched to using a power chair. Denise had to stop driving because her seat belt did not go around her belly. In addition she also had a hard time reaching for her seat belt.

Besides difficulty with walking, some women start having trouble when bending to lift objects. Sharon used a "reacher," a tool that is designed for taking objects from high shelves. She also pointed out that when a woman is pregnant and in a wheelchair, it is not as easy for her to carry things in her lap. In this case, attaching a lap tray or backpack to the wheelchair may help.

It is important to think about ways to adapt before mobility difficulties become serious. The interviewees used creativity and common sense in finding solutions. Paula said, "I felt off balance during the second trimester of my last pregnancy, so I used a baby buggy like a walker a lot of the time." Hannah could not carry her 2-year-old anymore when she was 5 months pregnant because the child weighed around 30 pounds.

Some women may need to start using an assistive device or a wheelchair, but this decision is not always easy. Psychological factors can weigh as heavily as physical problems. Many women feel that crutches and wheelchairs are symbols of disability. These assistive devices can help pregnant disabled women avoid the risk of being injured in a fall or fatigued by too much activity, however. Using an assistive device can save energy and make shopping easier. Caitlin said, "I started using my 4-wheeled walker because I had balance problems. "I had the walker, and used it for long distances prior to my pregnancies." Several of the interviewees wished that they had used a wheelchair, or started using one sooner. Hilary explained, "When I was a child, I was given a lot of positive feedback whenever I used my prosthesis, so using a wheelchair was hard on my self-image. When I consulted an orthopedist about pregnancy, he said I would need to use a wheelchair. I thought, 'Not me.' I waited until I really didn't have any other option. I was falling a lot, and it was astronomically easier to use the chair. I started using it earlier during my second pregnancy."

An important exception is the majority of women whose rheumatoid arthritis goes into remission during pregnancy. Jennifer and Roberta both found that walking was easier. Joan said her mobility and her ability to transfer all improved. She said, "I was more physically independent." Jennifer commented, "I complained about walking from the bedroom to the kitchen before I was pregnant. During pregnancy, I took long walks and enjoyed them."

FAINTNESS AND DIZZINESS

Faintness and dizziness are commonly caused by low blood pressure. Blood returns to the heart more slowly during pregnancy because pregnancy hormones relax the walls of the veins, and the uterus presses on several veins. Nadine had dizziness due to low blood pressure, and passed out at her doctor's office.

Some women notice that they feel faint in specific situations. For example, Amy felt faint after warm baths. She solved the problem by using cooler water. Others feel faint when they stand up after sitting or lying down. Try getting up more slowly, possibly using a support. Many women find that they can relieve dizziness by lying down, leaning back in a reclining chair, or bending forward with their heads lowered. Faintness and dizziness are the way the body adjusts to the increased volume of fluid during pregnancy.

Natalie had a fast heartbeat (*tachycardia*). Her obstetrician sent her to a cardiologist to check her heart, even though a fast heartbeat can be a symptom of pregnancy.

When Joan had tachycardia, she also experienced nausea and cold sweats. She was hospitalized to ensure that it was not preeclampsia, a dangerous medical disorder of pregnancy. Joan thought her problem was anxiety. She said, "I was scared because my heart was beating so fast." Joan's doctor said her fast heartbeat was normal. The problem might not have been her heart, but rather a symptom of *reflux*, a condition in which part of the esophagus touches part of the heart, resulting in the sensation of pounding, or rapid heartbeat.

Stephanie noticed that she felt faint after eating a large meal. She solved the problem by eating small, frequent meals. This is also a good strategy for preventing heartburn.

Sudden drops in blood sugar levels can also cause dizziness. Many women, including Pam, Stacy and Sylvia, found it helped to eat small, frequent meals in order to prevent extreme variations.

Orielle had hypoglycemia prior to pregnancy. She said, "The pregnancy threw my hypoglycemia for a loop. I would feel very lightheaded, like I would pass out and throw up. My blood sugar would drop without any warning, so I always carried food with me."

Stacy remarked that even when she is not pregnant, a maternity girdle improves her circulation. Wearing it when she was pregnant reduced her dizziness. Wearing elastic support stockings is another good alternative. Resting with the legs elevated several times a day can also help. Sonya would recline her chair and rest her head against the wall to help with her dizzy spells.

Sometimes anemia contributes to dizziness or faintness. Renee's dizziness improved after she started taking iron pills.

URINARY DIFFICULTIES

Many women have more trouble with urinary tract infections, incontinence, and stress incontinence during the second trimester. Stress incontinence is a condition in which urine leaks when pressure is put on the bladder from ordinary actions such as laughing, coughing, or sneezing. Disabled women who are prone to bladder infections will more than likely find that these symptoms are worsened during pregnancy. However, this may not occur in every trimester. Of the women who were interviewed more experienced bladder infections in the second then the third trimester. This may be related to the 60 percent increase in body fluid (especially blood volume) during pregnancy. It can take 3 full months to adjust to the this increase.

Hilary, Sharon, and Sasha all became more incontinent as their bladders were compressed by uterine growth. Using the bathroom more often does not seem to help most women. Heather said, "I leaked whenever I coughed or sneezed. Sometimes I had to go home from work to change clothes. It was wonderful to have an understanding boss."

For women with voluntary control of pelvic muscles, Kegel exercises may help to improve bladder control by strengthening muscles that hold the bladder in place (see Chapter 7). If other measures don't work, the best solution for many women may be to use absorbent pads or underwear. If you use waterproof underwear, watch for symptoms of vaginitis or skin irritation that can develop more easily when the genitals are kept warm and wet due to lack of air circulation. Using Depends™ may help keep the genitals dry. Caitlin was put on Urispas®, a medication to handle her stress incontinence. She said, "Urispas® worked for me; I took a very low dose of 100 mg a day."

Pregnancy increases the risk of bladder infections for all women. Women who are particularly susceptible should follow these simple preventive measures. Keep the genital area clean and dry and be especially careful to wash your hands and use proper techniques when using your catheter. Drink plenty of fluids (at least twice the usual intake). Sasha unintentionally increased her risk of bladder infections by treating her "same old, boring bladder" incontinence by drinking less fluid.

Watch for symptoms of bladder infections. If you develop fever, frequency, or urgency of urination, or pain and/or burning with urination, start drinking plenty of fluids and call your doctor. The doctor will ask you to bring a urine sample to the office or a clinical laboratory before prescribing an antibiotic.

Sherry Adele had bladder infections throughout both of her pregnancies. She got a *Pseudomonas* infection (species unknown) even though she was being monitored closely. She was referred to an infectious disease doctor. Fortunately, the infection did not trigger premature labor.

In this small sample, four women at particularly high risk developed kidney infections. Sally had kidney infections while not pregnant and only once during her first pregnancy. The infection cleared up after a few days of being hospitalized and treated with an antibiotic.

Sabine had to be hospitalized three times because of a kidney infection during the second trimester of her second pregnancy. Before her pregnancy, Sabine was able to keep her urinary illeostomy bag on for 5 days. It would not stay on, however, during pregnancy due to her changing shape. She went to an ostomy nurse for help, but nothing worked. Sabine had to change her bag every day. She said, "The illeostomy bag constantly filled up, and when it was full it pushed back up into the kidney. Sometimes this was also due to the tube being kinked and they would irrigate the bag." They put a catheter in her kidney and kept it in for the rest of her pregnancy. This cured her kidney infections.

Some women who were self-catheterized before pregnancy found this procedure more difficult during pregnancy. One woman who called Through The Looking Glass had injured herself while trying to self-catheterize because her view was obstructed. One possible solution to this problem is to use a mirror. Many types of assistive mirrors are available for use during catheterization. These mirrors can be ordered from rehabilitation catalogs. There is an assistive device that enables a person to watch while catheterizing. (See Figures 9-1 through 9-4 and Appendix D.)

Sophia Amelia said, "I found cathing more awkward, but not impossible. My bladder was kind of squished because it's tiny and has a section of bowel attached to it. I would have to stand up and move around a lot in order to empty it. I knew it was important to empty my bladder." During Sophia Amelia's second pregnancy, it felt as if her baby was sitting on her nonfunctioning kidney. She would position herself on her hands and knees "hoping that gravity would change the position of the baby."

Some women, who are bothered by the difficulty of self-cathing or by incontinence, may want to try using a Foley catheter (a catheter that remains in the urethra and bladder). Consider this decision carefully because an indwelling permanent catheter increases the risk of urinary infection. In addition, some researchers have found that spinal-cord-injured women who use an indwelling catheter during pregnancy often cannot discontinue using it after they give birth.

Sharon said, "I was dripping all the time and it was getting harder to reach around my belly to put the catheter in." Sharon's incontinence was so annoying that she decided to use a Foley catheter, but after her pregnancy she regretted the decision because she was not able to stop using it. (The use of a Foley catheter may result in the bladder losing its ability to hold urine.)

Sherry Adele was unable to hold her urine and had an indwelling catheter put in before the end of the first trimester. A Foley catheter takes time to adjust to. Sherry Adele said, "It wasn't the most pleasant of experiences." Unlike Sharon, Sherry Adele was able to return to self-cathing after delivery. This post-partum success may have been due to the fact she was given a new combination of medications that eased the spasticity of her bladder.

CONSTIPATION

Sabine had a tendency to have diarrhea prior to pregnancy. She was given Lomotil® for the diarrhea, but the dose had to be reduced when she became constipated during pregnancy. Rachel had to increase her dose of iron pills for iron deficiency anemia, but it made her constipated. She found that drinking four or five glasses of water was helpful. Signey's constipation was severe, and she was referred to a gastroenterologist specialist, who put her on a bowel program. She said, "Prior to being on the bowel program, I had some horrible episodes." This program included taking stool softeners—two in the morning and two at night, plus taking Citrucel® after dinner. Signey said, "The program made me go regularly, and I did not have painful bowel obstructions." Moira was borderline anemic, and was put on iron pills for 3 weeks. She did not experience constipation, possibly because she drank five or six glasses of water and juice every day.

NASAL CONGESTION

Hormonal changes and increased blood volume can cause the lining of the nostrils and sinuses to swell during pregnancy. The resulting "stuffy nose" is usually a minor nuisance, although some women have trouble distinguishing this condition from a cold or allergies. The one interviewee who recalled having this problem, Jennifer, said, "I managed to find nose drops that didn't have any harmful ingredients, but they were expensive." Many of the medications that relieve nasal congestion contain ingredients that may be harmful to the fetus, and should not be used without consulting a doctor.

Many women find that using a cool mist vaporizer, or inhaling steam from a hot shower or a cup of hot water, relieves their symptoms. Others feel more comfortable when they gently massage the area over their sinuses.

HEARTBURN

Heartburn is most commonly experienced during the third trimester. Some women with disabilities may have indigestion late in the second trimester, however. Heather Ann remarked, "I think I got heartburn early in my pregnancy because my pelvis is small and I carried high, which put more pressure on my stomach." Sonya was asked if reclining her chair helped with her heartburn. She said, "Nothing helped." She had to eat smaller meals "because the bigger I got, the less I could eat. The baby took up all the room." Sonya also said, "I could not get up and walk around to feel better." Using a table that maintains a person in a standing position might help reduce heartburn. Tina figured out that some of the foods she was eating made her heartburn worse (see Chapter 10).

BREATHING PROBLEMS

Respiratory problems are most commonly experienced during the third trimester, but some women with disabilities may have difficulty breathing in the second trimester. Chloe said, "It was harder to breathe. I would lie down more, which helped." Darlene found sitting with a pillow in the small of her back made it easier to breath. Nadine said, "I was short of breath right from the beginning, and would lie down and try to take deep breaths."

EDEMA

Julie recalled, "I had feet like an elephant." Some swelling can occur as early as the second trimester, as a result of the normal increase in blood volume. Even when you are not pregnant, some fluid escapes from your circulatory system into the space between the cells, which is called the *interstitial space*. Even more fluid may enter the interstitial space when the amount of blood increases during pregnancy. There is no need to worry about the mild, gradual swelling that makes your wedding ring a little tight or your shoes too tight at the end of the day. Caitlin and Shelby both bought larger shoes when they experienced edema. In addition, Caitlin elevated her feet whenever she could. Sudden or severe swelling may be a symptom of preeclampsia, a dangerous medical condition (see Chapter 10).

DISABILITY-SPECIFIC COMPLICATIONS

Nora said, "I felt weak starting during my second trimester. I had no idea if it was my disease [Charcot-Marie-Tooth], but immediately after the birth of my first child I felt better." Nora was interviewed 4 months after the birth of her second child. She said, "I felt weaker when I was pregnant, and I haven't felt strong again yet." Nora had a caesarean section with her second child, unlike the first one, which may have contributed to her fatigue.

Dysreflexia can cause problems with temperature regulation. Shelby had difficulty with her temperature. In one of her pregnancies, she was too hot to sleep, so she slept naked and used a cool cloth that she periodically sprayed with water.

Fetal Development

The placenta produces many pregnancy hormones, supplies nutrition and oxygen to the fetus, and filters fetal wastes. The placenta continues to grow during the second trimester. The fetus also grows much larger. The placenta weight increases from about ½ ounce to 1¾ pounds, and its length increases from 3 inches to about 13.

All the organ systems mature considerably. The skeleton begins to harden, and hair begins to grow in the fifth month. The increase in muscle mass and strength makes it possible for the mother to feel fetal movement. By the end of this trimester, the heart beats so strongly that it can sometimes be heard by pressing an ear against the mother's abdomen. In the sixth month, the eyelids open and close, the eyes move, and the tooth buds begin to form.

Some babies born at the end of the second trimester are well-enough developed to survive with intensive care, although they are far more vulnerable to health problems, especially respiratory problems.

Complications

The complications that may occur during the second trimester of pregnancy do not affect most women, although some of them can be serious. It is always important to watch for and recognize these signs and symptoms.

PREECLAMPSIA

Preeclampsia is increased blood pressure accompanied by *proteinuria*, and/or edema (swelling) after the twentieth week of pregnancy. Although the incidence of preeclampsia among all women is only about 5 percent, most often it affects women who are pregnant for the first time, especially older and younger women. Multiple pregnancies, preexisting vascular disease, and a family history of preeclampsia or eclampsia can also indicate an increased risk.

This condition is considered mild when proteinuria and some increase in blood pressure are the only symptoms. Severe preeclampsia, or eclampsia, can endanger both mother and fetus. These conditions can develop suddenly. (These conditions are described in detail in Chapter 10 because they are more likely to develop in the third trimester.) If you had edema or proteinuria from vascular or kidney disease before pregnancy, and these conditions worsen during the sixth month, preeclampsia is said to be superimposed upon the pre-existing problem.

A woman cannot know for certain that she has high blood pressure or protein in her urine. These problems are found during an office visit and lab tests. She can watch for swelling, however, which is often the first sign of preeclampsia. This is not the mild swelling many pregnant women experience, but rather swelling that is accompanied by a sudden weight gain of more than 2 pounds in a single week or more than 6 pounds in a month. Another sign to watch for is sudden swelling of your hands and face—even your eyelids can look puffy. Your fingers may become so swollen that suddenly your rings are painfully tight. Check for "pitting edema," which is when a pit or dent remains in the skin after pressing with your fingertip. Call your doctor and tell him you have an urgent problem if you experience severe swelling.

Clara had cerebral palsy on one side, and experienced pitting edema only in her dominant leg. This may have been caused by her dominant leg getting more use. Women with similar conditions should periodically elevate their dominant leg and apply cold compresses to relieve swelling.

Women who have preeclampsia must rest in bed for most of the day. You will need to see your doctor often so he can monitor your condition closely. If the problem does not improve, hospitalization will be necessary. Unfortunately, the most reliable medication for this condition cannot be taken by women with myasthenia gravis, because the medication can cause a dangerous exacerbation of muscle weakness.

If you have systemic lupus erythematosus (SLE), your doctor may order tests to determine whether your hypertension and proteinuria are caused by lupus exacerbation, preeclampsia, or both. A diagnosis of SLE can be difficult to make during pregnancy, and a thorough clinical and laboratory assessment must be relied upon (85).

If you have SLE, you will need to discuss possible side effects with your doctor. Make sure she helps you understand as clearly as possible how to differentiate between the symptoms of preeclampsia, SLE, and medication side effects.

It is also important to differentiate between the symptoms of preeclampsia and problems caused by disability. Carol had preeclampsia with both pregnancies, but only needed to be hospitalized during her second pregnancy. She had a perinatologist take over her case. Carol said, "The perinatologist checked my reflexes. If the reflex showed as hyperreflexive it was a sign of brain swelling. The area of the brain that is affected by cerebral palsy is hyperreflexive, and this can be a whole different issue when making a diagnosis. I tried to get the perinatologist to realize that what was happening to my legs was not a sign of any significance. I tried to make him realize that my legs were responding normally [for me]. I asked a physical therapist, who not only worked with me, but also worked at the hospital, to come out and address this. I wanted her and the perinatologist to focus on the reflexes in my upper body, as opposed to my lower body, because my upper body is not affected by cerebral palsy."

CERVICAL INCOMPETENCE

Cervical incompetence is a painless dilation of the cervix in the second trimester or early in the third trimester. The opened cervix is unable to retain the fetus in the uterus.

Bed rest was prescribed for Leslie, whose placenta was partially detached from the uterine lining. It was not yet known that her cervix was incompetent. She went into labor when she was allowed to sit up. Leslie explained that she did not know the signs of labor. She said, "I was in labor for 16 hours, thinking I had the flu. The contractions were one-sided, and I didn't realize I was in labor until the bag of water broke." Leslie gave birth to her son in the sixth month of pregnancy.

Because this type of dilation may be painless, and pelvic examinations are not routinely included in second trimester office visits, cervical incompetence may not be diagnosed until a woman has had more than one miscarriage. The primary treatment is bed rest. *Cerclage* may be performed; this is a procedure in which the uterus is sutured shut. A woman who has had cerclage must watch carefully for the signs and symptoms of labor, because her uterus might rupture if active labor begins before the sutures are removed.

MISCARRIAGE AND THREATENED MISCARRIAGE

Miscarriage and threatened miscarriage are rare in the second trimester, but may occur for a number of reasons, including fetal illness or death. Some women may need preterm delivery near the end of the second trimester. Many babies born this early cannot survive without intensive care, and early delivery will be considered only if there is a severe threat to fetal or maternal health.

If amniocentesis shows that the fetal lungs are immature, the mother can be given an injection of hormones that will cross the placenta into the fetal bloodstream. This may speed maturation of the lung tissue. A stress test can determine whether the fetus can tolerate labor. Labor will probably not be as uncomfortable for the mother as with a full-term baby.

Arlene's blood circulation was poor. As a result, her fetus did not receive enough oxygen and died early in the second trimester. Arlene said, "The first sign that something was wrong was when the doctor couldn't find the heartbeat. Then I had an amniocentesis to find out what was wrong. After the baby died, it was a month before I had a miscarriage. I had a mini-labor and delivery. Physically it was not bad."

During her second pregnancy, Sally started having preterm labor in her sixth month that continued until delivery. The contractions felt stronger when she was sitting; she also had dysreflexia symptoms during the contractions. The medicine used to stop the contractions was the same one she used to control dysreflexia. Sally was told to reduce her activity and relax. She reclined in her chair for at least an hour every afternoon and went to bed a few hours earlier. She went to work only in the mornings.

PLACENTA PREVIA AND PLACENTAL ABRUPTION

Placenta previa and placental abruption are dangerous to both fetus and mother. *Placental abruption* is partial or complete separation of the placenta from the uterine wall. In *placenta previa*, the placenta is placed low, possibly covering the cervix, so that it may separate from the uterine wall during cervical dilation or during labor (see Chapter 11.) These conditions can cause threatened miscarriage, miscarriage, or fetal death. Noreen's doctors thought she was at risk for placental abruption because of *hydramnios, also known as polyhydramnios*. Polyhydramnios refers to an excess of amniotic fluid; this condition is associated with fetal anomalies. Noreen gained 100 pounds, 75 pounds of which was amniotic fluid. She said, "I was very skinny except for my stomach, which made it hard to put on my seat belt."

The signs of placenta previa are painless bleeding and, sometimes, the passing of blood clots. Rachel started to bleed during the second trimester of her first pregnancy. The doctor thought she was having a miscarriage, and sent her home. The next day, Rachel was scheduled for an ultrasound to check on the viability of the fetus. She said, "When they did the ultrasound, they saw there was a perfectly healthy baby in there, and they determined that I had placenta previa. I was put on bed rest. By the third trimester, the placenta had moved up into the normal position, and I was able to have a vaginal birth." Ordinarily, with this type of bleeding, an ultrasound is scheduled on an urgent basis as soon as bleeding is reported.

In placental abruption, the bleeding is accompanied by severe pain, abdominal tenderness, or back pain. The bleeding may be visible or concealed in the uterus.

Leslie had a partial abruption in the second trimester of her first pregnancy. She recalled, "I had never experienced such pain in my life. When I got to the hospital, I ended up lying in an uncomfortable position, and stayed that way because it hurt too much to move. I was able to stay pregnant because the placenta was large and the abruption was only partial." Leslie's child was born in the seventh month.

Bed rest may prevent a miscarriage, but immediate delivery may be necessary to prevent further blood loss, especially in cases of placental abruption. The mother may need blood transfusions if a large amount of blood has already been lost.

INTRAUTERINE GROWTH RETARDATION

Intrauterine growth retardation (IUGR) is inadequate growth of the fetus. Placental abnormalities, multiple fetuses, and *hypoxia* (lack of oxygen) also contribute to IUGR.

IUGR can also result if the mother uses alcohol, tobacco, or illegal drugs while she is pregnant, and it may help if she stops.

IUGR is diagnosed by sonography. Little can be done to treat it in the second trimester. Improvements in her diet can help if she is undernourished or anemic. Bed rest may be advised.

IUGR may be caused by placental damage related to SLE. If a pregnant woman with SLE is not already taking medication to control her SLE, medication will probably be prescribed if her fetus is not growing normally.

Choosing a Childbirth Class

There are many different types of childbirth classes. Women with spinal cord injuries may wonder why they should take a childbirth class. Sharon remarked that she did not take a class because she did not think she needed one. Sheila was advised by her doctor that she did not need one. Yet, many women with spinal cord injuries give birth vaginally, and a few of them feel the discomfort of labor. Women who have lesions below the L-1 level feel labor pain. Those who have lesions between T-10 and T-12 generally do not, but they may experience increased clonus and spasticity during labor. In addition, women with higher complete or incomplete lesions have been known to feel labor pain. Childbirth classes also have much to offer besides information about coping with labor. They offer an opportunity to meet other pregnant women. But more importantly, you will have an opportunity to obtain information about medical procedures and medications, and also get help with decision-making regarding those procedures. In addition, the classes will provide information about deciding whether you are in true labor versus false labor, and knowing when to go to the hospital. The classes also discuss pregnancy discomforts, preparation for breast-feeding, and normal fetal development. Joy said, "I took the classes so I would know what was going to happen at the hospital."

Birthing classes can also prepare you for a caesarean section. Taryn Dion said, "I still feel the class helped me cope with the emergency caesarean section." Roberta commented, "I was glad I took a birthing class because I found out my baby was doing fine." You will learn coping skills at a birthing class.

Sophia Amelia was in labor for 8 hours with her first pregnancy. She went into labor unexpectedly the day before she was scheduled for a caesarean section. She had to wait for the caesarean because her obstetrician needed her urologist to be present. She ended up hyperventilating at one point. She said, "I had a labor and delivery nurse who got in my face and said, 'This is going to get a lot worse before it gets better.' I actually had to breathe into a paper bag for a while, but the pain wasn't too bad."

There are a number of ways to find a good childbirth class. Noelle checked a bulletin board at the hospital. Sara called a local school for adult education. You can also call a community recreation center, ask a friend or your physician for suggestions, or take a class offered by a local hospital or clinic. If several classes are available, the next step is to interview the instructors by telephone or in person. Ask each teacher how she feels about the use of medication. Simi thought she got poor advice from her teacher. Simi said, "The teacher told the class that anyone who used any kind of medication during childbirth was jeopardizing the health of their child. I didn't like the fact she was laying a guilt trip on me. I hated the instructor, but all the stuff they taught us about breathing worked." Felicia's sister-in-law teaches childbirth classes, and gave Felicia some guidelines. Felicia said, "I looked for a class that fit into my schedule and matched my philosophy. I looked for classes that did not demand the graduates to 'go natural.' I also looked for classes that taught relaxation, imagery, and techniques for coping with pain." Nora found a teacher who was willing to do a special class for her, because it was too hard for Nora to drive to the series of classes. She said, "We did a one-day special class, even though it cost more."

The teacher's personality and the organization of the class is sometimes more important than the method taught. Many teachers change their philosophies as they gain experience and continue their education, and different teachers individualize their classes in different ways. For example, one teacher might be interested in helping students experiment with different positions for giving birth; another might think it is important to have the students discuss the advantages and disadvantages of circumcising newborn boys.

Most childbirth educators teach either the *Bradley* method or the *LaMaze* method. Bradley teachers are trained and certified by the American Academy of Husband-Coached Childbirth; LaMaze Teachers by the American Society for Psychoprophylaxis in Obstetrics (ASPO). Books on these methods are available, and it may be easier to interview and choose a teacher after reading about the different methods.

It is important to talk to more than one instructor. Michelle interviewed two teachers, and chose the one she thought she could work with more easily. Stephanie said, "I looked until I found a teacher I thought had a positive attitude towards disability." The attitude of the interviewees toward their childbirth instructors paralleled their feelings about their obstetricians. They did not mind it when the instructors were unfamiliar with disability, as long as they were willing to explore ways of adapting. For example, Sara found a class in which she could exercise in her wheelchair. Sabine felt that she could make her own adaptations in a regular birthing class.

Both the Bradley and LaMaze methods emphasize teaching women about the labor process so that it becomes more familiar. Women who are not frightened can relax their muscles more easily, and they may feel less pain during childbirth, or at least find the pain bearable.

The LaMaze method emphasizes the intensive practice of specific methods for breathing and relaxation. The mother attempts to learn a new way of responding to pain and tension, so that she will react appropriately during childbirth. This method uses concentration on external objects as a way of distracting oneself from discomfort. The mother may be coached by a LaMaze instructor during the birth, or by a birthing partner who attended the class with her. Some women may find panting, one of the breathing techniques, difficult, but others may prefer it to deep breathing.

Bradley instruction emphasizes the naturalness of childbirth. The instructors emphasize the value of good health care and nutrition during pregnancy. The philosophy also encourages avoidance of medication and other medical interventions. This method relies on a simple breathing technique. The mother is taught to concentrate on internal sensations, rather than distracting herself during labor.

Women find advantages in both methods. Noelle, who preferred the Bradley method, explained, "Their philosophy really helped me." Clara said, "I chose the LaMaze method because looking inward only makes me tenser. I also liked having so many choices in breathing techniques." It may be helpful to ask the following questions when you interview a childbirth instructor:

- ❖ What method is taught? Not all advertisements state whether the teacher is a LaMaze or a Bradley instructor. The type of breathing used may be important to you. Noelle was simply unable to breathe deeply during her first labor, although she found deep breathing very relaxing during her second labor. Women who experience dysreflexia when they breathe deeply might not want to spend time in a class that emphasizes this method. You might want to make sure that you will learn a variety of techniques. The author recalls a student who disliked practicing shallow breathing in class, but she found this method useful during labor and was glad she had learned it.

- ❖ What are the philosophy of the teacher and the content of the class? Hearing the teacher explain the class philosophy can give you the best sense of whether you would enjoy working with that teacher. Class content should include any topics of concern to you. In addition to childbirth methods, the list might include information about general relaxation, exercise, breast-feeding, medical procedures, medication, caesarean delivery, fetal development, preparing older siblings for the birth, and the emotional concerns of new parents.

- ❖ How is the class organized? How much time does the teacher allot for lectures, small group discussions, and practice? Is the mix comfortable for you?

- ❖ How large is the class? Some people prefer the intimacy of a small class; others prefer a large class in which they can meet more people.

- ❖ Is other information available? Some people learn more if lectures and practice are reinforced by slides, videotapes, or printed materials.

- ❖ Are there ways to adapt the class to my disability? Many teachers enjoy the challenge of helping women find alternative ways to exercise or give birth. Hilary's teacher was happy to help her try to find a position in which she could receive a spinal injection.

Emotional Concerns

Pregnancy is a private matter during the first trimester. The only people who know are those the mother chooses to tell. During the second trimester, the pregnancy becomes visible, and women are confronted with curiosity, congratulations, and unsolicited opinions and advice from friends, family, and even total strangers. Because of widespread ignorance about disability, many people respond to the sight of a pregnant, disabled woman with surprise and even rudeness. Samantha commented, "It was hard for strangers to connect a wheelchair with pregnancy." Simi said, "People were weirded out. Some were curious; others were down-right rude." Patricia and Arlene had a similar experience, in that people simply asked questions because they were curious. Other women have met with behavior that was clearly inappropriate. Corrine, who walks with a limp, was approached by complete strangers asking, "Aren't you afraid your child will be disabled?" Sharon recalled that when she went to the emergency room with an ear infection and asked whether the prescribed medication was safe in pregnancy, the doctor asked her, "Do you know who the father is?" Oprah said, "The first time I took my daughter out, people assumed we were babysitting someone else's child."

Many people repress their questions and simply stare. Heather Ann recalled, "People stared a lot. Some people couldn't handle seeing a pregnant woman on crutches with only one leg. Don't let it bother you if strangers, friends, or family have difficulty understanding. Just do your own thing." Different women handled the staring in different ways. Sylvia spoke for many when she said, "How well I handled the stares and comments depended on my mood." Christina, who "just blocked out the stares," seemed to feel more uncomfortable than Portia, who said, "I usually get stares, so I didn't notice any difference when I was pregnant."

Some of the interviewees enjoyed having a chance to disprove misconceptions about disability. Samantha explained, "I enjoyed shooting down the idea that disabled people are asexual." Stacy liked to wear a T-shirt that said "Under Construction" because she enjoyed seeing the shocked expression on people's faces. Pam said, "When people stared at me, I just stuck my stomach out further." Nora said, "People would come up to me and ask how I could do this. They just don't understand."

Other women simply did not let themselves be affected by the reactions of strangers, like Noelle, who said, "When strangers looked at me like I shouldn't be pregnant, I didn't care because I was just so elated."

Of course, the interviewees cared much more about the reactions of their friends than the reactions of strangers. These reactions may include fear for the pregnant woman, admiration of her courage, or simple support. Paula said, "I enjoyed having people tell me what guts I had," but Celeste complained, "I got tired of hearing people worry that I had too much to struggle with."

Quite often, the chief concern the interviewees expressed was not related to their disability, but to the desire for emotional support. For example, Julie, who was not married, worried about how the people in her church would react. She was very happy when "they turned out to be a tremendous support." Arlene recalled, "It was nice that friends waited to see whether I would have an abortion or have the baby. I knew they would support any decision I made." Sasha felt that her family was fearful and overly concerned about her disability. She said she felt "vulnerable and betrayed" when they were not supportive of her pregnancy.

The feelings the interviewees expressed about pregnancy, body image, and self-esteem closely paralleled those of many able-bodied women. For example, Sybil said, "I felt good about myself. All my life, I had wanted a baby." Mary said, "I felt fulfilled as a woman." Sally said, "My body image improved. I had a sense of accomplishment." Signey said, "I was proud of my big belly." Tessa felt attractive, and said pregnancy boosted her confidence. Amanda was more self-conscious during her first pregnancy. She said, "I was much more aware of how other people perceived me as far as my abilities. I had the superwomen complex for a while. With my second, it didn't change much at all. But with the first one it was like returning to my teen years. I felt that I really had to overcompensate."

Joy said, "Pregnancy was an adventure. Prior to being pregnant, I had heard about how the body changes, but until you go through it yourself, it's hard to believe it. I really enjoyed each month and the changes."

Remarks about body image reflected typically contradictory feelings. Patricia, Roberta, and Jennifer all thought they were better looking when pregnant. Jennifer added that she also liked having a reason to buy new clothes. Some women thought they were more attractive because their breasts were larger. Simi said, "I thought it was great to be pregnant, but I did miss my lap. I didn't have any place to put things." Paula's comment was classic: "I had the special glow that all pregnant women have."

A few of the interviewees expressed the common feeling that pregnancy makes a woman look "fat and clumsy." Sheila regretted "losing her figure;" Stephanie thought her "huge stomach and spindly legs looked ridiculous;" and Sierra said, "I looked like a beach ball with crutches."

Feeling "as huge as a house and just as clumsy," as Heather Ann did, reflects the reality that mobility is reduced during pregnancy. Despite the problems with reduced mobility, however, the feeling that pregnancy represents normality was important to many of the interviewees. Corrine remarked, "Pregnancy was the first time my body worked; it was doing what it should." Christina said, "I felt better about myself because I was experiencing something all women do."

Some found a new sense of kinship with other women. As Celeste said, "It felt good to be a part of the sorority." Many of the interviewees enjoyed comparing notes with able-bodied women. Margie said, "It was fun." Tessa felt really lucky to have an easy pregnancy. She said, "I felt I deserved it after so many challenges. I realized I was healthy after all."

Some of the interviewees had problems during pregnancy, like Laura, who said, "Sometimes it was difficult being with women who had it easier." Sylvia had an unusually difficult pregnancy, and remembered feeling jealous of other women.

Amanda had two pregnancies, one easy and one difficult, which gave her perspective. She said, "With my first pregnancy I thought most of the other women were whiny because I had such a positive experience. With my second, I suddenly understood why they complained about their feet swelling and things like that. All of a sudden, those women weren't so grippey. We had things in common."

For women who are experiencing difficult pregnancies, the most serious issue is fear for the baby. Heather Ann, who had a threatened miscarriage, said, "Even though it turned out to be a positive experience, I was frightened. I kept wondering if my baby was moving enough." Dawn wished she could have found a support group for high-risk mothers. If you would like to find such a support group, ask local hospitals with maternity units, especially those with high-risk facilities. If there are no established support groups, consider starting one.

Be sure to discuss your fears with your doctor, because she will be able to help you keep your fears in perspective. Perhaps most important, she can tell you how to distinguish the ordinary discomforts of pregnancy from real danger signs.

Although it is not easy to cope with fear during a problem pregnancy, it can be worthwhile. Leslie said of her miscarriage during her second pregnancy, "It is the end of all the dreams you've had. I went to a support group, and I felt terrible for everyone in the class." Still, she decided to try a third pregnancy. She explained, "Otherwise, I would have always wondered if I could have done it. If I didn't try, I'd have no baby. If I tried, I'd have either a live or a dead baby. I did worry that the baby would be disabled if it was premature, but I was ready to take whatever came."

Closing Comments

The second trimester is the easiest of the three trimesters. The third trimester is the time when the baby begins to put on weight and so does the mother.

Nine Months of Change: The Third Trimester

W OMEN ARE FEELING BIG by the third trimester because the baby and the uterus continue to grow, possibly causing more discomfort. Only a small percentage of the interviewees had heartburn, urinary problems, or constipation, however. The majority of them experienced problems in the area of mobility, back pain, and edema. Most pregnant women are filled with joy and anticipation by the third trimester as the birth of the baby draws closer.

Office Visits

Office visits are more frequent during the third trimester. If your pregnancy is uncomplicated, your visits will be every 2 weeks until about the thirty-sixth week, and then they will be weekly. These visits follow much the same routine as second trimester visits, and will include a urinalysis and measurement of weight, blood pressure, fundal height, and fetal heart rate. During your physical examination, your doctor may check your hands and feet for edema, and your legs for varicose veins. At the twenty-eighth week, your blood sugar test may be repeated. This is a screening test for gestational diabetes, and further testing will be needed if results are not normal. Even if you test positive on the screening test, you still have only a 15 percent higher risk of diabetes. The Hg A1C test is the preferred standard fasting test for diabetes.

A vaginal swab taken between the thirty-fifth and thirty-seventh week can detect a streptococcal infection (group B). This type of infection can be treated with an intravenous antibiotic during labor. Streptococcal infection can cause death or disability in the newborn infant if it goes undetected and untreated.

After the thirty-second week, the doctor will include manually examine your uterus to determine the presentation of the fetus. *Presentation* is the term that is used to indicate which part of the fetus is pressing against the cervix; this could be the feet, head, or buttocks. An ultrasound examination may be ordered if your doctor suspects that the fetus

221

is not in a normal presentation. Holly knew her baby was in the breech position (feet first) because, "When she kicked me, it was much more painful because she kicked me in the cervix."

During the last few weeks of pregnancy, the cervix may be manually examined to determine whether it has started to dilate (open up). Your doctor will not necessarily examine your cervix, but she must judge the risks and benefits of doing so. The cervix will not be examined if the woman has placenta previa (see Chapter 11) because of the risk of causing bleeding. Women with spinal cord injuries are more likely to be examined by the thirty-second week because they have a higher risk of preterm labor, and because women with injuries at or above the T-12 level usually are not able to feel labor contractions. Women with a spinal cord injury may be examined as early as the twenty-eighth week. You may notice a small amount of brownish or pink discharge for a day or two after an internal examination. This discharge is usually nothing to be concerned about. A pink discharge or slightly blood-streaked mucus is sometimes a sign that labor will begin soon. Bright red spotting is a danger sign, and you should contact your doctor immediately.

Hannah needed internal exams because of her potential for preterm labor. Her doctors ignored her disability, however, and performed an internal exam with Hannah lying on her back and using the stirrups, instead of lying on her side. Lying flat on her back was quite painful because of her hip dysplegia.

Natalie's doctor used special accommodations. "She had me keep my braces and shoes on, and she put my feet up on the table. She said, "This is so much easier and more comfortable." Sydney needed some accommodation, and had a nurse hold her legs during an exam so they "didn't flop off the table."

It is a good idea to discuss with your doctor how to tell if you are in labor, or whether you are having Braxton-Hicks contractions (practice labor), especially if you have a spinal cord injury. Shanna did not realize that she was in labor because it was different from her first labor. Moreover, she had not been told how to recognize back labor. By taking a birthing class, you can learn how to distinguish true labor from non-productive contractions (see Chapter 11 for a discussion of back labor). Classes also offer the opportunity to explore your feelings surrounding birth.

If you and your doctor have not already developed a "birth plan," now is the time. Table 10-1 is a sample birth plan that has been adapted from one created by a couple in a childbirth class. Of course, your plan may contain different details. For example, you may want to have a warm bath available for the baby just after birth. To make it easier for the doctor to accept any special requirements you may have, add an addendum indicating that if an emergency situation arises that jeopardizes the safety of the mother or baby, you (and your partner) will cooperate completely with the decisions of the medical and nursing staff at the hospital. For example, the plan in Table 10-1 mentions allowing the presence of friends, relatives, and siblings in the delivery room. Find out in advance whether the hospital limits the number of people who may be present, and whether it requires siblings to take a special class before attending the birth.

TABLE 10-1
MARK AND JOLENE'S BIRTH PLAN

We, the parents realize that flexibility and a willingness to accept changes in our plan may be necessary. The following are our preferred options for a normal, natural labor and birth, and for possible variations from the normal.

Labor
A. Husband may be present throughout labor and delivery.
B. Mother to have only a "minishave" for possible episiotomy.
C. Freedom to walk and change positions.
D. Spontaneous labor—no induction or breaking of membranes.
E. Able to drink fluids—ice chips, juice, fruit popsicles.
F. Friends, relatives, and siblings may be present.

Birth
A. Birth in labor bed if possible.
B. No catheterization.
C. Episiotomy only if necessary; *local* anesthetic for pain of episiotomy.
D. Spontaneous delivery with no forceps.
E. Mirror to watch birth.
F. Tape recording and photos of birth.

After Birth
A. Baby on the mother's chest after birth until cord is cut.
B. Bonding and breast-feeding after baby is cleaned.

Baby
A. No glucose water given to baby.
B. Delay administration of eye drops.

In Case of Caesarean Birth
A. Husband present for moral support throughout delivery.
B. Father to hold baby, and mother to see baby if it is not in distress.
C. Mother allowed to breast-feed in delivery room if her and the baby's condition permit.

In Case of Premature/Sick Infant
A. Mother allowed to hold and see baby if the baby is not in distress.
B. Father and mother involved as much as possible in care of baby.
C. Mother to express colostrum to feed baby.

_____   _____
Parents' Signatures, Date   Doctor's Signature, Date

Below are some questions you may wish to discuss during an office visit during the third trimester:

❖ *Can my husband and I continue making love?* This question arises for many couples, and often the answer is "yes." If your doctor advises you to restrict sexual activity, he will give you a reason (for example, a woman who has placenta previa would be advised to avoid intercourse). If possible, ask this question when your husband is with you, so you can both hear the doctor's explanation and ask any further questions.

During Natalie's second pregnancy she spotted. She said, "I saw streaks of blood in my seventh month. I immediately went to my obstetrician. It turned out that I had bulging blood vessels in my vagina that had ruptured. These were caused by the normal increase of blood flow during pregnancy. We were restricted from having intercourse for the remainder of my pregnancy."

❖ *If I think I am in labor, when should I call the doctor?* Women are usually told to call their doctors when their contractions are 7 to 10 minutes apart and last 45 to 60 seconds. Your doctor may give you different instructions, however, especially if complications have been previously diagnosed.
❖ *If the doctor is unavailable, should I go to the hospital?* Women are usually advised to go to the hospital when contractions are 3 to 5 minutes apart and last 45 to 60 seconds. A number of circumstances could modify this rule. For example, if you live far from the hospital, when labor starts you may need to leave home earlier. Your doctor might advise you that if the "bag of water" breaks before you feel strong contractions, you should leave for the hospital without waiting.

Denise started spotting at 31 weeks, and went to her doctor for an evaluation. The doctor sent her home to rest and put her feet up, after telling her it was non-productive labor (false labor pains). Her mother called and asked how she was feeling. When Denise's mom heard about the cramping, she asked, 'How far apart are the pains, and are you spotting?'" Denise said, "I told her that the pains were 5 minutes apart. She asked why I had not gone to the hospital, and I replied, "I've never gone through this before, and I'm doing what the doctor told me to do." When we rushed to the hospital, the doctor said, 'You are in labor, even though you are only 31 weeks pregnant.'"

Felicia was having contractions 6 minutes apart, and they were getting more painful. She said, "My obstetrician told me that if I began to have frequent contractions, I should go into the hospital because I was so effaced [80 percent, as he discovered during a vaginal examination)."

Shanna delivered her baby at home on the toilet because she was not sure she was in labor. She felt her contractions the night before, but they were irregular. Her husband thought she should go to the hospital, but she did not want to go because she did want to be sent home. Shanna was able to sleep, even though she was uncomfortable. She said,

"I can't really describe it, but I woke up feeling weird. I felt that something was wrong. I had cramps, and my stomach dropped a lot. The first thing I did was go to the bathroom. I noticed I was bleeding, like period bleeding. So I knew something wasn't right." After questioning Shanna, it appeared that most of her pain was a backache. Back labor is difficult to time, and the contractions seem irregular (see Chapter 11). Women with spinal cord injuries may want to consider getting a home labor monitor, although monitors have not been found to be helpful for some women with other types of pregnancy difficulties.

Natalie's contractions started 4 hours after her water broke. Her contractions were 2 minutes apart when labor started.

- ❖ *Can you suggest a good pediatrician?* If your regular doctor is a family practitioner, she can become your baby's doctor. Your baby must have a physical examination before he can leave the hospital, and although this can be done by a staff physician, you may prefer to have it done by the person who will care for the baby ongoing. Give yourself plenty of time to find a pediatrician you can work with; start looking 4 to 6 weeks before the baby is due.
- ❖ If my baby needed special attention, would my baby be in the same hospital; for example, if my baby is premature?

Medical Procedures and Diagnostic Tests

RH ANTIBODY TREATMENT

If a woman has blood that is Rh negative, and she is exposed to the red blood cells of an Rh-positive fetus, she will develop antibodies to Rh-positive cells. In this case, the woman will be "sensitized." Sensitization is the same process as the development of immunity to disease after a vaccination. A woman can become sensitized during childbirth or miscarriage, from an ectopic pregnancy, or during a first pregnancy from placental bleeding. When a sensitized, Rh-negative woman is pregnant with an Rh-positive fetus, her antibodies will attack the fetal tissues. Prolonged exposure to these antibodies causes problems for the fetus.

If the blood tests that were done during the first office visit showed that an Rh negative woman is not sensitized, then at the twenty-eighth week she will be given an injection of Rh-immune globulin to suppress antibody formation and prevent Rh disease in the fetus. If she is already sensitized, amniocentesis will be performed regularly to measure the changing levels of antibodies in the amniotic fluid. Preterm delivery may be necessary if the level gets too high. Rh disease and the associated birth defects are increasingly rare because of these preventative procedures.

AMNIOCENTESIS

Amniotic fluid can be tested to assess fetal lung maturity and possible fetal distress, as well as assessing the presence of Rh antibodies.

Lea Rae had amniocentesis twice—once to make sure that the placenta was working, and the second time to see how healthy the baby's heart was. Diane had amniocentesis when she had twins. Diane said, "The only reason they did amniocentesis was because I was getting large, and they wanted to know how much longer I would last before I went into labor. They wanted to see how developed the baby's lungs were."

Your doctor may order a test that measures the lecithin-to-sphingomyelin (L/S) ratio when preterm delivery is being considered. This test is helpful in predicting fetal lung maturity, but it is insufficient as a stand-alone test. Your doctor may also order other tests (86).

Allison needed amniocentesis because the doctors saw antigens in her blood. Allison's leg was amputated after being in a car accident, and her doctors thought that the antigens in her blood might have resulted from the blood transfusion she received after her accident.

Amniocentesis can detect signs of fetal distress. In cases of post-term pregnancy, amniocentesis may be done so the fluid can be examined for the presence of *meconium* (fetal bowel waste). Meconium is a thick, tarry substance that can cause fetal distress and respiratory problems for the baby. Meconium stains or thickens the amniotic fluid, and may indicate that immediate delivery is necessary.

SONOGRAPHY

Ultrasound may be used to monitor fetal growth and activity, and as an adjunct to amniocentesis. It may also be used when there is concern that a post-term fetus will grow too large for vaginal delivery.

Sonography is used to assess the overall size of the fetus when growth retardation is suspected. Specific body parts can be measured for a more precise diagnosis. Darlene had many ultrasounds to monitor the growth of her fetus. She felt that the extra ultrasounds were ordered because medical personnel were "curious to see if the baby was a dwarf, even though we had not asked them about this." Not only was Darlene's sonogram misread by misdiagnosing that the baby had dwarfism, but the diagnosis was also discussed inappropriately. When the diagnosis was presented, the doctor said, "Unfortunately your baby is a dwarf." Darlene said, "It was really awful. I felt like he was saying how unfortunate that I am a dwarf."

A *biophysical profile* is a study that is used to assess the well-being of the fetus. Some physicians recommend this profile for use with fetuses at risk for developing heart block (in mothers with SLE who have SS-A and SS-B antibodies).

STRESS AND NON-STRESS TESTS

In a non-stress test, an external monitor is used to measure fetal heart rhythms. There are a number of indications for this test, including the following:

❖ Preterm labor
❖ Post-term pregnancy (perhaps the most common reason)
❖ Lack of fetal activity
❖ Signs of fetal distress
❖ Maternal complications, such as bleeding or high blood pressure, which might harm the fetus
❖ Multiple pregnancies
❖ Hydramnios (excess amniotic fluid)
❖ History of pregnancy complications

When Leslie experienced bleeding and pain after partial placental abruption, this test helped to determine that immediate delivery was not needed.

Non-stress testing may be repeated for continuing assessment of fetal health. Arlene had miscarriages in her first two pregnancies. She said that during her third pregnancy "they hooked me up from time to time to see if I was healthy. There were never any problems." When there is a risk of fetal heart block, monitoring may be done as often as once a week from the twenty-eighth to the thirty-fourth week. Thereafter, monitoring will be done twice a week from the thirty-fourth week to delivery.

Stress test monitoring is performed after uterine contractions have been intentionally initiated by nipple stimulation or IV injection of oxytocin, which is a hormone that, in larger doses, induces or augments labor. This test evaluates how well the fetus would withstand the stresses of labor and delivery.

Physical Changes

The physical changes of the third trimester are primarily a continuation of the processes that began in the first two trimesters—growth of the breasts and uterus, increase in blood volume, and other changes. Some women find that they either stop gaining weight, or gain weight more slowly. Many women notice the feeling of increased warmth, which is specific to the third trimester. This rise in temperature may be welcomed by women who have disabilities that impair circulation. Several of the interviewees commented, "It was the first time I felt really warm when it wasn't summertime."

INCREASE IN BLOOD VOLUME

The rise in temperature may be caused, in part, by the continuing increase in the blood supply. During the third trimester, blood volume is at least 40 percent greater than it was before pregnancy. This increase can contribute to edema and varicose veins, but it also has positive effects. Many of the interviewees noticed that despite their increased weight, they did not have pressure sores. They also commented that their skin was in better condition than it had ever been.

SKIN

Some, but not all, pregnant women develop "stretch marks," which are reddish streaks that may appear on the breasts, hips, or abdomen. Stretch marks are evidence that the skin is being stretched by the growth of underlying tissues. The abdominal skin is similar to elastic and, like elastic, it may not have enough "give." Although moisturizing creams can make you more comfortable if your skin is dry, expensive creams and exotic ingredients cannot prevent stretch marks. The appearance of stretch marks may bother you, but remember that they usually fade after pregnancy.

BREASTS

Your breast size may increase enough to make you uncomfortable, and if you do not normally wear a brassiere, you may need to start wearing one. Wearing a bra can prevent your breasts from bouncing around and aching. In addition, you can prevent the damp, sticky feeling underneath the breasts. If your disability makes it difficult for you to fasten a brassiere, try an athletic brassiere that fastens in front or pulls on over your head. You can also fasten your brassiere in front and then turn it around. Replacing hooks with snaps or a strip of Velcro™ may also help.

Your breasts may become more sensitive to touch or temperature. For example, your nipples may contract painfully in cold water, or feel uncomfortable in the shower.

Colostrum usually does not appear until after delivery. It may appear during the last several weeks of pregnancy, however. Do not worry if you notice a few drops of secretion or dried fluid on your nipples.

Some women's nipples become sore during the first weeks of breast-feeding, and women who are planning to breast-feed often try to toughen their nipples so that they will not be as sore at first. The following suggestions may help to desensitize your nipples:

❖ Cut holes in the cups of your brassiere, or wear a nursing brassiere with the flaps down, so that your clothing rubs against your nipples.
❖ Rub your nipples with a rough washcloth.
❖ Expose your nipples to air, but not to sunlight or a sun lamp, because dermatologists insist that *no* amount of sun exposure is safe.
❖ Gently but firmly squeeze and turn your nipples between your fingertips.

UTERUS AND CERVIX

Several changes occur in the uterus and cervix. The cervix begins to soften early in pregnancy, but it changes the most during the third trimester. The cervix normally feels about as firm as the tip of your nose. By the end of pregnancy, however, it will have become as soft as an ear lobe. The cervix may also begin to *efface* at about the thirty-eighth week, and may dilate as much as 2 cm. (about 3/4 inch) before labor begins. Dilation is a sign that labor may begin soon. If your doctor does a vaginal examination and finds that your cervix is dilated, you may want to make final preparations for childbirth such as arranging for transportation to the hospital or contacting a diaper service.

A woman whose cervix has dilated may also notice a blood-streaked mucus discharge as early as 2 weeks before labor begins. This "bloody show" often does not appear until after labor has started. If you notice such a discharge, call your doctor and watch for other signs of labor (see Chapter 11).

The uterus begins contracting continuously, although not regularly, at the beginning of pregnancy. These contractions are more noticeable by the seventh or eighth month. They may be quite uncomfortable during the last few weeks of pregnancy. They often feel stronger during a second pregnancy than a first. They usually last about 30 seconds, but may last as long as 2 minutes. These contractions are called *Braxton-Hicks* contractions. Braxton-Hicks contractions exercise the uterine muscles in preparation for labor, and may cause some effacement and dilation of the cervix. Many women take advantage of these contractions to practice the breathing and relaxation techniques they learned in birthing class. At times, Braxton-Hicks contractions can seem much like true labor. Call your doctor if you cannot distinguish between Braxton-Hicks and true contractions. Sydney experienced dysreflexia whenever she had Braxton-Hicks contractions.

Long labors, such as those over 12 hours, can be difficult. The Takoma Women's Health Center in Takoma, Maryland recommends the use of *prostaglandins* to shorten a long labor. Prostaglandins are synthetic versions of body chemicals that naturally induce labor contractions. Prostaglandins increase the ability of the muscles to become coordinated, and make them more receptive to contractions. The use of prostaglandins is controversial, but they may be used to "ripen" the cervix. An unripe cervix is long, firm, and unyielding; a ripe one is relatively shorter and softer. The cervix must be ripe before contractions can safely be induced. To ripen the cervix, a prostaglandin gel or suppository can be applied locally. The Health Center recommends the use of evening primrose oil, which contains linoleic acid that is converted into gamma linoleic acid (GLA), which is necessary for some prostaglandin synthesis. The Health Center has a specific program using this method.

Women who have spinal cord dysfunction may not feel labor contractions, and may be admitted to the hospital in the thirty-eighth week in order to avoid the risk of an unattended birth. They may be admitted earlier if there are signs of preterm labor. There are signs of labor that can be watched for at home, and it might be possible for women with spinal lesions to rent a home monitor to detect labor. Your doctor can advise you how often to check.

Another symptom of impending labor is "lightening." This term refers to the fetus dropping lower in the pelvis. The fundal height is lowered as well. Some women, especially first-time mothers, may experience lightening about 2 to 4 weeks before giving birth. The mother's abdomen will look different, and she may find that she breathes more easily and/or has fewer problems with heartburn and indigestion. Lightening can also cause various discomforts. Pressure from the fetal head can cause urinary difficulties, perineal pain, backaches, groin pain, and mobility difficulties.

Noelle said, "When the baby didn't drop in my second pregnancy, I was afraid I might need another C-section. I went to physical therapy, and used the standing table for half an hour, 3 times a week. The gravity helped; on the third day the baby dropped." Noelle may have worried needlessly, because in some pregnancies babies do not usually become engaged in the pelvis until after labor has begun.

The Discomforts of Pregnancy

UNUSUAL PROBLEMS

Sabine had a detached retina in her ninth month. She said, "I was sitting at the table, when I noticed a field cut in my vision. My doctor told me to get to the hospital fast. They diagnosed it quickly. I chose the procedure that was only 75 percent effective because I did not want to take the chance of an early delivery. The procedure was very painful, and I had to stay still. They saw me every day after that for a week, and then they gave the okay for my doctors to induce labor."

JOINTS

The gradual softening of joint tissues continues in the third trimester, contributing to the distinctive "waddling" walk of late pregnancy. Orielle's pelvic area was painful as her body prepared for birth, and her pelvic joints and ligaments began to loosen.

BREATHING DIFFICULTIES

By late pregnancy, the growth of the uterus pushes the diaphragm up about 4 cm. (1.5 inches). (The diaphragm is the muscle that expands the ribcage in breathing.) This can be a problem for many women. Women with dwarfism may be more vulnerable; three out of every four women who are dwarfs experienced breathing problems in the third trimester. Denise used a wedge under her head, neck, and back, which helped with shortness of breath. Dorothy said, "Breathing was hard; I could not exert myself. All I could do was sit around." Dorothy had a caesarean section a month early because of her breathing problems.

Orielle also had hard time breathing. Her difficulty was explained when she had X-rays of her chest taken by the anesthesiologist. She said, "When the anesthesiologist took the X-rays, he missed taking the picture of the lungs. He had to retake the X-rays higher up because my lungs were pushing up toward my collar bones."

Joan found it hard to breathe because she is small, and her baby was big. She said, "The baby did not have anywhere to go but up, and she would get stuck under my ribs. My husband would put his hands on top of my belly and push her down a little."

Lea Rae said, "It was harder to breathe when it started to get really cold. I was given two different types of inhalers, which helped a lot." Lea Rae was also given an increased dose of steroids.

Many women feel short of breath after exercise. A case study on this subject was reported by Carter and Bonckat regarding a woman with spinal muscular atrophy who required nighttime mechanical ventilator assistance (29).

Other women feel uncomfortable more of the time, like Noelle, who could not talk without stopping frequently to take a breath. Some women, like Carla, simply noticed that their breathing was shallower. Others, like Stephanie and Hilary, commented that breathing was actually painful.

Women who feel short of breath should experiment until they find a position in which they can breathe more comfortably. Stephanie said, "The baby's feet were constantly pressing on my diaphragm. The only way I could relieve the pain was to lie down." Some of the interviewees found that it was hard to breathe when lying down. Sheila solved this problem by sitting up when she slept. For some women, difficulty in breathing while lying down poses special problems. Leslie needed bed rest to prevent a miscarriage, but she was advised to lie flat with pillows under her knees. Unfortunately, this position caused her to feel short of breath. Noelle, who had difficulty breathing even in the first trimester of her pregnancies, found that she breathed most easily in a reclining position. She wishes she could have afforded a reclining wheelchair.

Women who breathe more comfortably in a reclining position should find out whether their medical insurance will pay for a reclining chair. Many insurance companies only pay for a new chair every 5 years. Your doctor can use the medical necessity of reducing respiratory problems as justification for a reclining wheelchair.

Some women, like Noelle, are more comfortable if they eat small meals, thereby avoiding the added pressure of a full stomach on their lungs.

Sometimes special breathing techniques are helpful. Sylvia breathed more easily when she inhaled deeply through her nose, and then exhaled through her mouth. If breathing is difficult in most positions, ask your doctor for a referral to a physical and/or respiratory therapist.

Severe problems may occur in women who have disabilities that ordinarily cause problems with breathing. For example, women with myasthenia gravis, dwarfism, severe scoliosis, or spinal cord injury affecting the diaphragm may be susceptible to respiratory infection. Lowered oxygen levels can endanger both mother and fetus if breathing is impaired.

Occasionally, a woman may find that breathing is easier in late pregnancy. Portia, for example, who commented, "The baby acted like a corset. The pressure made it easier for me to breathe and cough." Nicole said, "I did not have any problems with breathing, heartburn, or my bladder."

VAGINITIS

Although vaginal infections may occur at any time during pregnancy, none of the interviewees recalled having one before the third trimester. Women who are not pregnant can also develop vaginitis, but the hormone changes of pregnancy do increase susceptibility to infection. These infections should never be ignored. Not only do they cause discomfort, but they can also be passed on to babies during birth.

The discharge associated with vaginal infections is different from the normally thin, clear, or whitish discharge associated with pregnancy. The most common infection is called Candida, Monilia, or yeast. It produces a discharge that is thick and opaque, and many people say it looks like cottage cheese. It has a mild, characteristic odor. Clara remarked, "I knew I had a yeast infection because I recognized the smell." Another infection, Trichomonas, produces a thin, yellow-green, sometimes foamy, foul-smelling discharge.

Yeast organisms are always present in the vagina, but some conditions can cause them to multiply rapidly, causing discharge, mild to intense itching, irritation or burning, and redness. Women who experience the signs or symptoms of infection should call their doctor. The doctor can then examine them and, if necessary, prescribe locally applied medications—creams, gels, or suppositories that are inserted into the vagina. Yeast organisms thrive in warm, moist conditions. Women who keep their genitals clean and dry, and wear cotton underwear rather than synthetic, not only feel more comfortable, but they are likely to heal faster and reduce the change of re-infection. Some women find it is especially helpful to wear a skirt without any underwear during the day, and a nightgown rather than pajamas at night. Do not douche without instructions from your doctor.

Some antibiotics can increase susceptibility to yeast infection, and women who must use them should be alert for symptoms.

Symptoms of Trichomonas include pain, itching, and/or irritation at the vaginal opening. Pain is more likely to occur during intercourse. Again, women who experience these symptoms should call their doctor, who will prescribe the appropriate medication. Remember to ask your doctor about medication side effects. Trichomonas is easily transmitted between partners, and it is a good idea to have your partner examined and treated at the same time that you are.

Women who have reduced sensation may not be able to feel the irritation of vaginitis. Check for discharge or redness when bathing.

HEARTBURN AND RELATED DISCOMFORTS

Heartburn is a type of indigestion that has nothing to do with the heart. It occurs when stomach acids are forced from the stomach into the esophagus, which is the "tube" leading from the throat to the stomach. Irritation of the esophageal lining causes a burning sensation. Although this problem can occur earlier in pregnancy, it is most common in the third trimester, when pressure from the enlarged uterus is greater.

A related problem is reflux, a problem wherein a small amount of food is forced back into the esophagus. The amount may not be great enough to be considered vomiting. Some women find that reflux is more likely to occur after fetal movement. Whenever she eats, the mother may feel as though the fetus responds to the pressure from the stomach by kicking or stretching. Denise said, "I had to take Maalox™ every day because I had heartburn—big time. Nothing helped, even though I ate six small meals a day."

Orielle was prescribed two medicines to speed up her digestion: omeprazole (Prilosec®), and Propulsid®, which is used for gastroesophageal reflux disease.

One woman found that the treatment for her thrush, diphenhydramine (HCL) (Benadryl®), had an extra benefit: it reduced her reflux. Be sure to consult your doctor before trying this treatment.

Many women who have reflux avoid food that aggravates this condition. They avoid lemon juice, garlic, and tomatoes because they are more acidic. One to three acidophilus capsules may also be helpful for reflux, because acidophilus helps provide the healthy bacteria necessary for digestion. Try one capsule and increase slowly.

Hernia is another problem that may be associated with reflux. "Hiatal hernia occurs when the upper part of the stomach moves up into the chest through a small opening in the diaphragm (*diaphragmatic hiatus*)" (87). This type of hernia may cause vomiting, epigastric pain, and even bleeding. Another other type of hernia is diaphragmatic. "Diaphragmatic hernias need to be repaired during pregnancy, even if the patient is asymptomatic" (88).

Many women feel uncomfortable after full meals, even when they are not bothered by heartburn or reflux. Try the following suggestions to avoid or reduce heartburn and reflux:

❖ Eat small, frequent meals, so you do not become too full. Julie commented that this advice from her nutritionist was particularly helpful: "Take small bites and chew and swallow slowly."

❖ Sip cool water to "rinse" the esophagus, relieving irritation and washing digestive acids back into the stomach. Liquids may also help by diluting stomach acids. Heather felt more comfortable when she sipped milk or lemon-lime sodas, but other women may find soda irritating. Try drinking liquids at a different time than eating.

❖ Avoid eating mint, chocolate, and caffeine, because they relax the lower esophageal sphincter.

❖ Avoid gaining excess weight, which can increase pressure on the stomach.

❖ Do not wear tight clothing or a tight belt.

❖ Bend at the hips and knees, not the waist, when lifting objects and tying your shoes.

❖ Change sleeping and resting routines if necessary. Wait 2 hours after eating before going to bed. Raise the head of the bed about 6 inches, or sleep with several pillows. If you must rest during the day, do not lie flat. Julie preferred to be propped up at a 45° angle. She said, "I wish I'd had a recliner." Natasha preferred to lie on her left side with a pillow between her legs. As an added benefit, she never "woke up with a backache."

❖ Avoid cigarettes.

❖ Avoid stress during and after meals. Tension can make heartburn worse. If your heartburn occurs when you are under stress, find ways to solve the problem; for example, by changing your work schedule.

❖ Play soft background music while you eat to help you relax. Take a few minutes after eating to do some deep breathing or relaxation exercises, but do not lie down. Exercise several times a day. Raise your arms straight overhead, clasp your hands a moment, and then lower your arms to your side. This exercise temporarily relieves pressure, and may stimulate the fetus to change position. If you cannot do it independently, your husband or attendant can assist you.

Reflux can be a problem if it interferes with the absorption of oral medications. Discuss this with your doctor. Perhaps you can take medications between meals.

Constipation

As stated previously, constipation is having dry stools and straining during bowel movements. Do not worry if your bowel movements do not occur every day, as long as your stools are soft and pass easily. Constipation is a common discomfort during late pregnancy because pregnancy hormones relax the smooth muscles of the intestines (especially the colon), and decrease *peristalsis* (the regular muscle contractions of the bowel that propel the food). This makes digestion less efficient, and pressure from the enlarged uterus adds to the problem.

Women who have a disability that normally causes constipation may have worse problems during pregnancy. Women who have spinal cord injury may also have more difficulty with this problem because their bowel motility is already affected.

Fluid intake is critical for reducing constipation. Natasha increased her fluid intake from 8 oz. to 32 oz. per day. If your problem with constipation becomes severe, call your doctor right away to discuss whether you should use an enema or go to the office or the emergency room for disimpaction.

Iron supplements can be constipating, and several of the interviewees commented that they reduced or stopped taking iron in order to relieve constipation. Iron is an important nutrient, however. Rather than eliminating iron on your own, talk to your doctor about taking another type of iron or a lower dose. The absorption of iron can be enhanced by taking 500 mg of vitamin C.

Many of the interviewees eased or prevented their problems with constipation by drinking plenty of liquids and eating foods rich in fiber, including dried fruits, kidney beans (4 to 8 ounces a day), and garbanzo beans (chick peas) (see Appendix C). Stacy and Stephanie found that they had to use suppositories more frequently. None of the interviewees mentioned using exercise to reduce constipation, but women who can walk may find that it helps. Changing position more frequently or exercising may help relieve constipation (see Chapter 7). Resting your feet on a footstool may help reduce the strain during a bowel movement. Several of the interviewees mentioned using various types of laxatives, but laxatives can also cause problems, and you should talk with your doctor before using them. Hannah's doctor recommended Metamucil®, which worked for her.

Sylvia's problems were different than those of the other women. She explained, "I had an unpredictable bowel; it never responded to suppositories." At times, Sylvia had diarrhea, and often soiled while being transferred. She wore disposable underwear and tried to eat foods that would lessen the problem. Ongoing diarrhea can be a serious problem, leading to dehydration. Women with significant diarrhea should drink plenty of clear fluids to replace what is lost, and call their doctor.

Remember, too, that diarrhea can be a sign of labor. So, pay attention to any other symptoms that accompany diarrhea, and be sure to report them to your doctor.

Personal Hygiene

Denise had difficulty with personal hygiene. She said, "I had to go out and buy salad tongs so I could reach around to wipe myself." An alternative is a bidet, which can be attached to your toilet. It has a narrow line that squirts water for cleaning.

Amanda had problems pulling her underwear up or down during her second pregnancy because her balance was compromised. She would lean her head on the bathroom wall or use the grab bar in order to stabilize herself.

Hemorrhoids

Hemorrhoids are swollen veins in the anus. External hemorrhoids look like "blood blisters." They may be itchy or painful, especially during difficult bowel movements. They may even bleed.

Several factors can contribute to the development of hemorrhoids: pregnancy hormones may relax the walls of the veins; blood may pool in the lower body; or heredity may be responsible for weakness of the veins. Straining during bowel movements can also contribute to the development of hemorrhoids, or make existing hemorrhoids worse.

Stephanie commented, "I already had hemorrhoids. When I was pregnant, I had swelling all through the perineal area, and the hemorrhoids got worse." Cool Touch® is a cushion that stays cool. It comes in different shapes. This product is advertised as a great natural alternative for hemorrhoids, constipation, sleeping difficulty, and improving circulation.

Women who have hemorrhoids can use the following methods to reduce discomfort and avoid irritation, infection, and constipation. Straining during bowel movements can make hemorrhoids worse (see Chapter 6):

❖ Keep the perineum and anus clean. After each bowel movement, rinse with clear, warm water—not soap.
❖ Use white, unscented toilet paper.

❖ Ice packs or witch hazel compresses can relieve pain for some women. Ice did not help Stephanie, but it did help Felicia. (A bag of frozen peas can be used because it is flexible and forms to the area.)

❖ Warm compresses or warm soaks can help some women. If you cannot use a bathtub, try a sitz bath.

❖ Use a cushion to reduce pressure when sitting. Some women use a special inflatable, ring-shaped cushion.

❖ Preparation H® can be directly applied to hemorrhoids.

Felicia's hemorrhoids were so severe that she had a *hemorrhoidectomy* (removal of the hemorrhoid) 6 days before delivery. She said, "I had five thrombosed hemorrhoids. I had local anesthesia. I had no complications other than I really couldn't take pain meds. I took Tylenol®, but it was not strong enough to relieve the pain. I spent the next week battling pain, and becoming more and more exhausted. My blood pressure spiked, which I believed was also because of the pain. A hemorrhoid pillow and sitting on a bag of frozen peas helped.

Varicose Veins

Varicose veins are swollen veins, like hemorrhoids, but the problem is in the veins of the legs. They have the same causes as hemorrhoids. The leg veins may be only slightly more noticeable than usual, or they may look like swollen, twisting blue lines on the legs. They can be painless, mildly achy, or quite uncomfortable. Sometimes when the problem is severe, an *embolism* (blood clot) may develop in the varicose vein. Varicose veins usually improve after pregnancy, but may reappear or become worse in later pregnancies.

Women who have varicose veins can minimize the problem as follows:

❖ Avoid excessive weight gain.

❖ Avoid prolonged standing with knees locked. When sitting or lying down, elevate the legs to improve circulation.

❖ Wear support stockings all day if your doctor prescribes support stockings. Put them on before getting out of bed in the morning, and take them off just before going to sleep.

❖ Exercising as much as your disability allows will encourage better circulation. If your ability to exercise is limited, perhaps a physical therapist can provide passive exercise or massage to improve circulation.

Edema

Various studies have found that from 33 to 75 percent of able-bodied, pregnant women experience edema. Thirty percent of the interviewees had edema during the last trimester. Paula did not experience edema during her first pregnancy, which was before she became disabled, but she did have it in subsequent pregnancies.

Some swelling, especially in the feet, is quite common in the third trimester. Swelling of the hands is less common, but some women may need to remove their rings until the end of pregnancy. As explained previously, increased blood volume contributes to edema, and it will have increased by at least 45 percent by the third trimester. When the walls of the veins relax, and the uterus increases pressure on the leg veins, pooling of the blood can occur, which may contribute to edema.

One might expect that mobility impairment would make women more susceptible to edema, yet there was no such pattern among the interviewees. Sylvia had minimum swelling. Samantha said, "It wasn't as bad as I thought it would be." Stephanie commented, "I have always had edema, but it was just a little worse when I was pregnant."

Diane said, "My feet never touch the ground when I sit, so I try not to sit for long periods of time with my legs dangling." Joy said, "My feet were so swollen that I couldn't put my shoes on." She was able to find sandals with Velcro™, which worked until the middle of the eighth month.

Sally had swelling of her feet and ankles. She said, "I always have some swelling, but during pregnancy it was much worse." Reclining in her chair with her legs up did not help. Sally said, "They seemed to stay fat no matter what." Signey felt that a recliner helped to keep her feet elevated.

Natasha also experienced swelling in her feet. She normally has problems finding shoes because her shoes help compensate for drop foot. This became a bigger problem during pregnancy, resulting in her wearing only one pair of shoes during the third trimester. She said, "I figured it was going to be over soon. Why spend the money on more shoes. Natasha also experienced "pins and needles" in her feet.

Hilary felt better when she fastened her shoes more loosely. It may be worthwhile to buy inexpensive shoes that are more comfortable. Wearing elastic stockings helps some women. If you want to try them, first buy one pair, and make sure that it is not too hard to put them on and take them off.

Several of the interviewees felt that it was helpful to elevate their legs with pillows when they slept. Resting with your legs elevated also helps. Raising your legs higher than your body is best, but some disabilities make this difficult. Julie remarked, "I used a footstool; it was better than nothing."

During pregnancy, Allison carried extra prosthetic socks with her. She said, "I would start out in the morning not being able to wear my socks. As the day went on, the swelling reduced, and then I could put my socks on." Allison also fell. She said, "I slipped into a puddle of vomit, so after that I was really careful. I looked at the ground all the time."

It was not until the last 6 weeks of pregnancy that Natalie's feet began to swell. She said, "They kind of bubbled out around my brace at front part of my foot. They would really puff out when I took my brace off. I finally quit my job because I was standing on my feet up to 10 hours a day."

It is also important to differentiate the normal edema of pregnancy from disability symptoms and edema caused by medical treatment. Orielle had edema, partly because she was given steroids to ensure her son's lungs would be developed enough for an early delivery.

When Renee was awakened by swelling and pain, she realized it might be rheumatic inflammation. She reduced the pain by taking a hot bath. It is also important to differentiate between regular edema and preeclampsia.

Severe swelling can be a sign of preeclampsia. Pam recalled, "The swelling in my feet was so bad that my doctor thought I might have preeclampsia, but my blood pressure was normal." Call your doctor if you experience severe or sudden swelling. It is also wise to have your blood pressure checked regularly.

Painful or Tingling Hands

Sometimes swelling is severe enough to create pressure on the median nerve, resulting in carpal tunnel syndrome. This syndrome includes pain, tingling, and weakness in the wrist or hand, which makes it difficult to pick up objects. The syndrome is especially troublesome if the dominant hand is affected. Sometimes splinting helps relieve discomfort.

A differential diagnosis should be made between thoracic outlet syndrome (which occurs when the nerves in the neck are pinched) and carpal tunnel or edema. You do not have carpal tunnel syndrome if all your fingers are numb or burning, because the distribution of the median nerve is only to the thumb, index, finger, and middle finger. A differential diagnosis also should be made between carpal tunnel and a possible flare-up in women with lupus or arthritis.

Carpal tunnel syndrome is especially troublesome if both hands are affected. Andrea, Naomi, and Shelby had carpal tunnel syndrome. Naomi's disability caused her to have a predisposition to it. Andrea and Shelby's use of assistive devices caused their predisposition, because the assistive devices they used put pressure on their wrists, thereby putting them at risk for carpal tunnel syndrome. Andrea did not want to switch to using a wheelchair because she wanted to stay as physical as possible. Swimming, yoga, and other exercises are good alternatives for staying in shape (see Chapter 7).

Andrea now uses a manual chair more often. When she knows she will be going someplace that requires her to do a great deal of walking, she uses her manual chair or she rents a motorized scooter. Andrea's doctor would prefer that she use a power wheelchair at all times to prevent her condition from getting worse. Shelby needed surgery to correct her carpal tunnel symptoms. The surgery Naomi had after both of her deliveries was successful.

Vitamin B_6 deficiency is a common finding in carpal tunnel syndrome. The recommended dose is 100 to 200 mg per day. It can take up to 3 months before benefits are seen (61). As discussed in Chapter 6, vitamin B_6 can cause agitation or insomnia, and doses at 100 mg or above may cause permanent nerve damage.

Ask your doctor for a referral to an occupational therapist or physical therapy if hand weakness is making your normal daily activities more difficult. Raising your arms over your head can help relieve pain and swelling. Some women find massage or cool soaks helpful.

Natasha had swelling in her hands that resulted in her taking off one of her engagement rings and having the wedding band enlarged. The swelling in Sophia Amelia's hands made it difficult for her to push her chair because it was difficult to grip the wheel and her center of gravity had changed. Tessa was afraid that excess fluid retention would cause more pain in her arms, which could cause her to use her arms even less. Fortunately, this did not happen.

HEADACHES

During the third trimester, severe headaches may occur in women who have a shunt. This may be a result of the increasing size of the uterus as well as increases in intra-abdominal pressure (89). Holly said, "I had fewer headaches while I was pregnant with all three of my babies than I normally do. I analyzed this, and suspect that my shunt system worked better because of the higher pressure caused naturally by pregnancy."

URINARY PROBLEMS

The majority of women find that they have to urinate more frequently during the third trimester because of pressure from the enlarged uterus. Some begin to have problems with stress incontinence, which occurs when laughing, sneezing, or straining. Sudden fetal movements can also cause incontinence late in pregnancy. The flow of urine is sometimes so sudden that the mother cannot tell whether she has urinated or her "bag has broken." In this case, call your doctor and ask if you should come in for an examination. The doctor may ask you to watch for signs of labor.

Existing urinary problems may get worse, but sometimes the reason for urgency or frequency is unclear. Marsha, who took a vacation in Hawaii late in her pregnancy, said, "I couldn't tell whether the problem was from the heat, pressure from the baby, or exacerbation of multiple sclerosis."

Many of the interviewees coped with frequent urination by making sure that they were never far from a bathroom. Some of them also had difficulty with bladder control, and they stopped wearing pants or even underwear. This way, they could use the toilet as quickly as possible when the reached a bathroom. Signey said, "It was a balance between drinking enough water and getting to a bathroom in time. At the end, having the bedside commode helped a lot. I felt less restricted in terms of having to get to the bathroom in the middle of the night, and I was able to drink more."

Women who have catheters may have additional problems, because deposits of calcium crystals or pressure from the uterus may obstruct their catheters. Sylvia has a suprapubic catheter. She recalled, "I got a plugged catheter, and had to irrigate it twice a day.

The problem was worse when I drank milk, so I got calcium from other sources." Women who have catheters that are obstructed should not eliminate calcium from their diets without talking to their doctor or nutritionist about finding other sources. Fetal pressure caused urine to leak around Sylvia's catheter late in her pregnancy, so her doctor re-inserted it at a different angle.

Sydney had difficulty catheterizing while sitting on the toilet. If Shanna was out in the community and needed to catheterize, her husband had to go with her into the women's room. She did not have problems catheterizing when she was lying down on her bed.

Sabine's pregnant belly occluded her vision, and she could not change her ostomy bag. She had her husband change it.

Sara and Stacy retain urine, and needed to use a catheter until they gave birth. Stacy empties her bladder by manual pressure, but was unable to do so during late pregnancy. She said, "My obstetrician was concerned that if my bladder was full when I went into labor, it would interfere with the baby's descent. He inserted a catheter 3 days before the baby was born."

Women who have catheters and find blood in their urine should not be too anxious, because the problem may be mechanical irritation, but they should still tell their doctors. Stacy found blood in her urine after her catheter was inserted. Stephanie also noticed blood in her urine during the third trimester but, she said, "My doctor wasn't concerned" because the bleeding was caused by irritation from the catheter. Blood in the urine can also be a sign of bladder or kidney infection. You may want to ask your doctor to examine you for other signs of infection.

Women should be aware of the signs and symptoms of urinary and kidney infections and tell their doctors, because infections are most likely to occur during the third trimester. It has been reported that women with cerebral palsy have an increased incidence of kidney infection during the third trimester. Only one interviewee out of sixteen pregnancies had a urinary tract infection.

BACK AND LEG PAIN

You may begin to have back or leg pain in the third trimester because of the increased weight of the uterus and fetus. Joan was able to differentiate her arthritis back pain from pain that resulted from her pregnancy. Joy said, "The pain in my back was mostly from the way I stood because my big belly strained my back. The back support was helpful, and I also bought elastic panties for extra support."

Sophia Amelia took a bath to help relieve her backaches. She had a problem getting out of the bath, and needed her husband to help her transfer. Another woman found that getting into a reclining wheelchair relieved some of her back pain. The maternity back brace has reduced back pain for some women with a disability. Even if a brace reduces back pain, some women with limited mobility may want to get extra help for personal care and household work because pain can be exacerbated by activity. Using a pillow to support a new position can help reduce back pain.

Darlene sat with a pillow that helped her breathe, and also gave her hip and back support. Natalie had both back and hip pain. Many women feel more comfortable using a footstool when they sit. Sometimes, application of cold compresses can also help reduce the pain and inflammation. This may help with muscle pain, but it may not help with nerve pain. The Cool Touch™ cushion may also help.

The fetal head may put pressure on the sciatic nerve, causing *sciatica*. This nerve runs from the sacrum (lower spine) down the entire length of the leg and into the foot. Sciatic pain may be limited to the lower back and buttocks, or extend down the back of the leg. Carla remarked, "The pain made it difficult to walk. If I had it to do over, I would use a wheelchair." It is possible Heather felt sciatica as part of her phantom pain. She said, "The first time I was pregnant, I had muscle cramps in my stump and back. I also had phantom pain. I think it must have been my baby pressing on the nerve, because I didn't have any of these problems the second time." Holly said, "I had sciatica with my third child that caused me to lie down more."

Sierra had back pain so severe that she went to the hospital for relief. While she was at the hospital, they assessed whether she was having back labor or sciatic pain. The sciatic pain of pregnancy may be eased by the application of localized heat and finding comfortable positions when sitting and sleeping.

SLEEPLESSNESS

Many women have trouble sleeping during late pregnancy because they need to get up at night to urinate, and because it is difficult to find a comfortable sleeping position. As previously discussed in Chapter 9, the cardinal rule is, *never lie flat on your back*. The uterus presses on large veins in this position, interfering with circulation. It may also interfere with digestion, cause back strain, or make breathing difficult.

Sleeping on your stomach may also be difficult, but placing pillows under your breasts and hips may help. If you prefer to sleep sitting up, use a pillow as a backrest to avoid the discomfort of having pillows shift or slide out from under you. You can also take naps or rest during the day to catch up on sleep." If you sleep in a sitting or reclining position, it may be helpful to place pillows under your knees. This avoids stretching the sciatic nerve. Women with leg pain may find that this is the only way they can sleep really well.

Tessa found that sleeping on her side "seemed to compress her thoracic region, and further exacerbated her condition." She felt more comfortable sleeping "in a luxurious reclining chair." Renting a hospital bed may be an alternative. Pam and Sheila both said they wished that they had gotten hospital beds. Hannah said, "Towards the end of my pregnancy, I mostly slept on the couch propped up, more like lounging than lying." Pam elaborated, "I couldn't lie on my left side because of my shoulder fusion and spinal curvature, and I couldn't stay on my right side for long because the baby was more to the right and the pressure was uncomfortable. Pillows on either side just didn't help much. A water bed might have helped with the pressure points, but it's too hard to move on a water bed."

Some women sleep more comfortably when lying on their sides. Orielle slept in a reclining position by "using a billion pillows." Diane said, "I would always have a pillow on the side of me to help support my belly. Things always shift when you lie on your side."

Moira used eight pillows to get into the perfect position for sleep. She said, "I was slightly propped up in bed. Three pillows were under my head and shoulders. I slept slightly on my left side, and I had two pillows underneath my knees. I also held onto one pillow."

If you feel better sleeping on your side, try to sleep on your left side, because this position is best for good circulation. Place pillows between your legs, or place the top (right) leg somewhat in front of the bottom leg, supported by pillows. Michelle pointed out that, while pillows can add to comfort, they also make it difficult to move around.

Sleep will come more easily if you are relaxed and comfortable at bedtime. Do not eat too closely to bedtime. If you are having difficulty controlling your bladder, consider keeping a urinal under your bed, wearing absorbent underwear, or using a waterproof mattress-cover, so that anxiety about having an "accident" does not keep you awake. Keep the temperature of your bedroom at a comfortable level. Try taking a warm bath or doing stretching and relaxation exercises just before you go to bed. Schedule fewer activities if you find yourself overly tired during the day. Cheryl changed her work hours from full-time to half-time.

MOBILITY DIFFICULTIES

Even able-bodied women feel clumsier during the third trimester, because their center of gravity keeps changing as they gain weight. This makes it difficult to keep their sense of balance. The extra weight of pregnancy can also affect the ability to move, as well as the activities of daily living, such as bathing and dressing. Not all women experience these difficulties in the third trimester. Noreen felt better and was stronger for most of the third trimester, until the 34th week. She said, "I walked more. I went to the movies. I shopped for baby clothes. I didn't need as much help as I had previously. I did feel uncomfortable being so big." Noreen was put on steroids right before delivery. Holly felt her balance was affected only slightly in her first pregnancy. She was still able to work as a teacher and stay on her feet most of the day throughout her entire pregnancy.

Sherry Adele said, "I didn't have any problems with walking, I just couldn't walk as far." Deirdre's problem with balance started in the second trimester, but she got help in the third trimester. She said, "I had a home visit from a physical therapist who gave me some exercises to do until more physical therapy was authorized. The program included balance exercises."

Many disabled women are afraid of falling. Some women need adaptive equipment to making walking easier, but many are uncomfortable using or switching to adaptive equipment. Julie developed joint pain if she stood too long, so she sat on a high stool when doing things such as washing dishes. Jennifer said, "Walking was easier than standing. I got uncomfortable when I stood still. So I just walked back and forth whenever I had to wait in a line."

Several of the interviewees fell during the third trimester, and they reacted to the experience in a variety of ways. Celeste said, "I only fell once. It could have happened to anyone. It wasn't so bad." Julie said, "When I tripped over a rug, it really shook my confidence. I was afraid of falling again. I became much more cautious, and stopped work earlier than I had planned. I increased my attendant care and limited outside activities."

Naomi felt unsteady on her feet during her second pregnancy, plus her "hips felt wobbly." She lived in another area less receptive to the disabled and was not comfortable using a walker, as she had during her first pregnancy. During her second pregnancy, she avoided walking any distance and used handicap transportation within train stations. Moreover, she said, "I made people let me sit down on the metro."

Sabine also found that walking affected her during pregnancy. Her "good" leg was weakened. Her calf muscle got tight, and she had muscles spasms that were probably due to overuse. She found that walking with a cane helped.

Chloe needed help with standing and walking because she "felt top-heavy." Hannah, who walks with a noticeable limp, said, "It was hard to walk with my center of gravity changed. I did not do much walking. It had to be extremely important to get me to walk."

Many of the interviewees did not want to start using wheelchairs, but eventually they did. Some started using the chair more often. Hilary recalled, "The first time I was pregnant, I used my prostheses until I fell in the eighth month; then I started using a wheelchair. It was so much easier, that when I became pregnant the second time, I started using a chair much sooner. Some women may not use assistive equipment because it may not be offered as an option. Natalie fell six or seven times on the same day, and nobody discussed the issue of getting assistive equipment. This also happened to Andrea. She had such bad sciatic pain that she was unable to walk. Andrea suggests that women get a wheelchair if necessary. She said, "I had never thought of using the chair. I'd always been on my crutches, and it never dawned on me to use a wheelchair. If the doctor had suggested it, I probably would have listened a lot more. My husband encouraged me to use a wheelchair, but having two wheelchairs in one household was crowded." Andrea could have used her chair only out in the community.

Sierra also found it difficult get around. She said, "I would lie on the couch all the time because it was too hard to walk. What would normally be a 10-minute walk would take me a half an hour."

Although Nadine had never thought of using a wheelchair, when the question was raised, she said, "I probably would have gone out more. I was really stuck in the house at the end."

For some women, one alternative is to use a wheelchair for a few months. Using a wheelchair more of the time, or learning to use a wheelchair, can also cause problems. Sara recalled, "I only used a wheelchair for going long distances before I was pregnant. I used crutches until the seventh month. My balance was a problem, so I decided to use a chair. Once when I was going over a curb it flipped backwards." Sara was the only person whose wheelchair flipped while she was pregnant. If you regularly use a chair, it is worth noting that weight change can change the way the chair maneuvers. Some women felt that they might fall forward, especially when taking their chairs over curbs. Take the following precautions if you start using a manual wheelchair:

❖ Wear a seat belt. If your trunk stability is affected keep the belt under your belly
❖ Avoid taking the chair over curbs
❖ Use a driveway when you cannot find a curb cut
❖ Have an anti-tipping device installed, or have the chair re-adjusted
❖ Adjust the casters

Transfers

Sylvia preferred a cradle transfer when she was not pregnant. Using the cradle transfer made breathing more difficult during her last 2 months of pregnancy, however. She found that a pivot transfer was best for moving from her chair to her bed. Pam prefers to be grasped by the waist when she is lifted. She said, "I worried that pressure from the belt my assistant used might hurt the baby, but my doctor reassured me that the baby would be okay." A Hoyer Lift™ may be used to assist in transferring.

SITTING TO STANDING

Heather, Julie, and Christina all said that it became difficult to stand up from a chair or toilet. It may help to use a raised toilet seat. Use cushions to raise the seats of chairs because this will bring the center of gravity forward. Amy found a raised toilet seat helpful. (Appendix D contains information regarding the Uplift seat assist and a lift chair that is designed to help lift a person to the standing position.) In order for Nadine to get up from sitting in a chair, she would "sit on the edge and push off from the arms of the chair."

BED TRANSFER

Dawn said, "Moving from lying down to sitting up was a big hassle." Getting out of bed can be difficult, even for able-bodied women, if the bed is low. Chloe could not get on the floor. Moreover, she was unable to roll over in bed. Joan is unable to lean on her arms to get out of bed, so she normally does a quick sit-up. Her method of doing a sit-up was impossible with "a full belly." Nadine's solution to getting out of bed was to roll onto her side, then push up on her elbows and roll out to stand up. She said, "I'd be on my side resting on my elbows with my feet on the floor and my torso on the bed, and I would push up with my arms." (See Appendix D (Sammons Preston Catalog) regarding an adaptive device that allows a person to pull themselves into a sitting position. This "Bed Pull-Up," or "BedHoist," is attached to the bed.)

It is easier to move to a sitting position if you are sleeping with the support of pillows or a backrest. It may help to have a piece of sturdy furniture next to the bed and use it as support. If you have been sleeping on your side, try putting your legs over the side of the bed first, then use an arm or an object for support or leverage to help you come to a sitting position.

Shower or Tub

There are several problems in getting out of a bathtub:

- ❖ Difficulty maneuvering in a small space, especially if the tub has sliding doors.
- ❖ Changing to a standing position
- ❖ Stepping over the side of the tub
- ❖ Keeping your balance on the slippery surface

Getting in and out of the bathtub and moving in the tub was difficult for most of the interviewees, regardless of their degree of disability. Some women may decide to take sponge baths. Pam explained, "I couldn't sit in the tub without feeling like I might drown. I wished I had a shower or a completely tiled bathroom." Women who use wheelchairs often have more trouble transferring to the bathtub when they are pregnant. Sheila said, "It was scary. I needed more help to get in and out of the tub." Most of the interviewees avoided the problem of raising and lowering themselves by using a bath bench or a sturdy chair in the tub. Some women can swing their legs over the edge of the tub, and then use a bar to leverage themselves into a standing position. Other women get on their hands and knees, rise to a kneeling position, and then hold onto a grab bar. Both Dorothy and Orielle put a step stool in the bathtub. Hannah's solution was to take showers only when her husband was around to help.

Heather Ann bought an inexpensive plastic stool at a variety store to sit on in the bathtub. She said, "If my husband wasn't home, I would drain the water from the tub, and then sit on the side of the tub and grab the sink to get up." You may be able to add a hand-held shower attachment if you do not have a shower. Another solution is to use a shower stall. Place non-skid material on the floor of your bathtub or shower to prevent falls. Heather used a piece of indoor-outdoor carpet.

In addition to having difficulty getting in and out of the tub, Sherry Adele had trouble washing her hair, so she washed it while sitting in the tub.

CAR TRANSFER

Another problem that many of the interviewees experienced was difficulty getting in and out of cars. Hilary used two methods, depending on whether or not she was using her prostheses. She has no femurs, and her prostheses are somewhat like stilts. She said, "When I was wearing my prostheses, I got in the car about the same way a person with paraplegia does. I would put my crutches in the car, and then sit down on the front seat. I scooted backward a bit, grabbed my legs under the knees where my prostheses are attached, and then used my hands to pull my legs in. When I wasn't wearing my prostheses, I would begin by holding onto the steering wheel. Then I'd put my left foot in the car and, holding onto the wheel, I'd pull in my body and my right leg. At this point, I would be lying face down on the front seat. I pulled a little farther in, rolled over, and sat up. I rolled to sitting just the way an 11-month-old baby does."

Nora had a very healthy pregnancy, but said, "Transferring in and out of the car and bath got harder the last couple of weeks of pregnancy." She gave birth at 35 weeks.

Sherry Adele had problems standing up when getting out of the car. She pulled herself up using more of her upper body. Amanda did not have any trouble getting into the minivan because she could "put her butt on the seat and get in." Moira and Joy had no problems getting in and out of a SUV, but Moira said, "It just took little longer." This was not the case for Signey, who had more of a problem getting into a SUV.

Julie's solution was to use pillows as aids. She explained, "The pillow made it easier for me to slide off the seat of my wheelchair. I would then push back toward the passenger door to swing in my feet. Sometimes I would get stuck lying flat on the seat. If I was alone, I would use an extra pillow I kept on the passenger side for leverage."

Deirdre's backside was more sensitive, so she built her car seat back up by using egg crate foam on her seat and over her adapted back seat (Sacroease™).

Portia had five pregnancies. She said, "I used a sliding board even when I wasn't pregnant, and simply stopped driving when I couldn't fit behind the steering wheel. Another problem was that my wheelchair was so heavy I needed help getting it in and out of the car. I tended to stay home more during the last 3 months." Mostly I just went out with my husband." Carla, too, felt it was easier not to go out too often. She said, "I had my parents or my husband do the shopping." Simi said, "It was difficult getting the chair in and out of the car." The distance between Olivia and the steering wheel was too tight, so she pushed her seat farther back in order to get in and out easily. It is important to keep the seatbelt under your belly on your pelvic bones. Sophia Amelia had difficulty transferring inside a vehicle and from her wheelchair into the driver's seat. It was difficult for both Sienna and Sophia Amelia to drive because they had to sit so far back from the steering wheel.

Adaptive equipment is available to help with transferring in and out of a car. For example, a swivel cushion can help you swing your legs in and out. The CarCaddie™ is a piece of webbing strap that can be attached to a car window to help with leverage in getting out of a car.

Activities of Daily Living

Loss of balance and the size of the pregnant abdomen make it difficult to do tasks that require bending forward, such as adjusting a wheelchair or getting dressed. Women have varying degrees of difficulty with dressing. Darlene said, "I just lifted my foot up to put my shoes on." Lea Rae started wearing house slippers instead of shoes in the third trimester. When she did wear shoes, someone had to help her get them on. Nicole had another option; she used a personal care attendant to help her with household chores.

Shanna had a hard time righting herself. This caused her to stop picking things up off the floor. She got a reacher to "grab things off the floor." Orielle said, "I couldn't bend over to pick up anything." Her solution was to use her service dog to get things that she needed. Samantha pulled up her legs to put on her shoes; Julie used a footstool. Women who are able to balance well enough (possibly while holding onto a support) might try stepping into loafers.

Nancy had difficulty using her hands for activities such as writing and washing her face. She normally stabilizes the hand she is using by placing her opposite elbow on her armrest and grasping her forearm. When she was pregnant, however, she could not use the armrest because she needed to sit farther back in her wheelchair; she also had trouble reaching across her abdomen. A lap tray is useful in a situation such as this. You may need to consult an occupational or physical therapist.

Complications

GESTATIONAL DIABETES

The pancreas produces insulin, a hormone that facilitates the transfer of glucose (sugar) from the bloodstream into the cells of the body. During pregnancy, the cells become more resistant to the effects of insulin, in large part because of a hormone produced by the placenta. This causes many pregnant women to develop gestational diabetes.

Diabetes of pregnancy adversely affects both mother and fetus. Effects on the mother include a greatly increased risk of developing preeclampsia/eclampsia; increased susceptibility can lead to infection; and possibly difficulties in labor because the fetus grows too large. Possible effects on the fetus include birth injuries resulting from disproportion between a large fetus and the mother's pelvis, respiratory distress, metabolic problems, and birth defects.

Diabetes can be controlled by diet if it is mild, but more severe cases must be treated with medication. You will need to work closely with your doctor, and have frequent blood tests to monitor the effectiveness of your treatment. Gestational diabetes usually disappears at the end of pregnancy, but some women who have gestational diabetes become diabetic some years later.

The doctors discovered that Noreen had diabetes while she hospitalized in the last month of her pregnancy, despite her being on a diabetic diet and eating no sweets. She believes that the diabetes was probably due to steroids.

Sienna also had gestational diabetes and saw a dietician, who put her on a restricted diet the last 2 months of her pregnancy that eliminated sugar and limited fat intake.

At first, the doctors thought Felicia had gestational diabetes because of the results of her first blood tests. In subsequent tests, however, it turned out not to be true.

Preeclampsia/Eclampsia

Preeclampsia may begin or worsen during the third trimester. Signs that the problem is getting worse include the following:

❖ Sudden or excessive weight gain
❖ Sudden significant decrease in output of urine
❖ Puffiness of the hands or face
❖ Abdominal pain
❖ Persistent headaches
❖ Visual changes

Treatment for preeclampsia includes partial or complete bed rest. Medication may also be prescribed to lower your blood pressure. You may be hospitalized, as Laura was. Discuss your feelings with your doctor if you are reluctant to go to the hospital. Perhaps you can rest well at home, but that is not the only concern. It may be necessary to closely monitor your blood pressure, or watch for signs that you need medication to prevent or control seizures or high blood pressure. Seizures always require hospitalization.

Felicia said, "I developed borderline high blood pressure, but I did not have preeclampsia because I did not have all the symptoms. My blood pressure was reading at around 130 over 90. Then it became 140+ over 100+. At that point, it was considered high blood pressure. The doctors just monitored me. I had no other symptoms."

It is important to report any signs and symptoms to your doctor immediately, because the symptoms of preeclampsia and eclampsia may become suddenly severe and dangerous.

Ultimately, the only "cure" for eclampsia is delivery of the baby. Sometimes preterm delivery is necessary. Delivery may be delayed until tests show that the baby's lungs have matured. Immediate delivery of the baby may be necessary, however, if your blood pressure continues to increase, or if you have signs of placental or kidney failure.

If convulsions occur, preeclampsia has become eclampsia. Warning signs include:

❖ Severe headache
❖ Difficulty breathing
❖ Blurred vision
❖ Pain in the upper abdomen (stomach area)

If you are in the hospital and experience any of these symptoms, ring for a nurse immediately. If you are at home, call your doctor, but do not attempt to drive the car to his office or the hospital, because these symptoms indicate that convulsions may occur soon. You should also be aware that some of these symptoms may not be caused by preeclampsia. For example, Michelle's blurred vision was an MS exacerbation that was not associated with any other symptoms of preeclampsia. Severe headaches are also caused by dysreflexia. Severe headaches may also be a symptom of shunt failure, and it is important to check with your doctor.

DISABILITY EXACERBATIONS

Possible exacerbations of each disability are discussed in Chapter 3. Some disability symptoms are most likely to be exacerbated in the third trimester because of the effect of normal pregnancy changes. For example, uterine pressure on the lungs is greatest during this stage, and breathing difficulties are more likely to worsen. Women with diastrophic dwarfism are at risk for cardiac arrest, because the baby can become so large it can push the diaphragm up into the heart area. Denise was put in the hospital at 26 weeks so they could monitor the baby. Myasthenia gravis is more likely to be exacerbated in the third trimester. Kidney impairment, which is associated with more than one disability, is of special concern. If kidney function worsens and no reversible cause can be found, such as infection or dehydration, preterm delivery may be necessary.

Preparing for Labor

EXTERNAL VERSION

External version refers to a procedure in which the position, or presentation, of the fetus is changed. *Version*, when used in this way, means "turning." This can be difficult if the fetus is in a breech presentation. The physician may attempt to manipulate the fetus into a new position by pressing on the mother's abdomen. The procedure is usually performed during the thirty-sixth or thirty-seventh week. A sonography is used to locate the fetus; an external monitor is used to assess changes in fetal heart rate; and medication is given to relax the uterine muscles. The medication can make the procedure more effective and prevent contractions. It may also reduce any discomfort caused by the procedure.

This procedure may be contraindicated if you have hydrocephalus. External version involves a lot of abdominal pressure and may place your shunt system at risk. The doctor left the decision up to Holly as to whether she wanted to have a vaginal delivery, thereby putting her shunt system at risk for malfunction. Holly believed that her shunt malfunctioned after the vaginal delivery of her first child because of heavy abdominal pressure by a delivery nurse. Her past experience with abdominal pressure made it easy for her to decide not to have the external version procedure. She opted for a planned caesarean section, which went very well.

PERINEUM MASSAGE

The *perineum* is the area between the vagina and the anus. This area is meant to stretch during labor, but it is susceptible to tearing. An episiotomy may be done to avoid the risk of tearing. Many women, whether they are disabled or not, have found an episiotomy to be quite painful. One way to possibly avoid an episiotomy is to do perineum massage. It is recommended that the massage be started around the 34th week.

Some women find this massage quite uncomfortable, so go slowly and find the pace you feel the most comfortable with. Use natural oil such as almond, olive, vitamin E, or lubricant jelly. It may help to do the massage in a relaxed atmosphere while listening to music or anything else that that helps you relax. The massage needs to be done by a person who has the use of both hands. Otherwise, you may use a small vibrator. The first time you try the massage, have your partner place one or two of his fingers from each hand approximately two to three inches into the vaginal canal. It is important to communicate to your partner what you are feeling as the massage proceeds.

The next time, have your partner add pressure to the vaginal wall, moving the fingers down toward the back of the vaginal area next to the rectum then back up the sides in a rhythmic motion. Continue to apply steady pressure as the fingers move, and stop if it begins to hurt.

Next, try different pressures and speed of stroke to determine what feels good and works for your body. Allow the vaginal area to stretch open as much as possible comfortably. When you feel a burning or tingling sensation you will know you have stretched to the limit. Becoming familiar with the burning or tingling sensation will prepare you for the crowning of your newborn. Practice the breathing you learned in childbirth class during this massage. As you do the massage, you will find the vaginal wall responds easier (90).

An episiotomy is no longer a routine procedure. Many doctors are against it because some studies shows it is neither effective nor necessary. "It seems reasonable to conclude that episiotomy should not be performed routinely" (91).

Preterm and Post-Term Labor

PRETERM LABOR

Full-term labor occurs at 40 weeks after the estimated date of conception; this is the average length of pregnancy. Babies born about 2 weeks early or late are within the range of variation, and they are unlikely to differ from full-term infants in health or appearance. Often, labor only seems to be early or late when, in fact, the date of conception has been miscalculated. Preterm labor is defined as labor occurring before the thirty-seventh week of pregnancy; post-term labor is defined as labor occurring after the forty-second week. Sonography and hormone tests may be used to confirm a diagnosis of preterm or post-term labor. The causes of preterm labor include the following:

❖ Infections, such as urinary tract infection
❖ Cervical incompetence
❖ Placental abnormalities, such as placenta previa and placental abruption
❖ Chronic maternal illness, such as high blood pressure, kidney disease, and diabetes
❖ Use of some illegal drugs
❖ Distension of the uterus caused by excess amniotic fluid or multiple pregnancies
❖ Structural abnormalities of the uterus
❖ Fetal death in utero

Often the cause of preterm labor cannot be identified. Signey thought the pain she felt was her baby's head in her ribs, but in retrospect she thought it could have been preterm labor. Signey said, "The pain might have been contractions, but I really never felt any contractions. When I got admitted for preterm labor, they said I was having five contractions in less than a half an hour. Some of the pressure in my ribs was similar to what they called a contraction." Perhaps it was both the contractions *and* having the baby's head stuck up into the ribs.

Women with myasthenia gravis, systemic lupus erythematosus (SLE), and spinal cord injury are at increased risk for premature labor. The increased risk may result from other complications associated with disability. For example, a woman who has SLE and is in remission is less likely to have preterm labor than a woman who is not in remission. Sylvia's episode of premature labor was caused by dysreflexia and bowel problems. She may have had impacted feces. It is impossible to know in advance who will be vulnerable to preterm labor. For example, Sheila had persistent bladder infections throughout both of her pregnancies. During her second pregnancy, she used antibiotics and had less urinary discomfort. But it was in this pregnancy that she had an episode of preterm labor.

Hannah had preterm labor with both of her children, but she was not put on long-term bed rest with her second pregnancy. Hannah said about her second pregnancy, "It never turned serious enough to treat. It was a day or two of rest." Her doctor told her she had an irritable uterus. The term "irritable uterus" is actually a symptom, not a diagnosis. In addition, it is unknown what causes premature labor, although some possible causes may be an accident or an infection. Hannah's doctor thought that dehydration might have been the cause of her preterm labor, and had her increase the amount of water she was drinking from 3 quarts to 5 quarts a day. Hannah felt that the doctor treated her in the same way as all of the other pregnant women he worked with.

It is possible to have episodes of preterm labor, yet not give birth prematurely; only 10 percent of these episodes end in preterm delivery. Treatment may consist of bed rest and, sometimes, medications that suppress labor. Felicia was put on bed rest in the 34th week. Her contractions were 6 minutes apart, and the obstetrician's exam found her to be 80 percent effaced. Although she was 80 percent effaced, Felicia needed to be induced at 39 weeks because her blood pressure was spiking above 140/100.

Some women may have a reaction to medication. Signey was given magnesium sulfate while she was in the hospital for preterm labor, which apparently made her lungs fill with fluid.

Medications may be used to treat any underlying cause of preterm labor such as lupus flare, infection, or high blood pressure. If tests show the fetal lungs are immature, the mother may also be given a medication such as betamethasone, which speeds up fetal lung development, so that the baby will do better if he is born early. Hannah was put on bed rest during her first pregnancy, but it did not stop her preterm labor. So Hannah took terbutaline from 34 to 36 weeks. She said, "They wanted to keep me on it longer, but I refused. I felt as if I was on speed and couldn't sleep. Plus, I thought the baby had a good chance." Noreen was put on terbutaline and a small amount of steroids to help the baby's lungs develop. She was hospitalized because, "They were afraid that the baby or I would die at home because of placenta abruption."

Having a home maternal/fetal monitor to keep track of what is going on may help a woman avoid going to the hospital. A study of home fetal monitors failed to find them beneficial. It is unknown if the home monitor may help women with SCI especially at the T-10 to T-12 level to know if they are in labor. The recommendations against its use are made on grounds of costs and inconvenience (92). Sometimes the mother will be hospitalized.

Women with spinal cord injuries are likely to give birth prematurely, and they need to be monitored more closely. This may mean starting weekly doctor appointments sooner than other pregnant women. This precaution is especially important for women with injuries at T-12 who cannot feel labor contractions. Moreover, it is also important for women with injuries above T-6, because of the risk that dysreflexia will occur during labor, or be the sign that labor has begun.

One of the hazards of preterm labor is that the mother may not realize she is in labor. Leslie recalled, "I was in labor for 16 hours without realizing it because my contractions were one-sided, and I thought I had the flu. I didn't know what was happening until my bag of water broke."

Signs that labor may be starting are described in detail at the beginning of Chapter 11. Briefly, they include the following:

- ❖ Four or more contractions per hour that do not disappear with rest or change of activity (unlike Braxton-Hicks contractions)
- ❖ Contractions increasing in frequency and intensity that are similar to menstrual cramps. For example, Orielle said, "I knew I was in labor because of I could feel my stomach and my back tightening a bit. It was pretty consistent and seemed to be in a pattern, so I thought I was in labor."
- ❖ Low back pain that may radiate to the sides or the front, and that may not be relieved by position change
- ❖ Increase in vaginal discharge; the "bloody show" (watery, pink, or brown-tinged)
- ❖ A sudden gush of fluid or trickles of fluid, followed another gush after about an hour (the bag of water breaking)
- ❖ Diarrhea or indigestion

In women with spinal cord injury, symptoms may also include the following:

❖ Dysreflexia symptoms
❖ Internal discomforts that feel like indigestion or the need to have a bowel movement
❖ Muscle spasms or clonus

HOSPITALIZATION

Sophia Amelia had difficulty during a precautionary hospitalization for a urinary tract infection. She said, "I was unable to transfer off the toilet because it wasn't set up for me. I pulled the emergency cord, but no one responded. After an hour of waiting I decided to try to transfer by myself and I fell. My doctor was furious. In addition to neglect, Sophia Amelia also experienced prejudice from a nurse. The nurse asked where the father was. When the nurse found out that he was in another state, she asked Sophia Amelia who was going to take care of the baby. When Sophia Amelia told her that she was going to take care of the baby herself, the nurse called in a social worker. It was obvious that the nurse could not imagine someone in a wheelchair taking care of a baby. It may prove beneficial to do an in-service on your particular disability, because most labor and delivery and postpartum hospital staff are unfamiliar with disabilities.

Signey was hospitalized for 8 days for preterm labor. Most of the hospital staff had a hard time transferring her out of bed and onto the toilet because they did not have any experience with a disabled person. Sharon was hospitalized in her seventh month and the baby was born six weeks early. Her muscles stiffened and her spasms became more frequent because she was not given enough physical therapy. Sharon could have gotten a referral and a consultation for physical therapy (PT), because PT can help with ways to transfer. It can also reduce muscle spasm and tight muscles. Hannah also stated that bed rest made her stiffer in her back and hips.

POST-TERM PREGNANCY

The main problem associated with some post-term pregnancies is that the fetus grows so large that delivery is difficult. In post-term pregnancies, the aging placenta begins to function poorly, and fetal growth is retarded. Other changes may cause fetal distress.

If you appear to have a post-term pregnancy, your doctor must consider the possibility that the date of your last menstruation was miscalculated. You may have had ultrasound examinations earlier in pregnancy that confirmed the length of your pregnancy. If not, sonography or amniocentesis may be done at this time. Stress or non-stress tests and/or a biophysical profile may be used to assess the well-being of the fetus. Labor may be induced if the cervix is effaced and the fetus engaged.

Fetal Development

The fetus grows dramatically during the third trimester, from about 13 inches in length and 1¾ pounds in weight at the end of the twenty-fourth week, to 20 inches in length and 7 pounds in weight at the fortieth week. The appearance of the fetus changes as fat is deposited under the skin, the hair and nails continue grow, and the size and tone of the muscles increases. Only the mother can feel fetal movement during much of the second trimester. During the third trimester, the fetus does not *stop* moving, and the mother may invite other family members to put their hands on her abdomen to feel the baby kick.

During the last few weeks of pregnancy, when there is less room for the fetus to move, it may seem less active. If the amount of fetal movement changes gradually, you do not need to worry, but if you feel any concern, you certainly should bring it up with your doctor. A sudden increase or decrease in fetal activity may be a sign of fetal distress.

Development during the third trimester is significant, as the brain continues to grow. The fetus is able to suck its thumb and respond to light and sound. During this period, you may also notice a little lump appearing on your abdomen. This lump is the fetus stretching a limb, and the fetus will react by pulling away if you press it.

The body and the immune system of the fetus are both maturing. But even at full term, the immune system is immature, and the baby will be dependent on the mother's breast milk to provide antibodies after birth. As a result, premature babies are more susceptible to infection than full-term babies. It is important, therefore, to feed premature babies with breast milk if possible.

Lung development is a special concern during the third trimester. An inability to breathe, or difficulty in breathing, is the chief threat to the survival of premature babies. By the end of the seventh month, the bubble-like sacs at the surface of which oxygen is transferred to blood cells (*alveoli*) will have formed as well as the system of blood vessels in the lungs. A baby born at this time will have respiratory difficulties because the lungs are not producing the chemical that prevents the alveoli from collapsing upon contact with air. Therefore, doctors try to suppress preterm labor in order to allow time for the lungs to mature.

Emotional Concerns

Important emotional concerns in the third trimester include the following:

- ❖ Changes in sexual relationships
- ❖ Unhappiness about increased dependence
- ❖ Anticipation and fear about childbirth and motherhood

Most women experience some change in their sexual relationship when they become pregnant. Many couples experience a new sense of freedom, particularly during the first trimester. Many people feel more sexual desire and make love more frequently because they do not have to worry about contraception. For other couples, the discomforts of pregnancy may reduce desire. A woman who feels nauseated or short of breath may not feel sexy. Later in pregnancy, orgasm can cause uncomfortable contractions that feel somewhat like menstrual cramps.

A problem many couples encounter in the third trimester is difficulty finding a comfortable position. The problem may be worse for disabled women, whose choices may be limited by lack of mobility even when they are not pregnant. Amanda said, "My husband definitely had to be the balancer, because I had no balance whatsoever. I was terribly uncoordinated at that time." Heather said, "It was awkward. We tried different positions, but it was the most difficult during the seventh and eighth months." Sheila said, "After the seventh month, it was just too uncomfortable." Dawn felt that the problem was not one of awkwardness, but a "full" feeling that made insertion difficult. Possibly this problem arises for women whose babies are "engaged." Some women found that side-lying or sitting positions gave them more room to maneuver.

Some couples worry that lovemaking will harm the fetus or stimulate labor. There is almost never any need to worry, but if there is any doubt in your mind, do not hesitate to ask your doctor. She has answered similar questions hundreds of times, so there is no need to be embarrassed. Sophia Amelia thought that having intercourse could stimulate labor, but her sex drive was diminished from the sixth month on. You may be advised to avoid intercourse if you or your partner has an infection, or if you have signs or symptoms indicating a risk of preterm labor. Christina and Leslie were both advised to avoid intercourse when it became clear that they were at risk for miscarriage. If you must avoid intercourse, you can certainly show affection in other ways. Sylvia recalled, "We couldn't have sex in the last month because the baby was lying too low. We found other ways to satisfy our sex urges. Oral sex was a nice substitute."

Sometimes a couple's concerns have a more emotional basis. For example, a woman who feels that she looks less attractive may want to avoid nudity, even though she wants the reassurance of tenderness and romance. Concerns about how the new baby will affect the marriage may cause either partner to become uncomfortable with physical intimacy. Try to set aside time to discuss these feelings. Sharing them can deepen and enrich your relationship and prevent misunderstandings. In addition, there may be fewer chances to share feelings later when the new baby is absorbing your time and energy. Many couples feel it is helpful to join a support or discussion group for prospective parents. In these groups, they may talk about anything from infant-care tips to ideas for coping with interfering in-laws, depending on how the discussion group is structured. As couples become comfortable with each other, they may also discuss sexual relationships. It can be reassuring to learn that what you are feeling, whether it is increased desire or a complete loss of interest, is felt by others.

As a woman becomes slower and clumsier in late pregnancy, she may need to find more help for everyday tasks such as carrying groceries. For some women, the need for more help can cause a strain on their relationships. Pam felt that one reason she and her husband separated was that he was burned out from giving her extra help in late pregnancy. Try to find ways to get extra help. Perhaps a social worker can arrange for home help or additional attendant care, which is not ordinarily available. There are in-home support services in California but they are not available if you are married.

Natasha used to be embarrassed to ask for help when she dropped something in a store. When she was big and showing, however, she was able to use her pregnancy as a reason to ask for help. Other women may become upset when pregnancy begins to affect their independence skills. Take the attitude that if you are in control of a situation, you really are independent. For example, if you must ask someone to shop for you, take control by making out a detailed list so that you will have the groceries you want.

The opposite feeling can also occur. Natasha said, "I actually felt stronger, even though I was carrying around an extra 33 pounds. I was able to walk at pretty much the same rate and do household chores. It didn't slow me down at all."

Feelings about the impending birth intensify during the course of the third trimester. Although some women enjoy pregnancy so much they wish it would last forever, others feel like Arlene, who said, "I was just waiting for it to be over so I could have my normal body back." Many women fantasize that the baby will be born a week or so early, although in a first pregnancy the baby is more likely to be born a few days later than expected.

Some women fear the birth process, even though they are eager for the pregnancy to end. Patricia said, "I had an X-ray, and knew I could have a vaginal birth. I had two emotions at the same time. I was relieved that I didn't have to have a C-section, but I was apprehensive about labor and delivery. I kept trying not to think about how scary and painful labor might be." It really does help to discuss these fears in a birthing class, and with women who have already had children. Lea Rae was afraid of labor and delivery. She said, "I heard of women with diseases who died, or their babies died during childbirth." Lea Rae wanted a caesarean section because she thought it would be easier, but her doctor encouraged her to have a vaginal delivery, because having a caesarean section takes longer to heal.

Closing Comments

Regardless of having a disability or not, some women enjoy being pregnant. Those who enjoy pregnancy, enjoy it for many reasons. Many also feel that pregnancy lasts longer than the actual 9 months. Some express worries about being mothers. But most of all, women wonder about the birth of their baby.

All women have heard horror stories about labor, and they wonder whether they will be able to handle the pain of labor. They also wonder whether they will even recognize labor when it begins. The next three chapters will give you information that may help alleviate your fears, and give you options on methods to handle labor pain.

The Main Event: Labor and Delivery

The Course of Labor

Labor progresses in a series of well-defined stages: Stage 1 is labor, Stage II is delivery of the baby, and Stage III is delivery of the placenta. Stage 1 (labor) is subdivided into three phases. These phases are defined by changes in the condition and activity of the uterus. The length of labor varies from woman to woman. Even in the same woman, the labor of each of her pregnancies can vary.

The uterus is a pear-shaped, muscular organ. The cervix is the neck (bottom) of the uterus; it extends down into the top third of the vagina. The *os*, which means "mouth" in Latin, is a pinpoint hole in the center of the cervix. During Stage I of labor, the cervix becomes effaced (thinned) and dilated as it is pulled back into the uterus.

Stage I progresses through three phases. During the early phase, the cervix and the os dilate to 3 centimeters in diameter. At the end of Stage I, when the cervix is fully effaced and dilated to 10 centimeters in diameter, the interior of the uterus is continuous with the vagina.

When the early phase is prolonged, it is called *prodromal* or *latent* labor. During the active phase, the cervix dilates to 7 centimeters. The phase during which the cervix dilates from 7 to 10 centimeters is known as *transition* because it is the turning point between Stage I and Stage II (delivery).

During Stage II, the function of uterine contractions changes from opening the cervix to squeezing out the baby. This stage is completed with the baby's birth.

During Stage III, uterine contractions expel the placenta from the uterus. Finally, Stage IV refers to the first few hours after childbirth. During this time, bleeding from the area where the placenta was attached should lessen, and uterine contractions begin to close the cervix and return the uterus to its pre-pregnant size. The uterus continues to return to normal during the postpartum period (see Chapter 13).

Signs and Symptoms of Labor

The term *contraction* is used because the processes of labor and delivery are accomplished by rhythmical contractions of the uterine muscles.

Some women have read books or taken classes in which the pain of labor is minimized. Other women have heard horror stories about labor and delivery. In fact, there is a wide range of how women experience labor and delivery. For some women, labor is not very painful. In other cases, labor is the most severe pain they will ever experience. Contractions at the beginning of labor are usually not severe. Hannah said, "The contractions came on slow and there was no big pain with the first labor." Naomi, however, started contractions at 5 minutes apart, each lasting 1 minute in length. Therefore, there is no common way women feel or can tell that labor has started.

Selina started each of her labors with the shakes, which may have been a sign of dysreflexia. She did not have an epidural with her fourth child, and the shakes continued throughout labor and delivery. Pain is one of the causes of dysreflexia.

"Dysreflexia is caused by a variety of stimuli, including urethral, bladder, rectal, or cervical distention, catheterization, cervical dilation, uterine contractions, or examination of the pelvic structure. These stimuli may precipitate dangerous hypertension, which must be treated immediately. Spinal or epidural analgesia can prevent or avert dysreflexia, and should be instituted at the start of labor" (93).

Some women who have experienced pain because of their disabilities might not know they are in labor. Joan was in labor all day. She said, "By 3:00 P.M., my contractions were 5 minutes apart and 1 minute in length. I still thought I wasn't in labor because they didn't hurt."

Nikki did not know she was in labor with her first child until her doctor did a vaginal exam and found her cervix to be dilated to 4 cm. She was able to sleep through much of her labor with her fifth child.

It cannot be emphasized enough that *labor is an individual experience*. Both Chloe and Nora did not know their labor had begun because each started with a backache. Nora experienced low back pain while she was on her way to the hospital after her water had broken. She said, "I wasn't timing the contractions. Afterwards, I was glad my bag of water had broken because otherwise I would not have known I was in labor." If you are not sure whether your water has broken, one of the ways to differentiate between the amniotic fluid and urine is by smell. Some of the interviewees said this was easy.

Sasha's comment as to her level of pain was, "On a scale from 1 to 10, labor was a 5 or 6." Disabled women who have had painful injuries or surgeries might well agree with Sasha's assessment. Sabine said, "It also helped knowing that while my chronic pain went on for what seemed like forever, I knew this was not forever, and that helped me deal with it."

Some women—with or without disabilities—may become anxious about labor pain. Tessa worried about it, and was fearful and anxious concerning labor and delivery. Another issue related to labor pain is that women with spinal cord injuries may or may not feel it. Some women are surprised to find that they are able to feel labor pain. Women with injuries at T-10 to T-12, however, are highly unlikely to feel labor pain. For these women, it is important to watch for tightening and relaxation of the abdominal muscles. Shanna said, "My stomach was hard as a rock. We went to the movies and I didn't feel him kicking or moving. I called the doctor and was told to come in for an ultrasound. It was discovered that I had too little fluid, and they decided to induce me."

Selina's fifth labor was back labor. She said, "I really couldn't time the contractions. I just felt yucky. The day I went into labor, my belly was suddenly rock hard. It was hard to breathe and I couldn't hold a conversation. This wasn't like most of my other labors, when I had contractions that started on the side of the belly and went toward the belly button."

What a woman feels during labor depends on many factors outside of her control, including the position of the fetus, its size in proportion to her pelvic opening, and how long her labor lasts. Symptoms other than pain are also unpredictable. For example, the pain of excessive muscle stretching, including uterine stretching, often causes nausea. Clara falls frequently and becomes nauseated whenever she strains a muscle. She was sure that she would be nauseated during labor, but she was not.

The breathing and relaxation exercises taught in prenatal classes help many women to cope with labor pain and minimize the use of medications. It is worthwhile for every woman to learn these techniques, which can also be used to cope with pain in the years to come. Some women can handle the pain of labor, especially if it is of short duration. No one should be disappointed in themselves if they need pain medication.

Stage One

EARLY PHASE

It is not surprising that women wonder, "How will I know I'm really in labor?" There are many different signs and symptoms of early labor, many of them quite subtle. Weeks before labor begins in earnest, women may experience Braxton-Hicks contractions ("practice" contractions) that are surprisingly strong. Often, a woman in the last few weeks of pregnancy is told during a prenatal visit that her cervix is already slightly dilated. As she hears other women's stories, she learns that the sensations of early labor may not be what she expects. When Leslie was in the early phase, her contractions caused a dull, cramping feeling that she thought might be the flu. She remembers saying jokingly to her sister, "I'm probably in labor and too dumb to know it." Then she called her doctor and found out it was no joke!

Simi said, "I did not know I was in labor because I did not know what to expect. I thought I was having cramps. I told a co-worker whose wife gave birth 6 weeks before that I was having pulling and tugging in my muscles. He told me I was in labor, but I said, 'No, no, I'm not due for another week.' But I *was* in labor!"

Some women with disabilities may experience some atypical symptoms, and many women who have disabilities involving loss of sensation may not have the experience they expected. The sensory nerves to the uterus are between T-10 and T-12, and L-1 and S-2 to S-4, so women who have injuries that are below these levels will feel labor. Most women with injuries higher than T-10 usually do not feel labor. Those who do may have incomplete lesions. Samantha was sure she would feel labor contractions despite her disability. She had been experiencing Braxton-Hicks contractions, and her midwife told her that her cervix was slightly dilated. She never felt early labor, however. It began while she was asleep, and she suddenly woke up in the transitional phase. Some able-bodied women have had a similar experience. Other interviewees were surprised when they *did* feel labor contractions.

Of course, a good way to answer the question, "Am I in labor?" or even the question, "What is this discomfort I'm experiencing?" is to do what Leslie did. Call your doctor, midwife, or hospital and describe what you are feeling. Experiencing any of the signs and symptoms described here is certainly a good reason to call, but any other unusual or uncomfortable symptoms also merit a call to the doctor.

For some women, the first sign of labor is leakage of blood-tinged mucus, the "bloody show." The cervical os contains a plug of mucus, which becomes dislodged as the cervix dilates. Sometimes a few tiny blood vessels break as the cervix dilates, and the mucus plug will have a pinkish or brownish stain, or a few streaks of blood. Intercourse or a vaginal examination may result in some blood spotting up to 48 hours later, but otherwise, a show of brown or pink mucus is usually a sign that labor will begin soon. "Soon" means some time between a few hours and 2 weeks.

Selina had a bloody show with all five of her labors. She noticed it the day before she started labor. Of course, a bloody show may also appear with the first noticeable contractions. Carla remembers being awakened by "a crampy feeling," then finding the bloody show. *Bright red spotting is a danger sign that should always be reported to the doctor immediately.*

Thin liquid flowing from the vagina may be amniotic fluid. Between 10 and 20 percent of labors begin with rupture of the amniotic membrane, which is often called the "bag of water breaking." Sometimes there is an uncomfortable sensation of pressure before the membrane ruptures. Jennifer felt as if she needed to have a bowel movement, and her bag broke while she was on the toilet. Sometimes it is hard for a woman to be sure what is happening. The amniotic fluid may come out in a slow leak or a sudden gush.

Sierra woke up thinking that she had "peed" on herself. She said, "It kept coming out and didn't stop. Then I smelled my clothes, and I knew that my bag of water had broken." Mandy's bag of water broke with her second and third pregnancies. Mandy realized that her bag had broken "because before I started urinating, I was all wet." Lea Rae said, "I felt a release of water. I wet my seat. Even though I was urinating a lot, I knew at that point it was not urine. I went to the bathroom and saw a gel and a watery-like substance that was also red."

Natalie was already on the toilet when she heard a "pop." She and her mom looked in the toilet. They saw "stuff trickling." Natalie put a pad on. She said, "I could feel it gushing out while I was walking into the hospital. Natalie's contractions started 4 hours after her water broke, and they were 2 minutes apart when labor started.

Sometimes it is hard for a woman to be sure what is happening. When the fluid leaks through a small tear in the bag, the flow may be more continuous when she lies down. When she stands or sits, the baby's head presses against the cervix and may block the flow. Amniotic fluid is constantly being replaced, and one sign that the membranes have ruptured is another sudden gush of fluid about an hour after the first one. Women who have spinal cord injuries, and may have leakage around their catheters, will find it difficult to distinguish between amniotic fluid and urine. Litmus paper can be used to distinguish between them. Urine is acid and turns litmus paper red. Amniotic fluid tests base, whereas the litmus paper will be clear. Be aware that there can be urine and amniotic fluid present at the same time.

If there is a sign that the membranes have ruptured, whether a slow drip or a sudden gush of fluid, it is time to call the doctor. Do not wait to feel labor contractions. Your doctor can do a simple test to determine if there is amniotic fluid in the vagina. He will need to know what time the membranes ruptured. Most women whose first sign of labor is the breaking of the bag of water may have contractions within 12 hours. Your doctor will need to examine you for two reasons:

1. She will need to make sure that the baby's head is well engaged in the pelvis. If not, there is a chance that the umbilical cord, no longer supported by amniotic fluid, will slip down into the cervix. Then, later in labor, uterine contractions might press the baby's head against the cord, compressing it and interfering with the fetal oxygen supply.

2. The uterine environment is open to infection once the membranes have ruptured. If the gestational age is 36 weeks and the fetus is not in distress, the doctor may not induce delivery, in order to avoid the baby being premature. It is important to note that one of the dangers of the membranes being ruptured is infection in the mother and/or the baby. The doctor or midwife may watch for signs of infection by taking the mother's temperature or checking vaginal secretions for bacteria. If contractions have not begun within 24 hours, it may be necessary to induce labor (see "Medical Procedures").

Besides noting what time your membranes rupture, check the color of the fluid before calling the doctor. It should be a clear, pale yellow fluid. Cloudiness and brownish or greenish staining can be signs of fetal distress, and you should call your doctor immediately.

For most women, contractions are the first sign that labor has begun. Some women feel contractions intensely even in the early phase, and there is no doubt in their minds that labor has begun. Others have mild contractions at first, although it can be difficult to recognize them for what they are.

Julie had not attended a birth preparation class, and was thrown completely off guard. She "thought labor would be like in the movies with women screaming and pushing," so she thought her discomfort was the aftereffect of a fall in the eighth month of her pregnancy. Early contractions felt like gas pains to Portia and Sasha. Contractions that feel like gas pain or indigestion are sometimes accompanied by diarrhea. Patricia and Carla both said the sensation was "like menstrual cramps, only it hurt more." Lea Rae said, "They are the worst cramps you can have in your life. It was five times mega-cramps for all women who know what cramps are like."

Other women in early labor keep feeling as if they have to urinate, but they do not produce more than a few drops; others have a backache. Another occasional subtle symptom of early labor is change of mood and not knowing why. Some women become more irritable, short-tempered, or humorless.

As contractions continue, it may become more obvious that labor has begun. Portia commented that with her second child, as with her first, "it was impossible to tell labor pains from gas pains at first. I needed it to go on longer to make sure it was labor." Stacy thought she was having Braxton-Hicks contractions, but realized it was labor when "they didn't go away; they just intensified."

Labor often begins with cramps that do not stop. Try getting up and walking, transferring, or doing another activity. Take a shower, then rest. Labor has begun if the contractions continue.

Another way to make sure labor has begun is to time the contractions using a watch with a second hand. In false labor, contractions commonly occur at irregular intervals and last for varying amounts of time. In true labor, contractions are more likely to occur at increasingly regular intervals, which gradually grow shorter. For example, in false labor the intervals may be 10 minutes, 6 minutes, 15 minutes; in true early labor, the intervals may be 30 minutes, 30, 35, 30...25, 27, 25, 25...15, 15, 15. In true labor, it is more likely that each contraction will last the same amount of time—at least 45 seconds, with contractions gradually becoming longer as labor progresses. In timing contractions, it is important to note the time each contraction *begins*. An example of a written record is shown in Table 11-1.

TABLE 11-1
CONTRACTION CHART

Beginning of Contraction	End of Contraction	Duration	Spacing
8:40:30	8:41:20	50 sec	
8:51:20	8:52:10	50 sec	10 min 50 sec
9:01:10	9:03:00	50 sec	9 min 50 sec
.			
.			
.			
.			
9:45:00	9:45:45	45 sec	
9:50:00	9:50:50	50 sec	5 min

Note: *Duration* refers to the length of time of the contraction. *Spacing* refers to the time between the beginning of one contraction and the beginning of the next contraction.

The mother should be on her way to the birth center or hospital by the time the contractions are 5 minutes apart. Remember that this pattern is common, but it does not describe what happens to every woman. One of the author's students recalls that her first noticeable contractions were 5 minutes apart, and they continued to be 5 minutes apart throughout labor. "Expect the unexpected" certainly applies to the birthing experience!

It may be difficult to time contractions, because a contraction becomes more intense as it continues. A woman who does not feel her contraction at first may be recording contractions from peak to peak, not from beginning to beginning. This is probably what happened to a student in one of the author's birthing classes whose contractions seemed to be lasting only 30 seconds, just 2 hours before she gave birth.

Women with spinal dysfunction may experience labor differently. Those who have injury at the T-12 level or higher often cannot feel labor contractions as such. Women who have some internal sensation, such as the ability to feel bladder fullness, fetal movements, or Braxton-Hicks contractions while pregnant, may feel something during labor, but what they will feel cannot be predicted. Stephanie did not expect to feel her contractions as well as she did. She thought the sensation would be sufficiently dull to take the edge off, and she was surprised when it hurt more than she expected. Sharon described a feeling of pressure. Sheila said that when her second child was born, she felt an uncomfortable tightening and was able to time her contractions, although she did not feel contractions with her first child.

Women with spinal dysfunction may need to be alert for other signs or symptoms of labor. Sheila remembers that the night before her labor started, she felt an urge to urinate every 20 to 30 minutes, but she never passed much urine. Her amniotic membrane ruptured in the morning, and then she realized she was in labor. Looking back, she realizes that her urge to urinate must have been a response to labor contractions. Sheila remembers that just before her water broke, she looked down and noticed that her stomach "…had an odd, lopsided shape." Sharon, too, commented, "I saw my stomach stick out, then fall."

Shanna did not realize that she was in labor, which resulted in her giving birth at home on the toilet. When she sat on the toilet and found blood, she realized that she should go to the hospital immediately. She said, "I reached down to wipe and there was more blood, and I went to wipe again and felt this big gush of water. When I felt the water, that's when I knew I was in labor. Then I scooted to the edge of the toilet and tried to pull my pants up. My husband saw the baby being born and slipping into the toilet. He lifted me to the floor and then handed me the baby. The baby was blue and still attached to the placenta. Her mouth was wide open and there was nothing coming out, so I just sucked the water out of her. It was two sucks of water and then immediately she turned pink and there was a loud cry, and that's when I felt relief. It was an amazing experience."

During the last weeks of pregnancy, a woman with spinal cord dysfunction can respond to internal discomforts such as pressure, a feeling similar to indigestion, feeling as if she needs to have a bowel movement, a recurring need to urinate, or by watching her abdomen to see if it seems to be tightening and relaxing. If she is able to, she can rest her hand just below her navel and feel for tightening or hardening, or she can ask her spouse, friend, or attendant to check. Some women with spinal dysfunction never feel labor, and, therefore, it would be helpful if they made it a habit to look or feel for contractions a few times a day during the weeks preceding their due dates.

For some women, dysreflexia symptoms are a sign that labor has begun; this can occur in woman with lesions above T-6 to T-8. When a labor contraction increases pressure inside the uterus, these women experience the same changes caused by pressure from a full bowel or bladder—their blood pressure rises, accompanied by symptoms such sweating, headache, or muscle spasm.

Sheila's experience was slightly different with each birth. She had an excruciating headache with her first child. She lay down to rest, and when she sat up, her membrane ruptured, fluid gushed out, and her headache disappeared. The change was less dramatic with her second child. There was no gush of fluid, but rather a slow, steady leak accompanied by a milder headache. Sylvia's first signs of labor were unusually intense leg spasms.

Other surveys have found that women with spinal dysfunction sometimes experience increased leg and ankle spasms or clonus during labor. When Shelby went from Braxton Hicks contraction into active labor, her blood pressure elevated to 300 over 190! She said, "I was overwhelmed with fear until they got my blood pressure under control. Once it was under control, my pain was not as severe as what other women experience in labor."

Variations in Early Labor

One variation from the pattern we have been describing is *back labor*, in which the mother has constant lower back pain that becomes worse during contractions. It is often very painful. During back labor, the back of the fetus's head pushes against the mother's spine causing pain. It is unknown whether the pain of back labor is caused by the fetal head compressing the spinal nerves or if it is from pressure in this general area. Some women notice that their discomfort starts in the low back, and then spreads to the abdomen. Other women may have back labor and feel the contractions only in their back. Another indicator of back labor can be laboring for a long time without dilating. Tina was in labor for 8 hours. She went to the hospital but was sent back home, where she sat on her couch and took a lot of showers.

Position describes the way the fetus is facing in relation to the mother's body. On the other hand, *presentation* describes which part of the fetus is next to the cervix. In a *vertex* presentation, the head emerges first. In a *breech* presentation, the buttocks emerge first.

Amy said, "I never felt regular contractions." After questioning Shanna, it became apparent that most of her pain was a backache. Back labor is difficult to time and the contractions seem irregular."

Clara had back labor with her first child. She said, "I could never tell when a contraction was starting because the pain was continuous; it just never seemed to let up." Renee had back labor the second time she gave birth. She said, "It was more painful than the first time. The contractions went from peak to peak."

Holly found back labor debilitating. In retrospect, she decided she would have preferred caesarean section to labor and delivery. She was not given any pain medication.

A second variation is *precipitate labor*. Precipitate labor is much shorter than most labors, lasting less than 3 hours. Contractions in this type of labor are intense from the beginning, and may be only 5 minutes apart. Some labor seems precipitate because the cervix has been gradually dilating for several days, and the mother first notices contractions when she is close to transition. Otherwise, precipitate labor results from low resistance in the birth canal or unusually strong contractions. The cervix may dilate quickly. Clara's cervix dilated from 2.5 to 10 centimeters in diameter in 20 minutes.

Precipitate labor can present problems for both mother and fetus. The sudden, intense sensations may make it difficult for the mother to adapt to labor and use breathing techniques to cope with her pain. If the cervix, vagina, or perineum are firm and resistant to strong contractions, there may be tears or, in rare cases, uterine rupture. If these tissues are soft or well stretched, the mother probably will not experience complications. A resistant birth canal, however, may cause trauma to the baby's head. Another problem is that strong contractions, without much time to relax between them, may interfere with blood flow in the uterus, and thus with the fetal oxygen supply. A few women who have precipitate labor may experience injuries, and the baby may be born suddenly. It can even fall out and be injured if the mother is standing. These women may need attention at any moment. If a woman first becomes aware of labor because she experiences intense, closely spaced contractions, she may be starting a precipitate labor and should call her doctor or midwife right away. She should not be left alone.

A third variation is *dysfunctional labor* (also known as *dystocia*), which is any labor that progresses too slowly. Labor is dysfunctional if the early phase lasts more than 20 hours for a woman having her first child, or more than 14 hours for a woman who has had at least one child. Maternal exhaustion and increased risk of infection are just two of the problems presented by dysfunctional labor. There are several possible causes for dysfunctional labor, and appropriate treatment depends on the nature of the problem.

ACTIVE PHASE

A physical examination is often the only way to confirm that a woman is in the early phase of labor. Yet many women hesitate to call their doctor or hospital when they are in the early phase. Some are afraid they will be told they are not really in labor and they should go home. Others prefer to wait before dealing with the possibility of medical interventions. By the time a woman is in active labor—the phase in which the cervix is probably already effaced and dilated from 3 to 7 centimeters across—she needs to see her midwife or doctor immediately.

Stephanie noted the difference between early and active labor. She said, "That's when my husband started asking me if I wanted something for the pain." Jennifer said, "My husband knew it was time to go the hospital because I looked distressed and was doubling over with each contraction."

Most women are advised to call their doctor or hospital when their contractions are 5 minutes apart (from beginning to beginning). These contractions commonly last between 45 and 60 seconds. This guideline worked well for Stacy and Patricia, but not for some of the other interviewees.

One common sign to look for in active labor is mucus dripping from the vagina. It is also common for women in active labor to become more sensitive. In the active phase, most women need the breathing and relaxation techniques they learned in childbirth class. Sierra said, "The breathing really helped a lot."

A woman can become discouraged after being in early labor for a long time, but when she has a vaginal examination and is told that she is finally in active labor, the boost in morale can give her a fresh burst of energy.

The active phase of labor generally lasts approximately 4 to 5 hours. Sometimes the fetus spontaneously changes to a more favorable position for birth during this phase. If the active phase lasts too long, or if the position of the fetus does not change by the end of the active phase, intervention will be considered.

Transition

Transition is the part of the phase of labor when the cervix dilates 7 to 10 cm. A woman who experiences the specific signs or symptoms of transition can probably expect to be ready to push very soon. Here are some common symptoms of transition:

- ❖ More intense and frequent contractions
- ❖ An urge to push
- ❖ A sensation of rectal pressure (as if you need to have a bowel movement)
- ❖ Nausea, vomiting, belching, or hiccups
- ❖ Trembling—either all over or just in the legs
- ❖ Chills or hot and cold flashes
- ❖ Drowsiness
- ❖ Heavy perspiration
- ❖ Emotional changes
- ❖ Muscle cramps or clonus

Occasionally a woman will experience one of these symptoms before her cervix is dilated to 7 cm. Some women do not notice any real difference during transition. For example, one of the author's students commented after her cervix was fully dilated, "So that was transition? Boy that was easy!" Most women will experience one or more symptoms.

Transition is a difficult time for many women because contractions are spaced so closely together. Typically, contractions are 1 to 3 minutes apart and last 60 to 90 seconds. So, for example, if there are 2 minutes from the beginning of one contraction to the beginning of a second, and the first contraction lasts 90 seconds, there is only a 30-second rest period between contractions. For many women, the emotional reaction to transition is even more dramatic than the physical reaction. Women who are coping with the intense sensations of this stage can become irritable, sensitive to distractions, and quite uninhibited. Michelle was annoyed by the smell of apple juice in her room, by being touched, by the sensations caused by her identification bracelet, and by the feeling of cloth against her skin. She said, "I didn't want to wear any clothes, and that was a surprise because I'm usually so shy." Patricia was equally uninhibited about expressing the frustration and fear that can occur during this phase. She said, "I can remember wondering when it would be over. I was really frustrated that I couldn't push, and I kept thinking that they were lying to me. I usually don't let strangers see me cry or know that I'm in pain. But this time I wanted them to know I was in pain. I didn't care who saw me cry."

Shelby knew when she was in transition. She said, "Although I was aware that it was less challenging than for most other women, I still wanted to get out of it." When Samantha talked about this phase of her third labor, she said, "The contractions were right on top of each other, unlike my other labors, when I seemed to have some space between contractions. It was very intense." Samantha's remark is especially significant because her third labor occurred after her injury.

It is difficult to predict what labor will be like for women with spinal cord dysfunction. A woman who has a partial spinal cord injury may not have previously experienced autonomic dysreflexia, although she may experience it during labor. Therefore, it is important for the doctor to become aware of the symptoms and treatments for autonomic dysreflexia.

Many consider the true hallmark of transition to be a strong urge to push. Childbirth attendants are usually on the alert for this symptom. Jennifer remembers asking a nurse who had just checked on her, "When should I call you?" The nurse replied, "When you feel like pushing." This urge, or sometimes a feeling of rectal fullness, results from the fetal head pressing against the rectal nerve. This sensation is not mild, by any means. When Michelle said, "I needed all my concentration not to push," and Stacy said, "My need to push was too strong to control," they were both voicing common reactions.

Yet it is important not to push before the cervix is fully dilated. Some of the breathing techniques practiced in birthing class are specifically designed to help women who are not quite ready to push. Some women will be told not to push because of a cervical lip. When the cervix is completely effaced around most of its circumference, but one segment is still thick and distinct from the uterus, the thick segment looks like a lip. This lip of tissue can become bruised, swollen, or torn because of pressure from the fetal head if the mother starts pushing too soon. When the lip is drawn back into the uterus, the cervix is fully dilated and pushing can begin.

Half of the interviewees with a spinal cord injury experienced an urge to push. Possibly more of them would have felt this urge, but some of them had been given regional anesthesia to prevent dysreflexia. Sara, whose spinal cord dysfunction is caused by a tumor, may have felt the urge to push without recognizing it. She recalled, "I felt like I had to go to the bathroom, but nothing happened." Sasha was given general anesthesia while in transition, and does not remember if she experienced the urge to push. Most of the studies of pregnant women with spinal dysfunctions involve small numbers of women, and therefore the frequency of their urge to push cannot be compared with the frequency for able-bodied women. Lack of the urge to push also occurs in women who have had spinal anesthesia. Moira has MS, and was unaware that she was in labor. She did not have any urge to push. She said, "My OB told me 'You just had a contraction and with the next one I want you to push.' I asked him, 'I had a contraction? You better tell me when I have the next one.'"

In addition, some women *without* disabilities may not feel the urge to push. One of the reasons for the lack of this urge is that the fetus is not in a position to press against the rectal nerve during contractions.

Sheila had an unusual reaction to the pressure of the fetal head: her legs became numb. She said, "Usually I can do a standing pivot transfer to get into the car. But I couldn't do it then. My legs went numb and they were as limp as spaghetti."

Most of the other symptoms of transition are as variable for disabled women as they are for able-bodied women. Even muscle spasms were not too prevalent in the interviewees; they only occurred in a few labors.

Procedures for Stage I

Some of the following procedures are performed only by medical staff, while others can be handled by support people.

ROUTINE DIAGNOSTIC PROCEDURES

Pulse and Blood Pressure

At regular intervals, the midwife, nurse, or doctor will check the mother's pulse and blood pressure. They may palpate her abdomen to determine the position and presentation of the fetus. A stethoscope or Doppler™ may be placed against the mother's abdomen to check fetal heart rate.

Internal Examination

Occasionally, the mother will be manually examined internally. In the early phase, this examination is done to determine effacement and dilation of the cervix. In the active phase, it is done to assess the descent of the fetus. An internal examination must sometimes be done during a contraction, making the contraction more uncomfortable. Internal examinations are kept to a minimum to avoid causing infection, especially after the amniotic membrane has ruptured. The mother's temperature may be taken if she has symptoms of fever, or if a significant amount of time has elapsed since her membranes ruptured.

Introduction of an Intravenous Line

An intravenous line (IV) is an extremely fine plastic tube that is inserted into a vein in the hand or, less commonly, the arm. An IV may be used to introduce medications, as discussed below. They are used in many hospitals and alternative birth centers as a matter of routine.

Some women with disabilities must have an IV because they need to receive medications continuously, and labor interferes with the absorption of oral medication; for example, women who have myasthenia gravis.

Some women need an antibiotic because of an infection. Naomi needed an antibiotic to be given in an IV. She said, "Twenty-five percent of all women carry a bacterium called *beta strep* in the normal flora of their vagina. This particular bacterium, although harmless to most women, can cause a serious infection, such as meningitis, in a newborn passing through the vaginal canal. I am one of those women." Naomi is unable to take penicillin, but she can take erythromycin. The prophylactic treatment is to administer two IV doses of penicillin during labor to kill the bacteria just before delivery. Prior to her delivery, Naomi found a Web site that listed the neurotoxic drugs contraindicated for people with neuromuscular disease. Large dose of IV penicillin was listed. She discussed this with her doctor, and he said he would order erythromycin instead. Naomi continues, "But since my labor was so quick, he didn't have a chance to phone in the order for erythromycin, and the nurses had a standing order for penicillin. They kept offering me penicillin, but I refused. Fortunately, my doctor walked in and told them to give me erythromycin."

If a woman has been vomiting, an IV may be the best way to give her fluid and nutrients to replace the fluids lost during vomiting. Moreover, a woman who has been laboring a long time without eating or drinking may need an IV to replace fluids and electrolytes, and to help her keep up her strength. Women in these circumstances may welcome an IV despite the disadvantages.

One disadvantage is that use of an IV reduces a woman's mobility. The plastic tube is attached to a bottle or bag hanging from a tall pole, and even though the tube is taped against the skin so it cannot be dislodged easily, the woman is somewhat more restricted in her movements. For example, if she wants to turn onto her side, or lie down from a sitting position, she must do so without lying down on top of the IV line. Also, if she wants to get up and move around or go to the bathroom, she or her coach will have to push the pole along with her. Clara, who has hemiparesis, commented, "I'm really glad I didn't need an IV when I was in labor. Whenever I have surgery, they have to put the IV in my unaffected hand because it's too hard to get a good vein on the other side. Then it's really hard for me to change position." Heather Ann, who did have an IV during labor, said, "It was difficult to move. I was off balance." A woman who uses a wheelchair will need to make sure the IV line does not get tangled up while transferring. Many women with disabilities are likely to be much more comfortable if they are not given an IV. Although the sensation from an IV is hardly noticeable, some women are bothered by having one more thing that distracts them from coping with labor.

Another possible disadvantage is the difficulty in finding a vein. Amanda needed an IV in her hand for a pitocin drip. They called in the medical flight team because she does not have many veins in her hand. During her first labor, the anesthesiologist called Amanda's former anesthesiologist to find out how to get an IV in her hand. During her second labor, the medical flight team found it easy to find a vein because they usually have to put an IV in a person who is barely alive. Amanda did not find it hard going from lying to sitting, but she needed her mother or husband to feed her and help her use the bathroom independently.

Some people are concerned that a laboring woman who has an IV may be given medication without her knowledge. This concern can be resolved with good communication. The doctor or nurse can tell the mother what solutions are in the IV bag, or the mother or her coach can ask or look at the label.

Catheterization

If a woman has difficulty urinating and her bladder becomes too full, a fine plastic tube called a *catheter* may be inserted into the urethra, which leads from the bladder to the outside of the body. This tube is inserted so urine may be removed. Any discomfort involved is balanced by the reduction in discomfort from having an over-full bladder. An over-full bladder may interfere with descent of the fetus, or it can be injured when it is compressed by the descending fetus. Selina was able to catheterize herself before and after 5 centimeters.

Shanna had a Foley catheter inserted because it was too hard to urinate. She also found "it was more convenient to be in bed." She said, "My body felt tired and loose after the birth." Shanna said, "For my next labor, I do not want the Foley, and I will ask the nurses for help with catheterization."

In some situations, it is best to insert a catheter without waiting for the bladder to fill. Some physicians recommend routinely catheterizing laboring women who have spinal cord injuries above the T6 level in order to prevent dysreflexia.

Sabine experienced an unusual circumstance during her labor. Her urine bag was only changed in the morning. It stayed in place throughout the last 8 hours of labor and delivery. She said, "I emptied it. Actually, I think I was hooked up to a drainage bag."

Special Diagnostic Procedures

EXTERNAL MONITORING

External monitoring measures the fetal heart rate (FHR) and the frequency and duration of uterine contractions. Various patterns in the FHR give information about how the fetus is affected by the stress of labor. Changes in the frequency and duration of contractions provide information about how well the uterus is functioning.

External monitoring may be done for a variety of reasons. When a woman arrives at the hospital, she may be monitored for a short time to establish a baseline in order to learn how her fetus normally responds to contractions. Then, if the monitor is used again later in labor, the pattern of the FHR can be compared with the earlier pattern. Issues that arose during pregnancy, such as preeclampsia or twin pregnancies, are among the reasons why external monitoring may be started as soon as the mother arrives at the hospital. Sometimes, external monitoring may be necessary during the course of labor. For example, monitoring may be necessary if labor is not progressing, or if abnormal fetal heart tones were heard during a routine examination. Monitoring is also necessary when labor is induced or augmented. External monitoring has the advantage of providing more information than the routine methods described above, and it is noninvasive.

Two measuring devices are held against the mother's abdomen by plastic belts. One device, the *toco transducer*, is pressure sensitive and records uterine contractions. The other, an *ultrasound transducer*, senses and records fetal heartbeats. It is useful in determining how well the fetus is tolerating labor.

Monitoring the rate of contractions gives useful information about the progress of the labor, although it is only partial information. Also, the external monitor can help the labor coach. Instead of continually checking a watch, he can concentrate on the mother, only glancing at the recording occasionally to see if a contraction is about to begin. The mother may appreciate the help in knowing when a contraction will begin. Sabine liked monitoring. She said, "I could tell when the contraction began, and also when it was about to end." On the other hand, some people find that the coach becomes fascinated by the monitor and neglects the mother!

If the monitor shows the fetal heart rate is abnormal, the doctor can consider other diagnostic procedures, or take steps to resolve the problem. When the recording shows that the baby is doing well, the reassurance may help the mother to relax and cope with labor contractions.

Sometimes the belts the mother must wear are uncomfortable and need adjustment. This discomfort, like any other, may cause difficulty in coping with labor. Another problem is that the mother must lie still, because sudden movements interfere with the recording of the heart rate. Frequently, the mother is instructed to lie *supine* (on her back), because it may be possible to get better recordings in this position. Lying supine can in itself cause problems, because the weight of the uterus resting on major blood vessels can interfere with blood flow to the uterus, thereby reducing the amount of oxygen to the fetus and slowing the heart rate. The fetal heart rate may return to normal if the woman changes position to her left side. Disabled women who have spinal deformities that make it difficult or impossible to lie supine may need a pillow or other support, or may need to use another position.

The mother and medical staff can work out a schedule that permits her to adjust or remove the belts, move around, or change position from time to time. If staff changes occur while the woman is in labor, her coach or advocate may need to tell the new staff about any arrangements that have been made. The medical staff should check the monitor frequently. If the staff is delayed, and the mother has been moved or changed position, they should be told so they will know that some changes in the recording may have been caused by her movements.

Some birth professionals and consumers have expressed concern that the increased use of fetal monitors may have contributed to the increase in the rate of caesarean surgery. They worry that inaccurate diagnosis of fetal distress has led to unnecessary surgery in some cases. Yet, in other cases, external monitoring has certainly led to a correct diagnosis that might not have been made otherwise. Also, there are other factors contributing to the increase in caesarean surgery.

These concerns should be addressed. First, parents and medical staff can discuss whether electronic monitoring is appropriate. If the need for monitoring was not discussed before labor began, the mother or her coach should not hesitate to ask medical staff any questions that come to mind; for example, why does staff recommend monitoring, or can the monitoring be discontinued or stopped.

An external monitor should not be used with women who have spinal cord injuries at or above the T6 level until an epidural has been given, because the pressure of the belt could stimulate autonomic dysreflexia.

INTERNAL MONITORING

Internal monitoring measures FHR and the strength of the uterine contractions. To measure FHR, an electrode that is attached to recording equipment is inserted under the fetal scalp.

The device for measuring the strength of uterine contractions is an intrauterine pressure catheter. This is a tube filled with fluid that is threaded through the cervix. During uterine contractions, pressure on the amniotic fluid puts pressure on the fluid in the tube, which is connected to a pressure sensor attached to a recording device. In dysfunctional labor, the pressure catheter may be used to measure the strength of uterine contractions. It may also be used when labor is induced or augmented. Medication can be adjusted if uterine contractions are too strong.

The mother can move somewhat more freely with an internal monitor, because her movements will not affect the recording of the fetal heart rate. This method gives more accurate information than external monitoring. In addition, the intrauterine pressure catheter gives information that cannot be obtained in any other way.

There are disadvantages to these procedures, including a small risk that the fetal scalp will be injured or infected by the electrode. There is also a small risk that the tip of the pressure catheter will injure the placenta, or that the electrode or catheter will introduce infection. These risks can be limited by using good sterile technique and skillful procedure.

Internal monitoring is only possible if the cervix is partly dilated and the amniotic membranes have ruptured. Otherwise, an amniotomy (artificial rupture of membranes) will have to be performed. The advantages and disadvantages of amniotomy are discussed below.

FETAL SCALP BLOOD SAMPLING

Changes in fetal heart rate may leave doubt about whether or not the fetus is in distress. In these situations, a small sample of blood may be removed from the fetal scalp for analysis. The amount of oxygen and carbon dioxide in the blood, and its acidity or alkalinity, are measured. Sometimes these measurements are repeated.

By helping the physician to monitor the fetus more accurately, scalp blood sampling can help to assure that emergency procedures are performed only when necessary.

ULTRASOUND

As we explained in the previous chapter, ultrasound is a method for obtaining images by sound waves bouncing off the object under study. During labor, ultrasound examination can be used to determine the location of the placenta and the baby's presentation.

INTERVENTIONS IN LABOR

Amniotomy

Some medical texts suggest that amniotomy can be used in evaluating fetal well-being. The amniotic fluid can be examined for the presence of meconium (the baby's first bowel movement), a sign of fetal distress. It may also be examined for blood, a sign of premature placental separation. In either case, both are dangerous for mother and fetus, and the fetus may have to be delivered quickly by caesarean section.

One disadvantage of amniotomy is that it opens a pathway for infectious organisms to enter the uterine cavity. The risk of infection increases after 24 hours if the membranes have ruptured, either naturally or artificially. Thus, amniotomy starts a clock that cannot be turned back. On the other hand, if there is concern about fetal distress, it may be important to deliver the baby quickly.

Amniotomy may be done in preparation for internal monitoring. It can be dangerous, however, if the fetal head is not well engaged. When the head is not engaged and the amniotic fluid escapes, the umbilical cord may slip down into the space between the fetal head and the pelvic opening. Then, with each contraction, the cord can be compressed between the head and the pelvic bones.

Amniotomy may shorten labor. For the same reason, amniotomy may increase the pain of contractions. Patricia told us, "I had an amniotomy because the doctor said it would hurry up my labor, but it didn't improve the pain; in fact, the pain got worse." Felicia did not dilate after 6 hours of labor, in spite of being induced, so the doctors decided to do an amniotomy. After the amniotomy, Felicia went from 2 centimeters to 10 centimeters in 45 minutes. She said, "My entire body was shaking from the pain. I was out of my mind with the experience. I wish I'd had the epidural before they broke the bag of water. I learned that this is not an uncommon experience. I wish I'd had a birth plan and a copy of orders for an epidural (regional anesthesia). My fibromyalgia was not on anyone's radar screen. I was not treated by my obstetrician. I had two different doctors who did not know anything about my condition." Felicia's obstetrician was the only doctor who knew about her fibromyalgia, and he was not in the room.

Carol said, "My water was broken manually in both deliveries. This was fine the first time. The second time it caused so much pain that my spasticity became severe. The resident who broke my water then insisted I would need an epidural because my legs were spastic, even though she had created the problem in the first place."

Generally, most women do not find amniotomy painful. During Carol's second labor, the amniotomy may have produced a stronger contraction, thereby causing spasticity.

Amniotomy worked well for Michelle, who had a dysfunctional labor. Michelle's obstetrician was worried that continued labor would lead to exhaustion and worsening of her MS symptoms because women with MS are susceptible to fatigue. Her doctor performed an amniotomy after $2\frac{1}{2}$ days of labor, and the baby was delivered 5 hours later.

On the other hand, the amniotic membrane often ruptures spontaneously early in labor without harm to the fetus or the mother. The fetal head can mold better after the membrane ruptures, easing passage through the pelvic outlet.

Although Shanna's water broke naturally, she was at 4 centimeters when she was checked for the first time. The nurse was not going to do a pelvic exam because it was too soon, but because Shanna's water broke, the nurse checked her and found her to be at 10 centimeters.

Induction and Augmentation of Labor

Induction of labor is artificial stimulation of uterine contractions when labor has not begun spontaneously. Shanna was induced because she had a reduced amount of amniotic fluid. She was disappointed, and said, "I really wanted to experience what I'd seen in the movies. I wanted to say, 'It's time!' and be rushed to the hospital."

Charlotte was 2 weeks late so her doctor decided to induce labor, which immediately caused muscle spasms. A majority of people who have cerebral palsy find that pain triggers spasms. Regional anesthesia cannot be used until the active phase of labor. Therefore, you might want to ask your doctor about using muscle relaxers. In addition, holding the spasming limb away from the direction of the spasm helps the muscle relax.

Amanda was induced twice. Once because the baby was overdue by two weeks, and once because of fear that the baby would be too large. Amanda had an epidural after 48 hours of labor. She found the epidural so helpful that she had one during her second labor as well.

Augmentation involves stimulation of uterine contractions after labor has started. It is used when contractions have started and then stopped, or when contractions are weak.

Selina got stuck at 5 or 6 centimeters with all five of her labors. She said, "My labor would just continue with contractions 1 minute apart. They would give me a drop of pitocin. This tiny amount helped me dilate to 10 centimeters in an hour. They didn't want to bring on hard labor."

Natalie was given an epidural to help cope with the stronger contractions that were brought on by pitocin. When her contractions were 2 minutes apart, Natalie's doctor turned off the pitocin drip for a couple of hours. Then he turned it on again to "jump start my uterine contractions." Natalie went on to say, "I went from 4 centimeters to 9 centimeters in 1 hour when the doctor turned the pitocin back on."

Labor may be induced to treat some pregnancy complications (see Chapter 10). Labor will also be induced if contractions do not begin soon enough after the amniotic membranes have ruptured. In this instance, induction can be seen as a preventive measure, because surgical delivery may be considered if the baby is not born within 24 hours of membrane rupture. It has become a routine practice at many institutions to allow labor to continue for up to 36 hours after rupture of the membranes. Tina was induced after 30-plus hours because she was only 1 centimeter dilated. As of this writing, medical researchers are looking for a way to predict the likelihood that infection will develop after membrane rupture. Sabine was induced 2 weeks after her retina detached. She did not have high blood pressure, which is associated with a detached retina. She said, "I was not hypertensive. Sometimes people who are nearsighted are at risk for retinal detachment. The doctors were not afraid of the induction raising my blood pressure. My labor went a lot longer than I expected. I was only 1 to 2 centimeters after 24 hours, so they stopped the induction and told me to have dinner and go to sleep. The next day they started me up again. They were going to break my bag of waters if I hadn't made any progress by noon. I progressed fast after they broke the waters."

Labor must not be induced or augmented unless specific criteria are met. At least one indication for induction must be present, such as fetal post-maturity. There must be no contraindications, such as breech presentation. In a discussion between the author and Dr. Sandy Welner, who has since died, Dr. Welner stated that induction should be done only if the cervix is "ripe." She said, "When you induce a woman with a spinal cord injury, it is important to have a central monitoring line so you can have all the pressures that happen in the circulatory system carefully monitored, because something could change in a second. Since you are monitoring so precisely, and all the lines and tubes are in, if something happens, you do not have to worry about putting in a line. You have the access already established." When asked about epidurals, Dr. Welner said, "An epidural can be put in even before the woman is in labor. The spinal works quicker, but an epidural is better. With a spinal, you are likely to get a headache."

Natasha's doctor thought that her baby was getting too large. The doctors softened her cervix before they induced her. Deirdre's blood pressure was elevated, and she was encouraged to undergo induction. She said, "I was afraid if they induced labor or did any other procedures, I would need to have a caesarean."

In women with spinal cord injuries at or above T6, the longer, stronger contractions of induced labor seem to increase the risk of an episode of dysreflexia. The medical staff must be prepared to differentiate dysreflexia symptoms from preeclampsia symptoms because these conditions are managed differently. Ideally, a specialist will be available. The mother should tell staff immediately if she has dysreflexia symptoms. She should expect to have her blood pressure measured frequently during contractions, as well as between contractions. She may be given regional anesthesia or medications to control her blood pressure. Sally was happy to be induced with her first pregnancy. She said, "I was worried about going into labor and getting dysreflexia before I even got to the hospital. It was also an opportunity to have my high-risk doctor on duty that day." Unfortunately, Sally's high-risk doctor did not deliver her, and she had a resident (a doctor who is still in training) for her delivery. Sally said, "They did not give me a strong enough epidural with my first delivery. Their intention was to increase it as labor increased. But there was a lack of communication between doctors during the significant part of labor. They did not consider my particular needs. One doctor was unaware of my disability, and did not think it was prudent to increase the medication. This resulted in my blood pressure going very high." She demanded to see an anesthesiologist.

Pitocin is used to induce and augment labor after the cervix has ripened either spontaneously or after the use of prostaglandins. It is given intravenously, in a gradually increasing dose. When a maximum dose is reached, or effective contractions have begun, the oxytocin is then given at a steady rate. Medical staff will monitor contractions carefully to make sure the uterus is not being overstimulated. If contractions become too strong, the pitocin should be reduced or discontinued. The remaining pitocin will disappear from the mother's blood within an hour. If contractions are extremely uncomfortable, the mother or her coach can ask about reducing the dose of pitocin. The flow of pitocin may also be interrupted to see whether contractions will continue spontaneously. Sometimes pitocin administration fails to induce labor. Induction may be tried again after a day or two, depending on the circumstances, or surgical delivery may be necessary.

Intravenous pitocin is also used to stimulate contractions that have weakened or stopped after labor has begun. Just as there are specific indications for induction with pitocin, there are specific indications for augmentation. It must be determined that the contractions are not false labor, and other conditions must be met as well. For example, augmentation must not be done if the mother has certain health problems.

The advantages of induction and augmentation are that by shortening labor, these procedures may prevent infection, maternal exhaustion, or fetal distress. Successful augmentation of labor can prevent the need for surgical delivery.

Contractions may be strong from the beginning when labor is induced, rather than gradually increasing in intensity, as in most spontaneous labors. As a result, the laboring woman may not have the same opportunity to adapt gradually. Shanna said, "Every time it tightened, I couldn't breathe." Stimulation with pitocin tends to produce longer, stronger contractions than are typical in spontaneous labors, possibly making it more difficult for the mother to cope. Reactions vary. Corinne said of her second labor, "The labor pains were very bad. They were worse than the first labor." Mary said, "I expected it to be more traumatic."

The longer, stronger contractions of augmented labor have a greater potential for causing fetal hypoxia than spontaneous contractions.

Attempts to stimulate labor cannot be continued indefinitely. Whether labor is stimulated or spontaneous, forceps or vacuum extraction may be used to speed up delivery before the mother becomes too fatigued or the fetus becomes too distressed.

Complications of Labor

Complications of labor are variations from the normal course of labor that threaten the well-being of the mother or the fetus.

PREECLAMPSIA

Preeclampsia may be characterized by extremely high blood pressure, which is dangerous to both mother and fetus. In addition, it can progress to eclampsia during labor, and the mother may experience convulsions and possible coma. Treatment with medications to lower blood pressure and other emergency measures may be used. Caesarean delivery may also be necessary.

PROLONGATION OR ARREST OF LABOR

Insufficient Contractions

One cause of prolongation or arrest of labor is weak or uncoordinated uterine contractions. It is not always possible to determine the cause of insufficient contractions. Sometimes excessive or poorly timed doses of pain medication weaken contractions. A rigid cervix may also cause prolonged labor, because uterine contractions cannot dilate the cervix if appropriate changes in the cervix have not occurred. If the cervix is not rigid, then contractions may be stimulated by induction or augmentation.

Fetopelvic or Cephalopelvic Disproportion

Labor will also be prolonged if the size or shape of the pelvic girdle does not allow the fetus to pass through. This condition is known as *fetopelvic disproportion*. The problem may arise from the mother's individual anatomy, the presentation or position of the fetus, or the size of the fetus. The most favorable, and most common, fetal presentation is the *occiput anterior* (crown of the head first, fetus facing the mother's spine). Other presentations include *posterior presentation* (back of the fetus' head is pressing the spine), *brow presentation* (forehead first), and *breech presentations* (other parts of the body first, most commonly buttocks). Abnormal presentation can be a problem because the presenting part of the fetus does not fit well into the pelvic outlet.

Scoliosis or congenital hip or pelvic deformities can cause fetopelvic disproportion. This complication can cause maternal exhaustion, uterine injury, or fetal distress (defined below).

PLACENTA PREVIA AND PREMATURE PLACENTAL SEPARATION

The placenta is normally attached to the uterine wall in the upper part of the uterus. In less than one half of one percent of pregnancies, the placenta implants low in the uterus, with part of it over the cervix. *Placenta previa* may block the descent of the fetus, or the placenta may begin to tear away from the uterine wall as the cervix dilates. If the placenta separates from the uterine wall, maternal blood loss and fetal hypoxia and distress can be problems. Bleeding without pain is sometimes the first sign of placenta previa. Surgical delivery may be necessary if the placenta covers more than 30 percent of the fully dilated cervix. If placenta previa is less extreme, there may be a trial labor, during which the fetus is monitored and preparations are made to treat hypoxia and blood loss.

Premature placental separation, which is also called *placental abruption* or *abruptio placentae*, is a separation of the placenta from the uterine wall before the fetus is delivered. If blood does not escape through the cervix, then severe pain or fetal distress may be the first signs of placental separation.

UMBILICAL CORD COMPRESSION

Multiple pregnancies, fetopelvic disproportion, displacement of the umbilical cord, and other conditions may lead to compression of the umbilical cord between the fetus and the uterine wall. Compression of the cord is usually brief and intermittent, and there may be no harm to the fetus, but prolonged or continuous compression may cause fetal hypoxia and distress. Fetal distress is a sign of cord displacement and compression.

FETAL DISTRESS

Labor is always somewhat stressful to the fetus. The fetus is usually well able to tolerate some stress, however, reacting with moderate changes of heart rate. During contractions, the uterine muscles squeeze the blood vessels supplying the placenta, reducing the flow of oxygen to the fetus. Interference with the oxygen supply leads to *hypoxia*, a lack of oxygen.

There are several signs of fetal distress. Meconium in the amniotic fluid is an important indicator that the baby is in distress. Meconium is a tarry material, somewhat like feces, that is found in the digestive tract of the baby. Passage of meconium is reason for concern, because the fetus may breathe in (*aspirate*) meconium. This can cause hypoxia as well as other respiratory problems. Treatment of fetal distress can range from simply having the mother breathe oxygen, to emergency surgical delivery.

Another symptom of distress is extreme change in heart rate; the heart may beat either more quickly or more slowly. Change in fetal heart rate can be diagnosed by *auscultation* (listening with a stethoscope or Doppler™) or electronic monitoring. Sally's baby was monitored during her first labor. Sally had a sustained contraction that lasted 13 minutes, resulting in the baby's heart rate dropping. They gave her oxygen and decreased her pitocin, which resulted in normalization of the baby's heart rate.

Monitoring is important to track the condition of the baby. Amanda had difficulty keeping the oxygen monitor on her hand at the same time as the IV. She said, "They tried putting the monitor on my toes, but that didn't work, so they used my ear lobe. I don't know if it is a medically sound decision, but it worked."

If there is any question about the accuracy of diagnosis by monitoring, scalp blood sampling can differentiate between *stress* and *distress*. These procedures are discussed in the following section.

Methods for Coping with Labor Discomforts

A variety of methods have been developed to help women feel as comfortable and relaxed as possible during labor. Not every method is useful in every situation. For example, most women do not have back labor, and will not need suggestions for coping with it. The same woman may find light massage relaxing during one phase of labor, yet annoying during another phase. A method that helped during one labor may not help during another; for example, Noelle, who said, "With my first baby it really helped to have a focal point, but the second time I didn't use it." During Allison's first labor she found one object in the room to focus on. Nearly every woman will use at least one of these methods during her labor.

It is also helpful to pack the labor kit described in Table 11-2. Not every item will be used. Pack the labor kit a few weeks before the due date—nobody wants to be searching for socks and a mirror when it is time to leave for the hospital! Be sure to pack any special items that you might need; for example, Andrea wished she had brought a wedge pillow with her to put under her stump.

Most of the techniques for coping with labor can be included in one of the following categories: breathing techniques; other relaxation techniques; and relief of particular discomforts, such as cold feet or chapped lips.

THE ROLE OF THE COACH, OR DOULA

The most important roles for the coach, or doula, are to emotionally support the birthing mother, time contractions, and interact with hospital staff. Natasha was unsure her husband could get there on time because he was in the military. She said, "I was really afraid that he would miss the whole delivery, so when he got there it made me feel at ease. It really helped a lot."

Emotional support is very important, especially for those who have had past traumas associated with hospitals. Simi said, "Until I gave birth, I despised hospitals. It is a smell that hits you when you walk in the door. It brings back memories of being a child and being in the hospital and having a lot of surgeries and having no control. To me, walking into the hospital means losing all control over who touches you and what they might do to you. Hospitals mean pain and misery." Simi talked over her fears with her friends and her husband. She said, "My husband decided he was going to be my protector, and he

TABLE 11-2
LABOR KIT

Item	Purpose
Copies of medical information forms	If hospital misfiles this information, it will not have to be given all over again
Handouts on labor from birthing class	Reminds coach of coping methods
Stopwatch or watch with second hand, pen, paper	Timing and recording contractions
Money, including several coins	Coach's snacks, phones calls
Bag lunch or snacks	Food helps coach during long labor, coach may need to stay with mother
Massage items	Powder and body oil, bonger, vibrator, tennis balls, rolling pin for back labor
Focal point objects	Objects to focus the eyes on for relaxation, including an "emotionally satisfying object"
Spoon	For feeding ice chips
Washcloths	Help keep mother cool, wipe away sweat, help with massage
Breath spray	Freshen dry mouth or stale breath
Chapstick	Moisten dry lips
Sour lollipops	Sugar keeps up mother's strength, sour more refreshing than sweet, mother cannot choke on lollipop
Paper bag	Mother can breathe into bag if hyperventilating
Mirror	To let mother see birth
Glasses	Contact lenses should not be worn during labor
CD player, tape recorder, tapes, and headphones	Relaxing music or hypnosis tapes
Warm socks	To warm mother's feet if cold
Camera or video	Birth pictures
Telephone list	People to call after birth
Wedge and extra pillows, sheepskin, egg crate mattress	Comfort
Shower chair, Aqua Socks™, plastic lawn chair, commode chair	Comfort in hospital shower

Note: Pack all items 2-3 weeks before due date (except perishable food items).

wasn't going to leave me alone. If I was in pain and I didn't understand something, he would be the person to make the decisions. And that helped. He was the one who would be in control for both of us. When I couldn't concentrate on breathing, he would breathe. I would watch him, and then I would do what he was doing. When I got out of control, he would say, 'SIMI, LOOK AT ME.' We did all that stuff they taught us." Corrine said, "My husband didn't go to the birthing classes, but his presence was calming." Felicia's husband has aphasia, and is unable to express himself verbally. In spite of his disability, she said, "He played the role of my anchor. I was so scared and in so much pain. He reassured me and helped me to not completely lose it."

Sharon said, "I didn't need a coach, but it was good to have my sister there, even though we were just laughing." Stephanie thought both aspects of the coach's job were crucial. "He helped me breathe, he timed my contractions, and he helped me decide about pain medication." The coach can help the mother communicate with medical staff. For example, sometimes the mother is so intent on her labor that she does not hear something a nurse says, but when her coach repeats it, she will respond to the familiar voice. The coach may tell a doctor or nurse, "She'll answer your question in a minute, she just started a contraction." Some women who feel their husbands are not good with emotional support may want an additional person to act as a doula.

A coach who is familiar with disability can also help by letting medical staff know about the mother's special needs. People who are skillful at helping in childbirth may not have much experience with disability, and the coach may need to show them how to help the mother transfer, or remind them to help her change position to prevent pressure sores. Some coaches have an easy time. Jennifer quotes her husband, who had been expecting a long labor with many "trials and tribulations," as saying that her 5-hour labor was really "boring." For other coaches, especially those who assist in a long or difficult labor, the job can be tiring. Sierra said, "I had my coach get me something to drink. I was so thirsty. He would hold the cup and straw." Christina and Michelle made sure they had enough support by arranging for two coaches.

Christina said her second coach helped her husband to be more effective because "my husband was anxious, and my friend had a baby and knew what to expect." Coaches can give each other restroom and snack breaks. Simi's husband got hungry in the middle of the night and went out to get something to eat. The nurse took over during that time.

Another important role of the coach is timing the mother's contractions using a *stopwatch*. Sometimes a labor contraction feels like it will last forever. The coach can reassure the mother by telling her, "You're halfway through now. It's going to end in 15 seconds…10 seconds…5 seconds."

EATING

The advantage of eating during early labor is that food may help to keep up the mother's strength if the labor is long. If emergency surgery and general anesthesia become necessary later in labor, however, the woman will be at risk for coughing up and choking on any food remaining in her stomach. Therefore, get the doctor's permission to eat something light, such as gelatin, broth, or apple juice. You may also eat something light before going to the hospital.

ENEMAS

In the past, laboring women were automatically given enemas when they entered the hospital. This practice is now much less common. Medical experience has shown that fecal material in the bowel will not inhibit labor, and proper care eliminates any risk that the baby will get an infection from feces.

Some people feel that enemas speed up labor. Medical evidence shows, however, that, on average, women who have enemas labor just as long as women who do not have them. A better reason for having an enema is for comfort. An enema early in labor assures that a bowel movement will occur while it is still relatively comfortable. Also, many women feel more comfortable about pushing if they are not worried about fecal material coming out with each push. Women who have problems with constipation may want to have one last bowel movement before they give birth, because they may not have a bowel movement for a couple of days afterward. Women who are concerned about constipation can ask their doctor if it is advisable to have a prepackaged Fleet® enema ready to use at home when labor begins.

Women who have problems with dysreflexia should not use an enema, because the pressure of the enema might cause an episode.

MILD EXERCISE

Standing up and walking around are also helpful during early labor. Standing helps labor to progress, because gravity helps to maintain the pressure of the amniotic sac (or the fetal head) on the cervix. Mild exercise can help keep up the mother's spirits, but she may want to stop and lean on her coach or a piece of furniture during contractions. Walking is also helpful in later phases, but as labor intensifies, many women prefer standing still or sitting instead of walking around. Naomi used a walker. Deirdre said, "I walked up and down the hall with my walker to keep the contractions going. I also walked up and down the stairs. I had to have people on each arm to stay balanced. I wore my tennis shoes with orthodontics the whole time because of my weak ankles and plantar fasciitis. I used the Rollator™ (a four-wheeled walker) to walk around. I liked the Rollator™ because it had large wheels, which made it easier to push. The walker also had brakes, and I used them to stop when I had contractions. Moreover, it also had a seat."

Michelle and Renee also felt it was unpleasant to try to walk while in labor. Nadia wanted get up and she got out of bed, but she collapsed because the epidural left her legs numb and she was weak. Carla, on the other hand, usually does not like to walk, but she said, "I needed to walk during labor." Marsha could not walk, but commented, "Standing was less painful. I stood up and held onto a chair. My husband stood either behind me or at my side for support. I sat down in the chair between contractions." Medical staff will certainly encourage the mother to get up and walk around if labor slows down, so that gravity can make contractions more effective.

The mother should be encouraged to go to the bathroom about once an hour during every phase of labor. Then, instead of walking aimlessly, she has a specific place to go that is only a short distance away. She can change position from standing to sitting, and back to standing again. An empty bladder is more comfortable and less susceptible to injury. In addition, the mother's ability to urinate is an important sign that she is not becoming dehydrated.

BREATHING TECHNIQUES

Breathing properly helps the mother to relax and get enough oxygen for herself and the baby during uterine contractions. Relaxation techniques are every bit as important as other techniques for maintaining comfort. A woman who is tense or frightened is more sensitive to pain. The mother's fear and tension can affect uterine contractions and, indirectly, the baby's blood chemistry.

Breathing techniques are the most useful when they have been practiced in advance. A woman should practice every possible technique, because she may not know which breathing technique will help. The author recalls a student telling her that a breathing technique she had disliked in class was quite helpful when she was in labor. It is best to learn breathing techniques in a class where they can be demonstrated and practiced, not just described. Some women prefer to use the breathing techniques suggested for the early phase all through Stage I, while others need to use transition breathing techniques before they are in transition.

Breathing methods for labor help a woman to relax in the early and active phases because they help her focus on slow, rhythmical movement. Continuous rhythmical breathing gives her a sense of continuity between the times when the uterus is contracted and when it is relaxed. Cheryl said proper breathing was the most important technique she used to stay relaxed. Julie did not take childbirth classes, but she was taught how to breathe by the nurses at the hospital. She said these methods helped her handle contractions. Nora and Sabine also found breathing techniques helpful in handling labor contractions.

The two most useful breathing techniques for Stage I labor are *deep chest breathing* (also called *abdominal breathing*) and *ah-hee* breathing. Some women begin with deep chest breathing and change to ah-hee as labor intensifies. Other women are more comfortable using one technique throughout Stage 1. In deep chest breathing, the mother inhales slowly through her nose, and then exhales slowly through her mouth. She breathes so deeply that her abdomen and ribs visibly expand when she inhales.

Each breathing technique uses a *cleansing breath*. The cleansing breath is useful for a number of reasons. This extra-deep breath gives the mother a boost of extra oxygen.

Early in labor, when a regular rhythm of contractions is just starting, the mother can take a cleansing breath to signal to the coach that a contraction is beginning or ending. Later, when contractions occur more regularly, the coach can tell the mother to take a cleansing breath when the contraction is about to begin.

An alternative to deep chest breathing is *vocalization*. With this variant, the mother takes a deep breath, and then breathes out with a slow, deep groan. The sound provides an auditory focal point for many women, especially when other people in the room join in vocalizing. The effect is somewhat like the chanting heard during some religious ceremonies. Others simply find vocalizing more comfortable than other ways of pushing, like Stephanie, who said, "Groaning got me down more."

Ah-hee breathing is more rapid and shallow than deep chest breathing, and the woman needs to concentrate to keep from breathing increasingly faster and more shallowly. A good way to stay in control is to whisper "ahhhhh" while inhaling, and "heeeee" while exhaling. Another way to avoid hyperventilating during ah-hee breathing is to pause for one count between the "ah" and the "hee." The coach may have to remind the mother to slow down, especially if she starts feeling dizzy or nauseated, or if her hands and feet tingle. These can be symptoms of hyperventilation. If she hyperventilates, she can breathe into a *paper bag* until her symptoms disappear. Although this type of breathing requires concentration, many women prefer it. Noelle said, "I had a hard time relaxing during my first labor, and I couldn't deal with deep breathing." She preferred deep breathing during her second labor, however. Priscilla said she found slow breathing helpful early in labor, and that ah-hee at the end was also helpful. Ah-hee was the only method Clara liked. She explained, "I found it difficult to relax, and it was difficult to take a deep breath. Ah-hee took all of my attention, which I liked, because I was able to focus on the breathing instead of the pain or the effort to relax."

For women whose disabilities make deep breathing difficult, ah-hee breathing may be a useful alternative. If the labor nurse is worried because this shallower breathing seems to be happening too early in labor, the coach can explain that it is an adaptation to disability.

RELAXATION METHODS

Many different types of relaxation techniques are effective, and may help the mother to avoid using pain medication. Some women will start using relaxation methods during early labor; others may start using them in the active phase. Most of these methods involve either physical relaxation or visualization. A woman can use specific methods of muscle relaxation while she is resting in a comfortable position. As with breathing techniques, it helps to practice these relaxation methods before labor begins. Some people recommend practicing as much as 20 minutes daily to develop real skill in relaxation. Michelle said, "I had a special coach who helped me find out where I was tense, and then helped me get that part of my body to relax." Nora found a different method. She said, "I was not dilating very fast. Having my friends in the room helped me to relax and kept me from paying attention to the pain."

Sometimes there may not be a way to relax. Hannah's thigh muscles were in spasm, and relaxed only when she started pushing. Finding a comfortable position can help.

Progressive Relaxation

This method of relaxation teaches the pregnant woman to consciously relax in response to intentionally created muscle tension. She first tenses, then relaxes, one part of her body (for example, her right arm), then progresses to another part, until her whole body is relaxed. This can be done alone or with the help of a coach. Tense the body part just enough to increase awareness of specific muscles. Some disabled women, especially those with cerebral palsy, may find this technique too difficult. For some, it is simply impossible; once the limb is tense, it takes so much energy and concentration to relax that another relaxation method would obviously be better. For some women, tensing one limb will cause the other limbs to become tense and possibly spasm.

Massage and Acupressure

The coach can help the laboring woman in a more active way when using massage and acupressure. In massage, the coach gently but firmly kneads the tense area. Good places to massage are the feet, hands, neck, shoulders, and back. The neck and shoulders are especially important, because many people tense these areas when under stress. Tina was fine with only a foot massage. Massage can also help with muscle cramps. When using massage with a disabled woman, the rule is, "Go for the cramp."

The person giving the massage should have warm hands and be alert to the woman's feedback as to whether the massage is too firm, too gentle, or just right. Massage can be given more gently as the tense area relaxes.

The coach can use massage aids from the labor kit. *Powder* or *cornstarch* can be used to reduce friction. *Talcum powder* is less likely to cake on contact with body moisture. Cornstarch will cake, but some people prefer it because it has no odor. Some people prefer the dry, silky feeling of powders; others like the gliding feeling of lubrication with *massage oil* or *hand lotion*. Oil or lotion will soothe dry skin, too. If the coach's hands get tired, or if he is disabled, a mechanical massage aid such as a *vibrator*, *rolling pin*, or a *bonger* can be helpful. A bonger is a hollow rubber ball on a flexible metal rod set into a wooden handle. The coach gently taps ("bongs") the tense area with the ball. Do not rely only on a vibrator, because the buzzing sound may annoy the mother.

Squeeze the front of the thigh with both hands to help with thigh muscle cramps, which often occur during transition. To help with calf cramps, place the hands just below the knee, one on each side of the leg, and apply pressure. Another way to relieve a calf cramp is to bend the foot upward at the ankle, and keeping the leg straight, hold it until the cramp is gone. Having your legs massaged might feel good temporarily, even when they feel numb. Massaging the cramping calf muscle may not help, because it may feel sore for a while after the cramp is relieved.

Some women get more relief from acupressure than from massage. (The following descriptions of pressure points are approximate.) The coach will need to try several points in a small area, continuing to press different points until the woman says, "That's it!" First, try going slowly down the spine, pressing with the thumbs about one inch to each side of each vertebra. This works well with the woman lying on her side or sitting in front of the coach. Next, the coach can find the point that relieves tension in the neck and shoulders. This point is on the back of the neck, between the shoulders. The woman can lean her head slightly forward, resting her forehead on the coach's hand for stability, while the coach gently presses the thumb of one hand and the first finger of the other hand on different points up and down the neck until the right spot is found. Other pressure points are on the front of the body. Gently press along both sides of the hairline and the soft areas near the temples, working from the center of the forehead around to the back of the head and down toward the collarbones. Finally, a technique that may relieve pain during active labor and transition involves placing the fingers firmly on top of the head, with the thumb on the bridge of the nose, then gently pressing with the thumb. These techniques can also reduce pain and promote relaxation when practiced during pregnancy.

Touch Relaxation

Using this method, the coach uses touch rather than words to communicate with the laboring woman, calling her attention to the part of the body that needs to relax. The coach can touch an area that appears to be tense, such as the shoulders, or move slowly and systematically from one part of the body to another. Moving slowly is important for this technique to be effective. The coach's hands must be warm, since a touch from a cold hand is likely to startle the mother and make her tense her muscles. The appropriate touch is light; the coach simply rests her hand gently on the woman's arm, for example, until she sees or feels the tense muscles relax. This method may work better if it has been practiced beforehand, so the woman can learn to relax at her coach's touch. Some women do not want to be touched during labor, and will not like this method. A light touch is unpleasant for some women, but firm massage may be enjoyable. For others, relaxation through touch relaxation is wonderful. Hilary's disability made it difficult for her to be given a spinal injection. Her husband's verbal suggestions and gentle touch helped her to relax, and she takes pleasure in recalling his touch on her forehead and neck.

Effleurage is a variety of touch relaxation in which the abdomen is gently patted in a circular fashion. For some women, effleurage helps by bringing their attention to the surface of their body, away from their contractions. A woman can use effleurage on herself. Only a few of the women interviewed for this book tried effleurage, and none of them liked it. Renee explained, "It was very distracting." Yet many of the author's students have found effleurage helpful. It is certainly worth trying.

Visualization Techniques

Visualization techniques differ from other relaxation methods in that they concentrate the woman's attention on something outside of herself. One such technique is the use of a focal point. A focal point is anything a woman can focus her eyes on to aid her in concentrating. Some women prefer to use a picture that helps them think of their labor in a positive way, such as a picture of a dilated cervix or a baby. Others are very choosy about the focal point. Noelle brought along two pictures, and when she did not like one, she had her coach take it down and hang up the other. For some women, any focal point will do. Stacy said, "Simply concentrating on any object helped." Marsha said, "I stared at the wallpaper." Clara spontaneously invented a focal point during her second labor: "I suddenly remembered watching my LaMaze teacher moving her finger back and forth like a pendulum during breathing exercises. I started moving my finger the same way. Watching it helped me control my breathing, even though my labor was intense."

Using a focal point does not always help. Renee commented, "In my first labor, focusing on the baby was helpful, but during the second labor I was in too much pain to focus." Noelle, who had used two focal points during her first labor, found that during her second labor she needed to concentrate on herself rather than on an outside object. The best plan is to pack an *emotionally satisfying object* in the labor kit and be flexible about whether to use it.

Visualization uses imagery to assist in relaxation. Imagining a relaxing situation can help a person to relax. For example, a woman can imagine that she is at the beach resting on soft sand, feeling the sun's gentle warmth on her skin as her limbs grow heavier. She can privately imagine such images, or her coach can verbally paint a word picture, talking softly and slowly.

Another form of visualization that some women use is concentrating on positive images of labor. For example, the woman's coach can tell her, "Your contractions are working on your cervix. Your cervix is opening wider and wider, like a rose blooming."

Hypnosis

Hypnosis and self-hypnosis are similar to visualization, and use imagery or a focal point to achieve a trance state. Hypnosis does not work for everyone, but when it does work, it can effectively help a laboring woman stay relaxed and in control. Hypnosis is a skill that must be taught by a trained professional. Sometimes the professional will prepare a tape recording that can be used during labor. Clara said, "I couldn't do self-hypnosis. It's much more successful when my husband hypnotizes me. We had several sessions with a professional who taught us how. My first labor was very long. After 24 hours I felt quite discouraged, and was losing control. My husband was able to calm me down by hypnotizing me. I stayed in control for the rest of the labor and delivery—another 8 hours!"

Carol learned self-hypnosis for her first pregnancy, but induction interfered with her ability to use it. She said, "I had no time to adapt to the pain. I went from not having any contractions to having contractions 2 minutes apart. There was no time to get into self-hypnosis with that big of a change. Under those circumstances, I could get the rest of my body to relax, but I really couldn't get my legs to relax. Also, my regular doctor was out of town when the perinatologist decided to deliver my second baby. This made it much more difficult to deliver, because they didn't know me and really didn't understand CP like my regular doctor did.

Mimi had been encouraged to see a hypnotherapist, but she was not sure if it was helpful. The hypnosis probably was useful, however, because Mimi did not need any pain medication. This is unusual when labor is induced, because induction produces longer, stronger contractions, which are more painful. Moreover, Mimi had only 4½ hours of labor, and short labor can be more painful. She gave a lot of credit to a book called *Birthing from Within* (94). Mimi felt that listening to audiotapes in between contractions helped with relaxation. The hypnotherapist provided a tape and the music tapes came from home.

Music

Music can also help a laboring woman to relax. Noelle made a point of saying, "It really promoted relaxation during my second labor." Music may help in more than one way. Rhythmical music may help a woman to control her breathing; it can serve as a focal point; and music can create positive feelings in a way similar to visual imagery. Some studies have shown that women who listened to soft music during labor seemed better able to relax and feel positive about their experience afterwards. Music may also help birth attendants to relax. It may be useful to play music while practicing relaxation before labor. Some women use *headphones* to screen out distracting noises, but others feel isolated when they use headphones.

Warm Showers or Baths

Warm showers or baths can also aid in relaxation. Water baths for labor have been used in Russia, France, and England. There has been concern that laboring in water increases the risk of infection, but studies conducted in France have not shown any connection between water labor and infections. This practice differs widely in the United States. Whirlpool baths are being installed in labor suites in some hospitals; in others, the nurse has to get a doctor's permission to let a laboring woman take a shower or bath.

A warm water bath may help a woman relax partly by dilating surface blood vessels and increasing blood flow to muscles. Those who favor laboring in water theorize that contractions that are less painful will be more efficient. Also, women seem to feel that contractions are less painful when they labor in warm water. Laboring in a warm bath may have additional advantages for women with disabilities. Warm baths relieve muscle spasms, and women who are having problems with spasms may be helped by moving to a tub. Laboring in a bath can help women with arthritis avoid excess stress on their joints. In 2002, Tessa gave birth in a hospital that had a labor tub. She said that laboring in the tub was wonderful because the warm water muted the pain. Unfortunately, hospital staff would only let her stay in the tub for 45 minutes. Getting in and out of a bathtub can be cumbersome for some women. If you anticipate using a bathtub in the hospital, it is best to plan ahead as to how to get into and out of the tub while laboring, using support and avoiding injury.

An article published by Disability, Pregnancy & Parenthood International (DPPI) discusses a woman (Clare) with a chronic back condition whose first child was born by caesarean section (95). She was able to deliver her second child vaginally. Clare had a slow recovery from a caesarean section, and she wanted to try a vaginal birth with her next baby. Her midwives supported a vaginal birth, and thought that a water birth would help Clare by giving her freedom of movement and support.

One of the interviewees with multiple sclerosis said that using the tub "relaxed and relieved the pain, but after a while my MS symptoms started to reappear and I had to get out of the tub." Transferring to and from a slippery shower or tub may be too complicated or even risky for some women. To use a bath safely, the woman must be able to sit independently or she could slip under the water.

A warm shower helps to relieve the discomfort of back labor. The shower works best when the water flows directly onto the lower back. Clara was enthusiastic: "I found the shower incredibly relaxing. It really helped. I'll never forget how good it felt." Hannah stayed in the shower as long as she could stand during her first labor. She wished she could have had a *shower chair*. Some women might want to bring a *plastic lawn chair* or use *Aqua Socks*™. Nora wished she had either brought with her or arranged for a *commode chair* that could be used in the shower. Deirdre did not use a shower chair because she "needed people to hold her up." Amanda also loved showers, and was looking forward to being in the shower while she was in labor. Unfortunately, the shower at the hospital was inaccessible. Michelle disliked the shower because walking and standing were too uncomfortable for her. She might have been more comfortable with a chair in the shower. Some hospitals will provide chairs for this purpose. Good positioning may help if the shower is not available or a woman does not want to use one.

A Comfortable Position

One way to help keep muscles relaxed is simple: find a comfortable position. A number of positions may be useful during labor. It is best to change position approximately every 45 minutes in order to maintain comfort and help labor progress. Experiment with these positions:

- ❖ Standing
- ❖ Kneeling
- ❖ Getting on hands and knees
- ❖ Sitting upright
- ❖ Sitting partly reclined with the back at a 45° angle to bed
- ❖ Side-lying

Coaches can work together to help the laboring woman change positions. Deirdre had eight coaches who took turns helping her throughout her whole labor and delivery. Moreover, she had other coaches as backup reserve. Some of the responsibilities of the coaches were to reposition her, hold her legs, and help her walk. She could not move her legs without help. She said, "The people on my labor team helped to keep me from becoming overwhelmed. They were prepared in advance about what I would need to pull up my legs. There were people on each side." She also used the *extra pillows* that she had brought from home to help with positioning on the hospital bed.

Naomi's husband held her up because she preferred standing to sitting or kneeling. Regarding her second labor, Naomi said, "I preferred to labor standing and leaning slightly forward to support myself on the back of a chair until I got too tired. Then I would go to all fours on the bed or hanging on to the headboard."

For women with TOS, you might want to make sure that the positions you are in for labor do not put any undue strain on your arms. It is better for you to lean against your coach or the bed, but not on your arms.

The nurses made Simi get out of bed. She said, "My husband pushed me in the wheelchair. I had trouble getting out of the wheelchair, but I got help from my husband or the nurse. I also had trouble going to the bathroom. They did not want me to bear down, so they cathed me once. They felt I needed to get rid of the urine." Medical staff does not want laboring women to bear down, because the cervix can swell rather than dilate.

Sitting and standing may help labor progress by taking advantage of gravity. Naomi was able to kneel on the bed when she could not stand. Women who are more comfortable lying down should always lie on their left side, although this may be too difficult for some women. Andrea could not lie on her left side because it hurt too much, so she found other positions. Lying on the left side assures that the uterus does not press on major blood vessels and interfere with the oxygen supply to the baby. Side-lying will be more comfortable with the legs bent, the top (right) leg slightly forward, and a pillow between the legs or under the right knee.

Sitting, reclining, and side-lying are especially useful for women with disabilities. Side-lying can exacerbate disability in women with TOS, although Tessa was able to lie on her side during labor. It is important for women who have TOS to make sure that their arms are not tense after a contraction has ended. You may want the doula or your husband to make sure that your arms are not in one position too long; for example, having your arms bent at the elbow. Tina found that her favorite position was standing and leaning on her husband's shoulders.

Women who have difficulty changing positions should consider practicing with attendants or coaches beforehand so that when they are in labor, position changes can be made smoothly during the breaks between contractions. Samantha recalled, "I had my best friend and my husband help me change positions. They helped me to sit up and to turn onto my side." Sharon can usually turn onto her side by herself, but she felt she "needed to be careful because of the epidural catheter that was placed in my back in case I got dysreflexia," so she got help when turning onto her side.

Sometimes having an IV in the arm can make it difficult to change position. Natasha had difficulty because she was hooked up to multiple monitors, and because she was weak. She found a way to move by using the controls on the bed. Sally's husband and the nursing staff used a *rolling board* to help Sally change positions. A rolling board is generally used to transfer a person from one bed to another.

An ordinary hospital bed was helpful for some of the interviewees. Stacy grasped the handrails to help herself turn. A woman can get into a comfortable seated position using the controls of the bed, or move to a reclined position as a first step toward a side-lying position. Nora was able to roll onto her side when she was in the reclining position. She said, "It was useful for getting some of the pressure off my butt." Nora also sat in her chair to get some relief. Some of the interviewees with leg amputations felt that the most comfortable position was reclining with a pillow under the affected leg. Sally found the hospital bed too hard, so she asked for an *egg crate mattress*. They did not have an egg crate mattress, so they gave her a *sheepskin*. (Frequent position changes are needed to avoid skin breakdown.)

Noelle labored sitting in her wheelchair when she had her third child. She explained, "My husband was sick and couldn't help me transfer, so it was easier to just stay in my chair until I went to the delivery room. When they needed to do an exam, I just went over to a bed and somebody propped up my legs."

METHODS FOR RELIEVING SPECIFIC SYMPTOMS

Back Labor or Backache

Whether a woman has back labor caused by the pressure of the fetal head against the spinal nerves or simple muscle pain, the following techniques can be helpful.

The coach can place his thumbs in each of the dimples on either side of the lower back, just above the buttocks, and press firmly and steadily. The laboring woman will indicate whether the pressure is helpful. The only disadvantage of this method is that the coach's hands and arms may get tired. Some women are helped by constant pressure on the lower back, and there are many ways to apply the pressure. The coach can rest her palms on the woman's back and lean gently, or press a sock stuffed with *two tennis balls*, a *rolling pin*, or a *soft drink bottle* against the mother's back. You can also make a compress out of a *sock filled with rice*. You can microwave it so it is warm and put it on the lower back. If you want to make a bigger one, use a towel that is sewn up the sides and fill it with rice. Others like to use a hollow, plastic rolling pin filled with water. Some prefer the relaxing effect of hot water. The coach can also give firm massage, possibly using a vibrator or a bonger. Some women, including women with MS, usually prefer the numbing effect of cold water. One can also buy *cold compresses* at a drugstore to use on the back.

Sometimes a change of position relieves back pain. Renee got on all fours with her knees on a *beanbag* and her head on a *pillow*, so that her buttocks were higher than her head. She said this position "eased the pressure." Priscilla also used a position between kneeling and being on all fours during her first labor. Her knees were supported by a beanbag, and she faced the bed and held onto the rail. She said, "When I got into this position, the baby was sunny-side-up," (meaning the face rather than the back of the head was toward the front of Priscilla's body). "But getting into that position helped the baby turn, and that relieved the back labor." The change of position undoubtedly eased delivery as well. Women who cannot kneel or get on their hands and knees can try lying curled up (lie on the left side, not the right). Either of these positions makes it easy for the coach to apply pressure to the lower back.

Deirdre said, "My back was killing me, and I was moaning even when the contraction had ended. They (the nurses) gave me a *Thera-Band*™ *corset* that was really helpful. I wore it around my belly and my butt."

Dry Mouth or Thirst

Labor breathing is mouth breathing, so the woman in labor may easily get a dry mouth or chapped lips. Use *lip moistener* from the labor kit to soothe chapped lips. Use *breath spray* for a dry, cottony feeling in the mouth, or give the mother a *sour lollipop* or ice chips to suck. It is important to have a lollipop rather than a loose piece of candy, which might cause choking if the mother gasps. Of course, ice chips are great. You can also suck on a *washcloth* by wetting it with water or with ice chips.

Nausea

Nausea is most likely to occur during transition, but some women become nauseated at the end of a long early phase. Ice chips are often helpful. Sylvia said, "The ice chips helped so much they kept a tray nearby so I could get them easily." Noelle found that ice chips helped; having her face wiped with a cool, damp washcloth also felt good. Some women will vomit, so a basin should be kept nearby. Hospital staff will provide one.

Muscle Cramps

Muscle cramps are most likely to occur during transition. Besides massaging the cramped muscle, the coach can try holding and bracing the leg. Bracing is especially useful for the severe cramps and/or spasms some disabled women experience. Cramping may be less likely if range of motion is used throughout labor to help keep muscles loose. Christina had severe leg spasms during transition, and her three coaches took turns helping her. One coach would hold each leg while the third coach rested. Clara's worst spasms occurred during Stage II. They were so strong that her second coach could not hold her leg, but her husband managed by bracing Clara's foot against his chest and using both hands to turn it outward (Figure 11-1).

Noelle found an original way to relieve muscle spasms. She spent part of her time kneeling against a beanbag during one of her labors. She said, "Leaning against the beanbag was comfortable. Then I started having spasms, and my legs jumped with every contraction. We spread a sleeping bag on the floor, and I got down on all fours on the sleeping bag. The pressure on my knees stopped the spasms." Noelle's method might not work for all women, but is worth trying if other methods of relieving spasms do not work.

Hot and Cold Flashes

Flashes are most likely to happen during transition. Cover the woman with a light blanket if she is cold. Sometimes a laboring woman's feet are especially cold, and warm socks can help. Wipe her face and body with a damp washcloth to cool her if she is hot.

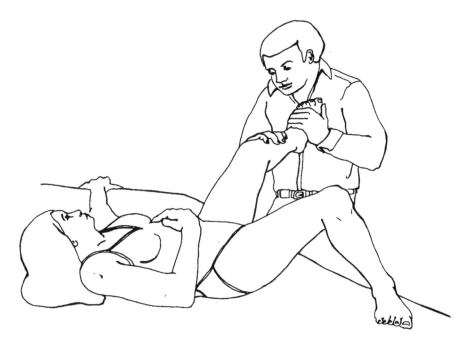

FIGURE 11-1   Birth position in which a leg in spasm is being supported.

Sleepiness

Sleepiness is most likely to happen during transition. For some women the ability to doze may give her the rest she needs. For others, sleeping may cause disorientation. If the women needs sleep, but gets disoriented during labor, it is useful to find a signal or message to help re-center her.

Anxiety

Sometimes a woman expresses her fear directly, but sometimes her inability to follow directions will be a sign that she is feeling afraid or out of control. These feelings are more common during transition. Wait until a contraction ends before attempting to calm her down. Some women are helped by a simple remark such as, "You'll be able to push soon," or, "You're in transition now and you'll feel better soon." It also helps to concentrate on just one contraction at a time. Tell her that breathing will help her feel better, and help her to breathe rhythmically by giving her instructions or breathing with her.

Urge to Push

Often a woman will want to push during transition, but she must avoid pushing until the cervix dilates completely. Holly was told not to push until her doctor arrived. Also, a woman may need to stop pushing briefly during Stage II in order to slow the descent of the baby and give the perineum time to stretch. A woman can avoid pushing by blowing out short puffs of air during contractions. Michelle said, "It was like blowing out a candle." It is impossible to bear down while blowing. (Some readers may want to pause and try it!) Deirdre said, "I needed to be told to push, and also to blow and to look up." If the urge to push becomes irresistible, and the mother stops blowing and starts pushing, the coach can try leaning closely and blowing in her face. Just as breathing in rhythm with the mother helps with deep chest breathing, blowing in her face may remind her to blow. For some women, the coach's closeness is a signal that "I won't leave you alone until you do what you need to do." Clara recalled, "I knew the only way my husband would get out of my space was for me to start blowing."

Pain Relief

A variety of analgesics, anesthetics, tranquilizers, and occasionally sedatives may be used to assist a woman in coping with the discomforts of labor and delivery.

ANALGESICS AND SEDATIVES

Sedatives may be offered to help a woman sleep during a prolonged early phase. Sometimes sedatives help to determine if a woman is experiencing Braxton-Hicks contractions or true early labor. If contractions have stopped by the time she awakens, it is assumed that she had Braxton-Hicks contractions. If contractions continue, and include effacement and dilation of the cervix, then it is hoped that the mother will be refreshed from her rest and better able to cope during the remainder of labor and delivery.

Sometimes tranquilizers are used to increase the effectiveness of analgesics because they lower pain perception as well as induce relaxation or even drowsiness. These may be given intravenously or by injection. Some women find the relaxing effects of these medications helpful. For example, Cheryl, who was given Demerol® (an analgesic) when her cervix was 5 centimeters dilated. She said, "I didn't ask for it, but it was offered because I was having really hard contractions. That one shot helped me get through labor without any more medication. It was really helpful; I almost fell asleep." Other women dislike the drowsiness, and find that it makes coping more difficult. Clara was given first morphine (an analgesic) and then Seconal® (a sedative) in an attempt to help her sleep during protracted labor. She said, "I kept waking up between contractions, completely confused." Tina was given morphine and Phentanyl® to help her sleep but it did not help, except "to take the edge off of the pain." These medications changed Tina's perception in such a way that she made a fist, resulting in a "flare." Sabine had a morphine pump that was not hooked up correctly, so she did not get the painkiller. Sabine said, "They finally fixed it and I got relief." Sierra said, "I was unable to have a spinal because of my spina bifida, so I was given meds that just made me sleepy, but it didn't help with the pain. Also, I needed help to get up."

Other women are helped by the pain-reducing effects of analgesics. Although some women find relaxation and breathing techniques adequate, others do not; for example, Stephanie, who said, "I gave up on the breathing. I needed something else. I also had other pain similar to phantom pain, and the Nisentil® dulled the pain." (Nisentil® is no longer available.)

Each type of pain medication has specific advantages and disadvantages. Sometimes analgesics cause increased restlessness, rather than relaxation. Some women have negative reactions, such as nausea, vomiting, or lowered blood pressure, to specific analgesics. Clara was given morphine to help her sleep, and to determine whether labor had really begun. Instead of sleeping, however, she suffered a long bout of nausea and vomiting. Analgesics are painkillers and usually do not make a person sleepy. If analgesics are administered too early in labor, they may interfere with the development of strong, effective contractions. On the other hand, the newborn may be sleepy and suckling or breathing may be depressed if they are administered too late in labor. Felicia was induced, so she wanted and needed an epidural. She is sensitive to narcotics so she did not take Phenobarbital®.

ANESTHETICS

Unlike analgesics, which alter pain perception, anesthesia blocks all sensation in the affected area, making it completely numb, except that some pressure sensation may remain. Local, regional, or general anesthesia may be used.

Local Anesthesia

The most common local anesthesia is a pudendal block, in which the anesthetic is injected through the vaginal wall into the pudendal nerve, numbing the vagina and perineum. It is useful for blocking out the pain of forceps, episiotomy, and episiotomy repair.

A paracervical block is a procedure that numbs the lower uterus using injections of anesthetic near the cervix. This method of anesthesia effectively reduces uterine discomfort, although it is used less and less because it can easily affect the fetus. Priscilla chose a paracervical block because she was worried about spinal anesthesia. She said, "My leg went numb. It was my good leg. Psychologically it was one of the scariest moments. It lasted 40 minutes and it seemed like an eternity." [This is not supposed to happen with a paracervical.] In a subsequent labor, Priscilla chose to use analgesics in early labor and was much more satisfied.

Regional Anesthesia

This is the most popular type of anesthesia used for labor and delivery. For regional anesthesia, medication is injected into the fluid surrounding the spinal cord (spinal anesthesia) or into the epidural space surrounding the spinal cord (epidural anesthesia). The dura is a membrane surrounding the spinal nerves and cerebrospinal fluid. For spinal anesthesia, a small, hollow needle is used to inject anesthetic through the dura into the cerebrospinal fluid. A needle is inserted into the epidural space for delivery of epidural anesthesia. This is a narrow "potential space," rich in blood vessels, that surrounds the dura. A thin plastic catheter is threaded through the needle, and then used for intermittent or continuous infusions of anesthetic into the epidural space. Regional anesthesia may not block all sensation. Felicia was unaware that anesthesia can be given in various strengths. She said, "I thought that once I was given an epidural I was protected. I did not understand that there was a gradient." Either epidural or spinal anesthesia may be used for surgical delivery (see Chapter 12).

Regional (usually epidural) anesthesia can be used during long or difficult labors to increase the comfort of the mother considerably. Roberta said of her epidural, "It was nice. Then my husband could enjoy my labor." Nadia was given an epidural to keep her comfortable 4 hours after inducing labor. She was able to preserve her strength, and it took only two pushes to deliver her child. Tessa's doula had raised an issue that having an epidural would eliminate the part of her body that was not affected by her disability. Yet, Tessa had no regrets about getting an epidural to help control labor pain.

One woman was at $3\frac{1}{2}$ centimeters for several hours, and then was given pitocin. The epidural was started an hour after the induction. She needed to sit still for the epidural, which turned out to be difficult because she went from $3\frac{1}{2}$ centimeters to 9 centimeters in 20 minutes. She said, "The epidural didn't help with the contractions, but it did help with pushing. I did not feel a lot of pain between 9 centimeters and the birth." A woman who has osteoporosis said, "It was hard to administer the epidural. The most difficult part was getting it in. When they put it in the first time, it didn't go in the right place. So they took it out and put it in again. It was the most painful thing I've ever had to go through." She also commented on the doctor: "He was a jerk. I told him I wanted to sit up during the procedure because it was better for me. He refused. He wanted to put it in while I was lying on my side. He told me to get into these weird positions that were killing my back." In this case, the anesthesia was not put in the right location because she still felt contractions. She said, "My doula helped me a lot with breathing and reminding me to relax. The deep breathing really helped."

Sabine was offered an epidural. She told the doctor, "'I don't want you trying that now.' Even though he knew I had spina bifida and had seen my X-rays, I did not want to risk it because I was told by other doctors I shouldn't have it."

Charlotte had problems getting an epidural, and also with the aftereffects of delivery. During labor, she had muscle spasms in her arm and leg, as well as labor pain. She could not hold still. The doctor tried several times to administer the epidural, and he became impatient. The anesthesiologist wanted Charlotte to sit bent over, which was a more difficult position for her than lying on her side. In the side-lying position, someone could hold her arm and leg to help control the spasms. After delivery, Charlotte's leg "blew up way too much." In addition the swelling of her leg, Charlotte continued to experience muscle spasms, which caused problems with walking. She needed therapy for walking after her delivery. The author asked Dr. Selma Calmes for an explanation as to the cause of the swelling in Charlotte's leg, and Dr. Calmes responded:

"(a) The swollen leg was most likely due to thrombophlebitis related to pregnancy and delivery. This is relatively common due to the effect of hormones and delivery. It is relatively hazardous due to the chance of a pulmonary embolus from the inflamed vein. Her OB physician should have explained the thrombophlebitis to her. There is risk for this in repeat pregnancies, so she should inform her current MD of her history. (b) It is possible to do epidurals with the patient lying on the side, and it seems this would help control her movements. She should mention this to the MD doing the epidural beforehand—that she had problems before, and she'll be more controlled when on her side. That should help the doctor place the epidural. (c) On what could control the spasms, I can't really help out here. I presume she has a doctor who is managing her health, and the doctor should be either aware of this or prescribing meds for her movements. It's difficult in labor, due to the need to avoid drugs that the baby would get. All the sedative meds given to the mother pass the placenta and depress the baby. Also, it may not be possible to control the spasms with medications."

The author has found other women with diplegic CP who have also reported difficulty walking after an epidural. A recent client of TLG was hospitalized for 2 extra weeks after her delivery. She was paralyzed for the first week after delivery; then she recovered fully. She remained hospitalized due to a rise in blood pressure.

Carol also experienced less spasticity after receiving an epidural during her first labor. She experienced a "rubbery leg" feeling, however. This lasted for a year after the birth of her first baby. Carol said, "I went to both a PT and an orthopedist. Neither of them could explain what had happened. Interestingly, the rubbery leg feeling stopped once I stopped nursing." With her second child, Carol had an epidural without ill effect.

Regional anesthesia may cause a drop in blood pressure. Although low blood pressure can be treated in most women, regional anesthesia is usually avoided in cases of placenta previa, severe preeclampsia or eclampsia, or severe fetal distress. Some physicians emphasize that regional anesthesia may benefit the infant by reducing maternal stress and indirectly assuring a good fetal oxygen supply. Others note that regional anesthesia may prolong labor, either by altering the pattern of uterine contractions or by affecting the mother's ability to push. The uterus is innervated by the autonomic nervous, and just as the heart works under anesthesia so will the uterus.

A woman's disability can affect the choice of appropriate pain medication. Although Selina did not have any problems with an epidural during her first three labors, she talked her doctor into not giving her an epidural for her fourth labor. Selina may have had dysreflexia symptoms (uncontrollable shaking). She had a drop of pitocin when she was at 5 centimeters. Without an epidural, it was inevitable that Selina experienced dangerously high blood pressure, which rose when her child was crowning. It did not drop until after the placenta was delivered. Selina was given an epidural as soon as she was admitted to the hospital for her fifth delivery.

Celeste, who had a vaginal delivery, was extremely dissatisfied with spinal anesthesia. She said, "The baby and I were both sick from medication. I had this dopey baby. I had difficulty urinating after having the baby. I decided to go natural with the second one." The small doses of medication used in spinal anesthesia do not make the baby drowsy, but sedatives do. What happened to Celeste is unusual, and her comment raises a second major concern about analgesics and anesthesia: the effect of sedatives on the fetus. Medication that is effective against labor pain can cross the placenta and affect the fetus.

Numerous studies have shown that if dosages are kept to a minimum and carefully timed, medications are unlikely to have a long-term effect on the baby. Still, medications can cause the baby to be sleepy and unresponsive at birth, and may temporarily depress the baby's breathing. Although epidural anesthesia is less likely than spinal anesthesia to cause postpartum headache, it is more difficult to administer and slower to take effect. There may be some leeway in deciding whether to use regional anesthesia, but the choice between spinal and epidural anesthesia depends on the expertise of the anesthesiologist. Regional anesthesia should be used to prevent dysreflexia in women with spinal cord injuries at T-6 or higher. Sally was given an epidural as soon as she arrived at the hospital to deliver her second child. She said, "We decided to do it nice and early." Epidural anesthesia is preferable to spinal anesthesia because it is slower to take effect, and blood pressure changes are monitored and controlled more easily. Although in the past it was thought that women who have progressive neurological disorders, such as MS, were often poor candidates for regional anesthesia, recent studies have found "that epidurals do not increase the risk of relapse or worsening disability in the postpartum period" (20).

Naomi said, "I was mortally afraid of having an epidural. I thought that it would affect my disability, especially if my diagnosis was spinal muscular atrophy. I came across something on the Web that said epidurals could affect the progression of Charcot-Marie-Tooth, which is another diagnosis I might have. I thought the epidural might affect any neuromuscular disease. So my OB had me set up an appointment with the anesthesiologist to discuss alternatives." Naomi was able to avoid all types of medication. In contrast, Natalie, who has a similar disability to Naomi, had an epidural without any negative effects. Natalie was able to walk with help to the bathroom the next morning, even though she had an epidural and a caesarean section.

Although Hannah was able to handle being induced for the first hour, she took an epidural for the rest of the labor. She said, "I've become a convert to using an epidural." Lea Rae was given an epidural that included an *epidural button*. She could press the button to control her own medicine. Lea Rae said, "They give me the same treatment when I have pain from lupus."

Spinal deformities, such as scoliosis, or an inability to flex the spine can make it difficult to administer regional anesthesia. Arthritic changes in the spine, or the enlarged vertebrae sometimes associated with cerebral palsy, also might make it difficult to administer regional anesthesia. Several women with cerebral palsy have contacted Through The Looking Glass to report that they had difficulty walking after an epidural.

As of 2002, the use of regional anesthesia to relieve the pain of labor has been considered the standard of care. Some women with disabilities have had problems with regional anesthesia, however. It might be prudent to talk in advance with one of the anesthesiologists at the hospital where you expect to deliver about the anesthesia that will be used for your delivery. Although it is unknown if an MRI is safe to have during pregnancy, it might be useful to have an MRI to alert the anesthesiologist to any potential problems.

Saddle block refers to anesthesia that numbs only the genital area—meaning the area that would normally be in contact with a riding saddle. The injection is given at the same site used for caesarean anesthesia, but a smaller amount of anesthetic is used. Often the injection will be given while the mother is in a sitting position, but some anesthesiologists prefer to have the mother lie on her side, so they can avoid "puddling" of the anesthetic in the sacral area.

General Anesthesia

General anesthesia was once common during vaginal delivery, and two of the interviewees were given such anesthesia. This type of anesthesia is used only in some caesarean deliveries. General anesthesia will be described in Chapter 12.

NONPHARMACEUTICAL PAIN REDUCTION

Transcutaneous electrical nerve stimulation (TENS) is a method of decreasing pain by electrical interference of nerve impulses to the brain. TENS has been used by physical therapists in treating certain types of muscle pain, especially chronic lower back pain. Many women with cerebral palsy will be familiar with the use of TENS in relieving muscle cramps. Recent studies show that TENS can be useful in controlling the pain associated with labor, especially back pain. A woman with multiple sclerosis wrote about her pregnancy and childbirth in the July 1999 issue of *Disability Pregnancy & Parenthood International* (96). She felt that the TENS unit did not relieve the pain of labor.

The TENS unit consists of electrodes attached to a handheld, battery-operated device. For controlling labor pain, two pairs of electrodes are placed alongside the lower spine. In this placement, TENS stimulation blocks pain in the uterus, cervix, and perineal region. The electrical stimulation creates a moderate tingling sensation. The unit can be operated continuously, or the mother or her coach can turn it on at the beginning of a contraction and off at the end.

The use of TENS does not appear to have side effects for the mother or the infant, although it may affect monitoring devices. Apgar scores of babies whose mothers used a TENS unit are comparable to those of babies whose mothers did not. If there is a possibility that a TENS unit has affected a fetal monitor reading, then *auscultation* (listening with a stethoscope) may be done to check the well being of the baby.

TENS may be useful in combination with other methods, even though its use is not widespread. It is not completely effective in controlling pain. For example, TENS is more helpful for back pain than for lower abdominal muscle pain. TENS has the possible advantage of avoiding or reducing the side effects of medication.

Stage II: Delivery of the Baby

This stage includes "pushing" and the delivery of the baby. Because the uterus is innervated by the autonomic nervous system, the ability to voluntarily "push" is not as important as it was once thought to be. Women with high spinal cord injuries have been able to give birth without voluntarily pushing. The second stage is described by how far the baby has moved down relative to the *ischial spines*, the protruding points on the pelvis. The space between the ischial spines is also called the *pelvic outlet*. It is the opening in the bony ring through which the baby must pass.

When the baby's head is 1 centimeter above the ischial spines, it is at the "-1 station." Level with the spines is the 0 station; 1 centimeter below the spines is the +1 station. At the +3 station, the baby's head is in the vagina. At the +5 station, the baby is *crowning* (the top of the head is emerging), and the baby will soon be born. A woman in Stage II labor may be told that her baby's head is (or is not) engaged; when the baby's head is engaged, the widest part of the head is between the ischial spines.

Stage II can last from less than 20 minutes to 3 hours for women who have had an epidural and are having their first baby. This average represents a great deal of variation, and although some women deliver their babies with just a few pushes, others may need to push for a few hours. Shanna pushed for only 10 minutes with her first delivery. Deirdre could not remember how long she pushed, but thinks it was between 2 and 4 hours. Many hospitals recommend a caesarean section after 3 hours of pushing, because pushing for a lengthy period of time puts stress on the baby.

For many women, the beginning of Stage II is a welcome relief, because instead of having to resist the urge to push, the mother is encouraged to push with each uterine contraction. Patricia said, "It felt so good to push." It is comparable to the relief of finally going to the bathroom after having to hold back. Patricia's frank comment, "It's just like taking a shit," reflected her earthy experience.

Other sensations during Stage II are caused by the stretching of the soft tissues of the cervix, vagina, and perineum as the baby descends. Women feel sensations of stretching or even tearing, or of burning and stinging. Leslie had a laceration of the cervix and uterus. She said, "It felt like I was being torn apart. I have a high pain threshold, and was even able to drive myself to the hospital when I had a ruptured ectopic pregnancy, but this pain was worse." Leslie wondered whether her birthing pain was intensified by her fear that something was wrong with her baby, who was born prematurely. Often, the burning, stretching sensation is strongest when the top of the baby's head begins to stretch the perineum, which is the skin and muscle between the vagina and anus. The woman may need to stop pushing at this point to allow the skin to stretch. Breathing through contractions at this time is often less difficult than during transition.

How a woman feels during Stage II is affected by how long she has been in labor and how long she has to push. Clara contrasted the births of her two children: "The second time, it felt like a torpedo going through me. I wasn't even aware I was pushing. I just knew another entity was coming through. I had to push an hour and a half with my first pregnancy. The doctor yelled at me to push harder when I thought I already was pushing hard enough. I don't remember a physical sensation so much as feeling inadequate." Christina, too, felt the exhaustion that is common for women who have labored more than 12 hours and then have to push for another 15 minutes or more. She remembers thinking, "I can't go on."

Sabine said, "I pushed for about 3 hours until they took me into the operating room (OR). The baby was not coming down. It was so painful. They tried suction when they first moved me to the OR, but that didn't work. Then they got the forceps and the doctor said, 'Now push with all your might. This is going to be the last push or else we will have to take the baby.' The whole nursing room staff was so helpful. They were all cheerleaders, including the neonatal nurses. They were waiting for the baby because I was on a morphine drip for labor pain. I just pushed like crazy and the baby finally came out." The doctors and Sabine both felt that she had difficulty pushing because of her disability. Other interviewees with similar disabilities did not have any problems with pushing. The morphine pump may have contributed to Sabine's problems during Stage II. Another hypothesis regarding her difficulty with the second stage of labor may have been that her uterine muscle may have become overly tired.

On the other hand, delivery should not be any more difficult for a woman with disabilities than it is for an able-bodied woman. Mary said simply, "It was easy; it only took 10 minutes." Paula's doctor, who was worried because he had never had a patient with post-polio syndrome, stayed with her during her entire labor. He told her afterwards, "There wasn't any resistance; it was easier than the average delivery." Tessa had only to push three times before the infant was born. Moira had only four pushes. Her husband held one leg and the nurse held the other one. It took one push to get the head out and three more for the rest of the baby.

Mandy thought that delivering her third child would be difficult because she was told that the medication used to induce labor would make her weak, but she said, "Even though I couldn't push, she was so small that she slipped right out."

Nadia was given IVIG (intravenous immunoglobulin) the day before delivery so she would have enough strength for labor. She was induced a week before her due date. The doctors wanted to start the medications for myasthenia gravis that could not be given while she was pregnant. She said, "I was super weak when they induced. They turned off the pitocin drip after 4 hours of labor. The muscles in my torso were affected, all of my pushing muscles. So they didn't know how much I would be able to push." Nadia never experienced an urge to push with any of her three children.

Some women with spinal dysfunction do not feel pushing contractions as such, but are able to follow instructions to bear down during Stage II. Sharon had no urge to push; her baby crowned after three or four pushes; and then delivery was completed with forceps. She said, "I could have pushed better if I'd been able to use my stomach muscles." Sheila, who was able to push with her second child, said, "I didn't feel different with the pushing, but I did feel the baby slip down."

Both Stacy and Samantha did some pushing, and then their attendants tried pressing on their abdomens in an attempt to make it more effective. *This procedure should never be done, because it can cause uterine rupture or involution (a condition in which the uterus goes inside out).* The uterus works well without this type of assistance because it is innervated by the autonomic nervous system, which is the same system that keeps the heart beating. Pressing on the abdomen can be dangerous, especially if you have hydrocephalus.

Holly said, "My baby got stuck near my tailbone." Her doctor never tried suction or forceps to facilitate her delivery. The nurse on duty pushed down on Holly's abdomen. Holly thinks this procedure caused a malfunctioning of her shunt 6 weeks after delivery. The shunt malfunction came on quickly, and she had it replaced the next day. Her doctor found blood in the shunt during surgery. Blood had never been found in her shunt systems during revision prior to this malfunction.

Flaccid perineal muscles do not resist fetal descent. In some women with spinal cord injury, the abdominal muscles spasm during labor, possibly massaging the uterus and assisting labor. The strength of the stomach muscles is less important to the outcome of labor than the strength of the uterine contractions. Some able-bodied women also have difficulty giving birth, and their difficulties are clearly related to weak or uncoordinated uterine contractions.

Nora said, "I did not think my muscles were strong enough to push out the baby. I did not think I was accomplishing much." Nadia also thought she, too, would have difficulty pushing her baby out. Nadia got encouragement from her OB, who told her how women with spinal cord injuries have been able to deliver vaginally. The vacuum helped a little bit, and then she pushed twice before her baby was born.

One special concern of disabled women at this stage is the transfer from a labor room to a delivery room. Many hospitals permit women to labor and deliver in the same room. If not, it is a good idea to let the woman's regular attendant show hospital staff how she normally transfers. Usually, a woman needs to stop pushing while changing rooms because she will not have the energy to explain how she needs to transfer.

Muscle spasms are also a concern during this stage. Sometimes able-bodied women suffer muscle cramps during Stage II, but women with disabilities may have more cramps, spasm, or clonus. The intensity of these spasms will vary. Sylvia said, "I had some spasm when I was pushing, but so much was happening that I didn't notice it." Sara said, "With the second labor, I wasn't pushing very long when the muscle spasm started. The spasm made it hard to keep my legs open, so they put me out." Two of the interviewees with spinal dysfunction and one with cerebral palsy experienced spasms during Stage II. Naomi did not have muscle spasms, but her foot went numb.

Women may experience intense physical and emotional reactions once the baby is born. Physical reactions such as trembling, uncontrollable shaking, fatigue, or a feeling of intense cold can occur.

Emotional reactions may depend on what is happening. Sharon, whose son had to be taken to an incubator, thought the coldness she felt after delivery was intensified by her loneliness, adding, "My sister wasn't there, and I needed someone to share the experience with." Sasha, who had to wait several hours to see her daughter, said, "I felt robbed. I was a basket case. But it felt so powerful when they finally put her in my arms."

Other interviewees felt excited, relieved, and amazed at their accomplishment. Celeste had been haunted during her first pregnancy by the fear that she would give birth to a dead baby; she simply could not believe that the baby on her chest was really her baby. She was less anxious during her second pregnancy, and when the baby was born, "…bonding started right away. I remember how nice and warm the baby felt." Amanda had to ask the nurse to bring her the baby right after delivery.

If the baby appears healthy and cries vigorously immediately after delivery, the doctor may give the baby to the mother before taking it for basic care. Otherwise, the baby will be examined before it is given to the mother. An Apgar score will assess the baby's condition (Table 11-3). The physical examination will help to determine gestational age and the status of the baby's heath, including whether the baby is premature or postmature. Mucus will be suctioned from the baby's nose and mouth, and it will be wiped clean and wrapped in a blanket. Before the baby leaves the delivery room, it will be given an identification bracelet, blood will be removed from the umbilical cord or heel for

TABLE 11-3
APGAR TEST

	Score		
	0	1	2
Appearance (color)[a]	Blue or pale	Body pink, feet and hands blue	Whole body pink
Pulse (heart rate)	Absent	Less than 100 beats per minute	More than 100 beats per minute
Grimace (response to irritation of sole of foot)	None	Grimaces ("makes a face")	Strong cry
Activity (muscle tone)	Limp	Some movement of limbs	Active movement
Respiration (breathing)	None	Slow, uneven	Good, crying

[a] For babies who are dark-complexioned at birth, the assessment is based on their lips, nail beds, and the soles of their feet.

Note: The Apgar test is a quick examination to assess the newborn's general well-being. It does not diagnose subtle health problems. The test was devised by Dr. Virginia Apgar, and the letters A-P-G-A-R stand for the five factors that are evaluated.

Apgar evaluation is done 1 minute after birth, and repeated 5 minutes after birth. A low score at 1 minute means the baby needs resuscitation. A low score at 5 minutes means the baby has a higher than average risk for health problems in the weeks after birth. A score of 7 to 10 means the baby is normal or only slightly depressed. A score of 4 to 6 means the infant is moderately depressed. A score of 0 to 3 indicates severe depression, and the infant will need resuscitation. The great majority of babies score 7 to 10.

testing, the stump of the umbilical cord will be clamped and bandaged, and in many states, medication will be put in the baby's eyes to help prevent the risk of blindness from infection by vaginal bacteria.

Holding the baby can be difficult for some disabled women, not only because they may be tired or shaking, but also they may feel insecure on the narrow delivery table. They may feel fearful of dropping the baby because of poor hand control. A little help from the father or nursing staff can assure that the first moments after birth are joyous.

Procedures for Stage II

Methods for coping during Stage II consist of finding a comfortable position and using appropriate breathing techniques.

FINDING A COMFORTABLE POSITION

Sitting with the back supported, squatting, and getting on the hands and knees can all be useful during this stage. Sometimes a woman will be encouraged to sit on a toilet to push. This method is useful when the baby gets stuck at the +2 station, which can happen when the baby's head is large in comparison to the pelvic opening. Women can seat on a nursing chair or use extra bars to help squat. Also, pushing out a baby feels much like having a bowel movement, and sitting on the toilet often makes pushing feel more familiar and comfortable.

Once the baby is at the +3 station (head in the vagina), a woman can try any of several positions while she pushes the baby to +5 (crowning), and then gives birth. She may try squatting, lying on her side with her upper leg in the air, sitting partially reclined with her back at a 45° angle and her legs supported by stirrups or held out to the side, seated in a birthing chair, or lying on her back on a delivery table with her legs raised, spread, and supported by stirrups. Nora could not use the stirrups, so someone held one of her legs; she had pillows under the other leg. Deirdre did not feel she could push in the side position. Her coaches were prepared to lift her leg and put it in another position. They also did range of motion before they put her foot into the stirrup. Some women lie on the delivery table while resting between contractions, then sit up with the coach's help while pushing.

There are advantages and disadvantages to using a delivery table. Some women feel restricted by the stirrups, others appreciate the help in keeping their legs supported and separated. Women may not be taken to the delivery table until the baby is crowning, because lying on the back is not a good position for laboring. Moving is difficult at this point, especially for women with mobility problems. Some hospitals have modified delivery tables with moveable handles. When the woman pushes, she presses down on the handles, partially sitting up. Pushing in this way may be more effective. Other hospitals provide birthing chairs, which offer the advantages of sitting up during labor and supporting the woman comfortably with her legs well spread. Delivery tables and birthing chairs are more comfortable for birth attendants than the ordinary beds available at home births and alternative birthing centers. When a woman is laboring or pushing in an ordinary bed, her attendants are likely to get backaches or sore knees from bending or kneeling, although they may be more comfortable if they sit on the bed with her.

A woman's disability will influence her choice of position. Squatting is not feasible for many disabled women. Some will be unable to balance; others need to avoid the stress on their joints. Using a birthing chair creates a position similar to a squat. Sitting on a toilet also has many of the advantages of squatting. Deirdre was able to squat by holding onto the Rollator™. Amanda thought that she might need a stirrup, but she did not use one because her hip is so rigid. She said, "I couldn't tell if my leg was up in the air." Someone held Allison's knee during her first labor so she could push. She kept her prosthesis on during her second labor, because "I wanted to press into something so I could push." For many disabled women, side-lying or partially reclined positions work well. Other women need help holding up their legs.

During Hannah's second delivery, the doctor recommended lying on her left side. She said, "It was a great accommodation to my disability. I could hold up my right leg on my own." Naomi put her top leg on someone's shoulder. She also tried kneeling with her legs far apart. Simi also delivered on her side, but she had her top leg resting in a stirrup. Sheila wanted someone to hold up her leg because it was more comfortable. Christina used a delivery table, but could not use the stirrups because she cannot bend her knees. Instead, two nurses helped by each holding one of her legs out to the side. Tessa was unable to hold up her legs, so she had the nurses bring them up and hold them in position. Sharon used the stirrups part of the time and had her legs held by the nurses part of the time. Other women found the delivery table and stirrups helpful, or even comfortable. Women who experienced leg spasms from using stirrups during prenatal examinations probably should avoid using them during labor. Try having friends support your back by holding you up or by sitting behind you.

Samantha gave birth at home. She sat more comfortably when her husband was behind her and she could lean on him for support. She held her thighs and someone else supported her lower legs. Celeste chose a side-lying position because she has difficulty spreading her legs. A nurse held up her top leg while she lay on her side and the delivery went well (Figure 11-2).

BREATHING TECHNIQUES

Two kinds of breathing may be used during Stage II: the *Valsalva maneuver* and gentle pushing. These two methods *begin* in the same way: First, breathe in deeply through the nose; then breathe out through the mouth. Next, breathe in through the nose and hold your breath. For the Valsalva maneuver, continue to hold your breath while bearing down. You will feel your throat close, enabling you to create maximum pressure on the uterus.

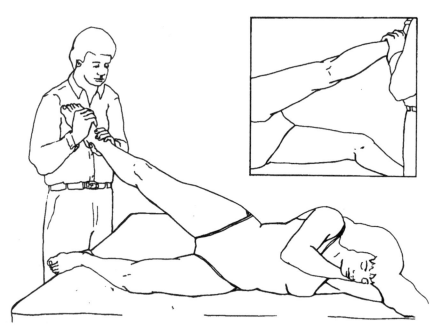

FIGURE 11-2 Side-lying birth position for women who cannot use stirrups or spread their legs wide enough for birth.

Women who have a shunt need to be aware of the potential problems of protracted Valsalva (closed glottal pushing) breathing, because it will increase intracranial pressure.

For gentle pushing, slowly let out a little air as you bear down. The sensation of letting out just a little air is like talking while holding your breath. Try quietly saying "eeeeeee" as you bear down. You will feel pressure in your throat as you push out the sound.

Some birth professionals favor gentle pushing because they worry that doing the Valsalva maneuver may increase the rise in blood pressure that occurs during contractions; others do not believe there is a problem. A woman may practice one type of pushing in birthing class, and then be shown another by her labor nurse. She may prefer the method the nurse shows her. If not, her coach can tell hospital staff, "She's comfortable with the way she's pushing now because that's the way she practiced in birthing class."

Sometimes it is necessary to stop pushing during Stage II. If a woman can avoid pushing during a few contractions, her perineum can stretch more slowly and she may be able to avoid an episiotomy. Or, if the umbilical cord has wrapped around the baby's neck, the mother may need to stop pushing while the doctor or midwife slips the loop of cord over the baby's head, or suctions mucus from the baby's mouth and nose. If the mother needs to stop pushing, she can "blow through" the contraction in the same way she did during transition. For some women, contractions will come close together. For others, there will be time to rest between contractions. Deep chest breathing may be used while resting.

Forceps Delivery and Vacuum Extraction

A doctor can assist birth by gently pulling the baby from the vaginal canal with forceps or a vacuum extractor. It is more common for suction to be used than forceps. The literature states that forceps or vacuum suction should not be used at mid-pelvic deliveries. The committees on obstetric practice believe that practitioners should be appropriately trained and familiar with the contraindications (97). A vacuum extractor is essentially a cup attached to a suction device that is placed over the baby's scalp.

There are several types of forceps. In general design, all of them are like a pair of tongs with curved, blunt blades. The inside of the curved blade is designed to fit the side of the fetal head, while the outside curve fits the contours of the mother's body. An episiotomy may be done before forceps are used, and local or regional anesthesia may be administered. The blades of the forceps are put in place one at a time, locked together, and then a gentle pulling motion is used to assist the baby's birth. "High" forceps procedures, in which the fetal head has not reached the pelvic floor, have been replaced by surgical delivery, which is much safer for both mother and baby. In "low" forceps procedures (also called *outlet forceps*) the fetal head is visible at the vaginal opening.

Forceps or vacuum extraction may be used if it appears that the uterine contractions are not strong enough to expel the baby. Shortening the second stage of labor in this way may prevent maternal exhaustion or fetal distress. Forceps or vacuum extraction may also help to prevent injuries to the fetus or mother when the perineum is unyielding, and episiotomy alone does not assist birth.

There are some advantages to using forceps and vacuum extractors. Some types of forceps may be used to alter the position of the fetal head, whereas the extractor can only be used for pulling. Although Nicole's babies were big, she was able to deliver all of them vaginally. Forceps were used in two of her three births.

The vacuum extractor is less likely to cause pain or injury to the mother. Each instrument may cause characteristic types of fetal injury—the most common and most minor are facial bruises from forceps and scalp bruises from the extractor. The doctor must carefully weigh the risks of using these instruments against the risks of allowing labor to continue. Risks can be limited by skillful use. Vacuum extraction has replaced the use of forceps in hospitals.

Felicia's baby was crowning, but she pushed for an hour with no luck. The baby was in the birth canal where the uterus was finished doing its job, so extra help was needed. Suction was used to deliver the baby. Unfortunately, Felicia's perineum was ripped. She said, "I wish they had done an episiotomy to reduce the risk of tear."

EPISIOTOMY

This procedure is not routinely performed anymore, except in rare circumstances. An *episiotomy* is an incision (cut) in the perineum, the skin and muscle between the vagina and the anus. The perineum needs to stretch to allow the baby to emerge from the mother's body. Often a midwife or doctor tells the mother to stop pushing and blow through a few contractions so that the baby's head will press on the perineum more gently, allowing more time for it to stretch. The birth attendant may help the perineum stretch by massaging it between contractions. If it appears that the perineum cannot stretch sufficiently, and if it is likely to tear instead, the doctor will perform an episiotomy. An episiotomy may also be done to speed up delivery if the fetus seems distressed, or to prepare for the use of forceps. One advantage of doing an episiotomy is that it may shorten the second stage of labor.

The disadvantage of an episiotomy is that the vaginal area will hurt much more during the weeks following birth than it would have if there had not been a cut or tear. Nikki said, "The episiotomy was the worst, because I was sitting on the cut all the time." Walking, sitting, urination, or bowel movements may be quite uncomfortable. The episiotomy may also itch or become infected.

Clara recalls that she wanted an episiotomy during childbirth. "When I had my second baby, the labor was fast and intense; it felt like a train going through me. I remember my husband started to tell the doctor that 'we were hoping to avoid an episiotomy,' and I said, 'Never mind that! Just get this baby out!'" Later, Clara felt some regret because the incision was sore, and walking and getting in and out of the bathtub were difficult.

If no anesthesia was given before the episiotomy became necessary, the procedure is done at a time when pressure numbs the perineum, or after a local anesthetic is injected. Medication will be injected before the episiotomy is repaired if it was made without anesthesia.

Stage III: Delivery of the Placenta

This stage is brief and mild for most women. New mothers are encouraged to stimulate Stage III contractions to expel the placenta by nursing their newborns, but sometimes the extra stimulation makes the contractions more painful. These contractions tend to be stronger after a second birth than after a first.

Stage III generally follows closely after Stage II. The placenta may slip out, or the mother may be told to give a few more pushes. Contractions sometimes stop just after birth. Although the placenta usually separates within 35 minutes after birth, up to 60 minutes may be allowed for its expulsion. The amount of time allowed depends on the mother's condition—especially on the amount of uterine bleeding. If the placenta is not delivered promptly, or part of the placenta is retained in the uterus, some intervention may be necessary. Only minor intervention is likely to be necessary if the placenta has separated from the uterine wall. This may include hand pressure on the fundus (the top of the uterus).

STAGE III MEDICATION

Pitocin or other medications may also be used after the placenta is delivered, because stimulating contractions can help to reduce bleeding at the site where the placenta was attached.

Stage IV: Postpartum

Stage IV is generally uneventful. Contractions continue during this stage in order to begin the process of restoring the uterus to its pre-pregnant size and shape. Some of these contractions may be uncomfortable, but usually they are not as painful as the contractions of labor and delivery.

If the woman had an episiotomy or tear, it will be repaired at this time. If the woman did not have anesthesia during labor, the doctor will inject a local anesthetic before starting the repair. Women who are paralyzed, but have some sensation, may want to remind the doctor to give them an injection. Stacy's obstetrician assumed that she had no perineal sensation because she was paralyzed. Stacy said, "Boy, those stitches hurt."

The mother will be encouraged to urinate at least once within a few hours after giving birth. If she gave birth in a birth center with an early release program, she must urinate before she goes home. If the bladder or urethra were irritated or injured during labor and urination is difficult, this problem must be diagnosed and treated. Tessa's disability is hidden, and the nurses did not understand her special need. Feeling had not yet fully returned in her legs, when the nurses asked Tessa to put her arms around them so they could support her while she walked to the bathroom. This was both difficult and painful. Tessa wished she had used a wheelchair to get to the bathroom or used a bedpan.

After delivery, Moira went to the recovery room, where she was given an I.V.I.G. infusion for 3 hours. She said, "They had it ready ahead of time. They put the IV in me and put the baby in the bassinette. My husband and the nurses took care of the baby while I was getting infused."

Closing Comments

Supportive medical staff and good communication are vital if the mother is to have a satisfying childbirth experience. Positive attitudes are important. Sylvia contrasted the "reassurance" of nurses who were experienced with disability with the "curiosity" of those who were not. Celeste recalled that when she gave birth, "There were a lot of people around because they hadn't seen a disabled woman deliver. They were expecting a difficult delivery. Also, they didn't know what to expect when I delivered in a side-lying position."

Although some women might be oblivious to such onlookers, others are disturbed. Some of the interviewees felt that a nurse's inexperience with disability is less important than a supportive attitude. Leslie recalled that, "I was more scared when my nurse was frightened and unsure of what to do when my blood pressure went up." Women with disabilities also worry that they will be over-treated. It is important for a disabled mother to understand the reasons for everything that happens. Noelle felt that she had a surgical delivery "because my doctor was freaked out by my disability." She was able to deliver vaginally with her subsequent pregnancies.

Having a birth plan can help. Nora had one nurse who stayed with her 25 hours. Deirdre said, "The staff was surprised that we brought in our own adaptations, but when they read my labor plan, which included my diagnosis, they understood."

An expectant mother can take steps to ensure that she will have good relationships with staff during childbirth. She can meet medical staff before she goes into labor so she will feel comfortable with them. She can work with her physician to make sure hospital staff has adequate information about her special needs. Lastly, she can bring a coach or advocate with her to the hospital who is prepared to provide information about her disability.

Another Way into the World: Caesarean Section

GIVING BIRTH BY CAESAREAN is not always necessary for women with disabilities, but it is quite common. Fifty-two of the interviewees had a caesarean birth (36 percent). This percentage has not really changed from the first edition of this book, in which it was stated that 39 percent of the interviewees had a caesarean. Research has shown that women with spinal cord injury are more likely to have a caesarean section.

About 22 percent of all babies are delivered by caesarean in the United States, making caesarean the most common major surgery in the country. The caesarean rate, while down from a peak of 25 percent of births 15 years ago, remains four times higher than it was in 1970. The U.S. Public Health Service and the World Health Organization say that the rate should be reduced to 15 percent.

The pros and cons of each individual case must be sorted out in order to decide whether a caesarean delivery is appropriate. The mother who has a caesarean may have a more difficult time during recovery. For example, a caesarean delivery can make it difficult for you to take care of your baby. This is particularly true if you have a bad back and have to depend on your stomach muscles. Movement will then be more difficult while the muscles heal from the surgery. On the positive side, there are the undesirable effects of allowing a problem pregnancy or a difficult labor to continue. There may be reasons to believe the caesarean birth will be safer for the baby. Concern for protecting the welfare of the mother and the baby is very important in some situations. For example, in the case of Oprah, "the doctors did not know if my pelvis would break. There was also a chance that the babies would have osteogenesis imperfecta (OI) and would be born with broken bones."

The special concerns of disabled women need to be examined carefully. It is important to compare the physical effects of the caesarean to the physical effects of labor on the mother. It is also important to compare the effects of labor on the baby to the effects of caesarean on the baby.

It is important for some disabled women to be assured that their disabilities did not weigh too heavily in the decision to perform a caesarean. Some of Noelle's disappointment that her first child was delivered by caesarean section stemmed from her belief that her doctor overreacted to her disability. In fact, she was able to deliver vaginally in subsequent pregnancies. The prospective mother is entitled to a clear explanation of the reasons for surgery, whether it was planned or unplanned. The explanation must differentiate between obstetric indications (pregnancy-related reasons, which might also apply to an able-bodied woman) and disability indications (reasons based directly or indirectly on disability). Sabine had switched her doctors, and her new doctors felt that it was important for her to avoid more surgery. On the other hand, her original doctor wanted her to have a caesarean. Sabine said, "He thought it was safer for some unknown reason."

For women who have shunts, a cesarean section may increase the risk of intraabdominal infection and adhesion formation around the distal end of the catheter. It is yet unclear on the best type of delivery because of the risk of intra-abdominal infection.

Mona thought it was important to ask about the amount of pain she might experience after a caesarean section, as well as the possible difficulties in changing position and transferring.

POSSIBLE FALSE ASSUMPTIONS

Some doctors seem to forget that the uterus is innervated by the autonomic nervous system. This means that muscles are not needed for pushing the baby out. Nancy and her doctor agreed that it might be hard for her to cope with the stresses of labor, considering her breathing difficulties and muscle weakness. Nancy also worried that her baby might be injured if her disability caused a prolonged labor. Yet, having a caesarean section is surgery, and may result in a long recovery. Moreover, general anesthesia can affect the lungs, impacting respiration. Many women have long labors that do not adversely affect their babies. An article based on two case studies showed that one woman who had a disability similar to Nancy was able to deliver vaginally (29). This article also stated that if the woman has a pelvis that may have been distorted because of her disability, the distortion will "determine the mode of delivery." Nina's doctors expected her to deliver vaginally, until tests determined that the baby was too big.

In the first edition of this book, it was stated that women whose disorders are exacerbated by fatigue face a difficult choice when labor is prolonged; for example, women with SLE or MS. Either the fatigue that follows protracted labor, or the fatigue associated with surgical recovery, could contribute to a flare-up of symptoms. The author now believes that this contains some elements of false thinking, because a caesarean is surgery and has its own complications. It may be true that women with certain disabilities will need to have a break during a long labor, but having medication may give them that break instead of a caesarean surgery.

Nadine Fiona, who has the limb-girdle form of muscular dystrophy, had a doctor who thought a caesarean section was appropriate because he thought she could not push. Natasha has the same disability as Nadine, but was able to delivery vaginally.

Sonya was given a caesarean section because her doctor believed that her Baclofen Pump™ required it. The author was referred to Dr. Richard Penn, a neurosurgeon at the University of Chicago, by the company that manufactures the pump. Dr. Penn believes there is no contraindication for a vaginal birth in women who have a Baclofen Pump™. The pump is used to control muscle spasms. Sonya has a high spinal cord injury, and her dysreflexia would have to be controlled during labor. The author asked Dr. Penn about the use of regional anesthesia, and Dr. Penn stated that there should be no problem using regional anesthesia to control dysreflexia during labor. He also said, "It does not matter whether the anesthesia is given either above or below the level of the catheter" (98).

Joan and Joy both have artificial hips, and their doctors did not want to risk possible dislocation of their hips during vaginal birth. Joan did not want to risk the dislocation of her hips during labor. LeAnn also had two hip replacements, and was encouraged to deliver vaginally; her hips did not dislocate. Questions were posed by the author to several artificial hip manufacturers asking whether women with hip replacement should or should not have a vaginal birth. None of these manufacturers were able to give any recommendations.

Sherry Adele preferred a caesarean section because she felt a vaginal birth "would put more stress and strain on her pelvic floor muscles and ligaments, which were already weak." This area may be stretched over three times as much as normal during a vaginal birth. A woman may experience stretching or tearing around the vaginal area, particularly the tissue that support her urethra and bladder neck. Incontinence may result if the urethra and bladder neck are not supported. In 1996, a British study confirmed that a vaginal birth can cause incontinence, but also that pregnancy can cause these same problems. During pregnancy, the hormones and/or the weight of the fetus (which puts extra pressure on the pelvic floor) can cause incontinence. These factors cause the pelvic floor to be relaxed, which, in turn, causes incontinence. This explains why women who have had a caesarean section also experience incontinence. The author concludes, therefore, that vaginal delivery is associated with weakening of pelvic organ support. This effect is greatest in deliveries using forceps. The observations from epidemiologic studies confirm that caesarean delivery has a protective effect against pelvic organ prolapse and incontinence later in life. All measurements showed significant increases in pelvic organ mobility between the third trimester and postpartum visits. These changes were not significantly related to length of gestation, history of induced labor, or duration of the first stage of labor (99).

"In women with OI who have normal pelvic dimensions, there does not appear to be a compelling reason to avoid labor or vaginal delivery" (8).

Disability indirectly leads to caesarean surgery for some women. For example, Sybil had a caesarean because her bladder had been removed before she was pregnant, and her doctor was concerned that the remaining scar tissue might cause problems during labor.

Sometimes surgery is scheduled because there is concern that a pregnancy complication will exacerbate the disability or cause a permanent medical problem if the pregnancy is allowed to continue. For example, Dawn had always had urinary problems, and when she developed a kidney infection, there was serious concern that she could be permanently affected.

Although women with disabilities are more likely than others to have caesarean sections, the decision for any woman, in any category of disability, will depend on individual circumstances. Although Sienna was overdue by a week, her doctor did not try to induce labor, but rather gave her a caesarean section. Her doctor may have been predisposed in his thinking that surgery is easier than a vaginal birth.

Women with SLE often have difficult pregnancies, and miscarriages are frequent. Laura's surgery was probably an indirect result of her disability. Blood tests showed that her placenta was not functioning, possibly because her disease was causing rejection of the placenta. Leslie also had many disability-related complications, but needed surgery for an obstetric reason: the fetus was in the transverse presentation.

Disability Indications for Caesarean Birth

As shown in Table 12-1, there is a broad range of reasons for which women with disabilities might need surgical delivery. For some women, disability leads to surgery in a direct way. Women with osteogenesis imperfecta have caesareans because everyone feels that labor and delivery can cause the pelvis to develop fractures and should therefore be avoided. Moreover, having a caesarean when your child can also have OI will prevent the baby's bones from breaking.

Caitlin was told that since her spasticity affected her vagina, it would also affect the cervix, and she needed a caesarean. She felt this was true because she had problems with sexual intimacy, and needed to use Milex Dilatators™ to be able to have sexual intercourse. Caitlin's obstetrician consulted a perinatologist, who felt that her spasticity would prevent the cervix from dilating. In fact, the perinatologist thought that labor would cause the cervix to become tighter. The author consulted with another obstetrician, who felt that the idea of the cervix becoming tighter was theoretical, and that Caitlin could have started labor to see what would happen. This is often referred to as "trial labor" or "trial of labor."

Although you may need a caesarean section, for whatever reason, you can always ask your doctor to wait until you go into labor before the surgery is performed. Of course, caesarean could then be considered if things do not go well.

All of the women with dwarfism who were interviewed for this book had caesareans. One reason Dorothy had an early caesarean was her difficulty with breathing. Darlene's doctors had another reason for doing a caesarean section. They could not determine if Darlene's pelvis was large enough for the baby to fit through. Darlene had not had an X-ray of her pelvis prior to her pregnancy, and had a scheduled caesarean. Although her baby was healthy, Darlene questions whether her baby might have been bigger and his lungs more developed if she had waited until she went into labor. Another disability that would require a caesarean section is when a woman with myasthenia gravis is having a crisis.

Although it is impossible to generalize about the effects of caesarean surgery on disabled women, it is clear that surgical delivery will not necessarily be safer or easier for the mother than vaginal delivery. It is important to remember the strong possibility that recovery from surgery may be more difficult for a woman with disabilities. Both the emotional and the physical aspects of surgical recovery can pose a challenge.

Obstetric Indiations for Caesarean Birth

The following sections discuss specific indications for caesarean delivery.

FETOPELVIC DISPROPORTION

This condition is responsible for a large percentage of caesarean deliveries. In women with fetopelvic disproportion, the fetus cannot pass through the birth canal, either because it is unusually large (*macrosomia*), or because the mother's pelvis is too small (*pelvic contraction*) or abnormally shaped.

Both macrosomia and pelvic contraction can be difficult to diagnose even with ultrasound examination. Usually, the diagnosis cannot be made until there has been a trial of labor. More frequent diagnosis of fetopelvic disproportion has contributed to the general increase in the caesarean birth rate.

Spine and hip deformities can also lead to disproportion. Some of the interviewees who had caesareans said that fetopelvic disproportion was the cause. Others mentioned spine or hip deformities, including Arlene (lordosis); Pam (scoliosis); Heather Ann, Amy, Andrea, and Hilary (small, misshapen pelvis); and Julie (spinal curvature). Julie also needed a caesarean because of arthritis in her hips, which prevented her from spreading her legs wide enough for delivery. Portia and Stephanie simply stated that their babies were too big. They did not mention any relationship to disability.

PLACENTA PREVIA

This condition is present when the placenta is lower in the uterus than the fetus, thus blocking the opening of the cervix. It may be discovered during an ultrasound examination following painless bleeding during labor. If such bleeding occurs, ultrasound examination is necessary because an internal pelvic examination could cause serious bleeding. When a large portion of the placenta covers the cervix, it will tear away from the uterine wall as the cervix dilates. The mother will then be in danger of bleeding to death, and the fetus may suffer brain damage or death from lack of oxygen.

ABRUPTIO PLACENTAE

Abruptio placentae, or placental abruption, refers to a separation of the placenta from the uterine wall before birth. Signs include bleeding and pain, in contrast to the painless bleeding of placenta previa. The dangers are the same as with placenta previa. Some women with certain disabilities may be at risk for placenta abruption. Noreen had an emergency caesarean because of this condition. She said, "After my water bag broke, the doctors realized the baby had *bradycardia* (slow heart rate). I didn't experience any pain, but I had trouble breathing."

CORD PROLAPSE IN EARLY LABOR

If part of the umbilical cord protrudes through the cervix, the cord will be compressed each time a contraction drives the fetal head against the cervix. The pressure on the cord will interfere with fetal blood circulation.

FETAL POSITION OR PRESENTATION

Some positions and presentations are always indications for surgery; for example, *transverse presentations* (fetus is sideways), or *breech* (feet first). The increasing use of caesarean surgery for breech presentations has contributed to the overall increase in the rate of caesarean births. Techniques for vaginal breech delivery can be difficult, and infants can be injured. Signey was given several reasons for having a caesarean section; some were because her disability and some were for other reasons. She said, "The neurosurgeon who originally treated me when I was first injured recommended a caesarean section because I have a *syrinx*. This is a fluid-filled cavity that is either in or beside my spinal cord. The added pressure from labor can worsen this condition. My obstetrician felt she would be better able to control the blood loss with this twin pregnancy. As it turned out, both of my twins were breech."

PREVIOUS CAESAREAN SURGERY

A large proportion of caesarean deliveries are repeat surgeries. The old rule, "Once a C-section, always a C-section," is no longer true, however. This issue will be explored later in this chapter (see "Vaginal Birth After Caesarean Section").

INSUFFICIENT CONTRACTIONS

Weak or uncoordinated contractions lead to a prolonged or arrested labor, and may be an indication for a caesarean delivery.

Preeclampsia/Eclampsia

Emergency surgery usually prevents or reduces eclampsia, which can endanger the lives of both mother and fetus.

Postmature Fetus

If pregnancy continues past the due date, tests will be performed to make sure that the placenta is functioning properly. Labor may be induced if the placenta is aging, and the fetus could suffer malnutrition or other problems. Caesarean surgery will be necessary if inducing labor is not safe.

Fetal Distress

This usually occurs when an inadequate placenta does not supply the fetus with enough oxygen. Distress may also be caused by mechanical difficulties, such as placental abruption or a short umbilical cord. It may be possible to relieve fetal distress by having the mother change position, or by giving her oxygen and/or fluids. An emergency caesarean may be needed if signs of distress persist. As the rate of caesarean deliveries has increased, the percentage of surgeries performed after a diagnosis of fetal distress has also risen. Often, infants delivered in these circumstances seemed completely healthy, with good Apgar scores. These facts raise the question as to whether fetal distress is often wrongly diagnosed. Some critics argue that increased use of fetal monitoring has led to mistaken diagnoses of fetal distress, indirectly causing many unnecessary surgeries. The relationship between use of fetal monitors and surgery rates is not a simple one. For example, results can be affected by the amount of experience hospital staff has with fetal monitors, the use of fetal monitoring in high-risk cases, and other factors. Also, the healthy appearance of a newborn may not mean that a diagnosis of distress was necessarily incorrect.

Maternal Immunization (Rh Disease)

If the mother has Rh negative blood and the fetus is Rh positive, the mother may develop antibodies that can destroy fetal blood cells. A caesarean may be performed immediately if fetal illness is diagnosed. In addition, if the mother does not get a RhoGAM shot after delivery, she may develop antibodies that can affect her next pregnancy.

Genital Herpes

The increased incidence of genital herpes has contributed to the overall increase in caesarean deliveries. If the mother has an active herpes infection during labor, there is a high risk that the infant will become infected during a vaginal birth. The risk to the baby is very high if it is the mother's first herpes infection. Most parents choose caesarean delivery because herpes infections are very dangerous to babies, often causing blindness and other serious problems.

Some books about childbirth suggest that tests for herpes infection be performed after the thirty-sixth week of pregnancy. The usual practice, however, is to watch for *active lesions* at the time of labor.

SOME MATERNAL ILLNESSES

Illnesses such as severe kidney problems and some types of diabetes may indicate the need for caesarean delivery.

What Happens During Caesarean Birth

PREPARATION

Whether caesarean birth is planned or unplanned, the preparations for surgery are essentially the same. Preparations for a planned surgery simply proceed at a slower pace.

For a planned surgery, the mother is admitted to the hospital in advance of the scheduled time, usually the same day. Blood and urine tests will be done while she is in her hospital room. The anesthesiologist will visit her to ask questions about her medical history, explain what will happen during anesthesia, and describe the possible side effects of anesthesia.

If the caesarean surgery is unplanned, blood tests will be done when the mother is admitted to the hospital, whether she is in labor or has troublesome symptoms such as pain or bleeding. The anesthesiologist will talk with her in the labor room or the operating room. The conversation will be brief if there is an emergency. The anesthesiologist might not know the woman's special needs because they have just met. Andrea needed to have support under her stump to even out her hips. She said, "The doctors and nurses did not have much empathy for my situation."

Andrea had to lie flat while she was on the operating room table waiting for the anesthesiologist. She said, "Having to lie flat made me feel as though my stump would split open at the seam (suture line). I had to beg them to release my leg so I could bend my knee to take the pressure off my stump. The doctor was angry that I wasn't prepared to get anesthetized."

Other preparations include washing the mother's abdomen and upper thighs, applying an antiseptic to these areas, and covering the areas around her abdomen with sterile drapes. The antiseptic may feel cold if it is applied before anesthetics are given. An intravenous (IV) line and a urinary catheter will be put in place. The catheter is a thin rubber tube that is put into the urethra to drain urine from the bladder. It may be put in after the anesthesia is started. Women who have general anesthesia will be given an endotracheal tube after they are unconscious; the tube will keep the throat from becoming obstructed, assuring proper breathing.

ANESTHESIA

Hopefully you will have met the anesthesiologist before delivery. The anesthesiologist may ask for information that is already in the medical records, but it is important to answer carefully, so that she can make sure she has the correct information. Julie had a rare allergic reaction to the anesthesia when she had her child. Somehow, she never mentioned this to a general surgeon years later. Fortunately, the anesthesiologist assisting this surgeon had also assisted Julie's obstetrician. He recognized Julie because her reaction to the medication was so unusual that he had never forgotten her. If the anesthesiologist had not known Julie, she might have been given the same anesthesia, and her reaction might have been stronger than the first time, possibly fatal.

Signey felt that shaking uncontrollably during the surgery was the result of the medication. She said, "I think they put morphine into the catheter. I had an incredibly itchy face for 24 hours or so after delivery." Itching is a side effect of morphine, but it is probably not an allergic reaction.

An important piece of information the anesthesiologist will need is any possible disability interaction with general anesthesia. For example, women who have juvenile arthritis may be at risk for subluxation of the neck because the ligaments get eroded at the C-1 and C-2 vertebrae, causing the neck to become unstable. Moreover, if the neck is hyperextended, there is a possibility that the head of the second vertebrae may press into the spinal cord causing quadriplegia.

Sienna's anesthesiologist had a difficult time administering her regional anesthesia. He tried at least three times before a second more experienced anesthesiologist was able to insert the needle in the right place. Sienna said, "The first anesthesiologist must have touched a nerve that went down my left leg, because each time he stuck me shooting pains went down that leg. The second anesthetist said the difficulty was due to scarring in the area and my inability to sufficiently round or arch my back." If the anesthesiologist is given either an X-ray or a MRI of your spine, you can probably avoid this problem. (It is unclear whether it is safe to have a MRI during pregnancy.) Sophia Amelia had a consult with the anesthesiologist during her second pregnancy, but both she and the anesthesiologist lacked important information. She said, "I have clusters of nerve endings that never went where they were supposed to, so I'm hypersensitive in certain places. This is why the spinal didn't take."

Joy was lucky that she did not have any problem with her spinal. It would have been safer to consult an anesthesiologist, because her arthritis could have impacted her spine. Naomi found information on the Web stating that epidurals might have negative effects on the progression of Charcot-Marie-Tooth. There can be misinformation on the Web, however, so it is important to talk with an anesthesiologist early on. Although Nadine Fiona does not have Charcot-Marie-Tooth, she had a similar reaction to the anesthesia.

She was given an epidural that did not work. She said, "The sensations were duller, but I could still feel." She was then given a spinal. They brought her into the delivery room, and she felt as though she could not breathe. She was hooked up to monitors, which said she was fine. Nadine Fiona, however, felt as though she was going to die. She said, "It was the scariest thing. I couldn't catch my breath; I couldn't talk; and I couldn't move my arms." She was given oxygen. The doctors told her everything was normal, including her blood pressure.

Either regional or general anesthesia will be used. Regional anesthesia can be "epidural" or "spinal" anesthesia. Obstetric anesthesia involves the baby as well as the mother, because the baby receives the anesthetics through the mother's blood. Since the late 1950s or early 1960s, it has been well documented that regional anesthesia (part of the body is numb; patient is not asleep) is safest for both mother and baby. Regional anesthesia for obstetrics is usually an epidural, which is done with local anesthesia, and with perhaps a small dose of narcotic added. A tiny catheter is placed in the *epidural space* of the lower back. This space is situated on or outside the *dura mater*, which is the material that surrounds the spinal cord. The medication can be given continuously. When to start the epidural varies somewhat throughout the country. Most obstetricians want labor to be well established before starting an epidural. The epidural can be used for both labor pain and for a caesarean if one becomes necessary. It can also be used for post-delivery pain. The use of epidural anesthesia for obstetrics is well established in the United States and is extremely safe.

Spinal anesthesia is often a good choice for a caesarean delivery if an epidural is not already in place. General anesthesia is only rarely used for caesareans or other obstetric surgical procedures because of its effect on the baby.

J. Carstoniu and colleagues wrote about the use of epidural anesthesia with a person with achondroplastic dwarfism (16). They stated, "The potential risk imposed by the spinal abnormalities and lack of clinical experience have probably deterred anesthetists from using spinal anesthesia." The article also stated, "There were no serious complications in the single case of a person with achondroplastic dwarfism having caesarean section under spinal anesthesia. The record indicated that the lumbar puncture was performed with difficulty and the patient became hypotensive following the block."

All of the interviewees with dwarfism had caesarean sections, but only half of them had epidurals. Not only did Darlene do research in finding an anesthesiologist, but the anesthesiologist also did research. Nevertheless, Darlene said, "They did not know the amount of anesthesia to use. I was getting close to feeling sick to my stomach."

Arianna said, "I did not want an epidural because I did not trust them one bit. I had a lot of problems with them (doctors and the hospital). They overdosed me on magnesium sulfate once during my pregnancy. That medication goes by body weight. They gave me way too much for my body weight, so I didn't trust them." In general, regional anesthesia is safer than general anesthesia. General anesthesia was probably a more comfortable option for Arianna because she had already experienced it.

Regional anesthesia can lower the blood pressure, and must be avoided in some situations. Epidural anesthesia may be preferable because it takes effect more slowly. Then, if the blood pressure goes down, the change is more gradual and controllable. Sydney had an epidural during her labor. She said, "Once they cranked up the medication in the epidural and added a narcotic to it during the actual C-section, I had a negative reaction. I got a splitting headache and the chills. I felt fine as soon as they cut it off. The hospital had something like a hair dryer that my husband used to pump in hot air under the blankets."

One disadvantage of spinal anesthesia is that some women may suffer "spinal headache," which lasts from several hours to several days after the birth. A more correct term is *post-dural puncture headache*, because the same headache may occur if an epidural needle accidentally punctures the dura. Sheila commented, "The headache was so bad that I refused the spinal for my second labor. I felt great after the second delivery. I was ready for anything. I used cold compresses and toughed it out." Laura's headache lasted 3 months. (Having a 3-month headache could have been caused by her disability rather than the anesthesia.) Dorothy is prone to migraine headaches, and experienced a migraine right after being prepped. There are treatments available for these types of headaches, but the headache from a spinal is usually improved by the third day and gone by the fifth.

Women with shunts need to be careful with regard to the use of epidural anesthesia. The placement of an epidural block should be accomplished with extreme care so as not to breech the dura, potentially contaminating the cerebrospinal fluid space and altering differential pressure.

Sherry Adele said, "I insisted on being awake. I had a spinal, but it took awhile to administer. It wasn't the easiest thing for the anesthesiologist. I saw him ahead of time and told him what I wanted." Chloe said, "They tried to do an epidural, but they couldn't get the needle in because my spine is fused." Orielle's anesthesiologist knew her from past surgeries. She said, "I liked him. He usually did not do C-sections, but he did do most of the OI patients. I was the first patient he ever had who had OI and was pregnant. He tried a spinal, but my back was too curved. They could only get one side of me numb, so they ended up knocking me out. I wanted someone who knew about OI."

For some women with Charcot-Marie-Tooth "distortion of maternal chest and lumbar spine increases the risk of malformation and makes epidural anesthesia more difficult" (24).

Diane had a regional anesthesia for each of her caesarean sections. She preferred to be given regional anesthesia in "the fetal position" rather than sitting bent over. She found it difficult to breathe in the sitting position, and it was hard for her to maintain that position.

The main advantage to regional anesthesia is that the mother is awake to see her baby's birth. She and the baby are less likely to feel groggy, and they may be able to spend more time together immediately after the birth.

General anesthesia uses a combination of medications that relax the muscles, block out pain, and make the woman sleepy. Some medications are given intravenously; others are gasses that are breathed in through a special mask.

General anesthesia can be administered quickly, and it takes effect quickly. It may be necessary in emergencies, or for some women whose disabilities prevent the use of regional anesthesia. Heather Ann's unusual experience led to emergency use of general anesthesia. She explained, "I had an epidural, and I was fine while they made the incision, but just as they took the baby out, it suddenly wore off. I was only numb from the knees down. The pain was terrible; it was a ripping feeling, like I was being torn in two. They had to put me out so they could finish." This occurred during Heather Ann's second delivery. Her experience during her first delivery had been quite different: "I was numb and there was no feeling, just a little pressure and a stretching sensation when they lifted the baby out."

Andrea had problems with regional anesthesia because her lumbar spine vertebras are "squished together," and the anesthesiologist had to go higher than he wanted. She said, "The result was that I was numb at my belly button and I could feel my stump. So I was numb where they were cutting. Then it wore off before they were finished with the surgery." General anesthesia may be the only option for some women.

General anesthesia has three main disadvantages. It is more likely to affect the baby, and there is some risk that the mother will vomit and breathe in food or stomach acid, resulting in pneumonia. To balance these disadvantages, surgery is performed as quickly as possible to minimize the baby's exposure to anesthesia, and emergency equipment is available to help the mother or infant if necessary. Still, there is no way to get around the third main disadvantage—the mother will not be awake for the birth of her baby.

THE SURGERY

Andrea had to transfer onto the operating table by herself, which was quite difficult. They also had her scoot on the table in the way that is the most difficult for her: by leading with her stump.

Caesarean delivery usually takes less than an hour. In many hospitals, a woman who has regional anesthesia may be joined by her husband and/or her labor coach after preparations for surgery are completed. They will be wearing sterile caps, masks, and gowns like those worn by the medical team.

She may be surprised to find that the operating table is somewhat tilted to the left; this tilted position helps maintain good blood pressure. The anesthetic will make her numb up to about the level of her nipples. She may not be able to feel her own breathing. Some women who have had caesarean surgery suggest that a woman who experiences this can say aloud, "I can't feel my breathing." A support person or the sound of her own voice will let her know: "If you're talking, you're breathing."

A screen will be placed above the abdomen to help keep the surgical area sterile, and to keep the parents from seeing the incision as it is being made. Once the cord is cut the doctor lifts the baby high enough for the parents to see. The baby's appearance may be a little startling. It helps to remember that vaginally-born babies can also have some blood smears, and that all newborns look bluish for a few seconds before they start breathing.

The anesthetic will block out any pain from the incision, but many women feel some discomfort from pulling or pressure when the baby is delivered. Heather recalled feeling "a little pressure and a stretching sensation" during her first caesarean delivery, but Leslie "couldn't feel a thing when they lifted the baby out." Dorothy said, "Although there wasn't any pain, it felt like strong pulling." The change in uterine pressure after the baby is born might make the mother feel dizzy or nauseous. Breathing oxygen through a mask can help with the dizziness.

After the baby is delivered, separate teams will care for mother and baby at the same time. It may be possible to watch as mucus is suctioned from the baby's nose and mouth, the umbilical cord is cut and clamped, and the baby is washed, dried, and wrapped in a warm blanket.

After the baby is removed from the uterus, amniotic fluid will be suctioned out. Any noise the suction equipment makes is nothing to worry about. The placenta will then be removed manually, and the doctor will examine the uterus and ovaries. Sterilization can be done at this time if the mother has requested it.

The most time-consuming part of the surgery begins next. The surgeon carefully sutures (stitches) the uterus, abdominal muscles, and skin, layer by layer, matching the edges of the incisions as closely as possible. The bladder, which was moved out of its normal position for the delivery, is also put back into place, and the incisions around it are stitched. The top layer of skin will be closed with self-dissolving stitches or metal clips, and covered with a gauze bandage. A new type of stitching is now available called "liquid stitches." According to an article in *USA Weekend* (59), "They are easier to use, do not hurt, and do not have to be removed because the adhesive disappears as the wound heals. Studies show Dermabond™ also is 99 percent effective in blocking infection."

CAESAREAN INCISIONS

Many women are concerned about the effect of caesarean delivery on their appearance. They may prefer a *bikini cut*, in which the skin incision and the resulting scar are in a horizontal line that is located where the pubic hair begins. The alternative is a *vertical incision* from just below the navel to just above the pubic hair. The vertical skin incision can overlie more than one type of uterine incision.

By far, the most common uterine incision is the *low transverse* incision, a horizontal incision in the lower portion of the uterus. (At times, a low vertical incision is made.) This type of surgery has real advantages, including less blood loss and better healing. The incisions are less likely to become infected, and fewer adhesions are likely to form. Also, a woman has a better chance of giving birth vaginally in later pregnancies, because there is less risk that the resulting scar on the uterus will separate during pregnancy or labor.

Sarah Pedersen's article describes one amputee in this way: "The brim of her socket rode very close to the incision site" (11). Therefore, she recommends that any above-knee amputee who needs a caesarean have the incision made a little higher.

Another type of incision is known as the *classical incision* because it was the most widely used type in the past. This incision on the uterus is a vertical cut at the midline that is higher than the low transverse incision. The classical incision can be made more quickly, which might be an advantage in some emergencies. In some cases, it is also the safer choice. For example, with some malpresentations, a low transverse incision may be too small for delivering the baby. In some cases of placenta previa, there is a risk that a low incision will start placental bleeding. The disadvantages of a classical incision are the possibility of more bleeding and a higher risk that the scar on the uterus will rupture during later pregnancies. Orielle's baby had OI. It was also in the transverse position, and a horizontal incision was used instead of a vertical incision. She said, "They opened me hip to hip because they knew he had OI. They wanted to lift him out carefully, so they opened me clear across." I had a huge incision.

Recovery

EARLY RECOVERY

The mother will spend the first few hours after surgery in the recovery room—until the effects of the anesthesia have worn off. Nurses will frequently check her breathing, pulse, temperature, and blood pressure. They will also check her incision and watch for excessive vaginal bleeding. The catheter will stay in place, and the nurses will measure urine output by checking the level of urine in the bag and replacing full bags. They will also feel her abdomen to make sure her uterus is beginning to *involute*. The uterus continues to contract after childbirth. These contractions begin the process of returning the uterus to its pre-pregnant size, a process called "involution." Postnatal contractions also help to stop bleeding at the site where the placenta was attached.

The IV line will stay in place, and the IV solution may include oxytocic, a synthetic hormone that stimulates contractions of the uterus. The surgical incisions will become painful as the anesthetic wears off, and the continuing uterine contractions might make the pain more intense. The oxytocic medication may be discontinued if these contractions become too painful.

The nurses will administer pain medications as the anesthesia wears off. Women who become nauseous from pain medication should tell the nurses, so they can be given additional medication for nausea. Report any sign of nausea immediately. It is important to prevent vomiting. Although Joan was in a lot of pain, she did not "want to take anything stronger than Motrin™." She said, "I needed to be alert for the baby. I wasn't going to be out of it because they had rooming in." There is a new method of pain relief without grogginess called ON-Q™. "It sends a local painkiller to the site of an incision. Unlike systemic narcotics and other pain relievers that can interfere with breast-feeding and bonding after a baby is delivered by caesarean section, ON-Q™ keeps the mom clear-headed, yet pain free. No dangerous drugs can get into the mother's milk, because ON-Q™

delivers the medicine right where the pain is, instead of circulating the drug through the whole body" (59).

Women who have had regional anesthesia will be watched for return of sensation and motion; the nurses may ask them to wiggle their toes, or to indicate whether they can feel a touch on their legs. These signs of returning sensation and motion cannot be used to verify that a spinal-cord-injured woman is recovering from anesthesia. Instead, the muscle tone and reflexes below the level of injury should have been evaluated during her pregnancy, and the anesthesiologist or nurse should watch for the return of the mother's usual spasticity and reflexes during recovery. As sensation returns to numb areas there may be a tingling feeling similar to the feeling in a foot that "wakes up" after it has been "asleep." Women who have had spinal anesthesia may be instructed to lie flat on their backs so they will be less likely to develop headaches. If lying flat is difficult, as it was for Heather, a woman can ask for a pillow for support, or she can ask the anesthesiologist for permission to lie on her side, if she did not already done so before surgery.

Some women also develop "spinal headaches," which are extremely uncomfortable. Laura described hers as "the worst headache I ever had." Drinking plenty of fluids will help, because the ultimate solution to the problem is replacement of the spinal fluid that has leaked out through the puncture. Until the headaches stop, the best way to relieve them is to lie down. Unfortunately, it is not possible to lie down all the time. Pain medications also help. Most spinal headaches disappear after a few days. Using a smaller needle can minimize the possibility of a headache. This may be overlooked if an epidural is used, because the epidural can go in farther.

Natasha had been told that she could be paralyzed longer than the expected time for women without muscular dystrophy. She said, "Luckily it wore off in a few hours instead of days." Denise had an endotracheal ("trach") tube down her throat during her second caesarean surgery. She said, "I had some kind of an allergic reaction to the trach tube; my throat swelled up and I had difficulty breathing. They gave me some medication that calmed this down. I also had a lot of pain. I couldn't even cry or say anything. My husband saw my tears, and was able to say, 'she doesn't normally react to things like that,' so they came over and gave me morphine."

Women who have had general anesthesia will feel confused when they awake, almost as if they are dreaming. All our interviewees used the word "groggy." Arlene said, "I was groggy. I could hear and remember what was said. They told me I gave birth to a girl. My mouth wasn't working and I couldn't respond." Often, a woman has only sketchy memories of what happened while she was recovering from general anesthesia. Nancy, who had given birth at ten o'clock in the morning, said she remembered being told that the baby was a girl, but she remembered almost nothing else that happened that day.

If the mother had regional anesthesia, her husband or friend can probably be with her in the recovery room. Sometimes she can have her baby with her, too. This depends on hospital policy and the baby's condition. The baby may need special care if it was premature or distressed, or depressed by anesthetics.

Even women who are not expecting a caesarean delivery might prefer to plan ahead for the possible separation of mother and baby. For example, should the partner be with the mother or the baby? Some couples feel that it is most important for the mother to have companionship, while others feel it is more important for the partner to be holding and cuddling the baby. When the mother has had general anesthesia, the partner cannot see her until she is conscious, but may be able to spend time with the baby. Later, any disappointment the mother feels about the separation from her baby may be eased by knowing that the partner and baby were together. Hilary liked knowing the details of what happened: "My husband bonded with her while I was still asleep. The hospital staff had him sit in a rocking chair so he could rock her." Noelle's husband tape-recorded their baby's cry while she was still unconscious. After she woke up, she still had to wait to see the baby, but she said, "Hearing the tape lessened my sadness a little."

The mother may be too tired or weak to hold the baby, even when the family can stay together. The father or partner, or a friend can hold the baby so that the mother can see it, or help her support the baby on her chest. Sybil, who could not hold her baby by herself until the third day after the birth, recalled, "I was very grateful to the nurse who helped me hold my baby."

THE HOSPITAL STAY

Women who have given birth surgically experience many of the same physical changes as those who give birth vaginally. Changes that all women experience, such as lactation, are discussed in Chapter 13. Here, we concentrate on recovery from the physical and emotional effects of caesarean surgery.

The progress women make during their first few days in the hospital can seem amazing. A woman who has just left the recovery room often needs to be lifted from the gurney to her bed. She still has her IV and catheter in place, and even deep breathing is painful. It seems hard to believe that in just a few days she will be eating, using the bathroom, and walking independently.

Some women may need to go to the ICU. Noreen, for example, was sent to the ICU because of severe weakness caused by myasthenia gravis.

Pain and discomfort are the most intense on the first day, and gradually decrease during the next few days. Amy said, "The first night I couldn't sit up and did not have any strength." Joan said, "I couldn't sit up by myself because my stomach muscles were cut. I had a hard time holding myself in an upright position for the first few days."

Not all women react to pain in the same way. Dawn recalled, "I found it difficult to move. The painkiller only helped a little. I only got painkiller four times a day; I wish it had been prescribed for me to take as needed." Arianna said, "I couldn't even move. It hurt to have somebody move me. They wanted me to get up the next day and I couldn't. Moving in the bed was enough movement for me. I experienced a lot more pain when they had to move me. They wanted me up, which meant they (the nurses) had to lift me into the wheelchair. When they picked me up, it felt like my stomach was being ripped open. I needed to feel totally stabilized so nothing was hanging; like my legs would hang, and that would pull on my stomach." It is important to talk to the nursing staff ahead of time in order to plan on the type of transfers you might need. Arianna said that after the first week it got a lot better. Hilary, on the other hand, did not want help moving from her gurney, and used her arms to maneuver into bed. Hilary said, "I didn't want any pain medications. I already felt too groggy from the anesthesia."

Most women are somewhere between the extremes that Hilary and Dawn represent. They find pain medications helpful, particularly in situations that intensify pain. For example, Pam commented, "The painkiller also helped with contractions." Some women may find that pain medications make them dizzy or nauseous. Women who are breast-feeding feel concerned that the medications will enter their milk and affect their babies. Noelle said, "It was hard to balance the pain medicine and nursing. I took it after nursing so she wouldn't be taking enough drugs to affect her." Women who are planning to breast-feed need to talk with their doctors about their concerns.

Women who simply feel more comfortable with less medication, like Hilary, can always tell their nurses they do not want any. It is also important to tell nurses when pain medication is not helping, because unusually severe pain can be a sign of problems. The first sign of an infection in Nancy's incision was persistent pain that was not relieved by medication.

Many women find that the same relaxation techniques that are useful during labor help them cope with surgical pain. Their nurses can also assist in maintaining comfort. One of the most useful ways is to gently but firmly press both hands and a pillow against the lower abdomen when moving, coughing, or walking. The support and pressure from the pillow will counteract the painful pulling on the incision. Dorothy said, "The nurses would come in once a day and push on my stomach right below the belly button. That was the most painful part." She felt that her "insides were falling out." Joan concurred: "I swear to God, the worst pain I ever experienced in my entire life—arthritis and all, everything—nothing has ever been worse than when they pushed on my uterus." Natalie said, "I couldn't lay my baby on my stomach. It just killed me. I could only hold him for a few minutes because it was hard to breathe. I wanted to hold him a lot, but I could only hold my baby high up on my chest."

Sometimes the pressure of the pillow against the abdomen may lessen the feeling that "things are going to fall out." It is helpful to find more than one comfortable position for resting, although changing positions can be painful. Many women find that it is most comfortable to lie on their sides, with their backs well supported by pillows, and a pillow between their slightly bent legs. This position can also be comfortable for breast-feeding. Sometimes a woman may need help with breast-feeding. Amy was unable to sit up because her stomach muscles were cut, so she needed help with breast-feeding and positioning. She said, "They just handed me the baby, but I couldn't do anything."

Nancy commented that some of her worst pain was caused by other people moving her because they had no way of knowing which movements jostled or pulled on her incision. Hilary was thinking of the same problem when she decided to move from the gurney by herself. She said, "It wasn't easy, but it was worth it. I knew it would hurt a lot more if other people tried to move me."

The muscles that are cut for a caesarean are the same muscles that Natasha uses for everything. She said, "It was already hard to get up, and then when I had to strain and pull on that incision and staples, it was that much worse. My husband had to pick me up off the toilet."

Here are some ways to avoid or reduce pain when others are going to help you:

❖ If you are planning a surgical birth, arrange to visit the maternity floor ahead of time. Discuss your needs with the nursing staff. Perhaps you or your attendant can show them ways of lifting and transferring.

❖ Even if you are not planning a surgical birth, try to arrange ahead of time to have your spouse, attendant, or a friend who has cared for you available to help in the hospital. Your friend may be able to give the nurse or nurses some tips, demonstrate ways of helping you, or help when the nurse is delayed in coming to your room.

❖ Try "talking through" a move step by step; tell the nurses what works best for you at home. Give feedback about what is most comfortable. This feedback encourages your nurse to offer reassurance. You may need to be reminded, "Don't worry, you can't really split open. You have several layers of stitches."

❖ Use assistive devices. The controls on hospital beds can be very helpful. Hilary said, "I couldn't use my prostheses, but I rigged up an assistive device in the hospital." She explained, "It's hard for people to help me walk because I'm so short. I walked to the bathroom by myself an hour and a half after I got to my room." Even if you use crutches rather than leaning on another person, have someone with you during your first few attempts to walk in case you get dizzy or lose your balance. One interviewee said, "The toilet seat wasn't high enough. I told them that I would not be able to get up. I have a hard time as it is. Although the doctor ordered a raised toilet seat, the nurses still had a hard time getting me up."

❖ Try to arrange to exercise when you are most comfortable; for example, about half an hour after pain medication is injected.

Whether you move on your own or with help, movement, deep breathing, and coughing will increase pain, but *they must not be avoided*. Breathing exercises help prevent pneumonia, which can be a complication of abdominal surgery. Exercise and walking maintain circulation, and help prevent pneumonia and the formation of blood clots in the leg veins. Although breathing and other exercises are painful at first, they do speed recovery. Breathing exercises are so important that women may even be encouraged to get started while they are still in the recovery room.

A good exercise to begin just a few hours after surgery is simply taking the deepest breath possible and holding it briefly. This is also a way to begin gently reconditioning the abdominal muscles. Later, begin coughing gently. There is no need to wait for the nurses to encourage this exercise, although they will. Nancy was taken to the ICU because she has breathing difficulties. The nurses in the ICU encouraged her to start coughing as soon as she arrived. Hospital staff may provide an assistive exercise device when coughing and breathing grow deeper. This device is made from clear plastic; blowing through a flexible tube moves a part inside that indicates how well you are breathing.

Whole body exercises can also begin while you are in bed. Gently stretch your limbs, tense and relax one limb at a time, and carefully roll to one side and back. Later, begin to exercise your lower abdominal muscles by pulling your heels toward your body, as if to put your feet flat on the bed with your knees making a "tent" under the covers. As the days go by, your feet can be brought closer and closer to your body. Most women walk at least once by the end of the first day after their surgery.

For women with disabilities, of course, the exercise may be different, and their experiences may even be different with each birth. Nancy was ready to use her wheelchair on the first day, but Arlene's nurses waited until the second day. Arlene commented, "It felt as though things were going to fall out. I had never had abdominal surgery before." Heather said, "It took me a whole day to get my balance back after my first baby. All I could do on the first day was sit on the edge of the bed. With my second delivery, I got up on my crutches the same day I delivered." Julie said, "My whole body was sore because of my dystonic reaction to the anesthetic, even my jaw. They got me up anyway. Within the first 24 hours they lifted me onto a rolling shower bench so I could take a shower. A nurse made me walk to the bathroom the next day. I remember how cruel I thought she was. I was in a lot of pain and running a high fever. But later I learned from my aunt, who is a nurse, how important it was for me to get up and start moving."

Nadine was up and walking 4 hours after delivery because they expected her to get up the same as everyone else. Nadine was upset because the nurses did not understand her special needs. She said, "When they brought the baby in, they would leave him across the room. I told them, 'Hey, you can't expect me to get out of bed and pick him up. You have to bring him to me. I can't even roll side to side.' They would ask if I wanted to keep him at night. All I could do was to give him a bottle. I needed a family member to help me because the nurses did not do anything."

Gradually, the walks last a little longer; the first few walks are only as far as the bathroom, then into the hallway, then farther. Each woman learns to find the right balance— just enough exercise to increase her strength, but not so much that she gets exhausted.

Although none of the interviewees mentioned problems with blood clots in their legs, it is possible that using a wheelchair will not be sufficient exercise for some women. Women who cannot walk may need to have their doctors prescribe passive exercise or special stockings.

Most women have a urinary catheter in place for the first 24 hours after surgery. Hilary was an exception. She explained: "My first doctor did not use catheters. Near the end of the operation, after he had the bladder in place, he pressed it gently so all the urine ran out. Later, I didn't have any problem going to the bathroom. I never did like catheters, so when I had my second baby and got the on-call doctor, I told him I wanted to go without one. He said we could try, but if I had any problems I'd have to have a catheter. I never needed it."

Some women, like Hilary, dislike having a urinary catheter. Noelle felt that her catheter caused the stress incontinence that bothered her after her baby was born. Pam said, "I couldn't wait until they took the catheter out." The catheter should not cause any discomfort, but it can get in the way of walking. Most women need a urinary catheter because their bladders do not function well after the trauma of surgery. Also, even if a woman is able to empty her bladder shortly after surgery, she may not be ready to walk to the bathroom. Getting up and down from the toilet or on and off a bedpan will be painful. The catheter will be removed after about 24 hours, although it may be reinserted if it is still difficult for the woman to empty her bladder.

The IV line also remains in place for about 24 hours, which may bother some women. Pam complained, "The IV made it hard to move my arms." Other women are annoyed because the IV gets in the way when they are walking or holding their babies. If the IV is in a woman's "good" arm, she can ask to have it moved to her other arm. A nurse should be told if the IV is painful, because there may be an infection or the needle may have moved out of place. IVs are necessary because after abdominal surgery the intestines stop functioning for about a day. During that time, most women cannot eat or drink, and must receive fluids, nutrients, and some medications by IV. Some women may be permitted to sip liquids on the same day as surgery.

Near the end of the first day, your nurse or doctor will occasionally put a stethoscope against your abdomen to listen for bowel sounds. You will be asked whether you have passed any gas. These are signs that the intestines are functioning again. Orielle said, "The worst pain was the air in my stomach from the C-section." The IV will be removed when your digestion is functioning again, and you will be allowed to sip clear liquids such as apple juice, broth, and gelatin. If clear liquids do not cause vomiting, the next meal may include full liquids like milk and custard. At the same time, some pain injections and other medications will be replaced by oral medications. Some women eat solid foods by the second day, others by the third. Most women welcome solid foods. They are starting to feel hungry, plus eating "real food" helps them to feel that they are truly recovering. It is still important to drink plenty of liquids, because fluids replace the blood lost in surgery, provide for milk production, and help prevent constipation.

As the digestive system begins returning to normal, many women have problems with gas pain and/or constipation. Mild exercise gives some relief from gas pain; some women find it helpful to sit in a rocking chair and rock gently. Lying on the side, slightly curled up, may be the most comfortable. Labor breathing and relaxation techniques help many women cope with gas pain and painful bowel movements. It also helps to press a pillow against the abdomen during a bowel movement. Many doctors routinely prescribe stool softeners, but if stools are still hard and dry after the first one or two bowel movements, ask a nurse for a stool softener.

If the skin was closed with metal staples, they will be removed by the doctor on the second or third day. There will be little or no discomfort when the staples are removed. Many women see their incisions for the first time when the stitches are removed. There may be some dry blood caked around the stitches, but these superficial scabs will fall off soon. Bruises around the incision will disappear in a few weeks, like any other bruise. The incision will look red and "angry," and the sight of it may be upsetting, but it can help to remember that the scar will eventually fade to a thin, white line like any other scar from a clean cut.

RECOVERY AT HOME

Leaving the Hospital

Sometimes you might not be ready to leave when the 3 days are up. Under the Newborn Federal Act of 1996, you can stay as long as 96 hours if you have had a caesarean section. Diane said she knew from previous surgeries that she would need a longer hospital stay, so she told the doctors what she needed and she was able to extend her stay.

A mother who has given birth by caesarean will have a complete physical examination before she is sent home. There should be no signs of infection in her lungs, uterus, bladder, or incision. Often, this last examination is done the day before she leaves the hospital. This last examination is a good time to bring up questions. Here are some issues you might want to discuss with your doctor:

❖ Ask the doctor about any symptoms that have been bothering you. Ask what is usually expected during recovery.

❖ Ask about any aspect of the surgery that continues to trouble you.

❖ Ask the doctor to explain any prescriptions, including why the prescription is necessary, how long to continue taking the medication, and what side effects to expect. Sometimes a doctor will order a partial prescription from the hospital pharmacy that can be refilled later at a less expensive pharmacy. If your prescription is not what you expected, call your doctor's office and find out whether it needs to be changed or refilled.

❖ Discuss whether you will need physical therapy or additional attendant care. Get a written prescription if necessary. You may not be given the prescription until you leave the hospital.

❖ Ask the doctor if there are any special instructions, such as restrictions on activity or watching for danger signs. Ask when you can resume any restricted activities.

❖ Find out when you should schedule your first follow-up visit to the doctor.

There will be quite a few details to take care of before leaving the hospital, including packing the possessions of the mother and the baby, doing the final paperwork, collecting prescriptions and doctor's instructions, and getting the baby from the nursery. The nurse will take the mother and baby to the hospital exit in a wheelchair.

Home Care

It is important for the mother to take good care of herself once she gets home. Certainly the same is true for any new mother, but remember that a caesarean mother is a new mother who is also recovering from surgery. Joan said, "The first few weeks after I got home, I needed help going from sitting to lying and vice versa because of my stomach muscles." It is especially important for new mothers to balance infant care and mild exercise with plenty of rest. Darlene planned ahead by telling people what she would need at home after a caesarean section. In addition, she also asked the doctor how long her recovery would take. She said, "I asked my friends for support. They cooked meals ahead of time." She also went to an acupuncturist, who helped her recover.

Nadine's right leg and foot were totally swollen. The doctor told her to keep her leg elevated, which she did. The swelling lasted 3 days. It took Nadine a month to recover. She was able to go out a little at a time during the last 2 weeks of the month.

Many doctors suggest some type of restriction on the mother's activity, at least until the follow-up office visit. For example, your doctor may advise you not to drive, not to lift heavy objects, not to climb stairs too often, or to avoid bending and lifting. It is important to follow this advice, because the mother who pushes herself too hard will suffer more pain and fatigue in the long run. Different people find different ways to follow this advice. For example, people who live in a two-story house might put an ice chest and hot plate for snacks in the bedroom, or set the mother up on the guest bed in the living room. If you have a low, old-fashioned cradle ready for the baby, you might borrow a friend's bassinet to use downstairs.

There is still a chance that uterine bleeding or infection will occur, although this possibility becomes smaller with each passing day. Watch for these warning signs:

❖ *Increased lower abdominal pain*

❖ *Pain, swelling, or oozing in the area of the incision.* Women who do not have sensation in this area should ask their attendants to inspect the incision when bathing them. Remember that the lower abdominal muscles and the incision are still uncomfortable. Muscles can get sore from too much work. The incision will hurt more if you bump into a piece of furniture or a toddler jumps into your lap. Remember, too, that the uterus contracts occasionally for a few weeks after the birth. These contractions are sometimes stimulated by breast-feeding. You should watch for unexplained or persistent pain, or increased discomfort.

❖ *Change in vaginal bleeding.* All women have a discharge that is called *lochia* for several weeks after giving birth. If the amount of discharge increases or the color darkens, you should report the change to your doctor.

❖ *Fever.* If you feel hot and feverish, take your temperature. If it is higher than 100.4°F, call the doctor or, if you do not have a regular doctor, call an emergency room. Women who have a temperature that is usually lower than the normal 98.6°F should call their doctors if their temperature goes higher than what is normal for them.

Some women develop bladder or urinary tract infections even after they leave the hospital. Any of these signs of bladder infection justifies a call to the doctor:

❖ Fever.
❖ Frequent or increased urination (urinating more frequently than at the time of discharge from the hospital).
❖ Often feeling the urge to urinate, then being unable to pass urine or only passing a few drops.
❖ Painful burning when urinating.

The incision should gradually become less sore and tender during the first few weeks after surgery. Wearing loose, airy clothes, with elastic at waist level (not hip level) will be more comfortable. Do not use tampons without your doctor's permission. Occasionally the incision will itch, sometimes intensely, but some itching now and then is a sign of healing. After 4 to 6 weeks have passed, the area around the incision will no longer be sore, but it may be slightly numb. The numbness may last many months.

Drinking plenty of fluids continues to be important, especially if you are breast-feeding. Fluids are important for the same reasons given above: replacing blood lost during surgery, making up for fluids lost in milk production, and constipation. A well-balanced diet also contributes to recovery. Complicated cooking will be too much of a challenge—just remember to eat simple, nutritious foods and to snack on fruits and vegetables instead of junk food. Eating plenty of fruits and vegetables also helps to prevent constipation, which is important because straining in the bathroom will continue to be uncomfortable.

Mobility will be affected because the abdominal muscles have been stretched by pregnancy and then injured by surgery. Other muscles, particularly the muscles of the lower back, may become sore from the strain of doing the work usually done by the abdominal muscles. Rest is good for any sore muscles, including abdominal muscles. Women with physical disabilities may need to work with an occupational or physical therapist to find alternate ways of moving, transferring, and doing household tasks. Some women may need to use a wheelchair or crutches temporarily. Sophia Amelia could not transfer for a month after the birth of her second baby. She could only bear weight on one leg, and experienced shooting pain in her leg from the spinal. Darlene experienced numbness in some part of her scar. She went to an acupuncturist to help with the numbness.

Gentle abdominal exercising can help speed recovery as your strength and mobility improve. Your doctor can help you decide when it is safe to begin.

Emotional Effects of Caesarean Birth

Women respond to caesarean birth with a variety of emotions, and the same woman may feel different emotions at different times. At one moment, she may be excited because she has given birth; at another moment, frustrated by her helplessness; and at still another moment, depressed by pain and fatigue. Sienna said, "I was having a rough time recovering from the numbness as well as having a great deal of abdominal discomfort. I could not sleep on my left side unless I propped my tummy on a pillow." She also said, "I felt debilitated and more disabled, and very limited in what I could do during the post-delivery recovery period."

Women may feel upset about having had surgery, or they may be concerned about the welfare of their babies. Natalie said, "I felt fine because the baby had been under distress and was now okay." Taryn Dion said, "It was more important to focus on the present rather than the idea that I didn't want an emergency C-section. I knew this was one moment in time; she was about to be born, but I just couldn't be present for it."

Some negative feelings are unavoidable. A number of factors influence a woman's feelings about caesarean birth: the type of anesthesia used, whether the surgery was anticipated or unanticipated, whether the mother felt she had a part in the decision to perform surgery, the presence or absence of a support person, the reactions of people important to the mother, and the physical effects of surgery. Sophia Amelia said, "I recovered quickly from the first one. I had the surgery and I got a wonderful return on it. I nursed my baby right away. I had a difficult recovery with the second one because of the spinal. It wasn't the C-section. It was the aftereffects of the spinal. It was difficult taking care of the baby and myself at the same time. I was in the hospital for an entire week with both of them. I also had digestive tract complications. It is pretty difficult to care for a newborn with an N/G tube and pump connected to you. Also, the pump didn't work half the time, and the nurses in labor and delivery had no experience with it, so they had to call down to other floors with questions."

Women who did not anticipate caesarean birth often feel disappointment. They may feel disappointed in themselves for "failing" to give birth vaginally, or because they had looked forward to certain kind of experience. Amy felt angry with the person who caused the car accident that had resulted in her disability. She said, "He took something away from me all over again. It felt almost like I got my legs cut off a second time. I had to relearn how to move again." Natasha was disappointed because she was unsure whether they had given her a fair chance. She said, "I wish they had waited a little longer to see if I could push him out." Natasha *had* been given a chance, however, because she not only labored for 6 hours, but also her baby's heart rate dropped. Noelle had not expected to give birth surgically, and she felt "robbed." Heather said, "I was emotionally prepared." Julie was glad she had attended a class on caesareans because the classes eliminated most of her fears, and she was mentally prepared for surgery. Hilary commented that because she took classes, "I knew all along what to expect." Learning about caesarean section beforehand may not be completely reassuring. Nancy carefully discussed all of her concerns with her doctor, but still felt anxious just before her surgery.

Classes are helpful even if they cannot eliminate all of a woman's fears. All women should take caesarean classes so they will know what to expect during and after surgery, and so they will be better prepared to cope with an unanticipated caesarean. Support people should also attend these classes for two reasons:

1. The hospitals that allow a support person to be present during surgery may require him to take the class.
2. The class will prepare her to give the mother the help she needs after surgery.

A caesarean class also prepares a woman to take part in the decision to have surgery. Stephanie did not feel upset about having had surgery because she felt involved in the decision. She added, "I'm a pragmatic person. Besides, my labor was quite uncomfortable."

Whether or not caesarean surgery was anticipated, concern for the safety of the baby may counteract a woman's negative feelings about surgery. For example, Laura said, "I was disappointed that I couldn't go natural, but I was glad the baby was alive." Julie, too, said, "I just thanked God I was alive and the baby was alive." According to some studies, women who have regional anesthesia feel more positive about caesarean birth than women who have general anesthesia. This result is not surprising, because women who have general anesthesia miss the experience of seeing their babies being born. Hilary and Sybil shared these feelings. Sybil said, "I didn't feel good about the C-section because I wanted to see my baby, like any other mother." Hilary, who had hoped to use hypnosis instead of anesthesia, said, "When I woke up, I was frustrated, and all I could do was cry. I didn't feel negative about having a C-section. It was just that I wanted to see the baby being born." Still, most of the interviewees were not too concerned about what kind of anesthesia they had. Denise had an unusual reaction during her first caesarean section. She said, "I could hear everything going on, but my body was paralyzed and I couldn't open my eyes. I couldn't do anything. It was weird. I felt I wasn't all the way put out. It was a really scary experience. I felt pressure, but no pain." Some of the interviewees pointed out that general anesthesia was needed for a specific reason. For example, Stephanie, who explained, "They were unsure how a spinal would interact with my spinal cord injury."

Julie was not disappointed, but she wondered whether she could have prevented her adverse reaction to the anesthesia. She had taken her caesarean class late and went into labor before she had time to talk to an anesthesiologist. She said, "I experienced a lot of pain, not only in my abdomen, but also my jaw and muscles were sore and weak. It's really important to talk to the anesthesiologist prior to surgery so he knows your body." Noelle said, "Next time, I would make sure I could get a spinal." She added, "I wish I had talked to the right people."

The physical effects of surgery can be upsetting. Taryn Dion said, "It was a very physically painful surgery, and I had some minor complications. The catheter caused some inflammation, which resulted in horrible spasms in my urethra. It was unbelievably painful." New mothers may be frustrated by helplessness and immobility, or by feeling more pain than they expected. Darlene had pain in her upper back and some cramping.

Pain tends to intensify other negative feelings as well. Some of the interviewees were also upset by the way the pain or loss of mobility affected their ability to care for their babies. Stephanie said, "The pain was so uncomfortable that I didn't want to see my baby. I was not disappointed about the caesarean. I just wanted to enjoy my baby." Carla said, "I was depressed because I couldn't move or do anything with my body. I had difficulty turning over. I had loss of mobility and couldn't see my baby." Heather compared her feelings about her two birth experiences in terms of her relationship to her babies: "The hospital staff didn't leave me alone with my first baby until I had my balance back. It was very different with my second. I had rooming-in within 18 hours of surgery, so I wasn't as upset as I was during my first delivery."

A woman's feelings about being intermittently separated from her baby can be influenced by the attitudes and behavior of the hospital staff. One of the author's students has never forgotten her annoyance with a nurse who told her—without first asking about her abilities—"We can't let you carry the baby because if you dropped it and it was hurt, the hospital might get sued." Supportive staff can relieve the mother's frustration and help her cope with practical difficulties. Recalling the nurse who helped her hold her baby softened Sybil's painful memories. Nancy was in intensive care because her disability causes breathing problems, and her doctor wanted to make sure that she did not develop pneumonia after surgery. She was able to have her baby brought to her, and she found that she could nurse by lying on her side supported by pillows.

Although the mother may be separated from her baby for only a few days, that separation can be painful. It is important for hospital staff to remember that a disabled woman feels as much need to spend time with her baby as an able-bodied woman, and she may be able to do more for her baby than they realize. Flexibility and imagination are important: Perhaps an obstetric nurse can simply ask nursery staff to bring the baby to cuddle with the mother when it is sleeping, and put up the sides of the mother's bed to protect the baby. The baby's father or partner, or a friend can help by arranging to be at the hospital to help while the baby visits the mother.

Perhaps the most painful situations are those in which the mother is anxious about her baby's welfare. Carla recalls, "I went crazy when I couldn't see my baby for a whole day because I was too groggy. I needed to know if my baby was normal." Reassurance is important for a woman in Carla's situation. Perhaps the best help a friend can give to the new mother is to leave her long enough to check on the baby—if only to look through the nursery window—and then come back and tell her, "Your baby is fine."

Julie spoke for many women when she said; "I was concerned because the baby was so drugged that he couldn't respond." It is helpful to remember that a sleepy baby is not necessarily in trouble. The aftereffects of anesthesia or pain medications in the mother's milk can make the baby sleepier, but these effects are temporary, just as they are for the mother. Any newborn baby spends a lot of time sleeping, and this normal pattern can contribute to the mother's feeling that the baby is "dopey."

Sometimes the mother is anxious because her baby really is ill. For some women, concern about the baby is an incentive to "get it together." Pam's baby was born 1 month early, and he was depressed by the anesthesia because he was premature. Pam commented, "I had to keep my wits about me because I was concerned about my son." For other women, worry about the baby is overwhelming. Leslie, whose baby was premature, recalled, "I was anxious about the baby. He was transferred to another hospital. It was hard for me to get out of bed because I wasn't motivated." Signey couldn't see one of her babies because he needed oxygen.

Noreen said, "When I woke up, I thought my son was dead. I didn't care about myself. My mom came in a few minutes later smiling, so I knew he lived." Noreen wasn't able to see him until 4 days later. Her baby was premature and she could see him, but she was not able to hold him for another 2 months. Most mothers are able to see their babies soon after the birth unless the mother is quite ill.

Again, anything hospital staff can do to help the mother spend time with her baby can be helpful. It is important for the mother to know that her relationship with her baby is appreciated, and that an effort is being made to help her spend time with the baby. Laura could not hold her baby for 4 days because the baby needed intensive care. Still, Laura felt that "the hospital worked in a humanitarian fashion" because "they made sure I saw my child 98 percent of the time. They made sure I didn't go it alone, especially since I didn't have a husband." Dorothy was upset because her baby needed intensive care.

Meanwhile, it is important for the mother to remember that by taking care of herself, she is helping her baby. Whether doing breathing exercises, or resting when necessary, everything she does to further her own recovery prepares her to care for her baby. Friends can help in a number of practical ways; for example, by donating blood if the baby needs transfusions, contacting a La Leche League milk bank to get breast milk for the baby, contacting caesarean support groups or support groups for parents of ill children, or finding books about caring for premature babies. The mother will feel less helpless when receiving this kind of practical support.

Aftereffects of Caesarean

Even when caesarean delivery is being considered for purely obstetric reasons, some disabled women may have concerns. Some women are worried how the anesthesia will affect their disability, or how the surgery will affect their recovery. Women who have not been in a long labor prior to the caesarean may have an easier recovery. Natalie said, "My second C-section was much easier to recuperate from. The first time, my obstetrician finally performed the surgery when I was physically exhausted from 21 hours of labor; it wiped me out." On the other hand, some women are relieved to know that the caesarean will prevent neurologic problems or other injuries to the baby.

A major concern is that recovery from surgery may be more difficult for a woman with disabilities. The most obvious problem is the effect of abdominal surgery on mobility, because the ability to change position, transfer, or walk can be affected. The effect will be brief for some women; for others, it will last for weeks. Heather Ann was able to use her crutches the same day she had surgery. Carla was more seriously affected: "It was difficult to move. My mobility was shot, and it took almost 6 weeks before I could walk holding onto the wall." Signey said, "After giving birth, the pain from the incision made it hard to get around. Initially moving at all was really painful. The first time I tried to stand—about 24 hours after giving birth—I couldn't put pressure on my feet, which made it impossible to do a pivot transfer. My husband had to support my whole weight. Progressively, I was able to put more pressure on my feet and stand on my own."

It took Sienna 3 to 4 months to be able to walk on her crutches. She was unable to bear any weight. It took a year or so before she regained the sensation in her leg. Sydney said, "There was no specific pain, but it definitely felt like a Mack truck had hit me when it was time to get out of bed. I felt much better by the third day. I had bloating of my abdomen when my bowels started working again."

Mobility limitations also influence other aspects of recovery. Women who cannot exercise may be more vulnerable to *emboli* (blood clots in the veins) and constipation, which is a common problem after abdominal surgery. Women with breathing difficulties may be more vulnerable to respiratory infection. For example, even though Nancy's nurses encouraged her to cough and do breathing exercises immediately after surgery she had to spend some time in the intensive care unit (ICU) as a safety precaution.

Although it is impossible to generalize about the effects of caesarean surgery on disabled women, it is clear that surgical delivery will not necessarily be safer or easier for the mother than vaginal delivery. It is important to remember the strong possibility that recovery from surgery may be more difficult for a woman with disabilities. Both the emotional and the physical aspects of surgical recovery can pose a challenge.

Vaginal Birth After Caesarean Section

"Once a C-section, always a C-section," was the standing rule for many years. For example, Portia had five children born by caesarean surgery. In the early 1950s, the first studies were performed suggesting that vaginal birth after caesarean ("VBAC") can be as safe as repeat caesarean birth. Additional studies in the 1960s and 1970s confirmed this finding. The increasing use of transverse incisions has contributed to the safety of VBAC, because the scar from a transverse incision is less likely to rupture during labor than the scar from a classical incision.

Although there is still some controversy about the safety of VBAC, doctors and hospitals are willing to discuss it with women who want to try having a VBAC. That does not mean a hospital or doctor willing to attempt VBAC will automatically agree to try it with any woman who asks. Noelle belonged to a prepaid health plan that considers every woman who has previously had a caesarean birth to be a candidate for vaginal birth. Yet, her doctors were reluctant to agree to a trial of labor when she wanted a vaginal birth.

The three most important factors affecting the decision to allow VBAC are as follows:

1. *The nature of the uterine incision.* As discussed previously, a classical (high vertical) incision is somewhat more likely to rupture during subsequent pregnancies than a low transverse or vertical incision. The decision to try VBAC may be altered during the course of pregnancy, or even after labor begins, if there are signs that the incision could rupture.
2. *The reason for the original surgery.* Perhaps the original indication for surgery is one that is unlikely to be repeated during a later pregnancy. For example, cord prolapse or placenta previa will not necessarily occur again. If the original indication is not present, the mother can try labor and, if no problems occur, she can give birth vaginally.
3. *The mother's current health and current obstetric considerations.* A problem could arise that is completely different from the one that made a previous labor difficult. For example, a woman might need surgery because of cord prolapse during one labor, and because of fetal distress during another.

Some women with disabilities will not be candidates for VBAC. Many disability indications, such as pelvic deformity, will not change from one pregnancy to the next. A disabled woman who has had surgery for obstetric reasons may want to try VBAC, however.

Two of the women who were interviewed for this book had a vaginal birth after caesarean surgery. Their experiences were different, and the contrasts are interesting. Noelle had surgery because her first labor was not progressing. She had only labored for 8 hours, and she felt that she might have given birth vaginally if she had been allowed to labor longer. She knows that many women are allowed to labor longer, and she had the impression that her doctor overreacted to her disability. She was interested in vaginal birth because "that's the normal way to have a baby." She added, "The C-section was so awful physically that to me it was worth it to try a vaginal birth."

When the doctors at Noelle's prepaid health plan expressed their reluctance to try a vaginal birth, she decided "it would be less of a hassle to get my prenatal care there and have the baby someplace else." Noelle found a teaching hospital where she could have a trial labor. She said, "The doctors thought I had a slim chance. They said, 'You're the one who will have to deal with the pain.' They didn't think of the pain I would have after surgery." She wrote a letter 2 weeks before her due date explaining her reasons for wanting a vaginal birth, and her doctors agreed to try.

Noelle succeeded in giving birth vaginally, and was glad she had done so. She explained, "I bounced back in 3 to 4 weeks after I delivered my second baby vaginally, but it took 3 to 4 months after the C-section. The medication for the C-section affected my balance and gave me a foggy head. Then there was the pain. I was really run down the first month. All that made it quite difficult to take care of the baby."

Leslie's experience was very different from Noelle's. She also wanted to try VBAC because she felt that it is normal to give birth vaginally. Leslie had needed surgery the first time because her baby was in a transverse presentation. She knew she was not likely to have that problem again. She had no problem convincing her doctor to allow her to deliver vaginally. Her doctor simply told her, "It's important for me to be around when you're in labor." Leslie experienced a cervical laceration with her second child, so, unlike Noelle, she felt that vaginal birth was more painful than caesarean birth. For Leslie, recovery from vaginal birth was just as difficult as recovery from surgical birth. She had uterine infections after both births and blood loss. Also, a lupus flare-up made recovery from the second (vaginal) birth difficult. Still, Leslie was glad to give birth vaginally because she felt "it was important to feel a part of the birth process."

The rate of rupture for *transverse low uterine segment* incisions during labor is extremely low—about one half of one percent (0.5 percent) in women with one previous transverse low uterine segment incision, and about 4 percent for women with more than one previous transverse low uterine segment incision (100). In the majority of cases, the risks associated with a VBAC are less than for a planned repeat caesarean section. The success rate for having a vaginal delivery following previous caesarean section is as high as 80 percent under the following conditions:

❖ Both the woman and her doctor(s) are knowledgeable and committed to giving VBAC a try.
❖ There are no clear reasons not to proceed with a trial of labor.
❖ VBAC is done in a hospital that provides obstetric care and is capable of performing an emergency caesarean section if required.

Some reasons for NOT having a trial of labor and/or a VBAC may include:

❖ A previous classical or inverted incision.
❖ Previous surgery involving the uterus, such as surgery to remove fibroid growths, if this surgery involved entry into the uterine cavity or extensive incision and repair of the uterus.
❖ A previous rupture of the uterus.
❖ An unusual position of the placenta.
❖ The baby is lying sideways.
❖ Other medical conditions in which labor would not be advised.

VBAC may be considered after consultation with an obstetrician and gynecologist in the following circumstances:

❖ A previous pregnancy resulted in a caesarean section because of dystocia. This may have occurred as a result of inefficient contractions or the baby's head was not flexed properly to allow for a vaginal birth. Having dystocia with one pregnancy does not mean that it will occur with another.
❖ A previous pregnancy resulted in a caesarean section because of *cephalo-pelvic disproportion* (CPD). This is a situation in which the baby was felt to be too large to pass through the opening in the mother's pelvis or the opening in the mother's pelvis

was felt to be too small for the baby to pass through. Having CPD with one pregnancy does not mean that it will occur with another.

❖ Your contractions are being made stronger or induced with the use of drugs.

❖ You are having twins or your baby is breech.

Closing Comments

One approach to caesarean delivery involves evaluating the appropriateness of this procedure in a general sense. This perspective involves asking such questions as, "Does the increase in the caesarean birth rate reflect a proper balance of concern for the mother and the baby?" "When should this procedure be used?"

A woman may feel disappointed even when she believes that caesarean delivery was appropriate, or even when the circumstances included good communication with her doctor and plenty of time to make a decision. These feelings, too, may depend on a particular perspective. During pregnancy and just afterward, childbirth does not seem like a beginning, but an ending—the climax to 9 months of planning, anticipation, and anxiety.

Yet, childbirth is only a beginning—a very brief beginning. The great majority of labors, whether they end in caesarean or vaginal delivery, last less than a day, while pregnancy lasts about 280 days and parenthood goes on forever. Most women find, as time goes by, that the way they gave birth seems unimportant in comparison to the joys of mothering.

Leslie's final comment on her birth experiences makes the perfect closing to this chapter about caesarean birth: "I was pleased and excited to have both kids and, in the end, it didn't matter."

After Delivery: The Postpartum Period

THE MOTHER'S BODY RETURNS to its pre-pregnant condition during the weeks following childbirth. In a sense, these weeks are the final phase of pregnancy, a phase commonly called the *postpartum period*, meaning "after the birth." It is traditionally considered to last 6 weeks, but can last longer for some women.

Many first-time mothers look forward to the end of pregnancy as a time when life goes back to normal. But as any woman who has already had a child knows, life never goes back to the way it was before you were pregnant. The new mother experiences many changes in her emotions and her relationships during this time. Just as her body gradually changed and adapted during pregnancy, the return to a nonpregnant condition is a gradual process accompanied by a number of physical symptoms. In this chapter, we will discuss the following topics:

- ❖ Medical care in the hospital and postpartum office visits.
- ❖ Physical changes, self-care, and postpartum complications.
- ❖ Emotional changes, including "postpartum depression."
- ❖ Sexuality and birth control.
- ❖ Breast-feeding: The choice between breast-feeding and bottle-feeding, suggestions for breast care, the art of breast-feeding, and combining breast and bottle-feeding.
- ❖ Suggestions disabled women can use in caring for infants.

Medical Care

HOSPITAL CARE

It is important to move as much as possible during recovery. The new mother will also be encouraged to use the bathroom. In fact, she must urinate at least once before she can

343

leave the hospital. Nurses will encourage her to urinate, and may ask her to use a bed-pan, or a "catcher" on the toilet, to measure the amount of urine produced. Routine medical care includes checking blood pressure, pulse, and temperature at least once before she leaves. Changes in these vital signs can be the first indication of infection or other complications. Medical staff will intermittently check the abdomen to assess the condition of the uterus, and to make sure that it has begun to contract down to normal size. The perineal area may be swollen, even if there was no episiotomy. The nurses will apply ice packs to reduce any swelling and lessen discomfort.

The obstetrician will do an examination and answer any questions, but nurses are also a link with the physician. For example, if a woman develops symptoms of infection, a nurse will telephone the doctor, describe the symptoms, and follow the doctor's instructions in giving medications or arranging for tests until the doctor can perform an examination. When the obstetrician visits, ask any questions you have about self-care, and when to schedule your next appointment. A pediatrician will examine the baby as well.

Your nurses can also give you advice or written information before you leave. They may offer you a kit to take home. Ask what is in the kit, and whether there is an extra charge, because it may contain items you already have at home, such as a thermometer, and you may prefer not to pay extra for another one.

Many programs include a home visit by a nurse 3 days after the birth. Usually, the nurse will be someone who did not attend the birth. Some pediatricians are willing to make a similar visit.

During this period, medical staff normally provides routine medical care, assistance with recovery from childbirth, and help with baby care and breast-feeding. Much of what nurses do to assist recovery may also be useful at home; for example, using ice packs to reduce perineal swelling.

Maternity nurses are a good source of advice and help in coping with postpartum physical changes, such as constipation. Nurses will also help with infant care, such as first attempts to nurse the baby as well as how to diaper. This kind of support and encouragement from nurses can make a new mother feel much more comfortable about caring for her baby. The emotional support nurses give is important, too. Sibyl recalled, "The nurse in the recovery room was excited for me. She made me feel really good."

Unfortunately some of the interviewees did not encounter supportive nurses. Natalie said, "The baby mostly stayed in the nursery unless my mom or husband was there. I could not get out of bed to take care of him. My doctor said, 'While you are in the hospital get as much rest as you can.' He recommended I leave the baby in the nursery." When the baby needed to be fed, Natalie would call for a nurse to come and get him. Natalie said, "I could not hang onto the glass bottles." When one nurse found out that Natalie had not fed the baby in the hospital, she questioned Natalie's competency. This nurse called in Natalie's pediatrician, who would not release Natalie and her baby until she fed him in the hospital. Her husband came in and fought for her rights. In this type of situation, it is important for hospital staff to understand why a new mother cannot use glass bottles. Natalie could have brought in bottles that were made of plastic and had a narrower base, because the narrower base made the bottles easier to hold.

Many women find that their postpartum hospital stay is different from their other hospital experiences. Obstetric nurses are responsible for the more generalized care of many patients, in contrast to rehabilitation nurses, who are responsible for the intensive care of a few patients. Obstetric nurses care for women who are recovering from caesarean surgery, and help women cope with postpartum discomforts. Their responsibilities do not usually include the specialized needs of women with disabilities. For example, helping a paralyzed woman change position several times a day is not within the usual responsibilities of an obstetric nurse. Your doctor should advise postpartum nursing staff that frequent position changes are needed to avoid skin breakdown.

This difference in nursing care made some of the interviewees feel that they did not have all the help they needed. Looking back on her hospital stay, Celeste said she would advise nurses to "be aware that a disabled woman may need more attention than other new mothers. Be patient and more understanding. I had trouble with nursing because I was left alone with my baby. Stay around and see if the woman needs extra help or support." On the other hand, some of the interviewees felt that their nurses offered more help than was necessary. Charlotte found the hospital nurses to be angry; perhaps they did not know how to help. The nurses were unfamiliar with one-handed techniques, so they were unable to help Charlotte with nursing. Women with unique problems could have an occupational therapist consult with maternity nursing staff.

Clara said, "Ask the woman what help she needs before you give it, both during labor and postpartum." Clearly, good communication between the disabled mother and nursing staff is important. If new mothers and nurses take the time to discuss any special concerns, they will have a more cooperative relationship. Nurses will be more efficient if they understand the disabled mother's special needs.

The difference in viewpoints between disabled mothers and their nurses can lead to misunderstandings. This occurred when Sharon, who had used an indwelling catheter when she was pregnant, began to catheterize herself in the hospital. Sharon was annoyed when a nurse criticized her technique. She said afterwards, "The nurse was so certain she was right and I didn't know anything. I don't have to use the same sterile technique a nurse uses. I've probably been cathing myself for more years than she has been a nurse." Sharon and her nurse were both right—many rehabilitation units teach a clean method of self-catheterization that is not sterile, but that is fine for use at home. In a hospital setting, however, sterile technique is important in preventing *nosocomial infection* (infection acquired in the hospital). Germs in the hospital are often more of a problem than those at home because they may be resistant to many antibiotics.

Other misunderstandings can occur when obstetric nurses are not familiar with the particular skills and problems of women with disabilities. These misunderstandings can be quite painful to the disabled mother. Marsha had problems with incontinence while she was pregnant, and she continued to have problems after her catheter was removed in the hospital. She said, "Some of my nurses got impatient or angry when I wet the bed. They seemed to think I wasn't bothering to get out of bed, when it was really an MS problem."

It is important to find ways to improve communication between disabled mothers and their nurses. Some of the interviewees suggested that the nurses receive special training before the disabled woman gives birth. Hilary said, "The obstetrician could have had a meeting with the hospital staff to coordinate plans." Jennifer suggested that nurses have sensitivity training in dealing with disabled persons. Work ahead of time with the maternity ward nurses so you can alert them to your needs.

A rehabilitation nurse can help coordinate planning before birth, or consult with maternity nurses after birth. Besides explaining the kind of care a mother with a disability might need, the rehabilitation nurse can suggest solutions for specific problems. For example, he can show nurses how to protect their own backs while helping a patient transfer, and how to use a local anesthetic jelly to avoid stimulating hyperreflexia when inserting a catheter. A rehabilitation nurse could have helped Marsha's nurses find ways to cope with her incontinence. They might have given Marsha absorbent underwear, or borrowed a mattress protector from the nursery and placed it under her hips. (A mattress protector is absorbent material with waterproof backing that helps keep sheets dry.) A rehabilitation nurse can also help staff to decide when to "bend the rules."

Sometimes medical staff may react in a certain way because of bias. Andrea said, "My doctor was concerned about me taking care of my second baby, because I had a disabled husband and another child. He told me he was not going to discharge me until I could prove to him that I had someone else at home besides my husband to help. I told him that he did not have a choice. I said, 'I'm leaving, goodbye.'" The doctor advised Andrea if she left without being discharged it would be "AMA," and she would then be held liable for the entire hospital bill for both herself and her baby. Andrea felt like she was being held hostage. She *had* to produce an able-bodied person, her mother, to prove to the doctor that she had ample help at home.

Other health professionals might also need to become involved. For example, an occupational therapist can help the mother find ways to care for her baby. A physical or occupational therapist can help provide passive exercise for the prevention of thrombophlebitis (blood clots in the veins) in women who have spinal cord dysfunctions. Physical and occupational therapists can help women who have been on bed rest during pregnancy to recover their coping skills and their strength in transferring. It may be necessary to get prior authorization for these services before the birth of your child.

Some of the interviewees suggested that extra help should be available. Stephanie said, "Make sure the hospital lets the husband room-in with the mother. They shouldn't just allow it, they should encourage it, because he can be such a big help. Some hospital rules really make life more difficult than it has to be." Hiring a special-duty nurse or arranging for a private room so the husband can "room-in" are expenses that may not be covered by the mother's insurance, and the hospital's social worker may need to participate in planning for special care.

LEAVING THE HOSPITAL

Most women who give birth will leave the hospital in less than a day. Some women may stay for up to 48 hours after a vaginal birth. A postpartum hospital stay rarely lasts more than 3 days, although women who develop complications, such as infections, may need to stay longer. You will be moved to another room in the hospital, and there will be an additional charge if you need to stay longer.

Your doctor will visit you before you leave the hospital and do a brief physical examination. It is important to discuss the doctor's recommendations for your care before your first postpartum office visit. Ask about any medications the doctor prescribes, and be sure to ask how long you should continue taking them.

It is important to discuss the possibility that you will experience pregnancy complications, or remission or exacerbation of your disability symptoms. Ask your doctor what signs and symptoms you should watch for, whether to call your obstetrician or your disability specialist when symptoms appear, and what tests might be done to differentiate between disability exacerbation and postpartum complications. Women who have spinal cord dysfunction usually find that their bladder control returns to whatever was normal for them before pregnancy. They are more susceptible to anemia, blood clots, and urinary infections in the postpartum period, however.

You should know the signs and symptoms of a uterine infection called *endomyometritis*. This infection can appear any time, but it generally occurs during the first 72 hours after delivery. Although it is rare, this type of infection can occur more than 1 week after delivery. A fever that occurs a week after delivery can also indicate *mastitis*, an inflammation of the breast. Another type of infection is *endomyometritis*; signs include: fever, a foul-smelling discharge, increased vaginal bleeding, low abdominal pain, and chills.

Nina was in the hospital for 1 week, which is standard in Sweden, the country in which she gave birth. On the second day she was home, however, she ran a high fever. She was unable to sit up, and was admitted to the hospital. The infection took its toll on Nina, and it was a month before she could be turned over without pain. Amanda had a strep infection with her second pregnancy, and it took her three times as long to recover as it did from her first pregnancy.

OFFICE VISITS

The first office visit takes place 3 to 6 weeks after the birth. If all is well at this time, it may not be necessary to see the doctor again until it is time for a yearly checkup. During this first visit, the doctor will do a general physical examination, and ask a number of questions about how you are doing. If the doctor is a family practitioner, consider scheduling a well-baby visit at the same time as the postpartum office visit. This is also the best time to discuss birth control. The physical examination will include these procedures:

Routine checkup: The doctor will check blood pressure, temperature, weight, and heart and lungs. Although blood pressure measurement is part of every routine examination, it is also important in choosing a birth control method. Blood pressure must be checked before hormones can be prescribed, because women with high blood pressure should not use hormones, including birth-control pills, patches, or implants.

Most women lose 17 to 20 pounds within 6 weeks of giving birth, including a loss of about 10 pounds at the time of birth. Women who feel that they should have lost more weight can talk to their doctors about diet.

Temperature measurement is important, because a high temperature may be a sign of postpartum infection.

Breast examination: The breasts will be examined for any abnormalities, masses (lumps or cysts), tenderness, or signs of infection. Women who are breast- feeding may want to ask questions about breast care at this time.

Examination of vagina and uterus: The size of the uterus will be assessed. The uterus should be reducing at a normal rate, and it should be close to pre-pregnant size by 6 weeks after the birth. The vagina and cervix will be examined. The cervix should be closing. The doctor will inspect any lacerations of the vagina or cervix to see that they are healing well. The doctor will assess the type and amount of discharge from the uterus, because discolored lochia, or too much lochia, can indicate infection or a retained piece of the placenta. (*Lochia* is defined below in "Changes in Body Systems.") The flow of lochia should have stopped by the fourth week after birth, allowing the doctor to do a routine Pap smear at the time of the first office visit.

Perineum: If there was a tear or an episiotomy, the perineum will be examined to assure that it is healing well.

Rectal examination: This examination is done as part of a general health assessment. The doctor will check for the presence of hemorrhoids, and make sure that any lacerations are healing.

Calves: The calves are examined for any signs of blood clots.

Blood test: Some doctors routinely test for anemia during the first postpartum visit. Others test only if the mother is extremely tired, or if she had been anemic during pregnancy or lost more blood than usual during delivery.

Evaluation of special health problems: Any special health problems that occurred during pregnancy are evaluated, such as varicose veins or diabetes of pregnancy.

You may want to ask your doctor some of the following questions:

When can my husband and I make love again? One family practitioner told us, "That is the most popular question." The doctor's reply will depend on how well the mother is healing. Most women can resume lovemaking within 3 to 6 weeks after giving birth.

What can I do about discomfort during lovemaking? (This answer to this question is discussed below in "The Sexual Relationship.")

What family-planning method should I use? (Birth control is discussed below in "Birth Control Methods.")

What about diet? Women who want to lose or gain weight should talk to their doctors about diet during the first office visit after they give birth. It is important to follow a nutritious diet even while losing weight, especially for women who are breast-feeding or who are anemic. Many people worry that doctors are not trained in nutrition, but this aspect of medical education has been improved. Also, many physicians employ a dietitian or a nurse with special training in nutrition; others will make a referral to a dietitian.

Questions in the following areas are more individual in nature:

Breast care: What can I do about sore nipples? This is a common question. Information about breast care can be found below in the sections on physical changes and breast-feeding, but it is always a good idea to discuss any concerns with your doctor. You can also discuss breast-feeding in terms of your baby's needs if your doctor is a family practitioner.

Medication: If any medications were stopped during pregnancy, they may be started again after the birth. Women who are breast-feeding need to discuss this with their doctors, because many medications pass into breast milk. Be sure to discuss all of the possibilities: Perhaps one medication was substituted for another during pregnancy, and it may be desirable to change back to the original medication; or a medication that was started during pregnancy can be continued if the woman prefers it, as was the case with Sylvia. Discuss whether the dose might be changed. Will it be necessary to see the doctor again, or call the doctor to discuss the dosage? Sometimes the dosage is based on a person's weight, so the dose will need to be changed because of the weight loss after pregnancy.

The relationship between pregnancy and exacerbation of autoimmune diseases is the subject of a number of studies. "It is important to recognize that some pregnant SLE patients experience disease exacerbations following delivery, it is generally recommended that medications be gradually tapered back to pre-pregnancy levels" (101).

Some studies have found that women with myasthenia gravis can either improve or experience exacerbation during the postpartum period. Women with this condition need to be aware that they might have an exacerbation. Although the long-term course of multiple sclerosis does not appear to be affected by pregnancy, women with MS are especially vulnerable to exacerbation postpartum. It might be more accurate to say that remission of rheumatoid arthritis ends with pregnancy, than to say that an exacerbation takes place; pain and stiffness do get worse. Symptoms of SLE may also become worse. Some women may hope to discontinue medications, but they must consult their doctors first. Many doctors prescribe corticosteroids or other anti-inflammatories to prevent SLE exacerbation, especially if symptoms were severe before pregnancy. Some women who have SLE need immunosuppressive medications during pregnancy, but the dosage should not be lowered abruptly.

Rehabilitation: If disability symptoms worsened during pregnancy, it may be possible to make some improvements after pregnancy is completed. Ask your doctor about an exercise program, or consider physical therapy if weakened muscles have affected mobility.

Other prescriptions or referrals: You may need a signed recommendation from your doctor to get the help you need, including increased attendant care, assistive devices, special medications, or temporary changes in medical or disability benefits. If you are not able to bring forms from your social worker or insurance company with you when you go to the doctor's office, your doctor may be able to obtain the forms for you, or tell you what you will need.

Normal Physical Changes

All the body systems that changed during pregnancy change again after birth. This section discusses the normal changes and minor problems that women experience, and ways to cope with them.

GENERALIZED CHANGES

There are a few changes that are noticeable to new mothers.

Weight Loss

Although a woman who has just given birth often finds that she still looks pregnant, the scales tell a different story. When giving birth, she loses approximately 12 pounds in a matter of hours. During the week after birth, she loses another 3 to 6 pounds as her body sheds the extra fluids retained during pregnancy. She may lose a few more pounds during the following weeks. Although many women are pleased to lose some weight after they are pregnant, they should not restrict their diets during the postpartum period, as explained below. Women who are concerned about losing too much or too little weight should discuss their concerns with their doctors during their postpartum office visit. Women who use a prosthesis may need to wait to be refitted and/or see if they return to their pre-pregnancy weight.

Fatigue

Many women feel tired during late pregnancy, but fatigue is often more of a problem during the postpartum period. New mothers feel exhausted, and while it may be hard to believe that the exhaustion is normal, it usually is. There are many reasons for fatigue, including:

The new infant: Most importantly, the effort of caring for a new infant can be tiring.

The birth process: Like other kinds of strenuous exercise, the work of giving birth can make a woman feel tired for days afterwards. The birth process is called *labor* for a good reason!

Emotional stress: Emotional stress causes fatigue. It is important to remember that any life change, even the joy of having a new baby, can be stressful. There may be other changes as well, such as coping with a jealous sibling or feeling frustration about unfinished housework. Many women feel uncomfortable about taking the rest they need. They worry about unfinished chores, or fear that they are "babying" themselves.

Sleep loss: Newborn babies have irregular sleep patterns. Being awakened by the baby several times a night is a major cause of fatigue, and may cause or trigger postpartum depression.

Anemia: Fatigue may be a symptom of anemia. Even the minor blood loss associated with birth can lead to anemia. And there is always some bleeding from the site where the placenta was attached, even if there are no other cuts or tears.

Many disabled women have learned to cope by forcing themselves to ignore fatigue. Although adequate exercise is important to postpartum recovery, adequate rest is equally important, and each woman will need to find her own way to balance rest and exercise. Sabine had to go to the hospital to see her baby, who stayed a few days longer than she did. She said, "I could hardly walk, but all that moving helped me get back to normal, although I used a cane."

Good nutrition in the postpartum period is as important as it was during pregnancy. Women who are breast-feeding need to follow a diet similar to what they ate while pregnant, so that they will get enough nutrients to nourish themselves and to produce milk. Some women need to eat iron-rich foods to help their bodies replace the blood lost during childbirth. All women will feel better if they follow a healthy, well-balanced diet. It is a good idea to ask your doctor about a vitamin supplement. If a postpartum blood test shows that you are anemic, your doctor will probably prescribe an iron supplement. Remember, vitamins can *add* to a well-balanced diet, but they cannot *replace* a diet of nutritious foods.

Often, a new mother feels that there is no time to cook the kind of food she needs. Yet, if she only snatches a snack here and an incomplete meal there, she will feel even more tired and more unable to care for herself and her baby. Here are some tips for keeping well nourished:

Make meals a priority: It is tempting to catch up on work when the baby is sleeping. You will feel better if you eat (or rest) first, and then take time for other tasks.

Take advantage of convenient appliances: If you cannot afford a microwave oven and/or a slow cooker, borrow them, or mention them to anyone who offers to give you a really special gift.

Cook simple meals: Save complicated recipes for a less hectic time.

Shop wisely: Begin in the produce and dairy sections of the store. Make it easy; have an apple, a glass or milk, or a tuna sandwich for a snack.

Use some convenience foods: Frozen vegetables may not be as pleasing as fresh vegetables, but frozen peas are better than peas growing moldy in the refrigerator because there is no time to shell them! It is also worthwhile to study and compare the nutritional value of each meal.

Cook ahead of time if possible: Double the recipe when making dishes such as stews and casseroles. It takes just a little more time, but part of the food can be frozen for another day. Stephanie suggested cooking and freezing several meals before the baby is born.

Let others help: If someone asks you, "What can I do to help?" tell them, "Bring healthy food!"

For many women, the help of others makes the difference between bearable fatigue and unbearable exhaustion. When Stacy was asked what advice she would give to other women, one of the first things she said was, "It is important to get help. Exhaustion was the main reason I was so depressed." Stephanie paid for professional help with childcare and housework. She said, "Extra help is essential." Margie commented, "After my first baby, I was so exhausted that my MS got worse. The main problem was blurry vision. After my second baby, I made sure to get plenty of help, and my MS didn't flare up."

When arranging for help, think about your individual needs and the talents of the people offering to help. If someone offers to help with the baby, and you would prefer help with housework, say so. A friend who is good at sewing could adapt baby clothes so that a mother with limited hand control can dress her baby; a friend with carpentry skills could lower a changing table to wheelchair height.

A hospital social worker may be able to make arrangements for at-home help before the new mother leaves for home, or her regular social worker may arrange a change of benefits. If a woman or her advocate checks with social workers before a scheduled visit to the doctor, she can bring the necessary forms to the first postpartum office visit. Hopefully, in the future women will be able to get extra help paid for through private insurance, Medicaid, disability insurance, or a local social service agency that provides home support services.

Sometimes fatigue is a sign of a physical or emotional problem. It is not always easy to tell when fatigue is a sign of other problems, because it is so common for women to be extremely tired during the weeks following birth. No woman should hesitate to tell her doctor about her concerns. The new mother may simply need a few words of encouragement and a reminder to rest, or she may need tests or medication.

Preventing fatigue is especially important for women with disabilities that are exacerbated by fatigue, including MS, SLE, and myasthenia gravis. If a woman has one of these disabilities, her doctor needs to determine whether she is experiencing a disease exacerbation. Her doctor must have complete information to know what she needs. Mary recalled, "My doctor made a point of telling me to have my mother or my mother-in-law come help out so I wouldn't get too tired." She also decided to bottle-feed her baby, rather than risk getting overly tired from breast-feeding. Michelle advises women with MS to breast-feed as little as possible. (This issue is discussed further in the section entitled "Breast-feeding.")

CHANGES IN BODY SYSTEMS

The Uterus

As previously discussed, the uterus returns to normal size in a process called *involution* after birth. Uterine contractions do not end when the baby is born. They become weaker and less frequent, but they continue for up to a week. These contractions are often called "afterpains." Some women feel so much discomfort from afterpains that they need to use the same breathing techniques they used during labor. Women who have had more than one child, or whose uterine muscles were stretched by a large pregnancy, may experience stronger afterpains. Oxytocin—the hormone that stimulates uterine contractions—is released when the baby suckles, causing many women to have sharper afterpains while they are breast-feeding. Sheila said, "When I nursed my baby, I could feel the contractions and it made me feel better because I knew my uterus was recovering."

The temporary sharp pain of a uterine contraction feels different from the constant pain that is a sign of bleeding or infection. During the first few days after giving birth, a woman with a spinal cord injury who is worried about uterine pain can reassure herself by placing her hand over her uterus to feel it contract, and then relax. A woman who still feels uterine pain more than a week after giving birth should call her doctor, because the pain could be a sign of infection.

During the first 2 days after birth, the uterine fundus (the top of the uterus) involutes to a level between the navel and the pubic hair. The uterus returns to its pre-pregnancy size after about 6 weeks.

As the uterus involutes, the muscle contractions squeeze the blood vessels. This helps to stop bleeding from the placental wound, and encourages the flow of lochia, which consists of blood, mucus, and other tissues left in the uterus after childbirth, including bits of the amniotic sac. For the first 2 to 4 days, the flow of lochia will be dark reddish brown and comparatively heavy, similar to menstrual flow. There may be some small clots. For the next 4 to 5 days, the lochia grows paler, a brownish pink color. During the next week or two, it fades to a brownish white, then a yellowish white. The flow of pale yellow fluid may continue on and off for up to 6 weeks.

Always use sanitary napkins to absorb the lochia. Tampons should not be used, because the uterus is vulnerable to infection during the healing process. Unusual changes in the color, odor, or the amount of lochia may be signs of renewed bleeding or infection. (The causes of excessive bleeding are discussed below in "Postpartum Complications.")

The Vagina

The vagina will be sore and stretched from the passage of the baby. Although the vaginal muscles regain some tone with the passage of time, they should be exercised to assure that they will become as firm as they were before pregnancy. Strong vaginal muscles are important for sexual satisfaction and for long-term health. The Kegel exercises we described in Chapter 7 can be started the day after the baby is born. It is enough to do a few gentle squeezes daily during the first few days. The number of repetitions can be gradually increased in the days and weeks that follow. Many women cannot even feel their muscles moving at first, but if they keep exercising daily, they will notice a change within a few weeks. Some women find that the best way to make sure they remember to do these exercises is to do them first thing in the morning, even before they open their eyes. Others do a few "Kegel's" every time they use the bathroom.

The lining of the vagina will be thinner, drier, and more sensitive. These changes are caused by *prolactin*, a hormone involved in milk production. For most women, the change is not noticeable except during sexual intercourse, which may be uncomfortable.

Women who do not breast-feed will find that this problem disappears in a few weeks, possibly before they start making love again. Women who breast-feed will continue to be sensitive for several months, however. Doctors sometimes prescribe a cream containing estrogen that can be inserted into the vagina. This hormone will cause the vaginal lining to grow thicker, but the amount given in the cream is too small to affect breast milk. Women who are susceptible to blood clots should discuss the use of estrogen with their doctors. A water-based lubricant, such as K-Y Jelly®, may be used as an alternative to make intercourse more comfortable. The spermicides used for birth control are also lubricating.

Episiotomies are generally not done anymore, but tears are still common. The perineum will need special care if there was an episiotomy or a tear. The perineum will be sore at first, and there may be some itching as the wound heals. An ice pack can be used for the first 24 to 36 hours in the hospital or at home. The ice pack should be waterproof, and wrapped in a clean, dry cloth. The cold will feel soothing, and will prevent or reduce swelling.

Heat can promote healing after the first day or so. An infrared heat lamp may be used in the hospital. A heat lamp used at home should have a timer as a safety feature to prevent burns. It can be used for 15 minutes, 3 times a day. Healing and comfort are also promoted by warm soaks, either in a clean, partially filled bathtub or a sitz bath. A sitz bath is a shallow pan that holds just enough water to cover the buttocks and perineum. It usually fits over the toilet bowl. The sitz bath may be used 5 to 10 minutes at a time, several times a day. Clara recalled, "I always felt better after using the sitz bath." It is best to dry the perineum completely after a warm soak.

Urination can be painful, because urine on the episiotomy wound can sting. Jennifer said, "Whenever I urinated, I poured water over the episiotomy at the same time." Clara said, "I would put some warm water in the tub before I urinated, then get in the tub right afterward. Sometimes I would pee in the shower or bath." Stacy said, "It was too hard to transfer into a tub, so the first week I would turn on the shower. Sitting in the warm shower while I urinated dulled the pain." Many hospitals provide a squeeze bottle that can be used to spray warm water on the perineum during and after urination.

Bowel movements can be painful if the cut or tear extends into the anus. Most doctors will prescribe a stool softener to prevent constipation, so that bowel movements will be less painful. Rinsing with plenty of warm water after a bowel movement will soothe pain, and help to prevent infection by cleaning the wound.

Some of the interviewees had trouble sitting or walking after having episiotomies. Clara said, "I think I had more trouble walking after my first delivery because I was torn up to the anus, and it was really sore." Stacy commented, "I had trouble transferring, mostly because I was weak, but also because the episiotomy was sore." Allison tore up to her anus during delivery, so afterward she could not find a comfortable position for sitting. In addition, her breasts were engorged. She said, "Sitting on a shower chair in a shower and letting the warm water pour all over my body made me feel better." Felicia found that sitting on a bag of frozen peas helped relieve her pain.

The Urinary Tract

Many women have difficulty urinating after giving birth. The problem may last for a few hours, or several days. The problem can arise for a number of reasons:

- ❖ The bladder may be bruised or swollen because of injury during childbirth.
- ❖ Urination may be painful because of an episiotomy or tears in the vaginal tract.
- ❖ Urine may be retained as an aftereffect of oxytocin use.
- ❖ Bladder sensation (the "urge" to urinate) may be reduced as an aftereffect of anesthesia.
- ❖ There may be a urinary tract infection.

It is important to urinate within a few hours after giving birth, and to continue urinating regularly. Otherwise, the bladder can become distended (over-filled), increasing the risk of urinary infection. It may be necessary to use a catheter if it is not possible to urinate, as Patricia, Christina, and Marsha did for several days after giving birth. Even when a woman begins to urinate spontaneously after removal of a catheter, her nurse may still use a catheter to remove any remaining urine. If too much urine remains in the bladder, a catheter may be left in place for another 12 to 24 hours. Using a catheter increases the risk of urinary infection, but this risk is smaller than the risk of not keeping the bladder drained.

Some women may have problems with incontinence (loss of bladder control) after childbirth, or after use of a catheter. If incontinence is normally not a problem, then it should be discussed with the doctor. Some women make sure they are never far from a bathroom until the problem is solved. Others wear special absorbent underwear.

Many women find that they have to urinate frequently from about the second day to the sixth day after giving birth. This increased need to urinate is not necessarily a sign of bladder infection. As we mentioned above, 3 to 6 pounds of extra fluid are lost after childbirth, and much of this fluid is eliminated in the urine. The symptoms of a bladder infection are different: one often feels the need to use the bathroom, but then produces only a few drops of urine.

Women with mobility problems who have occasional incontinence may need to keep a bedpan or bedside commode nearby, or sleep closer to the bathroom. Women with indwelling catheters may need to empty their urine bags more frequently.

The Digestive System

Quite often, women do not have a bowel movement for 1 to 2 days after delivery. Many women also experience constipation. The first bowel movements can be so uncomfortable that a woman may become afraid to go to the bathroom.

Plenty of fluid and fiber in the diet can help prevent constipation. It is also important to use the bathroom as soon as the need is felt. "Holding on" until it is convenient to use the bathroom can make the bowel movement more difficult and painful.

Some women find glycerin suppositories helpful, both for stimulating a bowel movement and for reducing strain. Women whose episiotomies make bowel movements painful are likely to find suppositories helpful. Many women find that the breathing and relaxation techniques that helped during labor also help during painful bowel movements.

Circulatory Changes

Many people are surprised to learn that two common postpartum changes are actually changes in the circulatory system.

The first is hemorrhoids, which are swollen blood vessels in the area of the anus. They resemble blood blisters. They are often painful, especially during bowel movements. Hemorrhoids are more likely to appear during pregnancy, and to improve after delivery. In some women, like Christina, they appear just after delivery.

The second symptom is only indirectly caused by changes in the circulatory system. As the amount of blood diminishes, and the body eliminates excess fluids, some women find that they sweat profusely at times during the 2 weeks after giving birth. Some perspire so heavily that they need to put towels on their pillows at night. Women who are quadriplegic may want to ask their doctors how to tell the difference between postpartum sweating and "quad sweats." Some women might like to buy a home blood pressure kit, and have their blood pressure checked when they start to perspire.

Some women become anemic after giving birth. A woman who is feeling tired should call her doctor and discuss whether she should take iron supplements.

The Breasts

Changes in the breasts are experienced by all women, whether or not they nurse their babies. (See "Breast-feeding" for a discussion of the advantages and disadvantages of breast-feeding and bottle-feeding, as well as advice on breast-feeding and breast care.)

During pregnancy, the breasts start changing in preparation for milk production. Often, the breasts even begin to produce colostrum (a thin, clear "pre-milk") during the last weeks of pregnancy. Every woman begins to produce colostrum by the second day after giving birth.

The milk comes in about 4 days after the birth, although it usually comes in even sooner after a second birth. Most women will have some problems with engorgement, a condition in which the breasts become swollen, painful, and hard. Sharon said, "When my milk came in, it felt like I had two stones on my chest." Cheryl said, "It felt like two bricks." Sometimes women with breast engorgement have a slight fever. Some women find that ice packs or cold compresses make their breasts more comfortable; others prefer a hot shower or a hot pad. Wearing a supportive bra also helps. Sometimes expressing a little milk relieves the discomfort, but women who do not plan to breast-feed should be careful to express only a small amount of milk, because if they express too much it will stimulate more milk production. Mild pain relievers are also helpful. Engorgement usually disappears within a day or two.

When the breasts are not stimulated by suckling, milk production gradually stops, often within a week.

Some women may wonder about having their doctors inject medications to stop milk production. Suppressing milk in this way is much less common than it was in the past. Often the injections only delay milk production, rather than suppress it. Also, these medications, like any other, should not be used without discussing possible side effects.

The Abdomen

When women imagine returning to their normal physical condition after the baby is born, they assume they will be able to wear the clothes they wore before they were pregnant—and see their own feet again without craning their necks! So it is always something of a shock when the abdomen does not look different just after childbirth. If stretch marks appeared during pregnancy, they will still be visible. The mother will look as if she is 4 or 5 months pregnant because of weight gain and stretched abdominal muscles. Stretch marks are similar to scars, and will gradually fade during the year or two following pregnancy. The abdomen will begin to look flatter as weight is lost. To some extent, the muscles will regain their tone during normal daily activities, such as walking and carrying the baby. If you are able to exercise, it is best to use the abdominal exercises described in Chapter 7 to help the muscles recover more quickly. Strong abdominal muscles will contribute to good posture and help prevent back discomfort. It is important to begin with gentle exercise, then change to more demanding exercise as the muscles grow stronger.

Some women develop a condition called *diastasis recti*, in which some of the abdominal muscles are separated. These vertical muscles are pushed apart by the pressure of the uterus. A mild separation is likely to heal with rest. If your abdominal muscles have been separated more extensively, do not try to exercise until the doctor indicates it is safe to do so. Always begin with exercises recommended by the doctor or physical therapist. Surgery may be suggested if it does not heal.

Postpartum Complications

Sometimes women experience postpartum changes that are not normal. These changes are signs or symptoms of complications. The most common complications are bleeding and infection. Sometimes thrombophlebitis (blood clots) occurs, but this is more common during pregnancy.

BLEEDING COMPLICATIONS

There are a number of reasons for postpartum bleeding. Sometimes the bleeding is caused by a laceration (cut or tear) in the cervix, vagina, or perineum. If these tissues were injured during birth, the doctor or nurse examining the mother will find bright red discharge, and/or too much bleeding. It may then be necessary to suture the injury to stop the bleeding.

If the uterus does not involute, there may be too much bleeding in the area where the placenta was attached. Normal involution compresses blood vessels and stops bleeding in the same way that pressure stops bleeding from an ordinary cut. Some of the causes of uterine bleeding are very unusual. Some reasons why the uterus fails to involute include the following:

❖ The uterine muscles were overly stretched by a large fetus or a multiple birth.
❖ The muscles were stressed by a prolonged or rapid labor.
❖ Contractions were affected by general anesthesia.
❖ The mother has fibroid tumors (a non-cancerous uterine growth).
❖ The mother has been weakened by illness or other problems.
❖ A part of the placenta is retained in the uterus. Although the placenta is examined for completeness after birth, sometimes it is unusually shaped, has an extra lobe, or part of it remains attached to the uterine wall.

Uterine bleeding is usually diagnosed easily. The doctor or nurse will often find bleeding that is not caused by a laceration, and an examination of the abdomen will reveal that the uterus is not involuting. Often, massage of the fundus (the top of the uterus) will stimulate good contractions. If massage is not effective, the mother may be given oxytocin.

If retained placenta is causing the problem, the placental material will have to be removed. Anesthesia may be necessary for this procedure. Pitocin may be given afterwards.

Rarely, a piece of retained placenta blocks blood flow, acting like a stopper in a bottle. When this happens, the first symptoms may be weakness from blood loss, or pain from the pressure of the blood leaking into the uterus. The mother may need to be treated for blood loss with intravenous fluid or blood transfusion in addition to having the retained placenta removed.

Leslie and Samantha both had postpartum bleeding complications. Leslie had a laceration, and Samantha had retained a lobe of the placenta. Each of them commented that it took them a long time to regain their strength.

POSTPARTUM INFECTIONS

Postpartum infections may occur in the uterus, the genital tract, a caesarean incision, or in the breast. Infection may be fairly easy to diagnose when there is pain in the infected area. The first signs of infection are sometimes symptoms such as fever or fatigue, and the doctor must examine the mother to find the cause of infection.

There are a number of possible causes for uterine infection. It may be introduced during examinations after the bag of water breaks, or during manipulation to help with delivery of the baby. Laceration of the cervix, vagina, or vulva as well as remaining fragments of the placenta or uterine lining may become infected. The infection may stay in one area (local infection), or it may be carried to other parts of the body (systemic).

In addition to the uterus, cervix, or vulva, the breasts may also become infected. Women who breast-feed can get an infection when germs from the baby's mouth enter the milk ducts. Women whose nipples crack are especially vulnerable to infection during the first weeks of breast-feeding. Breast infections may also be localized or systemic. Although it is rare, a continuing breast infection could be a symptom of breast cancer. Signs of postpartum infection include:

❖ Fever. Sometimes a woman is not even aware she has a fever. Even though Nancy was in pain, she did not think of taking her temperature until she noticed pus coming from her incision. The temperature should be taken if a new mother feels hot, dizzy, and weak, aches all over, or simply does not feel well. She should call her doctor if she has a fever; if she does not have a doctor, she should go to the emergency room or urgent care clinic.

   Some women ordinarily have temperatures lower than normal (98.6° F is "normal"), so when they tell a nurse or receptionist what their temperature is, it may seem that they do not really have a fever. It is important to say something such as, "My usual temperature is 97.3°, but now it is 99.0°."

❖ Pain or tenderness in the breast, lower abdomen (uterine infection), side, or in the area of an incision.

❖ Oozing, pus, or dampness in an incision. Women with severe infections of the uterus or surgical incisions may need to return to the hospital for treatment, including drainage of an infected incision, or administration of intravenous fluids and medications.

❖ Discolored, frothy, or bad-smelling lochia or vaginal discharge. These are signs of a uterine infection.

❖ Pain or difficulty in urination.

❖ A red, swollen, discolored, or tender area of the breast that is hot or hard to the touch (this will not feel like engorgement). These are signs of breast infection.

A culture may be done to identify the organism causing the infection so that the appropriate antibiotic can be ordered. The mother will need antibiotics unless her infection is localized and minor. She will also need to rest and drink plenty of fluids. Sometimes a woman will be advised to keep nursing while she has a breast infection. At other times, she may be advised to stop nursing temporarily. Use a breast pump to keep up milk production if you are asked to stop breast-feeding. Severe or repeated breast infections can mean that the mother must stop breast-feeding completely. In this case, women who feel breast-feeding is important can ask their pediatrician for suggestions about cleaning the baby's mouth.

Breast-Feeding

DECIDING WHETHER TO BREAST-FEED

In comparing the advantages and disadvantages of breast-feeding and bottle-feeding, there is no single right choice. In reading about feeding methods and talking to experienced mothers, you are likely to hear some strong opinions on the subject. Many people write and speak as though there is only one correct way to feed a baby, and the entire life of the baby will be affected by the choice. In fact, both breast-fed and bottle-fed babies grow into healthy children and adults. Also, the mother's needs are as much a part of the choice as the baby's needs. It is also important to remember that it may be possible to combine breast-feeding and bottle-feeding, and gain some of the advantages of each method.

ADVANTAGES OF BREAST-FEEDING

There are many advantages to breast-feeding:

- ❖ The baby receives colostrum from his mother's milk during the first few days after birth. The baby will have little appetite, and may only suck 1 or 2 teaspoonfuls at each feeding, but colostrum is quite nutritious. It has more protein and less sugar than breast milk or formula. Moreover, it contains antibodies that help to protect the baby from infection.
- ❖ Breast milk also contains many of the mother's antibodies, which help to protect the baby from infection, especially intestinal infections. This protection is most helpful during the first 6 to 12 months after birth, while the baby is developing the ability to resist infection.
- ❖ Breast milk is more digestible than formula, and allergies to breast milk are extremely rare.
- ❖ The baby's sucking stimulates the release of the hormone oxytocin, which allows the milk to flow more easily. It also stimulates the involution of the uterus during the first few weeks after childbirth.
- ❖ Some studies suggest that breast-feeding may lower the mother's risk of developing breast cancer.
- ❖ Breast-feeding saves money. There is no need to buy bottles, nipples, bottle warmers, formula, and brushes for cleaning bottles and nipples.
- ❖ Women with limited hand control may find it easier to breast-feed than to prepare bottles.
- ❖ Many women feel that breast-feeding is more convenient than bottle-feeding. They do not have to sterilize, fill, and heat bottles, or pack bottles and formula whenever they take the baby out of the house.

Many women get psychological satisfaction from breast-feeding, and enjoy it for a variety of reasons. Sonya, who has a high spinal cord injury, said, "I felt the only way I could bond with my baby was to breast-feed." Nina said, "I had this fixed idea that I should breast-feed. I was up in my wheelchair the same day as I had the C-section because I couldn't breast-feed lying down. It took 2 hours to get me into the wheelchair, crying the whole time." Some women enjoy the fact that they are the only person who can nurse their babies. It makes their relationship with the baby unique. Some women feel that breast-feeding is a sign that their bodies are working properly. Some women like breast-feeding because they feel that it is the most natural way to feed their babies. Others feel very womanly when they breast-feed their babies.

Although breast-feeding allows you to have a special relationship with your new infant, there are discomforts associated with breast-feeding. Luckily, there are ways to handle the discomforts.

Breast Care

Engorgement, infections, and sore or cracked nipples can all cause discomfort during the weeks after birth. There are two types of engorgement. The first is painful swelling caused by changes in the breast when the milk comes in. The second occurs when the breasts become over-filled with milk. This can happen if the baby waits longer than usual between feedings. Pumping or expressing some milk can relieve engorgement. It may be hard for the baby to take the nipple if the breasts are swollen. Try any combination of the following to ease engorgement: express a little milk before feeding the baby, gently tug on the nipple, or roll it between the fingers, so that the nipple takes a shape that fits the baby's mouth. Another way to relieve pain from engorgement is to breast-feed more often, but for shorter periods of time. Start off feeding for 5 minutes on each breast, then build up, so that by the fourth day the baby will be nursing 15 minutes on each side. Ice compresses may also help, though most women prefer moist heat.

A sleepy baby can also cause engorgement. It is perfectly all right to gently awaken a sleeping baby for nursing. It is good for both baby and mother to create a regular schedule. Some babies are difficult to wake up, however. Felicia's baby had a hard time latching on to the breast because he was too sleepy. It is possible that the Vicodin™ and Motrin™ she was taking for pain affected her baby.

Some women may have sore or cracked nipples. The position of the latch is crucial for comfortable nursing. When positioned correctly, the nipple goes deep into the baby's mouth to the junction of the baby's hard and soft palate. Here are some ways to care for the nipples:

Green cabbage: Natasha's nurses told her, "Refrigerate a green cabbage, and then pull a whole leaf from the cold cabbage. Put this leaf in your bra so it is between the breast and your bra. The cabbage has an enzyme that softens the breast." Natasha commented, "My nipple was inverted, but after one week with a cabbage leaf in my bra, my nipple popped out."

Protective cups: Some women like to wear protective cups over their nipples to keep clothing from rubbing their skin. This also protects clothing from stains until leaking stops naturally. Other women find that cups slow down healing by keeping their nipples damp. Cups may be helpful when it is necessary to go out, but at home it is better to wear a nursing bra with the flaps down. Exposing the nipples to the air helps keep them dry and promotes healing. Some women use a heat lamp for short periods of time.

Cracked nipple treatment: A combination of Mupirocin™ 2 percent ointment, Betamethasone™ 0.1 percent ointment, and Miconazole™ 2 percent or Clotrimazole™ 2 percent seem to help with candida, bacterial infections, and some dermatological conditions. Putting olive oil on your nipples is another treatment. Olive oil is an antifungal and basic moisturizer.

Deep breathing: Nursing when your nipples are sore is painful. The worst moment is when the baby "latches on." It helps to take a few deep, relaxing breaths before starting to nurse. Try using the deep breathing techniques of early labor for a minute or so until the pain fades.

Avoiding infection: It is possible to get a breast infection, even when the nipples are not sore. Germs enter more easily if the nipples are cracked. Watch for signs of breast infection if your nipples are cracked, and call the doctor if necessary.

Yeast infection: Medication is usually prescribed for a yeast infection.

THE ART OF BREAST-FEEDING

Breast-feeding can be very enjoyable for mother and baby, once it is an established pattern, but it does not always begin easily and naturally. Your first encounter with the art of breast-feeding will probably include hospital staff, some of whom may be knowledgeable about nursing, but they might not understand your special needs. Joan knew that she needed to adapt the nursing position from what she had been shown, but her nurse was not supportive in finding different positions that would work for Joan. After she went home from the hospital, Joan found that she could be successful nursing on her side (Figure 13-1).

Nina felt that breast-feeding was the one thing that she could do for her baby that no one else could do. She said, "I was so stressed, and so scared, that I think it was hard for my milk to come in. Then, because my milk did not come in, my baby cried all day and all night with only an occasional 5-minute break. He cried for 3 days. The nurse tried pumping my breast to the point of bleeding. It was really horrible. They gave him formula. He slept and I slept. I think that helped. Afterwards, my milk came in."

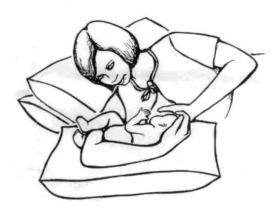

FIGURE 13-1   Side position for breast-feeding.

It can take several weeks for milk flow to become reliable and for the mother and baby to create a comfortable routine. Getting started may be frustrating at times, but a little patience at the beginning can be the start of a precious experience lasting for months or even years. One way to help your milk flow is to give yourself a break for a couple feedings during a day or two by having someone else give your baby a bottle. This break may give you time to sleep or rest so your milk can come in.

Here are some tips for successful breast-feeding:

Choose a comfortable brassiere: Some women prefer brassieres with flaps that can be lowered. (Note that women with limited hand control need flaps that fasten with Velcro™ rather than hooks.) Others prefer elastic athletic bras that can be pulled up and down over the breast. Your preference might change as time passes. An occupational therapist can help you make the best choice. Some women with both large breasts and TOS have found it difficult to find a comfortable bra. (The Bravado nursing/maternity bra is supportive and it feels comfortable, although it is hard to get on over the head. It does not dig into the shoulders.) Tina could not find an appropriate bra. Her solution was to have a friend adapt her regular bras for nursing.

Help the baby: Some babies need help in finding the nipple. Gently brush the nipple against the baby's cheek, and she will turn toward it. This is called *rooting*. Sometimes patience is needed, and if you let your baby root she will find the nipple on her own. The nipple and the areola (the dark area around the nipple) should be in the baby's mouth. Women with unusually large areolas may not be able to get the whole areola into the baby's mouth.

Women with large breasts may need to hold part of the breast away from the baby's face so the baby can breathe. The baby may stop after just a few sucks to breathe. In this case, you will want to hold the breast away from the baby's nose. Pressing on the breast to keep it away from the nose may cause the nipple to rub on the roof of the baby's mouth which may cause a blister on the nipple. A good technique to help keep the nose clear is to have the mom press the baby's hips close to the body. Women who do not have enough hand control to hold the breast can try cutting off the tip of the brassiere cup so that the areola is exposed, but the rest of the breast is held away from the baby's face.

Women with smaller breasts often find breast-feeding easier. Nancy commented, "I think my small breasts were an asset. My baby didn't have any trouble finding the nipple and clamping on by herself." Very young babies need to have their heads supported. You can support the baby's head by holding it in the crook of your arm. There are alternatives to the baby lying on your arm if you have a repetitive stress injury. Try using a pillow that is high enough to rest the baby's head on, and that allows the baby to easily reach the nipple and areola.

Find at least one comfortable position for nursing: For mothers who have had a caesarean section, the weight of the baby on the incision can cause pain. A new mother may experience so much pain and loss of mobility that she feels unable to hold her baby. Stephanie felt that her difficulty in finding a comfortable position was the most important problem to solve. She explained, "There really wasn't a comfortable position because I was in pain from the C-section and it made me less mobile."

Although Shelby did not have a caesarean, she also had difficulty in finding a comfortable position. She said, "It was difficult to get into positions that would be comfortable for me and the baby. I had a problem with both lying down and sitting up. I found out my milk flowed more easily when I was sitting rather then lying, but when I tried to breast-feed in my chair there were stresses and strains on my muscles. It was exhausting to hold up both my body and the baby's body at the same time. I had problems with my own trunk balance and finding a comfortable position for the baby. It was more challenging to sit up as the baby got heavier, because I still had to support my baby during breast-feeding. When I held myself up on my elbows, my baby was a counter pull on my body. My trunk wanted to come forward, but at the same time my child would also pull me forward. This was an immense amount of counterweight that I was not used to. It was like carrying a sack of potatoes. The result was my neck and shoulders hurt immensely." Fortunately, since the time when Shelby was nursing, there has been an increase in the types of commercially available nursing pillows. These pillows support the baby in a good nursing position.

The new mother, regardless of her disability, will probably need extra help soon after delivery, because many new mothers have problems holding and nursing their babies. Finding a comfortable position is a trial and error process. It may be best to get help from a lactation specialist.

Positioning the baby: It is important to change the baby's position slightly at each feeding so that a different part of the nipple gets the pressure from sucking; for example, prop the baby's pillow a little higher or lower. Some women prefer to use the "football hold" when the baby is nursing (in this position the baby remains facing in the same direction on both breasts). Thus, for example, the baby's feet point to the right when nursing at both breasts. Sonya said, "I would go to bed at 10 and start out lying on my left side to nurse the baby. Then I would wake up around 2 and holler for my husband, who has to sleep on the couch now. He would come in and roll me to the other side so I could continue nursing the baby. At 6 my attendant would come in and roll me to the other side, and I would switch the baby again. I switched sides about every 3 to 4 hours."

Some of the other interviewees also got help from nurses or attendants. Nancy said, "I needed help getting the baby into the right position on a pillow so she could find the nipple. Sometimes it was difficult to find the right position, and that was frustrating." Arlene's nurses also helped her find a way to use pillows to support her child while nursing. Christina's home health worker helped her experiment with different positions."

Other women struggled on their own. Clara commented, "It wasn't until I got home from the hospital that I found a really comfortable position for nursing. It was 3 days after delivery! I really needed an armchair with pillows supporting my baby to be successful." Many women find that sitting in an armchair or reclining chair is helpful, because the furniture supports their arms while they hold the baby. A footstool or recliner also helps with relaxing.

Many women feel it works well to lie on their sides with their babies lying beside them, possibly supported by pillows. Oprah said, "Lying on my side was especially helpful when the babies got bigger." Nancy found this position helpful when she went back to the hospital with an infection in her incision. When her baby came to her room, she could just turn on her side to nurse. Jennifer said it worked well to sleep with her baby because "when he woke up, I was able to turn over to give him a breast. It was a real energy saver."

But, for others, side-lying was difficult. Heather said, "I couldn't lay down and nurse him because I'm not balanced; I could roll over and fall on him. It meant I had to get up and sit with him in the middle of the night." Clara said, "I tried to nurse on my side, but it gave me a terrible backache."

Make sure there is a large glass or even a pitcher of water nearby before settling down to feed the baby: It is common for women to begin feeling thirsty a few minutes after they start feeding the baby. This reminds them of the importance of drinking plenty of fluids.

Releasing the nipple: When the baby is finished nursing, place a finger in the corner of the baby's mouth to release the suction on the nipple. Alternatively, the baby may spit the nipple out. If the baby lets go suddenly, or if the mother removes the breast without releasing suction first, the pull can be painful. It is important to let the baby finish the first breast. You can tell that the breast is empty because it will become softer, and the amount of fat in the milk will increase. After burping, the baby may or may not want the second breast.

Alternate breasts: A typical feeding will usually last 20 minutes. It is a good idea to empty one breast and then the other one. Alternate the breast used to begin each feeding. If one nipple is sorer than the other, or only one nipple is cracked, pump milk from the affected breast and let the baby nurse on the other side. Felicia found breast shields helped her cracked nipples.

DISADVANTAGES OF BREAST-FEEDING

Many women feel tied down by breast-feeding, especially during the first weeks of the baby's life, when they must nurse the baby every 2 hours. For newborns, the time between feedings may be only $1\frac{1}{2}$ hours.

Breast-feeding is quite demanding, and many women become exhausted when they must wake up for frequent night feedings. To assure that you have enough milk, do not nurse less than "eight times in each 24-hour period during the early days" (102).

Felicia felt she did not have enough milk. Her sister-in-law told her to take fenugreek, eat oatmeal, and to continue pumping. She said, "Eating oatmeal coupled with fenugreek seemed to be a good combination. I feel that the fenugreek really helped."

A German Commission E monograph recommends a daily intake of 6 grams of fenugreek. The suggested dosage is: 2 to 4 capsules, 3 times a day. Most capsules are 580 mg to 610 mg each. Some of the potential side effects of fenugreek are (103):

* Sweat and urine smells like maple syrup (this is common, and often a sign that you have reached the right dose).
* Loose stools that go away when fenugreek is discontinued.
* Hypoglycemia in some mothers.
* Can cause uterine contractions—do not use fenugreek if you are pregnant.

❖ Diabetic mothers should use fenugreek with caution, because it can lower blood glucose levels.

Many partners (and sometimes other family members) feel left out when they cannot help to feed the baby. There are other ways of bonding, however, such as bathing, dressing, and playing with the baby.

The mother may have to alter her diet. Occasionally the baby will have an allergic reaction to something the mother has eaten. In this case, the mother should try eliminating different items from her diet until the baby stops reacting. This process can be frustrating, and it is a real problem if the baby reacts to an important or favorite food.

For some women, it is stressful to plan a diet that includes all the nutrients needed for breast-feeding. After 9 months of pregnancy, it can be difficult for some women to continue to watch their diets closely.

Others feel concerned about losing weight. For example, a woman whose knees or ankles became more painful when she gained weight may want to lose it as quickly as possible. Fortunately, some women are able to lose weight while eating an adequate diet.

Breast-feeding can also interfere with a couple's sexual relationship, especially during the early weeks, when the baby nurses frequently. The parents may be interrupted when the baby wakes up, or they may feel inhibited because they worry that the baby might wake up at any moment. They may also be too tired to make love.

Prolactin—the hormone that stimulates milk production—causes the vaginal walls to become thinner and drier, affecting sexuality. The change in the vagina may make intercourse uncomfortable. Lubricants make intercourse less painful, although some couples are not comfortable with this solution.

Some women are embarrassed when their breasts leak and stain their clothing. Leaking stops after the first 2 or 3 months, but the wait may be too long for women who are easily embarrassed, or who must return to work after 6 weeks. Breast pads or shields may be used, but they are not always a good solution, because dampness can make the nipples uncomfortable.

Some women feel uncomfortable nursing in public. Others must cope with disapproval even when they are discreet.

Continuing to breast-feed after returning to work is not impossible, although some women find that their breasts simply stop producing milk if they wait too long between feedings. Some women are able to pump or manually express milk during breaks at work, but others are not. Not every workplace has a refrigerator where expressed milk can be stored. Some women use insulated bags to store their breast milk.

Factors Related to Disability

Disability can influence a woman's decision about how she will feed her baby. It is not always obvious which choice will be best for a woman with a particular disability. For example, women who have myasthenia gravis carry an antibody called *anti-acetyl-*

cholinesterase that can reach levels high enough to enter their milk and affect their babies. These women need to be tested to determine whether it is safe for them to breast-feed.

You may have to check further than your doctor for accurate information if you want to breast-feed. Nadia said, "During the last month of my pregnancy, I was under the impression that I would be unable to breast-feed. Then, 5 days after delivery, the doctors changed their minds and told me it would be okay to nurse."

Women with disabilities need to consider the following factors:

Exacerbation of disability: Although breast-feeding does not directly affect disability, it must be remembered that breast-feeding can be tiring. Women with disabilities that are exacerbated by fatigue such as SLE, MS, and myasthenia gravis, should stop breast-feeding if it becomes too tiring. Nadia's milk dried up at $5^{1}/_{2}$ months because of a myasthenia crisis. Stopping breast-feeding abruptly can cause postpartum depression, so taper off slowly. It is important to only stop one feeding at a time. You should drop a feeding no more often than every 4 to 5 days. For most mothers and babies the easiest feedings to drop are those in the middle of the day.

In a study of breast-feeding mothers with multiple sclerosis, the exacerbation rate was 38 percent; the exacerbation rate in non-breast-feeding mothers was 31 percent (104). A 1998 study found that breast-feeding did not increase the risk of relapse or of worsening disability in the postpartum period (20).

Women with MS also have concerns about avoiding fatigue and risking a flare-up of symptoms. Mary commented, "I didn't even try to nurse. My neurologist didn't think it would be a good idea." Margie said, "I nursed my first, but I bottle-fed my second because I needed the rest." She added that if she could make the decision again, she would have bottle-fed her first child. Michelle suggested a compromise: "When your milk is established, let someone else bottle-feed the baby at night so you can sleep. You can stop after the first few months because by then the baby has gotten the most benefit." Still, Michelle stressed the need to protect the mother's health. When she was asked how she would advise new mothers, she said, "Minimize breast-feeding. I thought it would be easy—a piece of cake. But I would get tired out and my milk supply would drop. I let myself get over-tired, and in the long run that didn't help the baby." There is no evidence that breast-feeding can cause an exacerbation of disability, but there is some evidence that being fatigued can cause an exacerbation.

A study by the University of Manchester in Manchester, England found that women with rheumatoid arthritis may have postpartum flare-ups. This is probably due to the increase of the milk-stimulating hormone prolactin. The researchers believe that "exposure to high levels of prolactin unaccompanied by correspondingly high levels of anti-inflammatory steroids could stimulate the development of RA in susceptible women" (105).

Joan went through 2 weeks of a flare-up before she gave up nursing. She said, "I needed to take the pills so I could play and interact with her." Joy, on the other hand, found that nursing did not exacerbate her symptoms.

According to the National Institute of Health, women with lupus may want to bottle-feed:

"Breast-feeding may not always be possible [for women with lupus] for the following reasons:

❖ A premature baby may not be able to suck adequately. Feeding your baby through a tube at first and then by bottle may be necessary. You may still be able to pump breast milk for your baby.

❖ You may not be able to produce enough milk if you are taking corticosteroids.

❖ Some medications can pass through your breast milk to your infant. It will be up to your doctor to decide whether breast-feeding is safe if you are taking any of these medications. Breast-feeding can be tiring, because breast-fed infants tend to eat more frequently than do bottle-fed infants. You may want to switch to a bottle and formula if breast-feeding becomes too tiring. Be confident that whichever method you choose to use to feed your baby, it will be the right decision for everyone concerned" (106).

It is not always obvious which choice a woman with a particular disability will chose. For example, Stacy and Sylvia are both quadriplegic, but they made different choices. Stacy felt breast-feeding would be too difficult. Sylvia said, "I was going to nurse come hell or high water. At first, looked like I might not be able to because I had inverted nipples, but I did!"

Commonly reported breast-feeding discomforts for nursing mothers are engorgement, infection, and the "let-down" reflex.

Breast-feeding may cause dysreflexia because it can be painful. Dysreflexia can be triggered by any physical discomfort. Therefore, women who have a spinal cord injury at T6 or above should be aware of any dysreflexia symptoms, and seek their doctor's advice about continuing to nurse. Sweating, hot flashes, and spasms are signs of dysreflexia.

Both Shelby and Sonya had dysreflexia when they breast-fed. Sonya said, "For the first 5 minutes during the first month, my nipples were really sore, and I could hardly stand the pain. When he first latched on, it caused me to spasm really hard. My husband would have to hold my arms until I relaxed so I wouldn't hurt the baby."

Women with a high spinal cord injury may have difficulty nursing because they do not produce enough breast milk. Having a limited milk supply may be due to the lack of sensation. Selina has a spinal cord injury at T4, and researched this topic. She thought it was important to nurse her children, but found she needed to supplement nursing with bottles because each of her babies stopped gaining weight. She found both the lactation specialist and the doctors were uninformed. Selina said, "My babies do well the first 2 weeks after birth. In fact, medically speaking, babies are supposed to return back to their birth weight by the time they are 2 weeks. Mine not only returned to their birth weight, but also superseded that weight. My milk tends to come in on the third or the fourth day like it is supposed to. I do feel definite fullness and tingling in my breasts. After a couple more days my breasts soften, and I just don't seem to have as much milk. The most important thing is that my babies have never lost weight. I never let it get to that point. We bought a baby scale, and if they didn't gain weight after 4 or 5 days I gave them a supplemental bottle. This usually happened by 6 weeks postpartum." When her fifth baby was $4\frac{1}{2}$ weeks old, Selina tried using an electric breast pump between feedings. Selina said, "The baby doesn't seem to be satisfied until I give her the supplemental breast milk in a bottle. I'm on Reglan™ right now. It is a drug used for stomach problems, but they found by doing research that it actually increases prolactin levels. But the problem I'm having with Reglan™ is it causes drowsiness." Selina found she had less milk when she stopped taking Reglan™. She said, "Breast-feeding is one of the most wonderful experiences of motherhood. Even though paralysis prevented me from providing all the milk my babies needed to thrive, I still believe there are many benefits to nursing beyond the nutrition aspect. I 'comfort nursed' my babies as long as they would let me. There is something about that closeness, skin to skin, that a pacifier cannot give."

Sydney has a T4/5 spinal cord injury with sensation above her right nipple and below her left nipple. She was able to nurse from only her left breast. She said, "My milk dried up in my right breast and shrank back to normal 2 to 3 weeks after delivery." Not all women who have spinal cord injuries and/or breast reduction experienced limited milk supply. According to *Disability Pregnancy & Parenthood International* (107), one woman who was a T-4/5 was successful in breast-feeding her twins. She said, "'I read that women with lesions above T4 might experience difficulty because the stimulus/response mechanism might be interrupted. I am a T4/5 and have little sensation in my right nipple. I couldn't always tell if the baby was latched on. I had to look to see if she was attached; my milk flow was unaffected.'"

Women who have had a breast reduction may also have difficulty with breast-feeding because innervations (nerve connections) may be disrupted (108).

Taryn Dion found that she did not produce much milk. She wasn't sure if it was due to her breast reduction or her baby being born prematurely.

Medication: Not all medications enter the milk and affect the baby, and those that do may not be concentrated enough to affect the baby. Research has identified the medications that are able to enter breast milk (see OTIS in Appendix D).

Of those medications that do enter breast milk, some cause only temporary problems. For example, if a woman develops a bladder infection, her doctor may be able to prescribe an antibiotic that is safe for the baby. The baby might have diarrhea temporarily, which would require giving the baby extra fluids and changing more diapers. This might be a problem for a severely disabled woman.

Other medications are dangerous for the baby, and the mother will have to bottle-feed her baby if a safer substitute is not available. There are some medications that must be resumed after delivery of the baby. Charlotte said, "I breast-fed for a week, then it was too much. I couldn't handle the spasms anymore. After a week, I went back on baclofen and stopped breast-feeding." Charlotte could have switched from taking baclofen in pill form to the pump, because baclofen does not cross the milk barrier when using a pump.

Mimi loves to breast-feed. She said, "I would be disappointed if I had to stop breast-feeding. I would like to do it for a year, but I may not be able to. Betaseron® is important for maintaining my health, but Betaseron® byproducts can get into the breast milk, and I don't want to risk my daughter's immune system." Initially, Mimi decided not to take Betaseron®, and she continued nursing. She said, "I learned from being a participant in a study that examined the effects of breast-feeding on MS that breast-feeding may protect against an exacerbation. So, I hope my physician will continue to support my decision to breast-feed." Mimi was still not taking any medication for her MS when her baby was 8 months old.

Moira was unable to breast-feed because there is no information on the effect of I.V.I.G. (intravenous immunoglobulin) on the baby.

OTHER LIMITATION ISSUES

Women with limited mobility can have other problems. Clara needed to have her husband bring the baby to her at night, because keeping her balance was difficult when she awoke from sleeping. If Clara had been a single parent, she might have needed to find an alternative to breast-feeding at night—perhaps giving the baby formula at bedtime so the baby would sleep through the night. Some bottle-fed babies do not sleep through the night, and their mothers have the same problem as Pam, who said, "It was difficult to find a position I could nurse in."

Amanda tried nursing for 5 days. She said, "It was the most horrible experience on earth. I had severe back pain. I tried all the positions as well as the different types of nursing pillows, but nothing worked." Amanda's babies also had difficulty latching on. One technique to help with latching onto the breast is: 1) place the infant in a good position on the breast; 2) give the infant a finger to suck on; and 3) after the infant is sucking the finger, switch to the breast.

Tina found that it was easier for her baby to latch on if she expressed a little milk before nursing. She also found that the baby would latch on successfully if she squeezed her nipple with two fingers in a downward direction and put the nipple toward the roof of the baby's mouth.

Selina found that the football hold worked well, because she has large breasts and numb hands. Naomi experienced difficulty when she breast-fed because of carpal tunnel. Her hands would go numb from supporting her baby's head with her hands. She said, "A lactation specialist told me to keep my wrist straight because this would help reduce the numbness. But that position was difficult to maintain because I had weakness in my fingers."

Taryn Dion found that using a breast pump aggravated her disability because holding the breast pump caused problems. Moreover, the vibration from the pump also caused problems. Assistive devices can be helpful. There is a bra made by Medela™ that has an attached pump, allowing the hands to be free. (Fine motor ability is necessary to attach the pump to the bra.) It is important to try different nursing pillows so you can find the best one to suit your needs. The La Leche League can give you recommendations on the many different types of pillows that are available.

Tina found a pillow at a back store that is in the shape of a "V" to support her baby's head, instead of her arms doing the job. She said, "The pillow was like a brace that held the baby in place." Tessa found that some of the contoured nursing pillows brought her arms up too high, causing more pain. Tessa also found that gazing at her baby during nursing caused pain. Tessa has better eye contact with her baby during other activities, such as diapering.

Women who are interested in breast-feeding, but who are worried about physical limitations, should first try breast-feeding. Changing from breast to bottle- feeding is easier than changing from bottle to breast-feeding.

Naomi had difficulty using a breast pump "because the vibration from the pump affected my hands." She was able to successfully breast-feed her second child for $4\frac{1}{2}$ months. She said, "I had carpal tunnel, but not as bad as the first time. The truth is that I was not that committed to breast-feeding. It's difficult to do it when you are out and about, especially when positioning is so important for comfort. It hurt my hands and arms if I didn't have a comfy armchair and nursing pillow. Also, my first child would get jealous and act out. I have seen other mothers read a book to the older child or somehow keep them entertained while breast-feeding an infant, but again, it was difficult for me because of carpal tunnel and weakened limbs in general. Bottles were faster and easier to manipulate. Also, pumping isn't pleasant at all. Once I stopped beating myself up about it, bottles and formula worked great for my family. My husband could feed the baby, and I didn't feel like I was missing out on time with my first child."

Infant Problems with Breast-feeding

Breast-feeding is not possible in some cases. For example, it can be difficult or impossible to breast-feed if the baby is hospitalized. The baby may be in isolation, or may be too weak to suck. Sometimes the baby is bottle-fed, and the mother can pump her breast milk for bottle-feeding, but the fatigue and stress of having a sick baby may interfere with milk production. The baby may have a cleft palate, which will interfere with sucking.

The baby may have a metabolic problem such as *phenylketonuria* (PKU). This condition is caused by an inability to digest the amino acid *phenylalanine*. All babies will have a blood test to detect PKU before leaving the hospital. Babies with PKU must go on special diets, or chemicals from incompletely digested phenylalanine will cause brain damage. These babies cannot nurse because breast milk contains phenylalanine. Occasionally, babies develop jaundice in response to a hormone in the mother's milk. Sometimes it is possible to solve this problem by giving babies water every day for several days, but sometimes the only solution is to stop breast-feeding.

Combining Breast- and Bottle-Feeding

For some women, the best approach is to combine feeding methods in some way, such as breast-feeding at first, then changing to bottle-feeding. This approach gives the baby the benefits of the immunity protection in breast milk, but delays the risk of an allergic reaction to formula. A second approach is to give both breast-feeding and bottle-feeding every day. This approach suits the needs of women who want to have the psychological benefits of breast-feeding, but need to avoid physical stress.

Consider formula feedings if you are feeling tired and overwhelmed, or your baby is not getting enough fluids. You can supplement breast-feeding by giving the baby a little sugar water, formula, or Gripe™, but be sure to nurse the baby at the next feeding so your milk production continues to be stimulated.

There are some disadvantages to bottle-feeding. Although some babies easily adjust to formula, others may react with an upset stomach, constipation, diarrhea, or diaper rash. A baby may be allergic to one or more types of formula, and it may be necessary to try several different formulas in order to find one that does not cause problems.

Many babies fall asleep sucking the bottle. Sleeping with the nipple in the baby's mouth causes formula to pool against the teeth, and the sugars in the formula can cause tooth decay. This problem is avoidable. If the bottle is left in the crib at night or during naptime it can be filled with water.

Sometimes women are advised to wait 6 weeks before introducing the bottle, so the baby will have time to become attached to the breast. Some babies, however, become so attached to the breast that they will not take a bottle. They seem to be bothered by the unfamiliar taste of the nipple or the formula. On the other hand, if women start bottle-feeding too soon, it may be more difficult for them to start regular milk production. They could have problems with engorgement, or trouble producing enough milk. Early on, babies are more likely to prefer the bottle because it is much easier to suck milk from the bottle. The baby may even start to reject the breast before the mother feels ready to stop nursing!

Clara had both experiences: "My first baby was so used to the breast that she just wouldn't take the bottle. It was too much trouble to fight with her, so she was completely breast-fed till she started solid foods. It was the opposite with my second baby. I thought I'd try giving him a bottle so my husband or the babysitter could feed him. After that, it was a struggle to get him to take the breast."

The baby may strongly prefer the bottle if you nurse infrequently. Wait a few days before replacing another feeding. The change from breast- to bottle-feeding needs to be gradual so the breasts and hormones will have time to adapt. After a month of breast-feeding, add only 1 to 2 bottles a day.

Bottle-feeding

Some of the advantages of bottle-feeding are related to the disadvantages of breast-feeding. At the beginning of breast-feeding, most mothers may experience discomforts such as sore nipples, or possibly breast infections and engorgement. Generally these problems are alleviated after the first couple of weeks. Another advantage of bottle-feeding is that others can do one or more of the night feedings.

Portia said, "Being disabled, I didn't need the extra burden of nursing a baby. Bottles were much easier." Bottle-feeding gives the mother more freedom and flexibility than breast-feeding. This is important because the mother can rest while other people feed the baby. Bottle-feeding can also be helpful for women who do not have flexible work schedules.

One advantage of formula is that is digested more slowly, which helps the baby sleep better. This is not an advantage if the baby is bothered by indigestion.

Prevention of Fatigue

Many women will not be able to choose a feeding method in advance, because the reality of caring for a baby is never the same as what they expected. Celeste commented, "I thought my problem would be carrying the baby, and that nursing would be easy. Nursing turned out to be a problem, too."

For some women, the physical demands of milk production, and holding the baby for every feeding, are too wearing. Night feedings can be difficult. Women who want to bottle-feed at night no longer have to get out of bed to get a bottle, because they can use Around the Clock™, a product that is kept on the bed stand. Around the Clock™ keeps the bottle cool until it needs to be warmed, and then warms it as needed.

Women who have difficulty holding a bottle can purchase baby bottles and bottle holders that enable the baby to drink without the bottle being held. This allows the mother to concentrate on finding a comfortable position to hold her baby.

BURPING TECHNIQUE

Whether they breast-feed or bottle-feed, most women with disabilities need a technique to help burp the baby. The over-the-shoulder burping position can be difficult or even impossible for many mothers with a disability because it requires muscle strength and coordination. This is a task that generally requires two arms. There are alternative positions and methods that are particularly useful for mothers who cannot reposition or bring their babies up on their shoulders for burping. TLG recommends the following "Sit & Lean" technique for burping:

The mother holds the baby on her lap, and faces the baby away from her body. Supporting the baby by placing one arm across the baby's chest, the mother then leans forward. This puts pressure on the baby's stomach and facilitates a burp (109).

Another technique that has been successful is to lay the baby across the mother's lap and pat the baby's back. Lay the baby on its right side and rolled slightly onto the mother's tummy.

There are also drops that help the baby produce a burp, which are manufactured under the trade names Mylicon™ and Gerber™.

Emotional Changes

The birth of a child is a major change in the life of the family. Relationships between the parents, and among parents, grandparents, and other family members, all change with the birth. Relationships with friends also change. Friends who already have children welcome the new parents into the club; childless friends worry that the new parents will talk about nothing but diapers and formula. The parents must adjust to a new identity and new responsibilities.

During the postpartum period there are many emotional changes, but this portion of the book will only focus on two major emotional changes: mood and the sexual relationship.

Mood Changes

Quite often, the first few weeks after birth are an emotional roller coaster. There are times when the new mother is filled with love and joy over the birth of her baby, and times when she is tired, frustrated, and depressed. Stacy recalled, "I felt so overwhelmed that I cried for the first 6 weeks. Then I felt better." It is so common for women to feel weepy and frustrated during the postpartum period that there is even a nickname for this feeling—the "baby blues."

It is important to remember that there are several physical reasons for the feelings that occur during the postpartum period. Besides lack of sleep, there are other discomforts that can wear down the resilience of new mothers, including sore nipples or strong afterpains. Changing hormone levels can also cause unpredictable mood swings.

It is a good idea to find ways to meet other new parents, perhaps by staying in touch with friends from birthing class, joining a parents' group at a community center, or starting a playgroup. You may be able to find solutions by sharing your feelings with other parents.

TLG has set up a parent-to-parent network for parents with disabilities under a grant from the National Institute for Disability Rehabilitation and Research, (which is under the U.S. Department of Education). This network has been matching parents up across the country since 1998. Hopefully, TLG will continue to have this service for many years to come (see Through the Looking Glass in Appendix D).

Physician T. Berry Brazelton has pointed out that it may be hard for parents to admit their most painful feeling—disappointment in the baby (110). Parents who visualized a soft, cuddly baby may be disappointed in their wriggly live wire. On the other hand, high-energy parents may feel irritated by a placid, sleepy baby. They may worry or feel guilty about their reaction until they have had time to learn to appreciate their baby's own unique individuality.

Some of the interviewees were disappointed by their first experiences of motherhood. Patricia said, "It wasn't exactly what it was cracked up to be." No matter how hard parents try to be realistic before the baby is born, it may come as a shock that it can be weeks before the baby even recognizes them. This problem, too, diminishes as time passes.

Marsha and Sharon were troubled by changes in their relationships. Marsha said, "It was difficult to relate to my husband as a lover, and embrace my new role as a mother at the same time. It was hard to switch between the two. It took several months to fuse both roles." Sharon was not married, and her child's father was not sure he wanted to continue the relationship. She said, "It was nerve-racking to think about it." Parent support groups may be helpful for couples whose relationships are troubled. Some parents find that professional counseling helps them adjust to their new situation.

Sometimes the new parents fear that the responsibility will be more than they can handle. Christina said, "I was overwhelmed at the hospital. But, the staff taught me to take care of the baby, so when I went home I wasn't really depressed." Other women feel comfortable in the hospital, where they have help, but become overwhelmed when they go home and are alone with the baby. Often, having someone come into the home to help with the baby makes the transition easier. The emotional support is as important as the practical support. Sharon recalled, "My mother came and stayed for a month. It really lifted my spirits. She helped me in an all-around, general way."

New mothers may feel sad about other changes in their lives. They may miss the freedom they had before they had to worry about babysitters and feeding schedules. They may even miss the way they looked before childbirth changed their bodies.

Sometimes new parents feel guilty about their negative feelings. They believe it is wrong to resent the baby for waking them up at night. Talking with other parents who obviously love their children can be helpful in coping with feelings of guilt and anger.

Finally, parents may be upset by worries about the baby. Even the healthiest baby can catch a cold, develop a rash, or cry for long periods of time, no matter what the parents do to comfort it. First-time parents can be the most upset. Cheryl said, "It was worse with the first one because I didn't know what to expect. With the second one, I was too busy to stop and think or feel." Women with disabilities may be even more frightened by any hint that something is wrong; for example, Carla, who said that she worried unnecessarily that minor symptoms were signs of disability.

Some women with disabilities do have babies with health problems, and concern for their babies adds to the emotional and physical pressures they feel. Their doctors and some hospital staff (for example, the hospital social worker) can help them contact organizations that provide information and support for parents of ill children.

For most women, the "baby blues" gradually disappear. Their hormones return to normal; they start getting more sleep; and they find ways of handling the changes in their lives. Some women develop more serious problems, however. They do not experience simple, temporary depression, but rather have *postpartum depression*. The "baby blues" should last only a couple of weeks. If the symptoms persist longer, it could indicate something more serious.

Postpartum depression is not always easy to recognize. Clara told us, "I read about postpartum depression some years after I had my first child, and many of the symptoms were just what I went through. At the same time, I learned I had a thyroid problem. I now know that hormonal problems can cause postpartum depression. I think I had postpartum depression and nobody recognized it at the time." Although a thyroid blood screening is now being done routinely during pregnancy, it should also be rechecked during the postpartum period.

No one should look at a list of symptoms and try to self-diagnose. If you experienced a depression before pregnancy, you are at a 30 percent higher risk for a postpartum depression (111). A woman can have one or two of the symptoms on the list below and not have postpartum depression. Another woman might experience symptoms that are not included in this list. A woman who is experiencing many of these symptoms, or other disturbing feelings, needs to tell her doctor. Someone who has postpartum depression may have trouble recognizing symptoms, or may not be able to bring herself to see her doctor. It is important to have someone close to her encourage her, or insist that she seek help.

The most important symptom of depression is sleep disturbance (other than waking to feed the baby at night). It is important to get five consecutive nights of sleep. One type of sleep disturbance is *initial insomnia*. In this case, you are not able to fall asleep when you first go to bed. If it takes more than half an hour to fall asleep, and the problem lasts longer than a month, or gets worse over time, it is insomnia.

Middle insomnia is more difficult to recognize because mothers are often awakened by their babies. Middle insomnia may be the problem if the baby is sleeping through the night, yet you often wake up for no reason, and then it takes more than half an hour to go back to sleep. Again, this would not happen just once or twice; it would be insomnia if the problem goes on for more than a month or grows worse over time. *Early insomnia* is insomnia that occurs early in the morning before your usual time for awakening.

It is a good idea to call the doctor if sleep disturbances are a problem, either alone or in combination with any of these symptoms:

❖ A feeling of being flooded with too many thoughts, as if your mind is going all the time and cannot stop.

❖ A sense of foreboding, that is, a constant feeling that something bad is about to happen. Feeling extremely depressed or wishing you were dead. Feeling a sense of hopelessness. Feelings of extreme shame—either feeling ashamed for no reason, or feeling ashamed about something that is usually just slightly embarrassing.

❖ Feeling unreasonably anxious or fearful about the baby. Clara said, "One of the reasons I think I had postpartum depression is that I worried much too much about my baby. I kept waking up at night to check my baby's breathing. I was sure I'd find her dead of SIDS." This may be considered a symptom of *postpartum panic*—a category of postpartum disorders.

❖ Excessive euphoria—exaggerated feelings of happiness. Extreme euphoria is not the usual joy people feel the first time the baby laughs or sits up. With extreme euphoria, the mother is so excited that she is too disorganized to take care of the baby. She may forget to feed the baby or change the diapers.

❖ Hearing a voice no one else hears, or seeing something no one else sees. If this happens, even once, it is important to see a doctor.

❖ An urge to hurt yourself or your baby. Many new parents will say something like, "When the baby wakes me up at night for the fifth time, I want to throw it out the window." But they know they do not really mean what they are saying. If you feel as though you might actually hurt yourself or the baby, call your doctor immediately.

A woman with symptoms of postpartum depression may need to see a psychiatrist. Some symptoms may be more obvious than others. At first, the woman and her doctor may think she simply has ordinary "baby blues." You should see a psychiatrist, however, if you do not feel comforted by your doctor's reassurances, or if you have severe symptoms such as hearing voices. It is important to see a psychiatrist rather than a psychologist or counselor, because a psychiatrist is also a medical doctor, and there may be a physical cause for the problem. Results from a pilot study suggest that low levels of estrogen may cause postpartum depression. The study also found that "estrogen replacement therapy may result in resolution of psychotic symptoms" (112). Although estrogen is not regarded as the sole treatment for postpartum mood disorders, it shows much promise. On the other hand, Depo-Provera™ may trigger postpartum depression. Unlike many other forms of birth control, which have both estrogen and progesterone components, Depo-Provera™ contains only progesterone and may adversely affect hormone balance during the postpartum period.

The psychiatrist may need to work with other specialists. Laura told us she suffered a severe depression after she gave birth. She assumed SLE caused the depression, and this may have been the case. A psychiatrist might have worked with Laura's rheumatologist to determine whether she was suffering from SLE (lupus) symptoms or postpartum depression.

THE SEXUAL RELATIONSHIP

Having a baby changes the marital relationship, including the sexual relationship. These changes can be positive if the new parents work together to solve their problems with creativity and patience.

Some couples feel that their sexual relationship begins to change during pregnancy; others feel that the change begins with the birth of their child. Since many couples continue making love even during the last weeks of pregnancy, the need to avoid intercourse during the weeks after birth can be a dramatic change. For some couples, waiting to make love is not difficult, at least for the first few weeks. Often the parents are tired from taking care of the baby, or from being awakened at night, so they are more interested in sleep than sex.

Sometimes, people unconsciously believe that their sex lives will go back to normal after a certain date. For example, if the mother's doctor tells her to wait for 6 weeks, she and her husband may believe that after exactly 42 days they will start making love as freely as ever. They may be disappointed if these expectations are not met.

Some common difficulties have simple solutions:

❖ One or both partners may feel deprived of affection when they cannot make love. It is important to find time to express affection in other ways, such as cuddling, kissing, and setting aside time to talk with each other.

❖ Reduce sexual frustration by caressing each other without having intercourse.

❖ Be aware that intercourse may be painful for the woman. The first attempts at intercourse must be slow and gentle if the woman has had an episiotomy. Wait a few days and try again if she is too sore. Marsha commented, "My episiotomy interfered with lovemaking at first because it wasn't healed, but when enough time passed, there was no problem."

❖ Many women find that kissing and caressing for a long time before beginning intercourse increases natural lubrication. Lubricants such as K-Y Jelly® are also helpful. Women who are breast-feeing may also find intercourse uncomfortable. As discussed previously, this type of discomfort is caused by hormonal changes.

❖ Often women who are breast-feeding do not want their husbands to kiss or caress their breasts. Even when their nipples are no longer sore, they may feel that after having their breasts handled by the baby all day they just want to be left alone. Try to have a positive outlook, and take the opportunity to look for sensitive areas you have not discovered before—perhaps the ear lobes, the nape of the neck, or the inner thighs.

❖ If one partner—usually the new mother—feels too tired to be interested in sex, it is all too easy for resentment to develop. She may feel that her husband is making unreasonable demands, or the husband may feel rejected. Try to work together to solve the underlying problem. Perhaps the husband can take over night feedings or some of the household chores, or a friend or neighbor can help. Perhaps the couple can decide together that it is better for them to let some tasks wait so they will have more energy for their relationship.

❖ Many people feel inhibited because the baby may wake up and interrupt them. Try hiring a babysitter on occasion. Some people leave the baby at the home of a relative or babysitter. Others leave the baby at home and go to a motel as a special treat.

❖ Sexual contact may be less satisfying because the couple do not "fit together" as well as they did before pregnancy. If the mother does Kegel exercises regularly, the muscle tone in her vagina will improve and lovemaking will be more satisfying. Meanwhile, the couple can experiment with different positions and caresses to find satisfaction.

Many of these problems will be solved naturally as time passes. For example, when the baby begins to sleep through the night, the parents begin to feel more relaxed about lovemaking.

A few women believe that sex is inappropriate once they become mothers. A man who complains about not making love often enough may be feeling jealous of having to share his wife's affection with their baby. When the new parents are able to discuss their feelings openly and cooperatively, the changes in their sexual relationship will become an opportunity for their friendship to grow deeper.

One important area of communication for new parents is the choice of birth control. Many people enjoy pregnancy because it is the one time that they do not have to worry about birth control. They may want to consider trying a new method after their child is born. Many women with disabilities erroneously assumed that they could not get pregnant, so after an unexpected pregnancy and birth, they must choose a birth control method for the first time.

Birth Control Methods

There are many good reasons to delay another pregnancy until at least a year after giving birth. Couples need to think ahead about a birth control method, so they will be prepared when the woman is ready to start making love again.

Couples tend to use the same method after pregnancy that they had used before pregnancy, but some women may need to change methods after giving birth. For example, a woman who was using birth control pills will need a different method if she breast-feeds her baby.

The reliability of a birth control method is measured by the percentage of women who do not become pregnant during a 1-year period. For example, if a particular birth control method is said to be 95 percent reliable, this means that 95 percent of the women in a study group did not become pregnant while using this method for 1 year. A range of reliability (for example, 80 to 99 percent) often reflects variations in the way people use their chosen methods. For any given method, some study groups have better results than other study groups. A higher percentage indicates a group that probably used the method more consistently; for example, *always* using spermicide with a diaphragm, or never forgetting to take a birth control pill. Each method of birth control has advantages and disadvantages. When choosing a birth control method, women who feel strongly about certain advantages or disadvantages need to discuss their concerns with a doctor or family planning practitioner. Medical professionals can provide recent information as to the reliability and safety of each method.

There are five types of birth control methods. Four methods are reversible, which means that a woman can become pregnant if she stops using them. The reversible methods include the so-called "natural" methods, barrier methods, intrauterine devices, and contraceptive hormones. The fifth birth control method, sterilization, is difficult to reverse and is usually permanent.

NATURAL METHODS

The natural methods are lactation, the rhythm method, and the symptothermal method—a variation of the rhythm method.

Breast-feeding Is Not a Reliable Method of Birth Control

Christina voiced a common misconception about lactation when she said, "I thought I couldn't get pregnant while I was nursing. I was sure I read it somewhere." It is true that during the first few months of lactation, the hormones that encourage milk production *may* prevent ovulation (release of an egg that is mature and ready to be fertilized). Even women who are breast-feeding begin to menstruate again about 6 months after giving birth. For some women, the first ovulation occurs earlier. A woman becomes fertile shortly before she starts menstruating again, so no one can be sure that she is safe just because she has not had her period.

The Rhythm Method

The *rhythm* method is a form of birth control in which a woman avoids sexual intercourse near the estimated time of ovulation. Many women choose this method because they dislike using other birth control methods; others choose it because of their religious beliefs. A disadvantage of the rhythm method is that it interferes with spontaneity—many people dislike making love by the calendar. This disadvantage is likely to be felt more strongly after a baby is born, because the baby may also interfere with spontaneity.

The simplest—and least reliable—form of the rhythm method involves keeping a record of the dates of menstruation, and estimating the time of ovulation as 14 days before the expected start of the next period. For example, if a woman menstruates every 28 days, she counts the first day of menstruation as Day 1, and she would expect to ovulate on Day 14. In this case, she should avoid intercourse from about a week before the estimated date of ovulation until a few days after.

No matter how "regular" a woman is, her time of ovulation can be affected by such factors as illness and stress. After she gives birth, the rhythm method will be useless until menstruation has resumed. Also, her menstrual cycle may be different from what it was before she was pregnant. It could be many months before the menstrual cycle becomes predictable. If a woman miscalculates and makes love shortly before ovulation, sperm deposited in her vagina could survive until she ovulates, and she could get pregnant. Sperm can survive in the woman for more than 3 days. As a result of these factors, the reliability of the rhythm method can be as low as 47 percent. In other words, some women who practice the simplest form of the rhythm method might as well flip a coin to decide if it is safe to make love.

Symptothermal Method

The symptothermal method is an improved form of the rhythm method. It is also known as "natural family planning" or "fertility awareness." This method involves keeping a daily record of the woman's temperature when she wakes up in the morning using a basal body temperature thermometer. This type of thermometer makes it easier to read smaller temperature changes than an ordinary thermometer. The recorded temperature is charted on a graph. When a woman ovulates, her temperature suddenly rises as much as one degree Fahrenheit, and continues to rise until her next period. She also watches for changes in her cervical mucus. When the mucus becomes thinner and clearer, it is a sign that she is about to ovulate. These changes can be subtle, and women who want to use the symptothermal method need to take a class at a family planning clinic.

Although the symptothermal method is more reliable than the simpler form of the rhythm method, it has similar disadvantages. A woman can make a mistake in calculating her time of ovulation if her temperature is affected by stress or illness, or if the texture of her cervical mucus is changed by a local infection. Besides the loss of spontaneity in lovemaking, many women dislike the routine of taking their temperature and checking their mucus. In addition, women with limited hand control may have difficulty taking their temperature, reaching into the vagina to collect mucus, or keeping records. Reliability of the symptothermal method can be as low as 80 percent.

CONTRACEPTIVE HORMONES

The major advantage of using *hormonal* birth control is effectiveness. This method can be more than 99 percent reliable when properly used. Some women also like this method because they know when they will menstruate. Another advantage is that the hormone method does not interfere with lovemaking in any way, unlike barrier methods and natural methods. Women who are not troubled by side effects may find this method convenient. Women whose disabilities make barrier methods awkward for them might also prefer the hormonal method.

Hormones can have both positive and negative side effects. One of the positive side effects is that menstrual flow may be reduced, and a woman is less likely to develop anemia with a lighter menstrual flow. Women who use hormones are also less vulnerable to certain types of pelvic infections. Hormones do not protect against sexually transmitted diseases such as herpes and gonorrhea, however.

Women who are breast-feeding cannot use hormones because they can enter the mother's milk; they can also interfere with milk production. Thus, some women base their choice of a birth control method on their decision about breast-feeding. Pam commented, "I chose the pill because I wasn't going to nurse."

Some women experience negative side effects from birth control pills, including weight gain, fluid retention, nausea, fatigue, and breakthrough bleeding (minor bleeding at unexpected times in the menstrual cycle). The only way a woman can know whether she will experience side effects is by trying hormones. She can expect hormones to affect her in the same way after she gives birth if she used them before she was pregnant, unless she changes to another type or brand of hormone.

Hormonal birth control comes in various forms:

Birth Control Pills

Birth control pills that contain both estrogen and progesterone seem to reduce the symptoms of rheumatoid arthritis (38). In addition, there is some evidence that the pill may also reduce MS disability symptoms (74).

Women with the following health problems should avoid birth control pills:

- ❖ Liver, kidney, or heart disease
- ❖ Family or personal history of blood clots or stroke

❖ Smoking (Smoking also increases your risk for blood clots, stroke, or heart attack.)
❖ Diabetes
❖ High blood pressure
❖ Sickle cell disease
❖ Other health problems, such as some kinds of cancer, or family history of cancer, as determined by your physician

Hormones may be contraindicated if a woman's disability causes a decrease in collateral circulation. For example, women who have paralysis—and some women with glaucoma and/or diabetes—have an increased risk of blood clots. Women with lupus may develop blood clots, and their lupus symptoms may worsen. Thus, women who have SLE are advised not to use birth control hormones. If they must use hormones, pills containing only progestin are considered the safest, because estrogen can cause lupus flares. There has been concern that the introduction of hormones into the female population may increase the risk of SLE.

Women who have cerebral palsy with speech involvement have experienced dry mouth after taking birth control hormones, which can make it even more difficult to talk. It is important to tell your doctor if you are taking anti-seizure medication, because many anti-seizure medications can affect the effectiveness of birth control pills. In addition, certain antibiotics may reduce the effectiveness of the pill.

Birth control hormones can sometimes cause high blood pressure and blood clots. Women who have spinal cord injuries that have caused such problems in the past should consult with a doctor familiar with their health histories when considering this method of birth control. If they do choose to use hormones, they should know the signs and symptoms of circulatory problems:

❖ Tenderness and swelling of the calves
❖ Severe abdominal or chest pain
❖ Shortness of breath
❖ Severe leg pain
❖ Severe headaches
❖ Eye problems such as blurred vision or flashing lights

A woman usually does not start taking birth control pills until after her postpartum visit at 3 to 6 weeks after birth. There are two different types of oral contraception. The older version of the pill contains estrogen and progesterone; the newer version usually contains only progestin. Both types are taken daily. Other types are taken daily for 3 weeks, stopped for 1 week, and then resumed again. Some women prefer pills that contain a smaller dose of hormones in order to minimize side effects. Small doses are less effective, however, and may cause irregular bleeding. Some case studies have reported that oral contraceptives can exacerbate systemic lupus erythematosus (SLE). Progestin-only birth control pills are a recommended alternative. There have been some studies suggesting that there is a protective association between oral contraceptives and rheumatoid arthritis (113).

Norplant® Hormonal Implant

Choose this alternative if you want a long-term (5 years) solution to contraception. Occasionally, it can be difficult for the doctor to insert the six rods that contain only progestin. Women who have contractures, spasticity, and/or athetoid movements should consider the difficulty of inserting the implant. Reversal (by removing the implant) is occasionally difficult, and requires paying for a doctor's visit. Some women experience frequent spotting. You may need to have the implant inserted into your leg if your disability affects your upper extremities. Norplant® can be felt under the skin, which some women find irritating. Some women "benefit from progesterone-only contraceptives, including Depo-Provera® and Norplant®" (114).

Depo-Provera®

Depo-Provera® is the brand name of a method of reversible birth control that is given as an intramuscular injection. It contains a hormone similar to progesterone that is called *depot-medroxyprogesterone acetate* (DMPA) (115). A shot of DMPA in the buttock or arm can prevent pregnancy for 12 weeks. Depo-Provera® keeps the ovaries from releasing eggs; thickens the cervical mucus to keep sperm from fertilizing eggs; and is 99.7 percent effective against pregnancy.

This contraceptive is associated with frequent amenorrhea (no periods), which can be a plus for some women. Joan chose this method because "it was really effective and there weren't any risks." She also thought this method to be a good choice because it lasts for 12 weeks. She later stated, "Depo did, in fact, have many risks. I was told there would no side effects from the shot, but then I suffered significant weight gain, migraine-type headaches, and an absolute lack of sexual desire. I went on the Internet to try to find out why I felt so bad. There were many women complaining of the same side effect, and worse, some had hair loss."

This form of contraception has been found to decrease the frequency of seizures. In addition, it does not seem to be affected by antibiotics or anti-seizure medications.

Some studies show progesterone can increase the chance of breast cancer. If breast cancer runs in your family, consult your doctor. Another possible side effect of Depo-Provera® is that it may trigger postpartum depression because of its effect on hormones. Your body may already be having difficulty readjusting the hormones from pregnancy and delivery. Suppressing them after the birth with Depo-Provera® may cause further problems.

Birth Control Patch (Ortho Evra®)

The birth control patch contains both estrogen and progestin. The hormones are transmitted through the skin and into the blood stream. The patch has to be replaced once a week on the same day. It can be worn on the buttocks, abdomen, upper torso, or upper arm. The common side effects are skin irritation, nausea, upper respiratory illness, menstrual cramps, and abdominal cramps. The possible serious risks are the same as with other hormone combinations.

BARRIER METHODS

Barrier methods involve the placement of an obstacle between the sperm and the cervix. Barrier methods include the diaphragm, cervical cap, sponge, condoms, and foam. These methods are the most effective when a physical barrier is combined with a spermicide (a chemical that destroys or inactivates sperm). Diaphragms are used with a spermicidal cream or jelly, which is applied separately. Sponges combine a physical and chemical barrier in one device. Different studies rate the reliability of barrier methods from 75 to 97 percent effective. Those who use the barrier methods correctly and regularly are able to achieve higher reliability.

The barrier method does not have any side effects, and it can be a good choice for women who are breast-feeding, and women who must avoid hormones for health reasons. Some people find the chemicals in the spermicide preparations irritating, and may need to try using a different brand. They may have to choose another method if all of the brands are irritating.

Condoms

The best-known barrier method is the condom, a special sheath that fits snuggly over the man's penis, preventing sperm from being deposited in the vagina. Unfortunately, the reliability of condoms can be as low as 75 percent. Condoms are more reliable when they are used in combination with a spermicide. Here are some tips for proper condom use:

❖ Use latex condoms, not condoms made from animal membranes. Latex condoms are more reliable and offer better protection against sexually transmitted diseases. The different brands of condoms have been tested for leakage. Ask a family planning practitioner or clinic for a list of the reliable brands, and use only the brands on the list.

❖ If one brand of condom seems to reduce pleasure, try another one. There is no point in buying condoms if you are tempted not to use them.

❖ The man should wear the condom throughout intercourse. Some sperm leaves the penis before the man ejaculates ("comes"), so do not wait until the man is close to orgasm (ready to "come") before putting on the condom.

❖ Do not use lubricants containing oils, because oil can cause latex to disintegrate. Many people mistakenly use lubricants that contain oil. Read the list of ingredients, or, better yet, ask your family planning practitioner to recommend a good water-based lubricant (one popular brand is K-Y Jelly®). Spermicidal creams and jellies can also be good lubricants.

❖ Use a spermicidal cream or jelly with the condom. Besides being good lubricants, they contain spermicides that make condoms more reliable.

❖ When putting on the condom, leave about a half-inch of space between the tip of the condom and the tip of the penis. This space catches the sperm, so the condom is less likely to break or leak when the man ejaculates.

❖ Do not let sperm spill from the condom into the vagina after orgasm. The man should withdraw before he loses his erection, while holding the condom to the base of his penis.

There are several advantages to using condoms. They are easily available and no prescription is needed. It was not long ago that you had to ask a pharmacist for condoms, because they were kept behind the counter. But now most drugstores and some supermarkets display them on open shelves. Condoms prevent transmission of venereal diseases and minor genital infections. For some people, it is easier to remember to use a condom than to remember to take a pill, because condoms are directly associated with lovemaking. Some women prefer condoms because they want their partners to share the responsibility for birth control.

One disadvantage of the condom method is that it can be easy to make a mistake. Sometimes people are tempted to have intercourse when no condom is available. This accounts for many condom "failures." Many men feel that condoms interfere with pleasure, others feel they do not. Some people feel that stopping to put on a condom makes lovemaking less pleasant, while others enjoy putting on the condom as part of lovemaking. If both partners have limited hand function, they may find it difficult to open the condom wrapper and put on the condom. Some women solve this problem by putting the condom on their husbands with their mouths.

Diaphragms

The diaphragm is a dome-shaped piece of rubber with a spring rim. The woman puts spermicidal cream or jelly in the center of the diaphragm, and inserts it into her vagina in such a way that it covers the cervix. Then she uses a special applicator to put more spermicide in her vagina. The diaphragm method is 80 to 95 percent reliable when properly fitted and used correctly. Here are some tips for using a diaphragm successfully:

❖ The diaphragm must be fitted to the individual user. Be sure to have a new diaphragm fitted at a postpartum examination. The size and shape of the vagina change after childbirth, so a diaphragm that was used before pregnancy will not be reliable after pregnancy.

❖ Do not use the diaphragm without spermicidal cream. One application of cream is only enough for one male climax. Reapply cream each time you have intercourse.

❖ Do not remove the diaphragm for at least 8 hours after intercourse. (This is easy to do if you make love at night—just go to sleep with the diaphragm in place.)

❖ After removing the diaphragm, wash and dry it carefully. Do not dust it with scented powders (a little cornstarch is all right). Store it in its case in a cool, dark place.

❖ Diaphragms should be inspected before each use for obvious tears. Periodically, hold the diaphragm up to the light and check for pin-sized holes. Replace it if necessary.

❖ Replace the diaphragm every year. In addition, make an appointment to have the diaphragm checked for fit after a weight gain or loss of 10 pounds or more.

❖ When the diaphragm is fitted, make sure it is comfortable and easy to insert. Diaphragms have two different types of rims. Try both kinds to see which feels better and which is easier to insert. Practice inserting and removing the diaphragm when it is prescribed, so your family planning practitioner can make sure you are inserting it properly. If your partner will be inserting or removing your diaphragm for you, have him practice in the doctor's office.

❖ If it is difficult to insert or remove the diaphragm while lying down, try crouching, sitting with one foot propped up, or sitting on a toilet.

❖ If your diaphragm is unavailable (perhaps because it was not packed before a trip), use a condom or sponge.

Some women prefer using diaphragms because they like to be in charge of their birth control method. Diaphragms are a good choice for people who dislike condoms. Some women feel that lovemaking is more pleasant when a diaphragm has been inserted ahead of time, and there is no need to stop to put on a condom. Others prefer having their partners insert the diaphragm as part of lovemaking.

Inserting or removing a diaphragm is difficult and awkward for some women. The difficulty may caused by the position of the uterus. This method can be difficult for some women with spine or pelvic deformities, and those with limited hand control. Hilary solved the problem by having her husband insert the diaphragm during lovemaking, then removing it herself while sitting on the toilet. Some women feel that the possibility of having their partner insert the diaphragm is an advantage, while others feel that relying on help is a disadvantage.

Women with weak pelvic muscles may not be able to use a diaphragm because of the possibility that it will slip out of position. Women who must empty their bladders by the Credé method (abdominal pressure) may dislodge their diaphragms. Selina had an increase in bladder infections when she used the diaphragm.

Some women feel that lovemaking during menstruation is more pleasant with a diaphragm because they prevent fluids from staining the sheets.

Some people feel that spermicides are advantageous because they are also lubricants. Others dislike them because they feel they are messy, especially when the diaphragm is removed. Some women remove their diaphragms while sitting on the toilet so that the melted spermicide does not run down their legs. Some women remove their diaphragms just before getting in the shower; others remove them in the shower.

Cervical Caps

Cervical caps are an alternative to diaphragms. The cap is smaller than a diaphragm, and fits more closely over the cervix. Some women feel the cap is more comfortable. A woman who has difficulty inserting a diaphragm will also have difficulty inserting a cervical cap.

Contraceptive Sponges

Contraceptive sponges are made of a synthetic, sponge-like material that has been impregnated (soaked) with spermicide. The spongy material acts as a physical barrier. The advantage of the sponge is that there is no need for a prescription—the same size fits any woman. But like the diaphragm, the sponge may be difficult for some women to insert or remove. Women who are able to insert the sponge themselves may feel that lovemaking is more spontaneous using a sponge than with a condom, because the sponge can be inserted well ahead of time. No additional spermicide is needed with the sponge, so lovemaking seems more spontaneous and less messy. It is recommended that the sponge never be left in place longer than a total of 30 hours. The sponge can cause irritation in some women.

Contraceptive Foam

Contraceptive foam, because of its texture, acts as a physical barrier as well as a spermicide. Women who are considering this method should ask their family planning practitioner for recent information about reliability. Women who want to use a barrier method, but have difficulty inserting a diaphragm or a sponge, may prefer foam.

INTRAUTERINE DEVICES

Commonly known as IUDs, intrauterine devices are small objects that are inserted into the uterus by a doctor. Usually, it is easier to insert an IUC in a woman who has had at least one child. A string attached to the IDU protrudes from the cervix, so that placement can be checked. A partner can do this if you cannot do it yourself.

The Dalkon Shield was a type of IUD that was once used, but it caused many problems and was removed from the market. There are two types of IUDs that are approved. One is the copper-containing IUC (CuT 380A). This device is not recommended for women who have problems with menstrual cramping and/or menstrual bleeding. The second device—the LNG IUC—is the most effective device available. The LNG IUD offers at least 7 years of protection and has noncontraceptive health benefits. Users have less menstrual flow and cramps (116).

"Women with an impaired immune response, such as multiple sclerosis or lupus, may be at greater risk for severe pelvic inflammatory disease (PID)" (117). The risk for infection is greatest during the first 3 weeks after insertion. Therefore, women with low immunity should be observed and screened closely. It has been theorized that the LNG IUC may be less likely to cause an infection resulting in PID, but there have not been any birth control studies that have included women with disabilities, making this theoretical.

It has been reported on some forum Web sites that women using the LNG (Mirena) have experienced weight gain, fatigue, and joint pain. On the other hand, no negative comments can be found on the Web concerning the copper IUC. The Mirena has been used in Europe for 10 years.

STERILIZATION

Sterilization is a surgical procedure that makes a person infertile. It is difficult, and sometimes impossible to reverse. Some researchers are working to develop surgical procedures for reversing sterilization, but even if such procedures become widely available, reversing sterilization will not always be reliable. Sterilization should be seen as permanent, and should only be chosen by people who are sure they do not want any more children. For these people, sterilization may be ideal. Sheila commented, "I'm really glad I did it. It gave me real peace of mind."

The advantages of sterilization are that it is more than 99 percent reliable, and it does not have the same risks or inconveniences as other birth control methods. Either partner can be sterilized.

Vasectomy

Sterilization of a man is called *vasectomy*. This procedure can be done in a doctor's office with a local anesthetic. An incision is made in the scrotum (the skin over the testicles or "balls"). Inside the scrotum are two tubes called the *vas deferens*. Each tube carries sperm from a testicle to the penis. The doctor removes a small section of each tube, seals the open ends, and then closes the incision. For a few days after surgery, the area around the incision will be uncomfortable. Some sperm may have been left in the part of the tube closest to the penis, so the couple will need to use another birth control method for a few weeks after surgery, or until a sperm count shows that the husband is completely sterile.

Very rarely, uncomfortable scar tissue forms after a vasectomy. Men who are worried about this should discuss their concerns with their doctors. Some men feel that somehow this surgery makes them less masculine. They, too, should discuss their concerns with their wives and doctors before having the surgery. Vasectomy does not affect male hormones or the ability to have sex. Men with vasectomies ejaculate normally, because most of the liquid that normally comes out is from the prostate gland, and that does not change after vasectomy.

Tubal Ligation

Sterilization of women is called *tubal ligation*. This procedure is performed on the fallopian tubes, which carry the ova (eggs) from the ovaries to the uterus. A section of each fallopian tube is either removed or clamped, preventing the eggs from being fertilized.

The two most common procedures are laparoscopic tubal ligation and mini-laparotomy. They are done in the hospital, but the woman enters and leaves the hospital on the same day the surgery is performed. Sometimes, she may stay one night. This surgery is comparatively minor, but usually requires general anesthesia. Women who are considering this method can read about anesthesia in Chapters 11 and 12, and discuss what they have learned with their doctors.

In a tubal ligation, a tiny incision is made just below the navel, and then gas is injected into the abdomen so that the internal organs are gently pushed apart. The doctor inserts instruments that make it possible to see into the abdomen and seal the fallopian tubes. Finally, the instruments and gas are removed, and the incision is sutured.

The woman will experience the usual aftereffects of anesthetic. The incision will be so tiny that it will be covered with an ordinary Band-Aid™. The scar will be barely visible after the incision heals. The shape of the navel may be changed slightly. Sometimes not all of the gas is removed from the abdomen, so some women may experience sharp pains for a few days until the gas is absorbed. Women should ask their doctors about these pains so they will know what to expect.

A mini-laparotomy can be done immediately after delivery or after the postpartum visit. If it is done just after delivery, the skin incision is made under the navel, because the uterine fundus and fallopian tubes are in that area. If it is done after the postpartum visit, the skin incision is made in the same area as the bikini cut for caesarean surgery, because the uterus and tubes will have shrunk back into the pelvis. In either case, the tubes are elevated out of the incision, each tube is tied in two places, and a section of tube between the ties is removed. The tubes are then placed back into the abdomen, and the skin incision is sutured. This incision is also so small that it can be covered with a Band-Aid™.

A tubal ligation can be performed during caesarean surgery. Arlene chose to be sterilized at the time of her delivery. She said, "I was getting older, and I was sure I didn't want to get pregnant again." Avoid making a last-minute decision about sterilization during caesarean birth, if possible, because it is important to take the time necessary to feel completely comfortable with the decision. Sybil was pressured into a last-minute decision that she later regretted.

Women who have been sterilized continue to menstruate. Some women have heavier periods. Also, 10 percent of women who have tubal ligations by any method develop irregular, painful periods within 3 years after the procedure. This post-tubal ligation syndrome may be due to partial impairment of the blood supply to the ovaries, which is caused by the cutting of blood vessels during surgery.

Infant Care with Adaptations for Disability

This chapter includes suggestions from the interviewees, but the majority of the information is based on the work done at Through The Looking Glass (TLG). Most of the women interviewed for this book did not receive services on parenting adaptation. They had a harder time. Many said that when their children were first born, they felt overwhelmed by the new responsibility. Stacy said, "I was scared to change diapers, dress the baby, nurse him, even to hold him."

Yet, when they were interviewed weeks, months, or years after giving birth, all of the women said that they were glad to be mothers. They said that they would make the same choice again, and they encourage other disabled women to have children. Although they remembered the postpartum period as a time of tears and frustration, their comments revealed that it was also a time of learning.

Many of the interviewees emphasized that babies learn to adapt to the mother's disability, and mothers are able to take advantage of that adaptability. Hilary commented, "As soon as my children were able to sit, before they crawled, they learned to scoot over to me." Sheila said, "I taught my babies from birth to help me when I picked them up. I would put one hand underneath the baby's back or tummy, and the other hand around the baby's wrist, and pull gently. They were eager to be held, and they were able to help. I discovered that even at 5 months, they could help a lot. I would take care of someone else's baby— these women weren't disabled—and because their babies didn't respond as my children did, I couldn't lift them up. My children were able to help even more as they got older."

At TLG, we have documented babies helping their parents with different baby care activities, from lifting their bottoms during diapering to crawling onto the diapering surface. There are some babies who take longer to adapt to the mother's disability. This may in part be due to inborn temperament, as well as to how the baby is taught. A good technique to help during diaper changing is to teach the baby to the lift his bottom. Put your hand under the baby's lower back and bottom. Lift the baby's back so her feet go above her head. If your hand is in the right area, the baby's bottom will easily lift up. At the same time say, "Bottom up." In this way, many babies gradually learn to lift their bottoms on command and without help (109).

Some women may need to arrange extra help to physically care for the baby. Nancy said that, at first, she had attendants available around the clock. Another way of coping with baby care if attendant care is not available, is to simplify housework and baby care. Hilary gave her favorite example: "I stacked all the clean sheets right under the crib so I wouldn't have to run around getting sheets every time the baby wet the bed."

FURNITURE AND EQUIPMENT

Since writing the first edition of this book, the author's opinion about baby furniture and equipment has changed. At the time the first edition was published, there was very little commercially available baby care equipment that parents with disabilities could easily use. The first edition included baby care solutions devised by some of the interviewees, but some of those solutions are no longer recommended. TLG's field-initiated research grants from NIDRR (National Institute of Disability Rehabilitation Research) have documented that many disabled parents tend to put themselves at risk for secondary injury in order to complete some tasks. Most parents with disabilities could benefit from some type of adaptive baby care equipment. Appropriate adaptive baby care equipment allows the parent to take care of their baby using good ergonomic positions. Moreover, adaptive equipment also seems to make baby care tasks less demanding. Baby care activities can cause physical problems for some women. Sydney was immobilized for 2 days soon after her child was born because she pulled her trapezius muscle when picking up and putting the baby in the crib. She could have benefited from a crib that has been adapted by TLG (see Appendix D). Sydney felt that she compensated for her lack of stomach muscles. At TLG, we have found that many parents put extra strain on their muscles when taking care of their babies.

Cribs with a gate opening are best avoided, because the baby can fall out if left unattended. TLG has designed a crib with a sliding side, so the parent can block the opening and, at the same time, have easy access.

Heather and Stephanie shopped carefully for well-designed changing tables. Stephanie: "I made sure the changing table was the correct height for me to get my wheelchair under." Heather said, "I needed something sturdy, one that wouldn't be wobbly, so I could lean up against it. The one that worked best was wooden." Some women prefer a table that has a built-in belt that holds the baby in place, leaving both hands free for changing the diaper and cleaning the baby. Many disabled parents diaper their babies on the floor because it feels more stable. Diapering on these surfaces can make transfers more difficult, however. It can also be stressful on the bodies of the parents.

Using a table as a place to diaper is a solution that TLG has found successful. Shelby used a desk for diapering. A table not only makes transferring the baby easier, it also places the parent in a good ergonomic position.

For more specifics on baby care equipment, please contact Through the Looking Glass at www.lookingglass.org, or by phone (510) 848-1112 or (800) 644 2666 (see also Appendix D).

CARRYING AND MOVING THE BABY

Naomi said, "By the time my baby was 6 months old, I developed excruciating pain in my shoulder and chest, probably from carrying her and being generally weaker in my upper extremities from neuromuscular disease. I needed physical therapy for several months." A possible method to prevent strained muscles is to get a referral to occupational therapy, preferably during pregnancy. Appropriate equipment can be arranged for in advance, and safer and more effective techniques will give you confidence.

From our research at TLG, we found that many of our interventions were focused around certain activities called *transitional tasks*, including: transfers, holding, carrying and moving, and positional changes. These tasks are crucial activities because they are the essential links between and within most baby care activities. These are the physical activities that begin and end a baby care task.

Holding is one of the main transitional tasks. Holding can mean that the baby is seated in a car seat that is placed on a table close to the mother. Taryn Dion used pillows as a way to hold the baby. She also tried using a Baby Bjorn™, but found that the straps compressed tender areas. She did not realize that the straps were hurting her until it was too late. Tessa found that she needed to invent her own front pack. Andrea also found that holding was an issue. Andrea needed to hold her baby on her left side for balance.

One of the most important activities is carrying the baby while moving. Each of the interviewees invented her own clever way of carrying her baby. Hilary said "I would carry my baby on my shoulder like a sack of potatoes, with one arm holding onto the baby's trunk. Since the baby was small, I could use the same hand to support her head. Then I'd use my other hand to hold onto a crutch, a piece of furniture, or the wall for support." Heather uses two crutches, but she also managed to carry her baby. She explained, "I used my upper arm and elbow to hold the crutch, then used my forearm to support my baby against my body, with my hand hooked in his armpit." Clara has some difficulty with balance. She found that she could carry her baby most securely when she hugged him against the front of her body. She said, "That way my chest and tummy supported the baby's back and head, and he could look around because he was facing forward." Although most people who are dwarfs generally find it difficult to carry a baby, Darlene enjoyed carrying her baby. Once her baby was big enough, she used a backpack to carry him when they were outside.

Pack-N-Ride™ by Basic Comfort, and PortaPak™ by Arm's Reach, are products that hold the baby in the same position as Clara did, plus they take the strain off the arms and shoulders. This product may not work for women with balance problems or low back pain.

The interviewees who could walk often used strollers or front packs to carry their babies. Darlene enjoyed walking around town using a stroller.

Heather found difficulties with these methods. She said, "The front pack didn't work because it felt like the baby was just hanging there. I just didn't like the sensation. Using my prosthesis didn't work either. I also tried to use a stroller, but it was difficult to bend down and lift the baby up. My crutches got in my way. The heavier stroller was more secure, but the lightweight stroller would go right out from under me." Several of the women liked using front packs and strollers; some even used wheeled bassinets or strollers to move their babies from room to room at home. Christina said, "Using an umbrella stroller was easier because my balance is a problem."

Unfortunately, parents with disabilities often buy commercially available baby care equipment that may not work for them. Through the Looking Glass has designed a stroller that is a safe and comfortable way to move the baby. We used a lightweight Rollator (a 4-wheeled walker) as the base, thereby making it possible for a person to maintain balance, and still have the ability to bear weight while moving the baby. A seat is secured to the Rollator so you can move your baby safely. For many women, the commercially available strollers are too low to transfer the baby comfortably, so having the seat open and at an appropriate height can make transfers easier. Many parents have used this stroller successfully. At TLG, the author worked with one woman who uses crutches and is unable to use a commercially available stroller, but with the adapted walker (stroller) she could take care of her baby.

Many of the interviewees who used wheelchairs held their babies on their laps. Celeste said, "I would hold the baby on my lap with one hand, and push the chair with the other." This is a laborious way to carry a baby and push a wheelchair. Sheila said, "When I used the footrest, I had more of a lap for both of my babies; I would also use receiving blankets to pad around them." For many women who cannot safely and comfortably seat the baby on their lap, a fanny pack can be a great solution until the baby blocks the mother's vision. Any commercially available front pack will probably work for women with good upper body coordination. In addition, there are several front packs that can be adapted for women who have limited coordination of the upper body. Christi Tuleja of TLG has designed a pillow with a waist strap and a recessed center that holds the baby. We have also adapted the Boppy™ to be used in carrying and moving a baby. A friend of the author, who became disabled, developed a unique way of carrying her newborn baby in her wheelchair. Janet used an infant seat, a luggage strap, and a cushion. The cushion is made out of a piece of foam and mat board. Janet places the padded side of the board on her lap, and rests the car seat sideways on the board. The luggage strap is used to attach the seat to her chair.

Some of the interviewees preferred not to hold their babies on their laps. Pam said, "I was afraid he could fall off." She solved this problem by strapping her baby to her body, commenting, "That way my hands were free." TLG has devised two different versions of a safe strapping method in which the baby and mother do not share the same strap.

Experiment with several types of front packs, baby slings, and strollers before making a purchase. When trying front packs and slings or strollers, ask these questions:

- ❖ How easy is it to get the baby in and out of the carrier?
- ❖ Will this carrier work when the baby is older?
- ❖ How easy is it to put the pack on and take it off, or put the baby in or out of the pack?
- ❖ If it is the kind of carrier that the mother puts on after the baby is inside, how easy is it to lift and put on with the baby inside?
- ❖ Will it be possible to use when the baby gains weight?
- ❖ Are the fasteners easy to manipulate?
- ❖ How does carrying a baby in front of your body affect your balance when walking?
- ❖ How will it affect your balance when the baby is heavier?
- ❖ Do the straps feel comfortable?
- ❖ Will your back and shoulders ache after you use the carrier?
- ❖ If possible, borrow one or more kinds of front packs and use them for 1 day each before deciding. (None of the interviewees used a backpack. A woman who is considering a backpack should also try several models.)

Ask these questions when choosing a stroller:

- ❖ If you need to lean on it for support, is it heavy enough to support your weight without starting to roll away?

❖ Is it lightweight enough to push easily, or to take in and out of the car?

❖ Does it have a brake you can use while putting the baby in or taking him out?

❖ How easy is it to use the brake?

❖ How easy is it to place the baby in the stroller or take her out?

❖ How well does the stroller turn, and how well does it roll on uneven surfaces?

❖ Can you maintain your balance?

❖ Is it easy to store?

❖ If it is collapsible, how easy is it to collapse and set up again?

❖ Can it be used to carry packages? Some strollers are so light that when a carrying bag is hanging from the handles, the whole stroller tilts over when the baby is lifted out.

Lifting a baby may require a separate piece of equipment. Stephanie found a new use for a type of harness that parents typically use so their toddlers will not run away. She said, "I dressed my baby in the harness and took off the straps. When I wanted to take her out of her walker, I could get a good grip on the harness and lift her up by it." At TLG, we have created a lifting harness that makes transferring the baby possible for some mothers, and easier for others.

Hilary pointed out that the idea of getting the children to help applies to the problem of getting them from place to place. She said, "I never carried either of them once they began to crawl. Sometimes I would have to coax them; other times I needed more patience. I even got them to crawl to me when I wanted to change their diapers. After a while they would follow me wherever I wanted them to go."

CHANGING DIAPERS

Some women may need help with caring for the baby's navel during the first 4 to 7 days after birth while it is healing. Occasionally, the area must be cleaned by gently dabbing with a swab dipped in alcohol. The mother's husband or attendant can do this if the mother does not have sufficient hand control. Also, the baby's diaper must be kept below the navel, because it is important to keep the area clean and dry to prevent infection.

Most of the interviewees felt that paper diapers work best because they are easier to use than cloth diapers and pins. Paper diapers that can be refastened are also available. Women who strongly prefer cloth diapers could look for diaper covers, which are designed to hold the diaper in place without pins. An "all in one" diaper holder can be adapted once, and then be reused. Sheila commented, "Sometimes it was hard to get the diapers tight enough. I used one hand, but sometimes I needed to use my teeth." Another way to tighten the diaper is by adapting the tabs with loops. There are one-handed techniques for tightening diapers by using the forearm between the baby's legs to stabilize the diaper, and moving the hand from one tab to the other. Diapering can be one of the most difficult tasks. As discussed previously, having the baby assist can be advantageous and make diapering easier.

Babies often do not want to lie still for diapering after they learn to roll over, which can cause a high degree of frustration for both the parent and the baby. At TLG, we have found that a toy mobile can be helpful in keeping a baby from moving around during diapering. The toy mobile uses interactive toys, which should be changed periodically so the baby does not get bored. TLG can provide information on one-handed techniques for changing a diaper. As previously discussed, many parents have taught their babies to lift their bottoms to assist in diapering.

BATHING BABIES

Several of the interviewees were uncomfortable with bathing their babies. Sheila found ways to carry her babies and change their diapers, but would ask her mother to bathe them. Clara explained, "I have good control of only one hand and arm, so I was scared the baby would slip away. I had my husband bathe them, or be there to help, until both of my babies were able to sit on their own. I would get in the bathtub, and he would give me the baby and then take it back. I finished my bath while he dried the baby."

Hilary used a baby seat. She explained, "I kept the baby in the seat while I got settled in the tub. Then I took the baby into the tub with me while I ran the water. After the bath, I did the whole thing in reverse—I'd let the water out, put the baby in the seat, and then get out of the tub."

There are bathtubs that make bathing easier for some people with certain disabilities. These tubs have inserts that keep the baby in a supported position. Moreover, there are adaptations that can be made to the baby's bathtub. The frustration of bathing a slippery, wriggly baby will soon become a laughable memory. The baby's adaptability and independence—and the mother's flexibility and creativity—will combine to make parenthood a joyous experience. When the baby has sitting balance, a bath seat can be used in a regular bathtub. When choosing a seat, try to see whether it will be easy to get the baby in and out. Once the baby is in the seat, how easy will it be to lift the seat into the tub and out again? Perhaps someone else can put the seat in the tub, and then the mother can bathe the baby. Is the seat designed so that the baby cannot slip out easily? Is it well balanced, so that it will not tilt over if the baby moves vigorously?

DRESSING

Snaps can be one of the hardest parts of dressing the baby; zippers and closings with Velcro™ are easier to use. Dressing the baby in a larger size can also make dressing easier.

Closing Comments

Portia commented that pregnancy is just one step on the way to motherhood. In the same way, infancy is just a step on the way to childhood. Newborn babies are dependent on their parents, and the responsibility for their care can be frightening. It helps to remember that most babies adapt quickly, adjusting their movements to their mother's so that she can lift and carry them more easily. There are also techniques available to help with baby care tasks and, as children get older, they will be able to assist with many activities, adding to the parent-child relationship.

Appendix A

Pregnancy Tables for Ninety Women

KEEP TWO CONSIDERATIONS in mind when reviewing the tables in Appendix A:

First, these tables are based on the interviewee's memories of their pregnancies and, therefore, the information may not be as accurate as it would have been if they had kept notes on their symptoms as they occurred. The reported incidence of some ordinary pregnancy changes, such as stuffy nose or breast soreness, is lower than average, and we suspect that, in many instances, the memory of some symptoms was eclipsed by the memory of other, more dramatic symptoms.

Second, the sample size is not large enough to answer several questions about specific disabilities. In particular, it is not known whether the interviewees whose symptoms were worse after pregnancy would have experienced the same degree of exacerbation if they had not been pregnant. The conclusions that can be drawn from these histories are confirmed by other studies, allowing for some basic recommendations to be made to disabled women and the professionals who work with them.

This appendix does not include further information on five women who were only partially interviewed. These pregnancy histories record the physical changes each woman experienced during each trimester of pregnancy. The tables also indicate whether a physical change was likely to have been due to disability, to pregnancy (including both normal pregnancy changes and complications), or to the interaction of disability and pregnancy. In some cases, it is difficult to know the cause of a symptom. For example, it is not possible to be certain whether one woman's pregnancy-associated edema would have been milder if they had been able to exercise. A question mark (?) in the table indicates that it was difficult to evaluate the cause of a physical change.

D   Disability-related physical change
P   Pregnancy-related changes
PD Changes related to interaction between pregnancy and disability
?   Difficult to determine cause of physical change
N   Neither

Amanda's Pregnancy History (Amniotic Band Syndrome)

Pregnancy: Age 24

Trimester	Cause	Physical Change
1st	P	Nausea
	N	Pain from ovarian cyst
	PD	Remission of arthritis symptoms in left hip
2nd	N	Surgery for ovarian cyst
	PD	Balance problems
	PD	Fell and cracked stump
3rd	PD	Energized
	PD	Started using a wheelchair

Pregnancy: Age 27

Trimester	Cause	Physical Change
1st		No specific changes recalled
2nd	PD	Difficulty with balance
	PD	Difficulty with activities of daily living
	PD	More tired
	PD	Increased pressure and pain on hip
	PD	Fell 2 or 3 times
3rd	PD	Balance was more affected
	PD	Fell 3 or 4 times
	PD	Difficult transfers in and out of the bathtub
	PD	Edema in foot and stump

Comments

Amanda fell in her first pregnancy after the flu and tripping on her skirt. Her stump healed three times faster than it did with other falls. Amanda carried her second pregnancy more forward, and her balance was affected sooner than her first pregnancy. She did not have relief from arthritic pain in her second pregnancy. She started to use a wheelchair sooner than during her first pregnancy. Amanda needed grab bars in the bathroom so she could pull up her undergarment. She delivered both of her children vaginally.

Amy's Pregnancy History (1) (Amputation)

Pregnancy: Age 29

Trimester	Cause	Physical Change
1st	P	Fatigue
	PD	Headaches
	P	Morning sickness
2nd	PD	Backache
	D	Phantom sensation
	PD	Hamstrings tight
	P	Spotting
3rd	PD	Hip pain
	PD	Back pain
	PD	Transferring became difficult
	D	Phantom pain
	P	Frequent urination

Comments

Swimming helped with her backache. She could not lie on her back because she could not stretch out her hamstrings. Amy switched from using a manual wheelchair to a power wheelchair because of thick carpet. She used a transfer board for the car, and a bathtub bench and a raised toilet seat. Her headaches may have been an interaction between her head injury and hormones. She uses a prosthesis for an hour at a time. Amy delivered by caesarean section because her pelvis was "contracted" from her first car accident.

Aftereffects

Backache increased, more headaches, and continued phantom sensations.

Andrea's Pregnancy History (2) (Amputation)

Pregnancy: Age 30

Trimester	Cause	Physical Change
1st	P	Morning sickness
	P	Fatigue
2nd	P	Fatigue
	PD	Balance problems
	PD	Edema
	D	Phantom pain
	P	Constipation
3rd	PD	Carpel tunnel, both wrists
	PD	Edema
	P	Hemorrhoids
	PD	Mobility problems
	P	Constipation

Pregnancy: Age 35

Trimester	Cause	Physical Change
1st	P	Same as first pregnancy: morning sickness and fatigue, although much better than the first pregnancy
2nd		Phantom pain
3rd		Sciatic pain (back pain)
		Carpal tunnel

Comments

Her foot and ankle were swollen, and she always wanted to elevate her leg. She wore a sandal. Andrea carried smaller with her second pregnancy, and gained less weight. Her carpal tunnel was not as bad as during her first pregnancy. Andrea wished she had used a wheelchair. It was Andrea's own stubbornness and the obstetrician's inability to listen or understand the interaction of sciatic pain and Andrea's inability to walk that caused her to deliver by caesarean section. She never progressed in labor. Andrea had to have emergency caesarean section with her first pregnancy because her cervix did not dilate. The doctors said it was because she had to labor on her right side instead of the traditional left side, because of her amputation. At no time during the pregnancy did her doctor inform her this might happen. She asked several times if he thought there would be a problem with labor due to her disability and was told no. The amputation didn't cause any problem with delivery. If she did not dilate it was probably due to the size of the baby.

Allison's Pregnancy History (2) (Amputation)

Pregnancy: Age 30

Trimester	Cause	Physical Change
1st	P	Morning sickness
2nd	D	Knee pain
	P	Dry skin
3rd	PD	Pain in her knees
	PD	Transfer in bathtub more difficult
	PD	Taking showers difficult
	PD	Mobility problems
	PD	Bed rest
	PD	Balance affected
	PD	Waddled when walking
	P	Stress incontinence
	P	Dry hair and dry skin

Pregnancy: Age 32

Trimester	Cause	Physical Change
1st	P	Morning sickness
	P	Fatigue
2nd	P	Fatigue
	P	Morning sickness
	PD	Pain in her knees
3rd	P	Fatigue
	PD	Pain in her knees
	P	Migraines
	PD	Transfer in bathtub more difficult
	PD	Taking showers more difficulty
	PD	Balance affected
	PD	Waddled when walking
	P	Stress incontinence
	PD	Edema in stump
	P	Dry hair and dry skin

Comments

With her first pregnancy, her morning sickness was in the afternoon and was manageable. Allison had an amniocentesis, which caused early labor, and was put on bed rest. During her second pregnancy, the prosthesis did not fit because of edema. She delivered both of her babies vaginally.

Arianna's Pregnancy History (1) (Arthrogryposis)

Pregnancy: Age 30

Trimester	Cause	Physical Change
1st	P	Morning sickness
	P	Fatigue
2nd	P	Fatigue
	PD	Balance problems
	PD	Edema
	D	Phantom pain
	P	Constipation
3rd	PD	Carpel tunnel both wrists
	PD	Edema
	P	Hemorrhoids
	PD	Mobility problems
	P	Constipation

Comments

Arianna's twins were by delivered by caesarean section.

Arlene's Pregnancy History (1) (Arthrogryposis)

Pregnancy: Age 36; miscarriage

Pregnancy: Age 36; miscarriage

Pregnancy: Age 37

Trimester	Cause	Physical Change
1st	D	Light-headed after hot baths
	PD	Swollen feet
	P	More constipation than usual; urinated frequently
2nd	PD	Swollen feet
	PD	Transferring became difficult
	P	Constipation; increased frequency of urination
3rd	PD	Swollen feet worst
	PD	Transferring still difficult, often avoided
	P	Constipation worst
	P	Further increase in frequency of urination
	PD	Pressure sore (abrasion)
All	P	Never felt cold

Comments

Arlene's doctor thought poor circulation may have contributed to her miscarriages. She advised Arlene to spend as much time as possible lying down with her legs raised, in an attempt to improve circulation to the uterus. Her light-headedness may also have been related to her circulatory problems. She delivered her baby by caesarean section.

Aftereffects

Occasional swollen feet since the pregnancy.

Caitlin's Pregnancy History (2) (Cerebral Palsy)

Pregnancy: Age 41

Trimester	Cause	Physical Change
1st	P	Fatigue
	P	Faintness
2nd	PD	Faintness and dizziness
	PD	Transferring and daily activities such as bathing and dressing became more difficult
3rd	PD	Mobility generally a problem; difficulty getting out of bed, rolling over in bed, and getting out of bathtub
	PD	Walking increasingly difficult
	PD	Balance: started falling
	PD	Edema
	PD	Right hip pain

Pregnancy: Age 42

Low hormone levels with miscarriage @ 6 weeks

Pregnancy: Age 44

Trimester	Cause	Physical Change
1st	P	Fatigue
	P	Morning sickness
	P	Faintness
	P	Bleeding
	PD	Stress incontinence
2nd	PD	Put on medication for the bladder
	PD	Balance: started falling
3rd		Same as first

Comments

Caitlin experienced more dizziness with her first pregnancy than with her second. She was put on an antispasmodic for her bladder. Caitlin has a mullerian anomaly, which is rare. Mullerian anomaly happens in utero. During normal embryonic development, fusion occurs between the two mullerian ducts forming the vagina, cervix, and uterine body. Mullerian anomaly can lead to urinary tract problems, and is unrelated to CP. She took Urispas® for bladder problems from the second month until the end of her pregnancy. She experienced edema in both legs, and had numbness on and off in her left leg. Her balance problems started earlier with the second pregnancy than with her first. During both pregnancies, Caitlin used a 4-wheeled walker (Rollator). She could not cross her legs, which caused problems with putting on her shoes. The left side of her uterus had never developed. She had pelvic pain, because of the baby's weight, and because she had a tipped uterus. Caitlin had a caesarean section because the doctors did not think she would dilate. They think that her spasticity also affects her vagina and uterus. The doctors did not know if the numbness in her left leg was due to two herniated discs or the epidural. Her children were delivered by caesarean section.

Carla's Pregnancy History (2) (Cerebral Palsy)

Pregnancy: Age 21

Trimester	Cause	Physical Change
1st	PD	Abdominal muscle cramps
	PD	Tight feeling in groin[a]
	PD	Sciatica
	P	Morning sickness
2nd	P	Heartburn
	PD	Leg cramps more intense
	PD	Walking and standing difficult
3rd	PD	Mobility generally a problem; difficulty getting out of bed, chairs, and bathtub
	PD	Walking increasingly difficult
	P	Edema
	P	Hemorrhoids

Pregnancy: Age unknown; miscarriage[b]

Pregnancy: Age 27

Trimester	Cause	Physical Change
1st	P	Same as first pregnancy, but morning sickness and sciatica worse
2nd		Same as first pregnancy
3rd		None reported

Comments

[a]It is difficult to say whether the tight feeling described by Carla and some of the other interviewees was due to their disabilities or to pregnancy. This sensation may have been a result of round ligament syndrome, which is common among able-bodied pregnant women. There are two round ligaments: one on the right and one on the left of the uterus. The uterus is suspended from the upper ends of the round ligaments, similar to a tent from tent ropes. The pelvic bones act like tent pegs on each side of the uterus, anchoring the uterus to the ligaments. The lower ends of the ligaments are attached to the pelvic rami. As the uterus grows, it stretches the ligaments. When the weight of the uterus is shifted, sometimes a woman feels a sharp pain due to the stretching of the ligaments. This stretching, and the consequent pain, can be caused by a simple movement such as rolling over in bed. These pains are known as *round ligament syndrome*. There is another possible explanation for Carla's groin discomfort. If a woman's disability causes hypertonicity in the muscles of the abdominal wall, these muscles may spasm when stressed by an increasingly heavy uterus. Carla had one child vaginally. She had a caesarean section with the other child because she stopped dilating.

[b]Carla's miscarriage was not caused by her disability, and it was not a pregnancy complication; it was caused by an unusual accident which injured her uterus.

Carol's Pregnancy History (2) (Cerebral Palsy)

Pregnancy: Age 31

Trimester	Cause	Physical Change
1st	P	Fatigue
2nd	P	Heartburn
	PD	Leg cramps more intense
	PD	Walking and standing difficult
	P	Hypertension
3rd	PD	Mobility generally a problem; difficulty getting out of bed, chairs, bathtub
	PD	Walking increasingly difficult
	PD	Edema
	P	Hypertension
	P	Hemorrhoids

Pregnancy: Age 34

Trimester	Cause	Physical Change
1st	P	Fatigue
	P	Morning sickness
	P	Faintness
2nd		Same as first pregnancy
	P	Hypertension worse than 1st pregnancy
3rd	P	Preeclampsia

Comments

Carol delivered at 32 weeks with her second pregnancy. Swimming helped bring down her blood pressure. Both swimming and hydrotherapy helped reduce her disability symptoms. During Carol's first pregnancy, she took time off work because of edema and the need to stay off her feet. During her second pregnancy, Carol's symptoms were more pronounced. She had both children by vaginal birth.

Celeste's Pregnancy History (2) (Cerebral Palsy)

Pregnancy: Age 29

Trimester	Cause	Physical Change
1st	?	Edema[a]
	P	Nausea
	P	Fatigue
2nd	PD	Edema
	P	Felt great during second trimester!
3rd	D	Anxiety[b]
	PD?	Edema

Pregnancy: Age 32

Trimester	Cause	Physical Change
1st	P	Same as previous pregnancy
2nd	P	Same as previous pregnancy

Comments

[a]Edema in the first trimester is unusual, and probably resulted from disability; in later trimesters, increased edema may have resulted from pregnancy alone. Celeste delivered both of her children vaginally.

Charlotte's Pregnancy History (1) (Cerebral Palsy)

Pregnancy: Age 27

Trimester	Cause	Physical Change
1st	P	Fatigue
2nd	PD	Balance affected
3rd	PD	Balance difficulty using steps
	P	Tying shoes
	P	Back pain
	P	High blood pressure (last month)

Comments

Charlotte delivered her child by caesarean section because of fetal distress.

Cheryl's Pregnancy History (1) (Cerebral Palsy)

Pregnancy: Age 28

Trimester	Cause	Physical Change
1st	P	Nausea
	P	Mood swings
	PD	Abdominal muscle cramps worse than usual
	P	Fatigue
	P	Cervical bleeding[a]
2nd	PD	Muscle spasms in back, thighs, and groin
	PD	Balance and walking more difficult
	P	Fatigue worse
3rd	PD	Muscle spasms in groin
	PD	Balance and walking still difficult
	P	Heartburn
	PD?	Shortness of breath[b]
	P	Urinating frequently
All		General health was excellent

Comments

Cheryl delivered vaginally.

[a]The bleeding caused concern that Cheryl was going to have a miscarriage. After a sonogram showed a normal pregnancy, it was found that a local irritation was causing bleeding from the cervical tissue.

[b]If her cerebral palsy affected her chest muscles, then her breathing capacity may have been diminished, making her more susceptible to shortness of breath during pregnancy.

Chloe's Pregnancy History (1) (Cerebral Palsy)

Pregnancy: Age 34

Trimester	Cause	Physical Change
1st	P	Fatigue
	P	Nausea
2nd	PD	Backaches
	P	Shortness of breath[a]
3rd	PD	Backaches
	PD	pneumonia/shortness of breath
	PD	Balancing, transferring, and daily activities such as bathing and dressing became more difficult
	P	Bladder infection
Unknown	P	Edema
	P	Tired more easily

Comments

[a]If her cerebral palsy affected her chest muscles, then her breathing capacity may have been diminished, making her more susceptible for having pneumonia during pregnancy. CP could make it difficult to cough. Chloe had a caesarean section because the baby was breech.

Christina's Pregnancy History (1) (Cerebral Palsy)

Pregnancy: Age 32

Trimester	Cause	Physical Change
1st	PD	Backaches
	PD	Muscle spasms
	P	Nausea
2nd	PD	Backaches
	PD	Muscle spasms
	P	Shortness of breath[a]
	P	Threatened miscarriage[b]
3rd	PD	Backaches
	PD	Muscle spasms
	PD?	Shortness of breath
	PD	Balancing, transferring, and daily activities such as bathing and dressing became more difficult

Comments

[a]If her cerebral palsy affected her chest muscles, then her breathing capacity may have been diminished, making her more susceptible to shortness of breath during pregnancy. Christina delivered vaginally.

[b]Christina's threatened miscarriage was caused by placenta previa, a pregnancy complication in which the placenta implants too low in the uterus. Placenta previa has nothing to do with disability. Christina was advised to rest in bed as much as possible. Lack of exercise caused some muscle atrophy and increased stiffness in the second and third trimesters.

Clara's Pregnancy History (2) (Cerebral Palsy)

Pregnancy: Age 30

Trimester	Cause	Physical Change
1st	P	Nausea
	P	Fatigue
2nd	PD	Muscle spasms
3rd	PD	Balance difficult; fell once; difficulty getting out of bathtub
	PD	Muscle spasms
All	P	Felt comfortably warm

Pregnancy: Age 34

Trimester	Cause	Physical Change
1st	P	Nausea
	P	Fatigue
2nd	PD	Muscle spasms
3rd	PD	Muscle spasms
	PD	Baby was low in pelvis, causing cramps in groin area that made walking difficult
	PD	Edema only in her nonaffected leg
	P	Vaginal infection
All	P	Felt warmer than usual

Comments
Clara delivered both her children vaginally.

Corrine's Pregnancy History (2) (Cerebral Palsy)

Pregnancy: Age 30

Trimester	Cause	Physical Change
1st	P	Nausea
	PD	Abdominal wall muscle cramps
2nd	PD	None recalled
3rd	PD	Physically awkward (had to take showers because getting in and out of bathtub was difficult)
	PD	Constant backaches
All	PD	Over course of pregnancy, posture became gradually more hunched over, and movement slower and more awkward

Pregnancy: Age 32

Same problems as first pregnancy, only more severe. Corrine delivered vaginally with both pregnancies.

Dierdre's Pregnancy History (1) (Degenerative Disc Disease)

Pregnancy: Age 43–44

Trimester	Cause	Physical Change
1st	P	Nausea
	P	Some fatigue
2nd	PD	Walking slowed down
	PD	Balance: fell more
	PD	Carpal tunnel symptoms reappeared
	PD	Back went out
	PD	Difficulty lifting legs up
	PD	Difficulty getting in and out of the bathtub and car
	PD	Difficulty putting socks on and off
	PD	Difficulty putting clothes on and off, and pulling pants up
	PD	Very tired
3rd	PD	More off balance
	PD	Less walking; more deconditioned
	PD	Walking difficulties
	P	Edema
	P	Blood pressure rose (last 3 weeks)
	PD	Sleeping disrupted

Comments

Deirdre started using her walker when she got out of bed during the night. She needed to urinate often. Getting in and out of bed often caused her back to go out. Her balance issues were worse than usual. She was immobilized the last 3 weeks of her pregnancy. She delivered her baby vaginally.

Darlene's Pregnancy History (1) (Dwarfism)

Pregnancy: Age 32

Trimester	Cause	Physical Change
1st	P	Morning sickness
2nd	PD	Hip pain
3rd	P	Indigestion
	PD	Backache
	P	Fatigue

Comments

Darlene only experienced minimal morning sickness. She controlled her hip and back pain with acupuncture. Darlene had backache that prevented her from sleeping on her back; she learned to sleep on her side. Darlene delivered by caesarean section because of fetopelvic disproportion (pelvis to small for fetus).

Diane's Pregnancy History (3) (Dwarfism)

Pregnancy: Age 27 (twins)

Pregnancy: Age 30

Pregnancy: Age 34

Trimester	Cause	Physical Change
1st	P	Hungry all the time
	P	Fatigue
2nd	PD	Bed rest
	PD	Hip pain
	PD	Edema
3rd	PD	Shortness of breath
	PD	Low backache
	PD	Mobility affected (waddled when walking)
	PD	Edema
	PD	Bed rest
	PD	Stopped driving

Comments

During her first pregnancy, Diane had contractions in the second trimester and was put on bed rest. Diane felt more movement of her babies in her 2nd and 3rd pregnancies because she had more room. With her second and third pregnancies, Diane did not experience much discomfort. She had only a little difficulty getting in and out of bed and walking. Diane delivered all of her children by caesarean section.

Denise's Pregnancy History (2) (Dwarfism)

Pregnancy: Age 21 early miscarriage 7 weeks

Pregnancy: Age 22 early miscarriage 10 weeks

Pregnancy: Age 23 Baby born prematurely and died

Pregnancy: Age 30

Trimester	Cause	Physical Change
1st	P	Spotting
	P	Morning sickness
	P	Anemic
	P	Fatigue
2nd	PD	Low back pain
	PD	Hip pain
	PD	Edema
	PD	Walking difficult
	PD	Impossible to reach for objects
	PD	Shortness of breath
	P	Morning sickness
3rd	PD	Shortness of breath
	PD	Heartburn
	PD	Low backache
	PD	Mobility affected
	PD	Edema

Comments

She had problems reaching for objects because her arms could not get around her belly. Denise could not drive her car. She also had problems reaching into cabinets. Other problems included the inability to carry lightweight objects as well as large items. She had warning signs with all four pregnancies, but it is impossible to tell if her disability caused the miscarriages. She spotted with all four pregnancies. Denise needed to be hospitalized at 26 weeks because of the danger the baby would press on her diaphragm and cause a heart attack. To prevent another miscarriage, Denise was put on bed rest. She felt that she should have been off her feet, because being on her feet contributed to her first miscarriage. She used a wheelchair in her last trimester. Denise had a caesarean section because her doctor did not want her to go into labor.

Dorothy's Pregnancy History (1) (Spondyloepiphyseal Dysplasia Congenita)

Pregnancy: Age 28

Trimester	Cause	Physical Change
1st	P	Morning sickness
	P	Hungry
2nd	PD	Respiratory problems
	PD	Edema
	PD	Difficulty dressing (putting socks on)
3rd	PD	Shortness of breath
	PD	Constipated
	PD	Balance
	PD	Transfer difficulty (in and out of bathtub)
	PD	Urinary incontinence
	PD	Difficulty dressing

Comments

Dorothy felt top heavy. Her baby was taken by caesarean section a month early because of her respiratory problems. She felt more immobile. Dorothy felt real good until the sixth month. She worked longer than she should have. She had extra amniotic fluid.

Dawn's Pregnancy History (1) (Dystonia)

Pregnancy: Age unknown; miscarriage[a]

Pregnancy: Age 27

Trimester	Cause	Physical Change
1st	P	Nausea
	P	Fatigue
2nd	PD	No specific changes recalled
3rd	PD	Urinated frequently
	PD	Hospitalized for kidney infections (problems persisted despite drinking plenty of water)
	O	Gastric ulcer
	PD	Backaches
	PD	Frequent muscle spasm
	P	Anemia

Comments

Dawn tripped so often she really could not walk at all. Transferring was not a problem, but getting out of the bathtub and sitting up from a lying down position were difficult.

Dawn delivered her baby by caesarean section.

[a]Dawn did not discuss this pregnancy because the baby died and the memory was painful.

Felicia's Pregnancy History (1) (Fibromyalgia)

Pregnancy: Age 36-37

Trimester	Cause	Physical Change
1st	P	Probable miscarriage of a twin
	P	Heavy bleeding @ 5 weeks
	P	Continued bleeding
	P	Morning sickness (throughout the day)
	PD	Terrible fatigue
	P	Back pain
2nd	PD	Asymptomatic except when working long days
	PD	Back pain made walking difficult
3rd	P	Hemorrhoids
	P	High blood pressure
	P	Early labor; cervix dilated at 34 weeks; bed rest prescribed
	P	Breast infection

Comments

Felicia had a vaginal birth.

Aftereffects

Felicia had a difficult delivery. She also had difficulty with breast-feeding during the first 3 weeks of the postpartum period, including cracked nipples, a breast infection, and thrush. She also experienced increased fatigue.

Hannah's Pregnancy History (2) (Hip Dysplegia)

Pregnancy: Age 24; miscarriage @ 10 weeks

Pregnancy: Age 28

Pregnancy: Age 30

Trimester	Cause	Physical Change
1st	P	Fatigue
2nd	PD	Arthritis in remission
	PD	Anemia
	PD	Constipation
3rd	P	Bed rest
	PD	More stiffness in hips and back
	P	Preterm labor (29 weeks)
	PD	Walking difficulties
	PD	Transfer problem
	P	Pitting edema
	P	Water retention

Comments

Second pregnancy: She was given iron because of anemia, which resulted in constipation. Hannah drank 5 quarts of water a day. Hannah's doctors felt her early labor was due to an irritable uterus. In her last 2 months of pregnancy, she put on 8 pounds in 10 days between visits to the doctor. Hannah's blood pressure did not rise, nor did she spill any protein.

Third pregnancy: She was not anemic and did not have to take iron, which resulted in her not being constipated. Her second pregnancy was the same as the first, except for a few exceptions: no medicine was needed, and extended bed rest was necessary to stop early labor. The early labor started at 34 weeks with the second. She had no edema. She found the last 6 weeks the worst. Breathing was difficult in the last trimester. Both babies were vaginal births.

Heather Ann's Pregnancy History (1) (Hip Dysplasia)

Pregnancy: Age 27

Trimester	Cause	Physical Change
1st	P	Heartburn
2nd	PD	Difficulty keeping balance
	P	Bladder control worse for remainder of pregnancy
	PD	Back pain and phantom pain worse
	P	Threatened miscarriage; bleeding, passing clots, and cervix dilating at 6 months (bed rest prescribed)
	P	Heartburn
3rd	PD	Balance worse; difficulty getting in and out of bathtub; began to use wheelchair outside of house
All	P	Heartburn
	PD	Muscle spasms in amputated leg more frequent
	P	Hair and nails healthier during pregnancy

Comments

When Heather was interviewed during her second pregnancy, she mentioned that she was much more comfortable than during her first pregnancy. She attributes this to being more relaxed because she knew what to expect. She commented, "I knew what my body would do; I knew my back would not be seriously affected." She had a caesarean section because of pelvic deformity.

Aftereffects

Heather's bladder control continues to be worse than before pregnancy; she urinates more frequently and has to go to the bathroom more often when she feels the urge.

Hilary's Pregnancy History (2) (Congenital Hip Deformity)

Pregnancy: Age 27

Trimester	Cause	Physical Change
1st	PD	Vertebrae slipped when lying down (had to realign joints before rising or movement was painful)[a]
2nd	PD	Balance became difficult
3rd	P	Edema
	PD?	Shortness of breath
	PD	Continued difficulty balancing
All	PD	Stress incontinence worse than usual

Pregnancy: Age 29

Symptoms were the same as with the first pregnancy, except that exacerbation of stress incontinence was even worse. Hilary decided to use a wheelchair during this pregnancy.

Comments

[a]This problem may have resulted from an interaction between Hilary's disability and the usual increase of joint mobility caused by pregnancy hormones. She had a caesarean section because of cephalopelvic disproportion.

Aftereffects

Hilary's back condition improved after the birth, but did not return to its original level.

Holly's Pregnancy History (3) (Congenital Hydrocephalus)

Pregnancy: Age 24

Pregnancy: Age 31

Pregnancy: Age 32

Trimester	Cause	Physical Change
1st	P	Morning sickness
	P	Distal end of shunt would stab[a]
2nd	P	Balance affected
	P	Fewer headaches
3rd	P	Balance affected
	P	Fewer headaches
	P	Distal end of shunt would stab

Pregnancy: Age 31

	P	Same as above

Comments

Her pregnancy at age 32 was the same as the pregnancy when she was 31. The trimesters of the second pregnancy were the same as the first pregnancy at age 24. The baby was lying on her sciatic nerve during the second and third trimesters. The baby was breech; Holly felt the baby kicking her cervix.

[a]Holly felt the reason the shunt stabbed her was the position of the baby in utero. Her shunt drains on the right side, and her babies preferred to lie on that side. In addition, the end of her VP shunt is low in the abdominal cavity where the uterus expands, especially during the first and third trimesters. She had fewer headaches with all three pregnancies. She knew that pregnancy raises intracranial pressure. She thought the reason she had fewer headaches during her pregnancies was because her shunt should have been at a little higher pressure. Holly's shunt was a problem for her first and third pregnancies.

Note: Holly's second pregnancy did not go to term because the baby had a fatal chromosomal disorder (trisomy 13). This fatal chromosomal disorder was found by a routine AFP test (low result), and then confirmed with a follow-up amniocentesis. Holly had two vaginal births and one caesarean section due to the baby's position.

Jennifer's Pregnancy History (1) (Juvenile Rheumatoid Arthritis)

Pregnancy: Age 30

Trimester	Cause	Physical Change
1st	P	Hungry all the time; felt sick when not eating enough
	PD	Started to enjoy walking[a]
2nd	P	Nasal congestion
	P	Leg cramps
	PD	Walked longer distances[b]
	P	Dropped objects often
3rd	P	Nasal congestion
	PD	Uncomfortable when sitting
	PD	Back pain
	PD	Increased skin sensitivity
	P	Feet swollen[c]
	P	Toe nails hurt[c]
	P	Edema
	P	Vaginal infection

Comments

[a]She used a wheelchair while at school, but walked more at other times.

[b]By the second trimester, the increase in how much she walked was dramatic: "I took walks for the first time in my life. Usually I complained when I needed to walk across the room."

[c]The pain of her swollen feet reminded Jennifer of the arthritic pain she often felt in her ankles, but it was most likely due to edema. The pain in her toe nails was probably another side effect of the swelling in her feet. She delivered vaginally.

Joan's Pregnancy History (1) (Juvenile Rheumatoid Arthritis)

Pregnancy: Age unknown; miscarriage (not believed to be related to disability)

Pregnancy: Age 22

Trimester	Cause	Physical Change
1st	PD	Disability went into remission
	P	Morning sickness
	P	Fatigue
	P	Spotting
	PD	Transferring improved
	P	Hair and skin better than ever
2nd	PD	Felt good
	P	Morning sickness (ended @ 5½ months)
	P	Nice hair
	PD	Transferring improved
	P	Hair and skin better than ever
3rd	PD	Breathing problem
	P	Backache
	PD	Transfers difficult (in and out of bed, car, and shower)
	PD	Difficulty dressing (pulling up panties and pants)
	P	Dizziness (low blood pressure)
	P	Hair and skin better than ever

Comments

Joan said her fatigue was "mind numbing." She knew she was pregnant because she had zero pain that lasted until postpartum. She had more mobility and energy because she was not restricted by pain, but she was so sick, she did not get to enjoy most of it. Joan stayed in bed most of time because of morning sickness. The baby was big and was riding high. Joan's skin was better than ever. Her bowels were more regular. Joan delivered by caesarean section because of fear that her hips could be dislocated.

Aftereffects

After she gave birth, Joan's arthritis pain returned 6 weeks postpartum.

Joy's Pregnancy History (1) (Juvenile Rheumatoid Arthritis)

Pregnancy: Age 35

Trimester	Cause	Physical Change
1st	P	Nausea
2nd	P	Felt great
		Flu
3rd	PD	Balance effected
	P	Incontinence
	PD	Back pain
	P	Feet swollen
	P	Edema in her legs

Comments

The pain of her swollen feet reminded Joy of the arthritic pain she often felt in her ankles, but it was most likely due to edema. She delivered by caesarean section because of hip replacement.

Julie's Pregnancy History (1) (Juvenile Rheumatoid Arthritis)

Pregnancy: Age 27

Trimester	Cause	Physical Change
1st		No specific changes recalled
2nd	PD	As weight increased, ankle pain became more severe than usual
	PD	As pregnancy progressed, some movements became more awkward and she had to change her way of getting in and out of cars
	P	Feet began to swell
3rd	PD	Ankles still more painful
		Fell and tore leg muscle in eighth month[a]
	PD	Hips more painful after fall
	P	Increased heartburn
	PD	Swollen feet
	PD	Pain in hips and tailbone
	PD	Standing and sitting difficult[b]
All		The level of arthritic pain in general remained unchanged

Comments

[a]Julie's arthritis did not cause her fall; she tripped on a throw rug. The fall caused a worsening of her arthritic pain.

[b]Julie adapted by sitting in different types of chairs at different times. For example, she sat on a high stool when she was washing dishes. She had a caesarean section.

Aftereffects
Julie's ankles bothered her more after she gave birth than they had before she was pregnant.

Laura's Pregnancy History (1) (Systemic Lupus Erythematosus)

Pregnancy: Age 37

Trimester	Cause	Physical Change
1st	P	Lupus mask darkened[a]
	D	Unpredictable joint pains
	P	Constipation
	P	Urinary infection
2nd	D	Joint pains continued
	PD	Difficulty breathing
	PD	Feeling ill (like having the flu)
3rd	D?	Food sensitivities developed
All	PD	Fatigue; mobility problems[b]; blood pressure labile

Comments
[a]The "lupus mask" is a reddish rash found on the faces of some people who have lupus. Chloasma, known as the "mask of pregnancy," occurs in some pregnant women. It consists of a darkening of areas of facial skin (with the same brown pigment found in a suntan or freckles). What seems to have happened is that chloasma darkened the same area of Laura's face which is affected by lupus mask. Her diagnosis switched between lupus and rheumatoid arthritis.

[b]Laura could not get around much, because she needed to move slowly and stop to rest, even after walking short distances.

In the third trimester, she was hospitalized for preeclampsia and treated with medication for blood pressure. Her baby was delivered by caesarean because of loss of placental function.

Aftereffects
She had seizures after she gave birth, and continued to have problems with fatigue and high blood pressure. Her seizures were mostly during the day. Second year postpartum, they were at night. By the third year, they were mostly at night and lessened. Her neurologist theorized that pregnancy triggered the seizures. When Laura was interviewed nine years later, her problems were fatigue and arthritis in her hands, shoulders, and knees; but no seizures.

Lea Rae's Pregnancy History (1) (Systemic Lupus Erythematosus)

Pregnancy: Age 38

Trimester	Cause	Physical Change
1st	P	Tired
	P	Nausea
	PD	Arthritis symptoms improved
2nd	P	Felt great
	P	Urinating more
3rd	PD	Difficulty breathing
	PD	Back pain
	PD	Edema in feet
	PD	Transferring in and out of car and bathtub
	PD	Difficulty putting on shoes
	PD	Exhausted

Comments

Lea Rae felt nauseous for 3 weeks and vomited twice. Although she felt tired, she said it was a different kind of tired. The baby was against her diaphragm, making it difficult to breathe, especially when it was cold outside. Lea Rae was able to walk with ease until the eighth month, when her feet swelled. Lea Rae delivered her child vaginally.

Leslie's Pregnancy History (3) (Systemic Lupus Erythematosus)

First Pregnancy: Age 26

Trimester	Cause	Physical Change
1st	P	Nausea
	D	Occasional blood spotting
2nd	D	Continued spotting (bed rest prescribed)
3rd	D	Premature birth with placental abruption[a]
All	PD	Psoriasis cleared up for duration of pregnancy
	D	Temperature fluctuations between 96° and 101°F
	PD	Remission of arthritic symptoms

Second Pregnancy: Age 29

Trimester	Cause	Physical Change
1st	P	Nausea
	D	Blood spotting
2nd	D	Felt pelvic pressure 4th month, miscarriage 5th month
All	PD	Psoriasis cleared up for duration of pregnancy
	D	Temperature fluctuations worse than during first pregnancy
	PD	Remission of arthritic symptoms

Third Pregnancy: Age 31

Trimester	Cause	Physical Change
1st	D	Temperature fluctuations (controlled with medication)
	D	Blood spotting
	P	Nausea
	PD	Partial miscarriage; one twin died (bed rest to end of term)
	P	Anemia after miscarriage to end of term
	P	Diabetes from 3rd month to end of term[b]
2nd	P	Yeast infection at end of trimester
	D	Less spotting with medication
	D	High blood pressure[c]
3rd	D	Temporary loss of vision in one eye[c]
	D	High blood pressure[c]
	D	Short-term memory impaired[c]
	D	Proteinuria[c]
	PD	Birth in seventh month
All	PD	Psoriasis cleared up for duration of pregnancy
	D	Temperature fluctuations in first trimester controlled by medication
	PD	Remission of arthritic symptoms

Comments

[a]The presence of lupus antibodies led to placental rejection.

[b]This appears to have been diabetes of pregnancy. Leslie did not need to use medication to control her diabetes, because she was able to do so with diet.

[c]Leslie said she had preeclampsia during her third pregnancy. These symptoms are also symptoms of SLE exacerbation, so it can be difficult to determine whether a woman is experiencing preeclampsia or SLE exacerbation. Since preeclampsia typically occurs in a first pregnancy, it seems likely that Leslie's problems were related to SLE. She delivered her first child by caesarean section because the baby was in a transverse position. Her other two babies were delivered by vaginal birth. In her second pregnancy, she lost a set of twins: one of the babies because of premature birth, the other by a miscarriage.

Aftereffects

At the end of each pregnancy, Leslie's psoriasis returned. After the third pregnancy, her vision began to return gradually. She had a flare-up of many other symptoms just after the third pregnancy, including difficulty walking, and the arthritis in her shoulders became so severe that it was hard for her to pick up her baby. She was bothered by fevers, nausea, and fatigue. At the time of her interview, when her daughter was 5 months old, she had only slight difficulty walking, and the arthritis in her shoulders and hands had improved.

Mandy's Pregnancy History (3) (Multiple Sclerosis)

Miscarriages: 7

Pregnancy: Age 14

Pregnancy: Age 28

Pregnancy: Age 36

Trimester	Cause	Physical Change
All	PD	Fatigue

Comments

Her miscarriages were due to a low level of the hormone progesterone. Mandy miscarried in the first trimester. She delivered vaginally with all three live births.

Aftereffects

After her first pregnancy, Mandy's felt exhausted after the delivery. She also experienced numbness in her legs. After the delivery of her second child, Mandy had numbness in her arms. After the delivery of her third child, Mandy had numbness in her hands and depression.

Margie's Pregnancy History (2) (Multiple Sclerosis)

Pregnancy: Age 27

Trimester	Cause	Physical Change
All	PD	Walking difficult, one leg dragged; bladder problems disappeared

Pregnancy: Age 30

Comments

Physical changes same as previous pregnancy.

Aftereffects

After her first pregnancy, Margie's MS worsened slightly. Her main problem was blurred vision. After her second pregnancy, she made sure she had extra help, and there was no exacerbation of MS. She delivered both of her babies vaginally.

Marsha's Pregnancy History (1) (Multiple Sclerosis)

Pregnancy: Age unknown; miscarriage

Pregnancy: Age 32

Trimester	Cause	Physical Change
All	D	Impaired mobility (needed to use two canes)
	PD	Bladder problems: alternated between urgency and incontinence

Aftereffects
Three years later, Marsha needed to use a wheelchair almost all the time. She delivered her baby vaginally.

Mary's Pregnancy History (1) (Multiple Sclerosis)

Pregnancy: Age unknown; miscarriage (caused by placenta previa)

Pregnancy: Age 31

Trimester	Cause	Physical Change
All	PD	Fatigue[a]
Unknown	PD	Poor bladder control[b]

Comments
[a]Mary said, "I used my walker, but sometimes I was so tired, I thought of using a wheelchair."

[b]Bladder control was so poor that she stayed close to home much of the time. She delivered her baby vaginally.

Aftereffects
Ten years later, Mary still tires easily and has considered using a wheelchair. She also had some muscle spasms.

Michelle's Pregnancy History (1) (Multiple Sclerosis)

Pregnancy: Age 35

Trimester	Cause	Physical Change
1st	PD	Tired more easily than usual
	P	Nausea
2nd	P	Low back pain
3rd	PD	Tired more easily than usual
	D	Vision more blurred
	D	Pins-and-needles sensation on right arm, leg, and scalp
	PD	Frequent muscle spasms for one week
All	PD	Increased urgency to urinate, but no incontinence
Unknown	P	Trouble sleeping

Comments
She delivered her baby vaginally.

Aftereffects
Two years after she gave birth, Michelle's hand and feet were somewhat numb.

Mimi's Pregnancy History (1) (Multiple Sclerosis)

Pregnancy: Age 35

Trimester	Cause	Physical Change
1st	P	Slight nausea
	P	Bladder infection
2nd	P	Intermittent heartburn
	PD	One instance of incontinence
	PD	Walked more
3rd	PD	Balance effected
	PD	Walk changed
	PD	One instance of incontinence
	P	More heartburn
	PD	More difficult to put shoes on
	P	Bladder infection

Comments
Mimi felt better when stopped taking Betaseron®. She had more energy during her pregnancy. In the second trimester, Mimi had more energy and enjoyed walking every day; in the third trimester, she walked less because it was more difficult. Mimi never experienced incontinence, except for the two incidences that occurred in the middle of the night. Mimi's gait got wider. She delivered vaginally.

Moira's Pregnancy History (1) (Multiple Sclerosis)

Pregnancy: Age 35

Trimester	Cause	Physical Changes
1st	P	Tired
	PD	Walking became unsteady
	P	No real problems
2nd	P	Borderline anemia
	PD	Tired
3rd	PD?	Back problems
	PD	Tired
	P	Huge
	PD	Balance effected

Comments

Moira had spasticity prior to pregnancy, but this was eliminated during pregnancy. She was tired her entire pregnancy. Moira felt great. Her husband helped her in the shower at 7½ months. Getting around was different thing. Moira delivered vaginally.

Mona's Pregnancy History (1) (Multiple Sclerosis)

Pregnancy: Age 33

Trimester	Cause	Physical Changes
1st	P	Nausea
	PD	Walking became unsteady
2nd	P	Anemia
	PD	Could walk longer distances
	PD	Balance improved
3rd	PD	Needed walker
	PD	Had less energy
	PD	Spasticity continued

Comments

Mona had spasticity prior to pregnancy, but it worsened during pregnancy. She was not tired from the first trimester until the first half of the second trimester. Mona felt the first trimester was more "bothersome," because "everything was new and there were a lot of changes." Mona was put on iron supplements in her second trimester, and she had more energy. She got around more. During the third trimester, it was more difficult to get around. Mona had a caesarean section because her baby was breech.

Naomi's Pregnancy History (2) (Charcot-Marie-Tooth)

Pregnancy: Age 35

Trimester	Cause	Physical Change
1st	P	Fatigue
	P	Hungry
	P	Little nausea
	PD	Carpal tunnel (6 weeks)
2nd	PD	Carpal tunnel
	PD	Balance affected
3rd	PD	Carpal tunnel
	PD	Used a walker
	PD	Drop foot worse
	PD	Difficulty carrying things
	D	Transfer hard (in and out of bathtub)

Pregnancy: Age 37-38

Trimester	Cause	Physical Change
1st	P	Lethargic and did not feel well
	P	Barely any nausea
	PD	Mild carpal tunnel
2nd	PD	Very lethargic
	PD	Mild carpal tunnel
	PD	Avoided walking long distances
3rd	PD	Had more energy
	P	Gestational diabetes diagnosed
	PD	Carpal tunnel worse
	P	Mild sciatica right leg
	PD	Unsteady on feet; hips wobbly

Comments

Naomi got cortisone shots for her carpal tunnel. She fell and sprained her fingers. She had a vaginal birth in her second pregnancy. Naomi felt "out of it." this was probably due to gestational diabetes. In the second trimester, she avoided walking long distances, and did not use a walker because she felt uncomfortable using it in public. Naomi did not have any problems other than expected when getting up from a chair. She did not have any problems getting in and out of the bathtub or car. She delivered her children vaginally.

Aftereffects

Naomi was able to walk for many blocks without using an assistive device other than her leg braces. Naomi had excruciating shoulder/chest pain, probably from carrying her baby and being generally weaker in her upper extremities because of her disability. Physical therapy was needed for several months. The pain diminished after 4 months of physical therapy.

Natalie's Pregnancy History (2) (Charcot-Marie-Tooth)

Pregnancy: Age 26-27

Trimester	Cause	Physical Change
1st	P	Morning sickness
	P	Fatigue
	P	Spotting
2nd	P	Felt great
	P	Starved
	PD	Felt weaker difficulty getting in and out of bathtub and car
	PD	Waddled when walking
	PD	Backache
3rd	PD	Drop foot worse
	PD	Difficulty getting in and out of bathtub and car
	PD	Felt weaker
	PD	Feet ache (edema)
	P	Bladder infection
	P	Lost sleep
	P	Fast heartbeat and nausea

Comments

Natalie felt she had a healthy pregnancy. She did not feel her baby kick. The cardiologist said her tachycardia (fast heart beat) was due to the increase in blood volume and hormones, which is common. Her baby rode low. Another doctor felt that the baby was lying on the sciatic nerve, causing her to fall. Natalie had edema the last 6 weeks of her pregnancy. She experienced edema after the birth of her baby. She delivered by caesarean section because of fetal distress.

During her second pregnancy, Natalie had swelling of her feet during the last 8 weeks of pregnancy. She delivered her second baby vaginally.

Aftereffects

Five months post-delivery, Natalie saw no negative effects from the first pregnancy. She recovered sooner from her second pregnancy.

Nora's Pregnancy History (1) (Charcot-Marie-Tooth)

Pregnancy: Age 28

Trimester	Cause	Physical Change
1st	P	Morning sickness
	P	Fatigue
	P	Difficult to rest (psychologically difficult)
	P	Nose bleeds
2nd	P	More growth in both hair and nails
	PD	Felt weaker
	P	Nose bleeds
3rd	PD	All transfers difficult (in and out of bathtub and car)
	PD	Felt weaker
	P	Nose bleeds

Comments

Nora felt she had a healthy pregnancy. She could not tell if she was getting weaker, or if her weakness was because of weight gain. She was able to transfer during the first trimester. Nora needed to stay home more because of difficulty transferring on and off the toilet. She delivered her baby vaginally 5 weeks early (35 weeks).

Noelle's Pregnancy History (1) (Friedreich's Ataxia)

Pregnancy: Age 25

Trimester	Cause	Physical Change
1st		No specific changes recalled
2nd	P	Shortness of breath after large meals
	PD	Sharp pains with fetal movement[a]
3rd	P	Heartburn
	PD	Increased scoliosis and backache
	PD	Stress incontinence worsened
	P	Constipation
All	D	Disability symptoms slowly worsened throughout pregnancy; bladder problems increased; leg cramps became more frequent; [b]increased mobility difficulties

Comments

[a]Noelle considered this pain to be a normal, if uncommon, pregnancy discomfort.

[b]She retained enough leg strength to transfer, but needed support when standing or getting in and out of the shower.

Aftereffects

During the 6 months after childbirth, Noelle's disability symptoms returned to what they had been before pregnancy. Later worsening of symptoms can be attributed to the expected progression of her disorder.

During a conversation several years after her interview, Noelle had had a second child, and was pregnant for the third time. Her first child was delivered surgically, and her second was born vaginally. Noelle commented, "I often wonder whether I really needed to have that C-section the first time." She also commented that she recovered much more quickly after vaginal delivery.

Nikki's Pregnancy History (7) (Friedreich's Ataxia)

Early miscarriages (4)

Pregnancy: Age 25

Pregnancy: Age 27

Pregnancy: Age 29

Pregnancy: Age 33

Pregnancy: Age 35

Pregnancy: Age 37

Pregnancy: Age 39

Trimester	Cause	Physical Change
1st	P	Morning sickness
	P	Exhausted
2nd		Felt great
3rd	PD	Shortness of breath
	PD	Mobility impaired (difficulty rolling over)
	PD	Difficulty transferring (on and off the toilet and bathtub)

Comments

Nikki experienced heartburn, and felt more nervous during the night with the last three pregnancies. She used a walker during her first pregnancy. She found it difficult to use the walker. Nikki was independent in using bathroom facilities. She started using a wheelchair because she fell and was afraid of hurting the baby. Nikki experienced muscle spasms at night. She had shortness of breath in the third trimester with all her pregnancies. This happened at night and sometimes during the day. Nikki delivered all seven of her children vaginally.

Aftereffects

Nikki returned back to normal after a few months.

Nadine Fiona's Pregnancy History (1) (Limb-Girdle Dystrophy)

Pregnancy: Age 21

Trimester	Cause	Physical Changes
1st	P	Morning sickness
	P	Fatigued
	P	Light-headed
	D	Fibromyalgia (worsened)
	D	Short of breath
	P	Heart racing
	P	Trouble sleeping
	P	Light-headedness (low blood pressure)
2nd	P	Morning sickness (fourth month)
	PD	Fatigued lessened
	PD	Transfers difficult (seated to standing)
	PD	Balance affected
	PD	Walking more difficult
	P	Low blood pressure (light-headed)
	P	Fibromyalgia in remission
	PD	Short of breath
3rd	PD	Edema
	PD	Transfers difficult (seated to standing; in and out of bed and bathtub)
	PD	Balance worsened
	PD	Walking more difficult
	PD	Fibromyalgia in remission
	PD	Back weaker
	PD	Stopped driving
	PD	Short of breath
	P	Light-headedness (low blood pressure)

Comments
Nadine Fiona felt sick all day. She felt her bigger belly threw her off balance and made walking more difficult. She had a caesarean section.

Aftereffects
Her fibromyalgia returned.

Natasha's Pregnancy History (1) (Limb-Girdle Dystrophy)

Pregnancy: Age 20

Trimester	Cause	Physical Change
1st	P	Morning sickness
	P	Fatigue
2nd	P	Fatigue lessened
	PD	Transfers difficult (seated to standing)
	PD	Balance affected
3rd	PD	Edema (hands and feet)
	PD	Backache (diminished)
	PD	Balance affected
	P	Constipated
	P	Heartburn
	PD	Waking more difficult
	P	Hair and skin better than ever

Comments

Going from seated to standing, Natasha needed to twist and turn to compensate for lack of muscle strength. This caused a feeling of pressure on the spine. She had a more difficult time choosing shoes because of foot drop and edema. Natasha never woke up with a backache if she slept on her side with a pillow. She had a caesarean section because of fetal distress.

Aftereffects

Natasha's pregnancy made her weaker. She felt that her inability to go from seated to standing without assistance was not caused by the pregnancy, but by the natural progression of her disability, which had started prior to pregnancy.

Nicole's Pregnancy History (3) (Limb-Girdle Dystrophy)

Pregnancy: Age 18

Miscarriage: Age 20

Pregnancy: Age 21

Trimester	Cause	Physical Change
1st	P	Morning sickness
2nd	P	Morning sickness
	PD	Transfers difficult
3rd	P	Morning sickness
	PD	Transfers difficult

Comments

The cause of the miscarriage is unknown.

1st pregnancy: Nicole went from walking to using a wheelchair full time.

1st, 2nd, and 3rd pregnancies: Nicole was only a little sick with morning sickness, otherwise there were not any differences between the pregnancies. Her babies were vaginally delivered.

Nadia's Pregnancy History (1) (Myasthenia Gravis)

Pregnancy: Age 34

Trimester	Cause	Physical Change
1st	P	Fatigue
	P	Morning sickness
	O	Sinus infection
2nd	PD	Extreme fatigue
	O	Sinus infection
3rd	PD	Facial weakness
	D	Double vision
	D	Difficulty smiling

Comments

Nadia felt was aware of her first symptoms of myasthenia gravis during her second trimester. Nadia had double vision and arm weakness in her second trimester. She had no problems with walking and transferring. Half of her face was paralyzed. She was able to deliver vaginally.

Noreen's Pregnancy History (1) (Myasthenia Gravis)

Pregnancy: Age 27

Trimester	Cause	Physical Change
1st	PD	Extreme fatigue
	P	Morning sickness
	PD	Depressed
2nd	PD	Extreme fatigue
	PD	Trouble walking: implanted fascia; burning pain in fascia
3rd	PD	Improved; felt stronger
	PD	Developed diabetes

Comments

Noreen had polyhydramnios (too much amniotic fluid). She was hospitalized in the 34th week for this problem. She became weak, and went to stay with her parents in order get support. She was able to go shopping in her third trimester. She had a caesarean section because of placenta abruptio.

Nancy's Pregnancy History (1) (Spinal Muscular Atrophy)

Pregnancy: Age 22; elective abortion

Pregnancy: Age 24

Trimester	Cause	Physical Change
1st	PD	Fatigue (end of trimester)
2nd	PD	Bronchitis (three times)
	PD	Difficulty transferring by end of trimester, especially in shower; low back pain
3rd	P	Bladder infection
	PD	Continued difficulty transferring
	PD	Low back pain continued; lower back stiff
	PD	Difficulty balancing; used arms for stabilizing
Unknown	PD?	Breathing more difficult
	PD	Back pain worse

Comments

Delivered by caesarean section; possibly due to misinformation.

Aftereffects

Two years after she gave birth, Nancy's breathing difficulties and back pain remained worse than they had been before pregnancy.

Nina's Pregnancy History (1) (Spinal Muscular Atrophy)

Pregnancy: Age 21

Trimester	Cause	Physical Changes
1st	P	Morning sickness
	PD	Backache
2nd	P	Morning sickness (4th month)
3rd	PD	Transfers difficult (being rolled over, and onto the toilet)

Comments

Nina felt sick all day. She got antinausea medication that stopped the vomiting. She had a caesarean section because the baby was too big to be delivered vaginally. Nina's husband does much of her personal care, including transfers into the bathtub and rolling her over in bed. Nina did her own transfers to the toilet, but got a personal care assistant who did her personal care after pregnancy. Her baby was delivered by caesarean section.

Olivia's Pregnancy History (1) (Osteogenesis Imperfecta)

Pregnancy: Age 36

Trimester	Cause	Physical Change
1st	P	Nausea
2nd & 3rd	P	Felt great

Comments

Olivia delivered by caesarean section.

Oprah's Pregnancy History (2) (Osteogenesis Imperfecta)

Pregnancy: Age 25

Trimester	Cause	Physical Change
1st	P	insomnia
2nd	*see below	
3rd	D	Broken hip (crutches slipped)
	P	Heartburn
*All	P	Morning sickness
All	P	Migraines dissipated
All	P	Heartburn

Pregnancy: Age 27

Trimester	Cause	Physical Change
1st	P	Insomnia
All	P	Felt great
All	P	Migraines dissipated
All	PD	Walking

Comments

Oprah gained 15 and 18 pounds during her pregnancies, respectively. This may have contributed to her not experiencing any mobility problems. She walked with both pregnancies. She also did not have any problems with self-care. Oprah thought that that staying active helped with decreasing breaks. She delivered both of her children by caesarean section. Her second child was born 4 weeks early because she went into labor; medication could not stop the early labor. Her second child weighed four pounds eleven ounces.

Orielle's Pregnancy History (1) (Osteogenesis Imperfecta)

Pregnancy: Age 34

Trimester	Cause	Physical Change
1st	P	Morning sickness
2nd		Flu
		Hypoglycemia worsened
3rd	PD	Difficult breathing
	PD	Pelvis area painful
	PD	Difficulty transferring (bed, car, and bathtub)
	PD	Difficulty with the activities of daily living: could not tie shoes laces or do laundry
	PD	Difficulty picking things up off the floor

Comments

Oriel had hypoglycemia that came on fast; she got a headache and was light-headed. She was the most uncomfortable when the baby was small and under her ribs. As the body prepares for birth, the ligaments loosen as well as the interpubic disc, which impacts the diameters of the pelvic area. Her pelvic area was painful.

Aftereffects

Oriel's back improved. She had scoliosis, which improved by 10 degrees.

Pam's Pregnancy History (1) (Post-Polio Syndrome)

Pregnancy: Age 26

Trimester	Cause	Physical Change
1st	P	Fatigue
	P	Nausea
2nd	P	Continued nausea
	PD	Weight of pregnancy caused stretching of implanted fascia and burning pain in fascia
3rd	P	Badly swollen feet
	PD	Pain in fascia increased
	P	Urinating frequently
	PD	Constant aching in right hip[a]
	PD	Some decrease in mobility (rolling over became more difficult; could not sit up in bathtub)
All	P	Fewer bladder problems than usual, but continuous problems with edema

Comments

[a]Pam could not lie on her left side because of her scoliosis and shoulder fusion. Her baby was positioned to the right, so while she was pregnant, there was more pressure when she lay on her right side. The extra weight led to the aching in her hip. She had a caesarean section because not only was her baby was bigger than her pelvis, but also her pelvis was deformed.

Patricia's Pregnancy History (1) (Post-Polio Syndrome)

Pregnancy: Age 20

Trimester	Cause	Physical Change
1st	P	Fatigue
2nd		No specific changes recalled
3rd	P	Heartburn
All	P	Occasional hemorrhoids

Comments
Patricia delivered vaginally.

Paula's Pregnancy History (2) (Post-Polio Syndrome)

Pregnancy: Age 25

Trimester	Cause	Physical Change
1st	P	Morning sickness
2nd	P	Morning sickness continued
3rd	P	Urinated frequently

Pregnancy: Age 27; miscarriage due to polio infection (first trimester)

Pregnancy: Age 29

Trimester	Cause	Physical Change
1st	P	Morning sickness
2nd	P	Morning sickness
	PD	Difficulty balancing (getting in and out of car)
	PD	Swollen legs
	PD	Aching in hips and back
	PD	Muscle spasms
3rd	P	Urinated frequently
	PD	Problems with balance

Pregnancy: Age 31

Comments

Symptoms same as previous pregnancy. Paula delivered vaginally.

Portia's Pregnancy History (5) (Post-Polio Syndrome)

Portia did not remember her pregnancies, so this table was eliminated.

She had five pregnancies from age 23; last pregnancies were at age 36. All five were delivered by caesarean section.

Pricilla's Pregnancy History (2) (Post-Polio Syndrome)

Pregnancy: Age 27

Trimester	Cause	Physical Change
1st	P	Fatigue
2nd		No specific changes recalled
3rd	P	Anemia

Pregnancy: Age 37

Trimester	Cause	Physical Change
1st	P	Fatigue
2nd		No specific changes recalled
3rd	P	Heartburn

Comments

Pregnancy did not seem to impair Priscilla's mobility. She delivered both of her children vaginally.

Aftereffects

She feels she has gotten much stronger since her second child was born. She started taking yoga classes.

Rachel's Pregnancy History (2) (Rheumatoid Arthritis)

Pregnancy: Age 31

Trimester	Cause	Physical Change
1st	P	Morning sickness
2nd	P	Placenta previa
3rd	P	Placenta moved into the normal position

Comments

Rachel did not have any rheumatoid arthritis symptoms prior to getting pregnant. Symptoms started during pregnancy and lasted until her child was two. She was anemic before pregnancy, and continued to be anemic during pregnancy. She delivered her child vaginally.

Pregnancy: Age 34

Trimester	Cause	Physical Change
1st	P	Morning sickness
	D	Increased difficulty walking
	D	One knee got synovitis and became more "bent"
	D	Tops of her feet affected
2nd	D	Flare-up worsened
	D	Could not bear any weight on her right leg
	P	Constipation (because increased iron pills)

Comments

Her first child was born vaginally. Her arthritis symptom occurred when her baby was 2 years old. She had a positive pregnancy blood test with her second pregnancy. She was also tested for the RA factor, which came back negative. She had never had negative RA results before. In fact, she was having an arthritic flare-up. The reason it came back negative was because she was pregnant. Her morning sickness did not include any sensitivity to taste and smell. She was anemic before pregnancy, and she continued to be anemic during pregnancy.

Renee's Pregnancy History (2) (Rheumatoid Arthritis)

Pregnancy: Age 22

Trimester	Cause	Physical Change
1st	D	Leg became stiff and sore[a]
2nd	D	Increased difficulty walking
	D	Arthritis diagnosed; unable to move one leg
	PD	Difficulty getting in and out of bathtub
3rd	D	Increased difficulty walking
	P	Occasional dizziness in afternoon (improved with iron tablets)
	PD	Difficulty sitting (driving became difficult)

Pregnancy: Age 26

Trimester	Cause	Physical Change
1st	D	No arthritic pain
2nd	D	Increased difficulty walking
	D	Arthritic pain increased
	PD	More difficulty getting in and out of bathtub than in previous pregnancy
3rd	D	Increased difficulty walking
	D	Arthritic pain increased

Comments

[a]First symptoms of arthritis occurred; leg became increasingly sore and stiff throughout pregnancy. Arthritic pain was worse with emotional stress. She delivered both of her children vaginally.

Aftereffects

After Renee's first child was born, her leg improved somewhat, but it was still stiff and painful.

Roberta's Pregnancy History (1) (Rheumatoid Arthritis)

Pregnancy: Age 28

Trimester	Cause	Physical Change
1st	D	Arthritic pain worsened; stiffness in hands, shoulders, and knees in the morning[a]
2nd	PD	Pain and stiffness improved
3rd	PD	Further improvement in arthritic pain
All	PD	Continuous problems with bladder and urinary tract infections
Unknown	P	Experienced muscle cramps about five times

Comments

[a]Roberta said, "My arthritis improved about 95 percent. I felt as if I could walk forever. I felt better than usual and I had lots of energy." She delivered her child vaginally.

Sophia Amelia's Pregnancy History (2) (Sacral Agenesis)

Pregnancy: Age 24

Trimester	Cause	Physical Change
1st	P	Morning sickness
	P	Difficulty sleeping
	P	Migraine
	P	Started having breasts
	PD	Bladder infection
	P	Constipation
	P	Gas pains
2nd	P	Morning sickness (subsiding)
	P	Gas pains
	P	Migraine (subsiding)
	PD	Bladder infection
	PD	Edema in feet
3rd	P	Heartburn
	P	Gas pains
	PD	Difficulty transferring out of bed (easier to go from up to down)
	PD	Balance difficulty
	PD	Back pain
	PD	Edema in feet

Pregnancy: Age 29

Trimester	Cause	Physical Change
1st	P	Morning sickness (less severe than the first)
	P	Heartburn
	PD	Bladder infection
	P	Constipation
2nd	P	Heartburn
	PD	Severe kidney pain
	PD	Balance difficulty
	PD	Back pain
	PD	Edema in hands
3rd	P	Heartburn
	PD	Difficulty transferring out of bed (easier to go from up to down)
	PD	Stopped driving (difficulty getting from wheelchair to driver's seat)
	PD	Back pain
	PD	Getting on and off the toilet
	PD	Edema in hands
	PD	Difficulty pushing her chair

Comments

She delivered both children by caesarean because she has a dislocated pelvis and hip.

Sabine's Pregnancy History (2) (Spinal Bifida)

Pregnancy: Age 39; miscarriage

Trimester	Cause	Physical Change
1st	P	Fatigue
2nd	D	Radicular pain

Pregnancy: Age 45

Trimester	Cause	Physical Change
1st	P	Morning sickness
	P	Fatigue
2nd	PD	Kidney infections
	PD	Difficult to keep ostomy bag attached to the skin
3rd	PD	Mobility problems (used canes)
	PD	Edema (both feet)
	PD	Detached retina
	PD	Difficult to keep ostomy bag attached to the skin

Comments

Sabine's radicular pain followed the dermatome at T-6, 7, and 8 level. She did not have pressure sores, heartburn, or respiratory problems. She had a splint on her leg. Sabine's good leg gave out during pregnancy. She experienced calf tightness. Sabine delivered her child vaginally.

Sasha's Pregnancy History (1) (Spinal Bifida)

Pregnancy: Age 24

Trimester	Cause	Physical Change
1st	P	Fatigue
2nd	P	Heartburn (developed hiatus hernia)
	PD	Difficulty walking (began using crutches)[a]
	PD	Difficulty getting in and out of car
	PD	Problems with pressure sores, which disappeared for remainder of term[b]
3rd	P	Continued heartburn
	PD	Continued difficulty walking
	P	Edema
	PD	Back pain
All	PD	Bladder problems worse than usual; constant dripping

Comments

[a]When interviewed, Sasha said she wished that during the second trimester she had started using a wheelchair all the time. She thinks she would have been much more comfortable. Sasha delivered her baby vaginally.

[b]This was the first time that Sasha was not troubled by pressure sores.

Sherry Adele's Pregnancy History (1) (Spinal Bifida)

Pregnancy: Age 31

Trimester	Cause	Physical Change
1st	P	Fatigue
	P	Hives
	PD	Foley catheter
2nd	PD	Bladder infection
	PD	Difficulty going from sitting to standing
3rd	P	Continued heartburn
	PD	Continued difficulty walking
	P	Edema
	PD	Back pain

Pregnancy: Age 34

Trimester	Cause	Physical Change
1st	P	Fatigue
	P	Morning sickness
2nd	P	Heartburn (developed hiatus hernia)
	PD	Bladder infection (Pseudomonas)
	PD	Foley catheter
	PD	Bathing a problem
	PD	Difficulty going from sitting to standing
3rd	PD	Difficulty walking
	PD	Skin improved

Comments

Sherry Adele's stump improved. As soon as she conceived, she broke out in hives. Then she broke out again 6 months post-delivery. Having an indwelling catheter did not change her bladder capacity after pregnancy. She was given a medication cocktail after her second pregnancy, which reduced the spasticity of her bladder. She had a prolapsed uterus, resulting in a hysterectomy. She delivered her babies by caesarean section because she felt that labor would put more strain on her ligaments and muscles.

Sienna's Pregnancy History (1) (Spinal Bifida)

Three miscarriages

Pregnancy: Age 33

Trimester	Cause	Physical Change
1st	P	Morning sickness
	PD	Bladder infection
2nd	PD	Decrease of back pain
	PD	
3rd	PD	Left hip pain
	P	Fibroids (8th and 9th months)
	PD	Difficult mobility (walking and driving)
	P	Gestational diabetes

Comments

Her blood tests indicated lupus-like traits, which may have caused the earlier miscarriages. She had regional anesthesia, resulting in a long recovery period. It took Sienna 3 to 4 months to be able to walk on her crutches. She was unable to carry any weight. She could not even carry a purse. It took a year or so before she regained the sensation in her leg. Sienna had an unplanned caesarean section because she was overdue; the doctor did not induce.

Sierra's Pregnancy History (1) (Spinal Bifida)

Pregnancy: Age 22

Trimester	Cause	Physical Change
1st	P	Morning sickness
	P	Bladder infection twice
2nd	P	Morning sickness
3rd	PD	Mobility problems (hard to walk)
	PD	Breathing difficulties
	P	Heartburn
	PD	Transfer problems (getting off the couch and out of the bathtub)
	PD	Urinating urgency
	PD	Severe back pain (last week of pregnancy)

Comments

Morning sickness lasted until seventh month. She threw up every day. Sierra usually does not have bladder infections. She delivered vaginally. Her child has mild CP; cause unknown.

Simi's Pregnancy History (1) (Spinal Bifida)

Pregnancy: Age 32

Trimester	Cause	Physical Change
1st	P	Fatigue
	P	Morning sickness
2nd	PD	Transfer problems (in and out of bathtub)
3rd	PD	Mobility problems
	PD	Edema
	PD	Transfer problems (in and out of car and bathtub)

Comments

She had morning sickness and constipation, and threw up every day. Simi has not had any bladder infections since she was 19, and did not have any during her pregnancy. Simi delivered vaginally.

Aftereffects

Her bladder went numb after delivery, but returned to normal 9 months later.

Sybil's Pregnancy History (1) (Spinal Bifida)

Pregnancy: Age 22

Trimester	Cause	Physical Change
1st	P	Morning sickness
2nd	PD	Back pain
	PD	Kidney infection
3rd	PD	Continued back pain
	P	Edema
	PD	Difficulty transferring from bed to chair and from chair to bathtub
	PD	Difficulty bending, particularly when putting on shoes
	PD	Difficulty using crutches (began using wheelchair)
All	PD	Muscle spasms in legs worsened
Unknown	P	Sleeplessness

Comment

Sybil delivered her baby by caesarean section because she has a urostomy.

Sally's Pregnancy History (2) (Spinal Cord Injury)

Pregnancy: Age 30

Trimester	Cause	Physical Change
1st	P	Tired easily
2nd	P	Skin broke out (pimples on back)
	PD	Kidney infection (6th month)
	PD	Bladder infection
	PD	Spasm diminished
	PD	Transfers were more difficult
3rd	P	Edema (feet and ankles)
	PD	Spasm diminished
	PD	Bladder infection

Pregnancy: Age 34

1st	P	Tired easily
2nd	P	Skin broke out (pimples on face)
	PD	Bladder infection
	PD	Transfers were more difficult
	PD	Preterm labor (controlled by medication)
3rd	PD	Dysreflexia
	P	Edema (feet and ankles)
	PD	Spasm diminished
	PD	Bladder infection

Comments

Sally said getting bigger made it more difficult to position herself in her chair. It was also more difficult for her attendants to transfer her. She uses her spasms to help with a standing transfer, but this diminished during pregnancy. She had about three bladder infections with each pregnancy; this was not an unusual increase. (Sally usually has bladder infections when she is not pregnant.) She delivered both of her children vaginally.

Comments

First pregnancy: She was hospitalized for kidney infection. The kidney infection cleared up during the hospitalization.

Second pregnancy: Sally worked only in the mornings, in order to help control preterm labor. She rested whenever she felt contractions. Her contractions only happened when she was sitting. Sally felt that her recliner wheelchair helped control the preterm labor. She took the same medication as that used to treat high blood pressure, which is another symptom of dysreflexia.

Samantha's Pregnancy History (3) (Spinal Cord Injury)

Pregnancy: Age 15 (non-disabled)

Trimester	Cause	Physical Change
1st	P	Bladder infections
2nd		None recalled
3rd	P	Edema

Pregnancy: Age 17 (non-disabled)

Trimester	Cause	Physical Change
1st	P	Bladder infections
2nd		None recorded
3rd	P	Edema

Pregnancy: Age 27

Trimester	Cause	Physical Change
1st	P	Bladder infections
	P	Morning sickness
2nd	PD	Difficulty transferring into van
	PD	Could not bend over to reach floor
3rd	PD	Increased difficulty transferring into van; difficulty transferring into bed
	PD	Pressure sore
	PD	Backaches
	P	Edema not as severe as in previous pregnancies

Comments

Samantha delivered vaginally.

Shanna's Pregnancy History (2) (Spinal Cord Injury)

Pregnancy: Age 23-24

Trimester	Cause	Physical Change
1st	P	Felt tired
	PD	Back pain
	P	Migraines
	PD	Heartburn
	P	Feeling queasy
	PD	Swollen feet
2nd	PD	Back pain
	PD	Shortness of breath
	PD	Problems with balance
	PD	Difficulty bending to pick things up
	PD	Swollen feet
	PD	Difficult to catheterize
	PD	Difficulty transferring
3rd	PD	Difficulty bending to pick things up
	PD	Back pain increases
	PD	Difficulty transferring
	P	Shortness of breath
	PD	Difficult to catheterize
	P	Bladder infection
	PD	Problems with balance
	PD	Swollen feet

Pregnancy: Age 25-26

Trimester	Cause	Physical Change
1st	P	Felt a little tired
	P	Felt queasy when she did not eat
2nd	P	Felt more of the baby kicking
	P	Started showing in the fifth month
3rd	P	Bed rest because of early labor
	PD	Spasms in her legs if not drinking enough water
	PD	Difficulty transferring in and out of shower
	P	Gaining weight
	P	Difficulty sleeping
	PD	Problems with balance
	PD	Swollen feet

Comments

Shanna had a NDI device (neuro-stimulator) that reduced her bladder infections until the last week of pregnancy. She had to remove the device because it was dislodged by the pregnancy. The ER should not have touched this neuro-control device. During her first pregnancy, Shanna could catheterize only if she was lying down. She was active during her second pregnancy until the seventh month, when the baby dropped. She delivered both of her babies vaginally.

Sharon's Pregnancy History (1) (Spinal Cord Injury)

Pregnancy: Age 34

Trimester	Cause	Physical Change
1st	P	Tired easily
	P	Stomach aches
	PD	Difficulty inserting catheter[a]
2nd	PD	Difficulty transferring into bathtub
	PD	Difficulty maneuvering wheelchair into car
	PD	Increased difficulty bending and picking things up
	PD	Urine constantly dripping[b]
	PD	Chronic bladder infection
3rd	P	Hospitalized for premature labor in seventh month (baby was born 6 weeks early)
	D	Muscle stiffness and increased muscle spasms (due to insufficient physical therapy in hospital)
	P	Swollen ankles
	PD	Backaches
	P	Improved circulation in upper body; felt warmer than usual
	PD	Phlebitis in legs reappeared
All		Condition of hair and skin improved

Comments

[a]Pressure from the growing uterus may have compressed the bladder outlet enough to make insertion of the catheter more difficult.

[b]Sharon started using the Foley catheter, which remains in place constantly. When Sharon requested an indwelling catheter, her doctor expressed concern that she would not be able to discontinue using it later. Sharon decided to try using the indwelling catheter because of the difficulties she was having. After giving birth, she found she had to continue using it. Her doctor's concern was justified. She delivered her baby vaginally.

Shelia's Pregnancy History (2) (Spinal Cord Injury)

Pregnancy: Age 24

Trimester	Cause	Physical Change
1st		No specific changes recalled
2nd	PD	Muscle spasms[a]
	PD	Began having difficulty transferring in and out of bed
	PD	Difficulty breathing
	P	Edema
3rd	P	Anemia
	PD	Muscle spasms
	PD	Difficulty transferring to bathtub
	PD	Unable to find comfortable position for intercourse
	PD	Difficulty bending when dressing
All	PD	Persistent bladder infections[b]
	P	Nausea

Pregnancy: Age 29

Trimester	Cause	Physical Change
1st	P	Fatigue[c]
2nd	PD	Muscle spasms
3rd	PD	Episode of premature labor[d]
All	PD	Persistent bladder infections[d]

Comments

[a]During Sheila's first pregnancy, a physical therapist did leg stretches, which helped reduce her muscle spasms. Sheila wishes she had had the same therapy during her second pregnancy.

[b]During her first pregnancy, Sheila's bladder infections were recurrent, and she only used antibiotics when she had an active infection. During her second pregnancy, a bladder infection caused uterine contractions in the seventh month. She was advised to use antibiotics continuously until she gave birth. She later remarked that she was much more comfortable when she used antibiotics continuously, and she wishes she had done so during her first pregnancy.

[c]Sheila thinks that she felt so tired early in her second pregnancy because she was feeling upset; the pregnancy was unplanned, and her husband was not as supportive as he had been during the first pregnancy.

[d]Her disability did not directly cause premature labor.

She delivered both babies vaginally.

Shelby's Pregnancy History (2) (Spinal Cord Injury)

Pregnancy: Age 35

Trimester	Cause	Physical Change
1st	P	Morning sickness
	PD	Severe spasticity
	PD	Temperature regulation (summer months)
2nd	PD	Difficulty with self-catheterization
	PD	Respiratory
	PD	Bowel activity increased
	P	Skin improved
	PD	Edema (feet)
	PD	Carpal tunnel
	D	More frequent spasms
3rd	PD	Respiratory
	PD	Difficulty with self-catheterization
	PD	Carpal tunnel
	PD	Bowel activity increased
	P	Skin improved
	PD	Pitting edema (feet)
	P	Weight gain (40-45 lbs.)
	P	Big breast
	PD	Dysreflexia
	D	More frequent spasms
	PD	Pressure sore (abrasions)

Pregnancy: Age 37

Trimester	Cause	Physical Change
1st	P	Morning sickness
	PD	Severe spasticity
2nd	PD	Respiratory
	D	Spasms more frequently
	PD	Bowel activity increased
	P	Skin improved
	PD	Difficulty with self-catheterization
	PD	Pitting edema (feet)
3rd	PD	Respiratory
	D	Spasm more frequently
	PD	Bowel activity increased
	PD	Dysreflexia
	PD	Temperature regulation (hotter summer months)
	P	Skin improved
	PD	Difficulty with self-catheterization
	PD	Pitting edema (feet)
	P	Weight gain (30-40 lbs.)

Comments

With all of her pregnancies, Shelby had severe muscle spasticity that threw her out of her chair. The severe type of spasm ended at the first trimester, but although they reduced in severity, they increased in frequency. She had an extensor trunk spasm. She did not get the shivers and feel cold after she lay down. The respiratory problems were the most dramatic when lying down. She needed to change her bowel program to every day instead of every other day. She was able to do most of her transfers all the way through pregnancy. Shelby was unable to transfer from the passenger side of the car, but she could still transfer on the driver's side. Dysreflexia was triggered by Braxton-Hicks contractions. Shelby used suppositories prior to pregnancy, and kept the same regimen while pregnant.

Shelby's carpal tunnel was probably due to transferring and pushing her wheelchair. She needed to have bilateral surgeries. She did not fit into her wheelchair because of weight gain, and had her hips pressed up against the frame. It was more like an abrasion, and it healed quickly. She delivered both babies vaginally.

Signey's Pregnancy History (1) (Spinal Cord Injury)

Pregnancy: Age 37-38

Trimester	Cause	Physical Change
1st	P	Fatigue
	P	Nausea
2nd	PD	Balance unsteady
	PD	Difficulty walking
	PD	Using the wheelchair
	PD	Constipation
3rd	PD	Started to use a raised toilet seat
	PD	Used a bedside commode (at night)
	PD	Difficulty transferring into the car
	P	Hospitalized for 8 days for premature labor in 8th month
	P	Preeclampsia (baby was born 6 weeks early)
	P	Fluid in her lung from being treated with magnesium sulfate for preterm labor
	P	Swollen ankles and swollen feet (edema)

Comments

Signey did not have any urinary tract infections. Because she was pregnant with twins, it was not unusual to go into early labor. Moreover, it was recommended by her original neurosurgeon. In addition, it was easier for the obstetrician to control blood loss from the birth of twins. She delivered her twins by caesarean section.

Sonya's Pregnancy History (1) (Spinal Cord Injury)

Pregnancy: Age unknown; miscarriage (end of first trimester)

Pregnancy: Age 26; miscarriage (first trimester)

Pregnancy: Age 29

Trimester	Cause	Physical Change
1st	P	Fatigue
	P	Morning sickness
	D	Leg pain
	D	Insomnia
	PD	Muscle spasms
2nd	PD	Muscle spasms
	PD	Heartburn
	PD	Dizzy spells
3rd	PD	Urinary tract infection
	PD	Shoulder/upper back pain
		Flu
all	P	Fatigue
	P	Morning sickness
	D	Leg pain
	D	Insomnia
	PD	Muscle spasms

Comments

During this pregnancy, a physical therapist did leg stretches with Sonya, which helped reduce spasms. Sonya had morning sickness during the 1st trimester with her first child, and occasional morning sickness during the 1st trimester with her second pregnancy. Her spasticity was worse in the second trimester, in spite of a *slight* increase in baclofen. She would recline her chair and rest her head against the wall to help with dizzy spells. She was hospitalized for a urinary tract infection. Her breasts got bigger. She got physical therapy. She delivered her baby by caesarean section because the anesthesiologist was unaware that a spinal could be given to someone who has a Baclofen Pump™.

Stacy's Pregnancy History (1) (Spinal Cord Injury)

Pregnancy: Age 24

Trimester	Cause	Physical Change
1st	P	Felt tired[a]
	PD	Back pain
2nd	P	Still tired
	PD	No back pain[b]
	PD	Felt faint at times
	PD	Problems with balance: did not walk for fear of falling
3rd	PD	Difficulty bending to pick things up
	PD	Back pain
	PD	Difficulty transferring
	PD	Could not stand
	P	Difficulty breathing when lying on back
	PD	Increased constipation
	PD	Bladder never emptied completely
	PD	Urinary bleeding (possibly caused by irritation from catheter)

Comments

[a]Although Stacy said she often felt tired when she was pregnant, she also said she frequently pushed her wheelchair for 60 laps on a 200 meter track!

[b]During the second trimester, Stacy's back pain was alleviated by the use of a maternity girdle. Stacy delivered vaginally.

Stephanie's Pregnancy History (1) (Spinal Cord Injury)

Pregnancy: Age unknown; miscarriage (12th week)

Pregnancy: Age 31

Trimester	Cause	Physical Change
1st	P	Fatigue
	P	Faintness
2nd	P	Hemorrhoids
	P	Vaginal swelling
	P	Continued faintness
	PD	Mobility so reduced that she began using wheelchair all the time
	PD	Difficulty transferring in and out of car
	PD	Low back pain
3rd	P	Chest ached from upward pressure of uterus
	D	Urinary bleeding[a]
	P	Urinating more frequently
	P	Increased edema
	PD	Continued lower back pain
	PD	Aching in lower pelvis

Comments
[a]Her doctor suggested that the bleeding was caused by her catheter irritating the urinary tract more than usual. Stephanie delivered by caesarean section because of the shape of her pelvis. It is unclear whether her pelvic shape is congenital or caused by her car accident.

Sydney's Pregnancy History (1) (Spinal Cord Injury)

Pregnancy: Age 33; miscarriage (9th week)

Pregnancy: Age 34

Trimester	Cause	Physical Change
1st	P	Fatigue
	P	Faintness
	P	Hunger
2nd	P	Continued faintness
	PD	Transfers more difficult
3rd	D	Urinary tract infection
	PD	Balance changed
	PD	Increase of dysreflexia
	P	Constipation
	PD	Catherization more difficult
	PD	Spasms increased

Comments

During her second trimester, Sydney became faint when driving a car, and she stopped driving until post-delivery. Sydney described her spasms as "bouncy legs." She said, "I've never really had the need for stool softeners, even during pregnancy. She delivered by caesarean section because she had hip contractors and fetal distress.

Sylvia's Pregnancy History (1) (Spinal Cord Injury)

Pregnancy: Age 23

Trimester	Cause	Physical Change
1st	P	Morning sickness
	P	Mood swings
	P	Anemia
2nd	P	Light-headedness
	PD	Bowels relaxed (unpredictable bowel movements to end of term)
	P	Anemia
3rd	PD	Problems with breathing
	P	Anemia worsened
	PD	Episode of premature labor ($6\frac{1}{2}$ months)[a]
All	D	Episodes of dysreflexia, which were often worse when bowel or bladder was full
	PD	Muscle spasms more intense
	PD	Increased mobility difficulties [b]

Comments

[a]Premature labor was precipitated by dysreflexia and bowel problems. Also, the baby was low in the pelvis and the doctor manually changed its position.

[b]Balancing became more difficult as pregnancy progressed, especially because the baby was carried low. Maintaining balance while transferring and sitting became increasingly difficult. Sylvia delivered vaginally; forceps were used because the baby's shoulder was caught.

Aftereffects

Sylvia needed a blood transfusion after the baby was born.

Selina Tracy's Pregnancy History (5) (Spinal Tumor)

Pregnancy: Age 20

Pregnancy: Age 28

Pregnancy: Age 30

Pregnancy: Age 31

Pregnancy: Age 34

Trimester	Cause	Physical Change
1st	P	Slight nausea
2nd	PD	Muscle spasms increased
	PD	Bladder infections
3rd	PD	Numbness in hands
	PD	Transfer difficulty (especially bathtub and shower, the bed, floor to chair or couch, couch to chair, and in and out of car)
	PD	Equilibrium off

Pregnancy: Age 34

Trimester	Cause	Physical Change
1st	P	Morning sickness
2nd	PD	Muscle spasms less severe than previous pregnancies
	PD	Bladder infections
3rd	PD	Equilibrium off
	PD	Transfer difficulty (especially bathtub and shower, the bed, floor to chair or couch, or couch to chair)

Comments

Selina Tracy did not have problems getting her chair into her car, because she had a chair carrier topsider. Transfer into the car was not difficult with her fourth and fifth children because they bought a van. She has a bed on a pedestal. She uses a bathtub bench. Selina found her weight gain difficult. Since her children were close together, it was difficult to lose weight, making transfers difficult. She was on bed rest with her second pregnancy because she was carrying the baby really low. When she is not pregnant, she gets a bladder infection only periodically. She experienced spasms with all five of her pregnancies. She delivered all five pregnancies vaginally.

Sara's Pregnancy History (2) (Spinal Tumor)

Pregnancy: Age 22

Trimester	Cause	Physical Change
1st	P	Morning sickness
	P	Frequent urination
2nd	PD	Muscle spasms increased
	PD	Some days urinated frequently, retained urine on others (stayed close to home)
	P	Numbness in hands[a]
	P	Shooting pains in hands and feet[a]
3rd	PD	Began falling; started using wheelchair in 7th month
	PD	Retained urine

Pregnancy: Age 26

Trimester	Cause	Physical Change
1st	P	Morning sickness
	PD	Frequent urination
	P	Threatened miscarriage
2nd	PD	Muscle spasms less severe than previous pregnancy
	PD	Some days urinated frequently, retained urine on others (stayed close to home)
	P	Numbness in hands[a]
	P	Shooting pains in hands and feet[a]
	PD	Began falling; started using wheelchair in 7th month
3rd	PD	Bowels became impacted several times
	PD	Retained urine
	PD	Back pain
	PD?	Edema

Comments

[a]Although Sara did not identify them as such, the numbness and/or pain in her extremities are common symptoms of edema. This was probably caused by edema in Sara's case, because she remembers being told late in her second pregnancy that she had edema.

[b]Sara was hospitalized in the 8th month because her doctor did not know what to expect. She saw her doctor every other day. Sara delivered both of her babies vaginally.

Taryn Dion's Pregnancy History (1) (Thoracic Outlet Syndrome)

Pregnancy: Age 38

Trimester	Cause	Physical Change
1st	P	Very nauseous[a]
	P	Tired
2nd	P	Tired
3rd	PD	Difficulty getting out bathtub
	P	Tired

Comments

Taryn Dion had an emergency caesarean section because of preeclampsia and the fetus was in a breech position.

Tessa's Pregnancy History (1) (Thoracic Outlet Syndrome)

Pregnancy: Age 37

Trimester	Cause	Physical Change
1st	P	Nausea
	P	Irritable
	P	Calf spasm
2nd		No problems
3rd	PD	Pain in shoulder
	PD	Sleep problems
	PD	Difficulty with toe care
	PD	Could not stand

Comments

Tessa delivered vaginally.

Tina's Pregnancy History (1) (Thoracic Outlet Syndrome)

Pregnancy: Age 37

Trimester	Cause	Physical Change
1st	P	Heartburn
	P	Sensitive to smells
	P	Food sensitivity
	P	Bronchitis
2nd	P	Heartburn
	P	Sensitive to smells
	P	Rash
3rd	PD	Sleeping problems (shoulder pain when sleeping on side)
	P	Difficulty bending down
	P	Mastitis
	P	Tired

Comments

Tina delivered vaginally.

Appendix

Pregnancy Discomfort Tables

Table B-1
Discomforts Reported for Ninety Pregnancies of 143.5 Women

Symptom	Trimester			Comments
	1	2	3	
Abdominal muscle cramping/stretching	5	3	1	
Anemia	4	4	5	
Appetite affected:				
increased	6	1	0	
sensitivity	2	1	0	
Back, pelvic, or joint pain	11	22	36	
Backache improved	0	2	1	
Carpel Tunnel/numb/ painful hands/TOS	2	6	6	
Constipation	5	6	10	
Bowels increased	0	2	1	
Difficulty dressing	0	2	10	
Edema	4	16	43	One case; not known which trimester.
Emotional extremes/ anxiety	5	0	1	
Energy boost	0	4	1	
Faintness/Fatigue	61	26	12	One due to low blood pressure in third trimester

(continues)

Table B-1 (continued)

Symptom	Trimester 1	2	3	Comments
Felt warmer	0	2	4	
Gestational diabetes	1	1	4	
Headaches/Migraines	3	1	1	
Improved headaches	2	5	4	
Heartburn	6	15	16	One developed hiatus hernia in third trimester.
Hemorrhoids	1	2	6	
Hip pain	0	5	8	One due to fall.
Hypertension/ high blood pressure	1	4	4	
Low blood pressure	1	1	1	
Indigestion	0	0	1	
Kidney infection/pain	0	4	1	Two women used an ostomy bag that by-passed the bladder. One person had sacral agenesis.
Leg spasms/muscle tightness	9	38	18	
Spasms improve	0	1	2	
Nausea	83	18	7	
Nose bleeds/stuffiness/ infection	2	3	2	
Placenta Previa	0	1	0	
Postpartum/breast infection	0	0	1	
Preeclampsia	0	0	5	One lost vision in one eye, developed short-term memory problems, and had a live birth at 7 months.
Respiratory issues	2	20	16	
Skin/hair improved	3	7	7	
Skin/hair issues	1	3	3	One had hives in first trimester.
Sleeplessness	5	2	9	
Sore breasts	0	0	0	
Urinary infection	9	15	10	In the second trimester, 12 out of the 15 women had spinal cord dysfunction.

Table B-1 (*continued*)

Symptom	Trimester			Comments
	1	2	3	
Urinary problems:				
frequency/incontinence	11	16	25	One person; only happened once in second trimester, and once in middle of the night during second trimester. Another retained urine. Difficult to catheterize is counted here and in "other" category in "disability related symptoms (2 tics).
Vaginal discharge/spotting	7	3	0	
Vaginal infection	0	1	3	
Vaginal swelling	0	1	0	
Other	1	3	8	Includes breast infection, fast heartbeat, detached retina, phlebitis, fluid in lungs from magnesium sulfate treatment, tying shoes, stopped driving, and other.
Miscarriage or Early Labor				
Abortion	1	0	0	
Episode of premature labor	0	3	9	In second trimester, baby born at 6.5 months. In third trimester, baby born 6 weeks early; this is not unusual for twins. Another came on time.
Premature birth	0	0	3	One due to placenta abruption, live birth. Another due to respiratory problems.
Miscarriage	15	3	1	Two counts of miscarriage not known which trimester they occurred. One had heavy bleeding.
Threatened miscarriage	1	2	0	
Disability Related Symptoms				
Dysreflexia	1	2	4	
Exacerbation of symptoms	3	3	2	
MS exacerbation	0	0	1	Includes blurred vision and numbness in arms, legs, and scalp.

(continues)

Table B-1 (*continued*)

Symptom	Trimester			Comments
	1	2	3	
Phantom pain/ stump issues	0	6	2	
Pressure sores	0	0	3	
Prosthesis use	0	0	0	
Impaired mobility: balance/transfers	12	61	84	Includes about six people having trouble picking things up in the third trimester.
Remission of symptoms	9	12	7	Except when working long days.
Start using equipment	1	4	8	Includes wheelchair, walker, cane, and raised toilet seat.
Other	8	10	15	Includes temperature fluctuation (one controlled by medication), mild seizures, lupus mask darkened, shunt, foot drop, weak legs, weakness, fibromyalgia, facial weakness, double vision, broken hip, difficulty driving, difficulty pushing wheelchair, radicular pain, difficulty keeping ostomy bag attached, difficult to catheterize (double counted, see urinary problems).

Table B-2
Discomforts Reported for 33 Pregnancies of 22 Women

Symptom	Trimester			Comments
	1	2	3	
Abdominal muscle cramping/stretching	1	0	0	
Anemia	1	1	2	
Appetite affected: Increased	1	0	0	
Back, pelvic, or joint pain	2	5	11	
Backache improved	0	2	0	
Carpel Tunnel/numb/ painful hands/TOS	0	2	2	
Constipation	3	2	4	
Bowels increased	0	2	1	
Difficulty dressing	0	0	1	
Edema	1	8	17	
Emotional extremes/ Anxiety	1	0	0	
Faintness/Fatigue	17	5	0	
Felt warmer	0	0	1	
Gas pains	1	1	1	
Gestational diabetes	0	0	1	
Headaches/Migraines	2	1	0	
Heartburn	2	5	5	
Hemorrhoids	0	1	0	
Hip pain	0	0	1	
Kidney infection/pain	0	4	1	Two women used an ostomy bag that by-passed the bladder. One person had sacral agenesis. One person had SCI quad.
Leg spasms/muscle tightness	11	16	11	
Spasms improve	0	1	2	
Nausea	21	5	3	
Preeclampsia	0	0	1	
Respiratory issues	0	3	5	
Skin/hair improved	1	4	4	Includes hives and pimples.
Skin/hair issues	1	2	0	
Sleeplessness	2	1	2	

(continues)

Table B-2 (*continued*)

Symptom	Trimester			Comments
	1	2	3	
Urinary infection	6	12	7	Total of 16 pregnancies of women with T6 and above in each trimester
Urinary problems:				
frequency/incontinence	3	3	6	
Vaginal swelling	0	1	0	
Other	1	0	1	Includes temperature regulation issues.
Miscarriage or Early Labor				
Episode of premature labor	0	2	5	One baby was six weeks early; 16 pregnancies of women with T6 and above
Miscarriage	5	0	0	
Disability Related Symptoms				
Dysreflexia	1	2	4	Out of 16 pregnancy of women with T6 and above
Exacerbation of symptoms	0	1	0	Radicular pain
Impaired mobility:				
balance/transfers	2	14	25	
Remission of symptoms	0	1	0	Pressure sore improved
Other	2	5	11	

In first trimester, one person had a Foley catheter inserted, and another had difficulty being catheterized. In the second trimester, one person had an ostomy bag that was hard to attach, another had trouble keeping the Foley catheter on, and another was catheterized. In the third trimester, one person had a detached retina; another had phlebitis; another was catheterized; and one had trouble keeping her ostomy bag attached.

Notes: Seven women with spina bifida had nine pregnancies.
        Fourteen women with spinal cord injuries had 21 pregnancies.
        One woman with sacral agenesis had two pregnancies.

35 percent of the women had a bladder infection in the second trimester, the most common time for bladder infections to occur.

Table B-3 (Neuro-Muscular)
Discomforts Reported for 21 Pregnancies of 12 Women

Symptom	Trimester 1	2	3	Comments
Abdominal muscle cramping/stretching	1	0	0	
Appetite affected: increased	1	1	0	
Back, pelvic or joint pain	1	1	4	
Carpel Tunnel/numb/ painful hands/TOS	2	2	2	
Constipation	0	0	2	
Edema	0	1	3	
Emotional extremes/ anxiety	2	0	3	
Faintness/Fatigue	10	5	1	
Fast Heart rate	1	0	1	
Heartburn	0	3	5	
Leg spasms/muscle tightness	1	2	1	
Nausea	13	5	0	
Nose bleeds/stuffiness/ infection	1	1	2	
Respiratory issues	1	10	2	
Skin/hair improved	1	2	1	
Sleeplessness	1	0	4	
Urinary infection	0	0	2	
Urinary problems: frequency/incontinence	0	0	1	
Vaginal discharge/spotting	1	0	0	
Miscarriage or Early Labor: 0				
Disability Related Symptoms				
Exacerbation of symptoms	1	1	5	

In third trimester, two people experienced foot drop, two people felt weaker, and one person had double vision and facial weakness. One person experienced fibromyalgia in the first trimester, which lessened in the second trimester.

Impaired mobility: balance/transfers	4	11	12	

Table B-4 (Autoimmune)
Discomforts Reported for 13.5 Pregnancies of 10 Women

Symptom	Trimester			Comments
	1	2	3	
Amanda was not included because her arthritis was not due to autoimmune problems.				
Anemia	1	0	1	
Appetite affected:				
increased	1	0	0	
sensitivity	0	0	1	
Back, pelvic	1	1	4	
or joint pain				
Carpel Tunnel/numb/	0	0	1	
painful hands/TOS				
Constipation	1	1	0	
Difficulty dressing	0	0	2	
Edema	0	2	3	
Faintness/Fatigue	3	1	4	
Gestational diabetes	1	1	1	
Hip Pain	0	0	1	
Hypertension/	1	2	1	
high blood pressure				
Leg spasms/muscle	1	2	0	
tightness				
Nausea	8	2	0	
Nose bleeds/stuffiness/	0	1	0	
infection				
Placenta Previa	1	0	0	
Preeclampsia	0	0	1	
Respiratory issues	0	1	2	
Skin/hair improved	2	3	3	
Skin/hair issues	0	0	1	
Urinary infection	2	1	1	
Urinary problems:				
frequency/incontinence	0	1	1	
Vaginal discharge/	3	1	0	
spotting				
Vaginal infection	0	1	1	
Miscarriage or Early Labor				
Premature birth	0	0	2	
Miscarriage	1	1	0	One twin miscarried.

Table B-4 (*continued*)

Symptom	Trimester			Comments
	1	2	3	
Disability Related Symptoms				
Exacerbation of symptoms	1	0	0	
Impaired mobility:				
balance/transfers	1	5	8	
Remission of symptoms	9	5	2	
Temperature				
fluctuation	2	2	1	
temperature improved				
with meds	1	0	0	
Other	1	1	0	Includes lupus mask and seizures.

Table B-5 (Cerebral Palsy)
Discomforts Reported for 16 Pregnancies of 10 Women

Symptom	Trimester 1	2	3	Comments
Abdominal muscle cramping/stretching	5	0	0	
Back, pelvic, or joint pain	5	3	7	
Difficulty dressing	0	0	1	
Edema	2	2	9	
Emotional extremes/ anxiety	1	1	1	
Faintness/fatigue	11	2	0	
Felt warmer	2	2	2	
Heartburn	1	3	1	
Hemorrhoids	0	0	4	
Hip pain	0	0	1	
Hypertension/ high blood pressure	0	2	3	
Leg spasms/muscle tightness	2	5	3	
Nausea	11	0	0	
Preeclampsia	0	0	1	
Respiratory issues	0	2	3	
Sleeplessness	0	0	1	
Urinary infection	0	0	1	
Urinary problems: frequency/incontinence	1	0	1	
Vaginal discharge/ spotting	2	0	0	
Vaginal infection	0	1	0	
Miscarriage or Early Labor				
Miscarriage	1	0	0	
Threatened miscarriage	0	1	0	
Disability Related Symptoms				
Impaired mobility: balance/transfers	0	7	13	

Table B-6 (MS)
Discomforts Reported for 8 Pregnancies of 8 Women

	Trimester			
Symptom	1	2	3	Comments
Anemia	0	2	0	
Back, pelvic, or joint pain	0	1	1	
Difficulty dressing	0	0	1	
Faintness/Fatigue	4	3	5	
Heartburn	0	1	1	
Nausea	3	0	0	
Sleeplessness	0	0	1	
Urinary infection	1	0	1	
Urinary problems: frequency/incontinence	2	3	3	

Miscarriage or Early Labor: 0

Disability Related Symptoms

MS exacerbation	0	0	2	One person had numbness and tingling on one side and vision problems. Another experienced muscle spasms.
Impaired mobility: balance/transfers	5	3	6	
Remission of symptoms	1	3	1	
Start using equipment	0	0	1	

Chart on Labor and Deliveries

(Where categories had 3 or more women)

AMPUTATIONS

3 women; 5 pregnancies
3 caesarean sections and 2 vaginal births

CEREBRAL PALSY

10 women and 16 pregnancies
C- Section
Chloe had a caesarean section because the baby was breech.
Caitlin had a caesarean section because the doctors did not think she could dilate.
Carla stopped dilating. Charlotte's baby was in distress.

VAGINAL

(2 Carol) (1 Carla) (2 Celeste) (1 Cheryl) (1 Christina) (2 Clara)
(2 Corrine) =11 Vaginal

DWARFISM

4 women and 5 pregnancies
All but 1 baby was born by C-section.
The baby born vaginally was premature and died.

JRA AND ARTHRITIS AND LUPUS

10 women and 13 pregnancies
Jennifer delivered her baby vaginally.
Joan delivered by caesarean section because of fear that her hips could be dislocated.
Joy delivered by caesarean section because of hip replacement.
Julie had a caesarean section.
Rachel delivered her child vaginally; 0 hip replacement.
Rene delivered both of her children vaginally; 0 hip replacement.
Roberta delivered her child vaginally; 0 hip replacement.
Lea Rae delivered vaginally and had a hip replacement.
Laura delivered her baby by caesarean because of loss of placental function.
Leslie delivered her first child by caesarean section because the baby was in a transverse position. Her other two babies were delivered by vaginal birth.

MULTIPLE SCLEROSIS

8 women and 8 pregnancies
7 out of 8 gave birth vaginally
Mona had a caesarean section because her baby was breech.

NEUROMUSCULAR

12 women and 21 pregnancies

Six women delivered 15 babies vaginally. Natalie gave birth to one of her children vaginally. Six women delivered 6 babies by caesarean section. Two babies were delivered caesarean section because of fetal distress; Natasha's and Natalie's because of fetal distress. Two women delivered their children by caesarean section because of lack of knowledge. One woman delivered her child by caesarean section because of placenta abruptio. One woman delivered her child by caesarean section because of inability to dilate.

OSTEOGENESIS IMPERFECTA (OI)

3 women and 5 pregnancies

All three women delivered by caesarean section because of fear of the pelvis would break during delivery, or if the baby had OI, his bones would break during birth.

POST-POLIO

5 women and 9 pregnancies

Three women delivered their children vaginally (Patricia, Paula, and Pricilla).

Two women delivered their children by caesarean section.

Pam and Portia both delivered their children by caesarean section because the babies were too large.

SPINAL CORD DYSFUNCTION

22 women and 33 pregnancies

8 women delivered 10 babies by caesarean section (Sophia, Sherry Adele, Sienna, Sybil, Signey, Sonya, Stephanie, and Sydney); 14 women delivered 23 babies vaginally. It seemed that some of the caesareans were done out of ignorance: Sonya's doctor was unaware that the Baclofen Pump™ could be used with spinal anesthesia. Sienna's doctor never tried medical intervention for a vaginal birth.

THORACIC OUTLET SYNDROME

1 woman delivered by caesarean section and 2 delivered vaginally.

Taryn Dion had preeclampsia and her baby was in distress.

Appendix C

Diet Plan and Suggested Food Lists

THE FOLLOWING MEAL PLAN is adapted from the Dietary Guidelines and Daily Food Guide in *Nutrition During Pregnancy and the Postpartum Period: A Manual for Health Care Professionals*, published by the California Department of Health Services. A woman who uses this plan will meet all her nutritional requirements. It is different in some respects from other diet plans you may have seen. A short explanation should help you feel comfortable with this plan and use it wisely.

Rather than making suggestions for what you should eat at each meal. Information on the food groups and serving sizes (Table A) is provided to allow you greater flexibility in planning meals according to your individual needs. For example, if you are eating small, frequent meals to cope with indigestion (as suggested in Chapter 6), you might want to include some suggested servings in between-meal snacks. You might prefer to have more protein servings at breakfast, and fewer at dinner, to avoid getting heartburn from a heavy evening meal. If you are troubled with muscle cramps at night, you might eat some calcium-rich foods as a bedtime snack, to see if the calcium alleviates the cramping.

Another difference from many diet plans is that the number of portions may seem high. This is because the portion sizes given in this meal plan are smaller than in others. Using smaller portions adds flexibility and variety to your diet, which is especially helpful during the first trimester when food is so often unappealing. The smaller portions will also help you in planning several small meals a day, which can help prevent many pregnancy discomforts.

The amount of protein provided in this meal plan is greater than the minimum daily requirement. Eating additional protein is the only way to obtain enough vitamin B_6, iron, and zinc from food.

Tables B–H list a variety of foods in each food group. Enough choices are listed to help you plan interesting, enjoyable meals. These lists will help you safely meet all of your nutritional needs if you have allergies. They also make it possible to plan meals that are relatively high or low in calories. The key difference is in how well you follow the advice to limit fats and sweets. For example, cooked yams are rich in vitamin A, but canned yams that contain sugar will supply more calories than a plain, baked yam, which is naturally sweet. If you choose lean meat, fish, and vegetable proteins, and avoid fried foods and sugary foods, you probably will not consume too many calories. If you need to gain weight, do not eat more fatty or sweet foods, but more breads and cereals. Your doctor or nutritionist can advise you.

Because fiber is now known to be an important part of your diet, fiber-rich foods are marked accordingly. The inclusion of several ethnic foods, such as tortillas, chitterlings, and tofu, should help make sensible eating enjoyable eating.

I have eliminated charts listing foods rich in some nutrients, such as magnesium, because they contain foods which are included on other lists, and have expanded the list of sweeteners to include names that are frequently included on food labels; for example, "sucrose" for sugar.

Table A
Daily Food Guide for Women

Food Group	Minimum Number of Servings		
	Nonpregnant Adolescent Female	Nonpregnant Adult Female	Pregnant/Lactating Adolescent/Adult Female
Protein foods	6[a]	6[a]	8[b]
Milk products	3	2	4
Breads, cereals, grains	6[c]	6[c]	6[c]
Fruits and vegetables			
Vitamin C-rich	1	1	2
Vitamin A-rich	1	1	1
Other	3	3	3
Fats and sweets	Use sparingly		
Water[d]			

[a]Equivalent in protein to 6 oz of animal protein; at least one of these servings should be from the vegetable protein list.

[b]Equivalent in protein to 8 oz of animal protein; at least two of these servings should be from the vegetable protein list.

[c]At least four of these servings should be from whole grains.

[d]Eight 8-oz servings per day are recommended for all groups.

Table B
Protein Foods

Type of Protein	Serving Size[a]
Animal: Low in Fat (< 5 g/serving)	
Beef: lean cuts (round, sirloin, flank steak)	1 oz cooked
Chicken	1 oz cooked
Clams	3 medium raw or 1/4 cup canned, drained
Crab	1 1/2 oz or 1/3 cup
Duck	1 oz cooked
Fish: fresh or frozen	1 oz cooked
Fish, canned: salmon, tuna	1 oz or 1/8 cup
Fish, canned: sardines	3 medium or 1 oz drained
Hogmaws (pork stomach)	1 1/2 oz cooked
Lobster	1 1/2 oz cooked
Organ meats: heart, kidney, liver	1 oz cooked
Oysters	6 medium, 3 oz, or 1/3 cup raw or canned
Pork: ham roast	1 oz cooked
Pork: loin, roast, chop	1 oz cooked
Rabbit	1 oz cooked
Scallops	2 medium or 1 oz cooked
Shrimp	2 large, 1 oz cooked, or 1/3 cup breaded
Turkey	1 oz cooked
Tripe (cow stomach)	1 oz cooked
Veal: ground, cube, roast, chop	1 oz cooked
Animal: High in Fat (≥ 5 g/serving)	
Beef: ground, cube, roast, steak, chuck	1 oz cooked
Beef: short rib	1 small
Chitterlings (hog intestines)	3 oz cooked
Eggs	1 large
Fish sticks, breaded	2 medium
Frankfurters	2 medium
Lamb: ground, cube, roast, chop	1 oz cooked
Luncheon meat: bologna, ham, liverwurst	2 slices or 2 oz
Organ meats: sweetbreads	1 oz cooked
Oysters, fried	7 medium
Pig feet	2 oz cooked
Pork: ground, roast, chop	1 oz cooked

(continues)

Table B (continued)

Type of Protein	Serving Size[a]
Pork: spareribs	2 small ribs
Sausage	3 small links or 2 oz cooked
Tongue	1 oz cooked
Vegetable: Low in Fat (<5 g/serving)	
Beans: garbanzo, kidney, navy, pinto, baked, pork and beans (FF)	1/2 cup cooked
Lentils (F)	1/2 cup cooked or 3/4 cup lentil soup
Peas, split (FF)	1/2 cup cooked or 3/4 cup split pea soup
Soybeans	1/4 cup cooked
Soybeans, roasted	2 1/2 tbsp
Soybeans, fermented (tempeh)	1/4 cup or 2 oz
Soybean curd (tofu) (F)	3 oz
Yeast, nutritional	tbsp
Vegetable: High in Fat (≥5 g/serving)	
Baked beans with franks (FF)	1/2 cup
Chile con carne (FF)	1/2 cup
Falafel (garbanzo croquette)	3 patties
Hummus (garbanzo-sesame dip) (F)	1/2 cup
Nuts: almonds, mixed nuts, walnuts (F)	1 1/2 oz or 1/3 cup
Nut butter: cashew, sesame	3 tbsp
Nut butter: peanut	2 tbsp
Peanuts (F)	1 oz or 1/4 cup
Seeds: pumpkin, sunflower	1 oz or 1/4 cup

[a]Each serving provides a minimum of 6 g of protein.

Abbreviations: F, Moderately rich in fiber (1 to 3.9 g/serving); FF, rich in fiber (≥ 4 g/serving).

Table C
Calcium-rich Foods: Milk Products

Milk Products	Serving Size
Low in Fat (< 5 g/serving)	
Milk: nonfat dry milk powder	1/3 cup
Milk: nonfat or nonfat dry reconstituted	1 cup
Milk: nonfat, evaporated	1/2 cup
Milk: buttermilk or lowfat	1 cup
Yogurt: nonfat or lowfat, plain or fruit-flavored	6 oz
High in Fat (≥ 5 g/serving)	
Cheese: brick-type or semi-soft (except bleu, Camembert, cream)	1 1/2 oz or 1/3 cup grated
Cheese: cottage (creamed or lowfat)	2 cups
Cheese: hard, grated (e.g., Parmesan, Romano)	4 tbsp
Cheese: ricotta (from whole or part-skim milk)	1/2 cup
Cheese: spread or cheese food (e.g., Velveeta)	2 oz
Cream soups made with milk	1 1/2 cups
Custard (flan)	1 cup
Ice cream	1 1/2 cups
Ice milk	1 1/2 cups
Milk: whole or chocolate	1 cup
Milk: whole, evaporated	1/2 cup
Milkshake	1 cup homemade or 1 average commercial
Pudding	1 cup
Yogurt: whole (plain or fruit-flavored)	8 oz
Yogurt: frozen	1 1/2 cups

Table D
Calcium-rich Foods: Nondairy Products[a]

---

5 medium sardines (2 1/2 oz)
1/2 cup canned salmon (with bones)
9 oz tofu (must be processed with a calcium salt)
4 oz almonds
1/4 cup tahini (sesame butter)
2 cups baked beans or pork and beans
7 corn tortillas (treated with lime or calcium carbonate, as is masa harina)
5 medium oranges
1 1/2 cups broccoli, fresh cooked
1 1/2 cups turnip, cooked
2 cups bok choy, collard or dandelion greens, cooked
3 cups kale or mustard greens, cooked
2 tbsp blackstrap molasses

---

[a]Each serving is approximately equivalent in calcium to one serving from the milk products group (250–300 mg calcium) in Table C.

Note: Other dark, leafy greens, such as spinach, are not good sources of calcium because they contain a chemical that binds the calcium and makes it unavailable.

Table E
Breads, Cereals, and Grains

Whole-Grain	Serving Size
Bread: whole-wheat, cracked wheat, pumpernickel (F)	1 slice
Bran, unprocessed (FF)	1/2 cup
Bran cereals, flaked	1 oz or 3/4 cup
Bulgur, cooked (FF)	1/2 cup
Cereals, cooked: oatmeal, Wheatena, Malt-O-Meal, Roman Meal (F)	1/2 cup
Cereals, ready-to-eat:	
Cheerios, Wheaties (F)	1 oz or 3/4 cup
Cereals, puffed (F)	1 oz or 2 cups
Crackers, fat added: Triscuits (F)	1 oz or 8
Crackers, fat added: Wheat Thins (F)	1 oz or 12
Crackers, no fat added: Kavali, Wasa (F)	3/4 oz or 2–4 slices
Grapenuts (F)	1 oz or 1/4 cup
Granola	1/2 cup
Muffin: bran or whole-wheat (F)	1
Pasta, whole-wheat: macaroni, noodles, spaghetti (F)	1/2 cup cooked
Popcorn (F)	2 cups
Rice, brown (F)	1/2 cup cooked
Rice cake	3
Rye Crisp (F)	4 (2" x 3 1/2" crackers)
Shredded Wheat (F)	1 oz, 1 biscuit, or 3/4 cup
Tortilla, corn	1 small (6" diameter)
Wheat germ (FF)	1 oz or 4 tbsp

Enriched	Serving Size
Bagel	1/2
Bread	1 slice
Bread sticks, crisp	2 (4" x 1/2")
Bun: frankfurter or hamburger	1/2
Cereals, cooked: Cream of Rice, Cream of Wheat, Maypo	1/2 cup
Cereals, ready-to-eat	1 oz or 3/4 cup
Cornbread (F)	1 piece (2" square)
Crackers, fat added: Ritz	1 oz or 8
Crackers, no fat added: soda crackers	1 oz or 8
Croutons	1/2 cup
Dumpling	1 small
Grits	1/2 cup cooked

(continues)

Table E (continued)

Whole-Grain	Serving Size
Graham crackers (FF)	4 (2 1/2" squares)
Muffin, biscuit, dumpling	1
Muffin, English	1/2
Pancake	1 medium
Pasta: macaroni, noodles, spaghetti	1/2 cup cooked
Pita	1/2 (6" diameter)
Rice, white	1/2 cup cooked
Roll, dinner	1 small
Stuffing	1/4 cup
Tortilla, flour	1 small or 1/2 large
Waffle	1 (4 1/2" x 4 1/2")

Abbreviations: F, Moderately rich in fiber (1 to 3.9 g/serving); FF, rich in fiber (≥ 4 g/serving).

Note: Brand names are cited as examples only and do not imply endorsement or superiority over products with similar nutrient characteristics.

Table F
Vitamin C-rich Fruits and Vegetables

Product	Serving Size[a]
Juices	
Orange	6 oz
Grapefruit, lemon	6 oz
Fruit juices enriched with vitamin C	6 oz
Tomato Juice	6 oz
Vegetable juice cocktail	6 oz
Fruits	
Cantaloupe (F)	1/4 medium or 1/2 cup cubed
Grapefruit (F)	1/2 medium
Guava	1 medium
Kiwi	1 medium
Lemon	1 medium
Mango (F)	1 medium
Orange (F)	1 medium
Papaya	1/4 medium
Strawberries (F)	1/2 cup
Tangerine (FF)	2 medium
Vegetables	
Broccoli (F)	1/2 cup raw or cooked
Brussels sprouts (F)	3 medium or 1/2 cup cooked
Cabbage (F)	1 cup raw or 1/2 cup cooked
Cauliflower (F)	1/2 cup raw or cooked
Peppers: hot, chili	2 tbsp raw or 1/2 cup canned/bottled
Peppers: sweet	1/2 raw or 1/2 cup cooked
Snow peas	1/2 cup raw or cooked
Tomatoes: green, red (FF)	2 medium raw
Tomato paste	1/2 cup
Tomato puree	1/2 cup

[a]Each serving provides a minimum of 30 mg of vitamin C.

Abbreviations: F, Moderately rich in fiber (1 to 3.9 g/serving); FF, rich in
fiber (≥ 4 g/serving).

Note: Although fresh, frozen, or canned fruits and vegetables may be eaten, fresh is preferable.

Table G
Vitamin A-rich Fruits and Vegetables

Product	Serving Size [a]
Juices	
Apricot nectar	6 oz
Vegetable juice cocktail	6 oz
Fruits	
Apricots (F)	3 medium raw or 1/4 cup dried
Cantaloupe (F)	1/4 medium or 1/2 cup cubed
Mango (F)	1/4 medium or 1/2 cup cubed
Papaya	1/2 medium or 3/4 cup cubed
Vegetables	
Bok Choy	1/2 cup cooked
Beet greens	1/2 cup cooked
Carrots (F)	1/2 cup or 1 small
Chard, swiss	1/2 cup cooked
Collards (F)	1/2 cup cooked
Dandelion greens (F)	1/2 cup cooked
Kale (F)	1/2 cup cooked
Mustard greens (F)	1/2 cup cooked
Parsley (F)	1 cup raw or 1/2 cup cooked
Peppers: hot, chili	2 tbsp raw or cooked
Pumpkin (F)	1/2 cup cooked
Onions, green	1/2 cup chopped
Spinach (F)	1 cup raw or 1/2 cup cooked
Squash, winter (F)	1/2 cup cooked
Sweet potato (F)	1/2 cup cooked
Tomatoes, red (F)	2 medium raw
Yams (see note below) (F)	1/2 cup cooked

[a]Each serving provides a minimum of 2,000 IU of vitamin A.

Abbreviations: F, Moderately rich in fiber (1 to 3.9 g/serving).

Note: The yams commonly available in U.S. markets are actually sweet potatoes and thus rich in vitamin A. True tropical yams are not deep yellow or orange and are not rich in vitamin A.

Table H
Other Fruits and Vegetables[a]

Products	Serving Size
Juices	
Apple	6 oz
Cranberry	6 oz
Grape	6 oz
Pineapple	6 oz
Prune	6 oz
Fruits	
Apple (F)	1 medium or 1/4 cup dried
Applesauce (F)	1/2 cup
Avocado	1/2 medium
Banana (F)	1 medium
Blackberries (FF)	1/2 cup
Blueberries (F)	1/2 cup
Cherries (F)	1/2 cup
Dates (F)	4
Figs (F)	1/2 cup fresh or 1/4 cup dried
Fruit cocktail	1/2 cup
Grapes	1/2 cup or 15 small
Kumquats	1 medium
Nectarine (F)	1 medium
Peach (F)	1 medium or 1/2 cup sliced or canned
Pear (F)	1 medium or 1/2 cup sliced or canned
Persimmon	1 medium
Pineapple (F)	1/2 cup
Plums (F)	2 medium
Pomegranate	1 medium
Prunes (FF)	1/2 cup cooked or 1/4 cup dried
Raisins (F)	1/4 cup
Raspberries (FF)	1/2 cup
Watermelon	1/2 cup

(continues)

Table H (*continued*)

Products	Serving Size
Vegetables	
Artichoke (FF)	1/2 medium
Asparagus (F)	6 medium stalks or 1/2 cup cooked
Bamboo shoots	1/2 cup
Bean sprouts: alfalfa, mung (F)	1 cup raw or 1/2 cup cooked
Beans: green, wax (F)	1/2 cup
Beans: lima (FF)	1/2 cup
Beets (F)	1/2 cup
Celery (F)	1/2 cup
Corn (F)	1/2 cup or 6" cob
Cucumber	1/2 cup
Eggplant (F)	1/2 cup
Hominy	1/2 cup
Jicama	1/2 cup
Kale (F)	1/2 cup
Lettuce	1 cup raw
Mushrooms	1/2 cup
Okra (F)	1/2 cup
Onion (F)	1/2 cup
Parsnip (F)	1/2 cup
Peas: green (FF)	1/2 cup
Potatoes: red, white, russet (F)	1/2 cup
Radishes	1/2 cup
Seaweed	1/2 cup
Summer squash (F)	1/2 cup
Tomatillos	1/2 cup
Turnip (F)	1/2 cup
Zucchini (F)	1/2 cup

aFoods in this group contribute varying amounts of fiber and other nutrients.
Abbreviations: F, Moderately rich in fiber (1 to 3.9 g/serving); FF, rich in fiber (≥ 4 g/serving).

Table I
Fats, Sweets, and Other Foods That Should Be Limited

Unsaturated Fats
  Margarine (listing liquid oil as first ingredient on label)
  Mayonnaise
  Oils, vegetable (except palm and coconut)
  Olives
  Salad dressing (oil-based)
Saturated Fats
  Butter
  Bacon
  Coconut
  Coconut oil
  Coffee whitener
  Cream, coffee
  Cream, sour
  Cream, whipping
  Cream cheese
  Lard
  Margarine (not listing liquid oil as first ingredient on label)
  Palm oil
  Salad dressing
  Salt pork
  Shortening
Sweeteners

Corn syrup	Sucrose	Fructose
Honey	Dextrose	High-fructose corn sweetener
Molasses	Levulose	
Sugar	Maltose	

Sweets
  Candy
  Cake
  Cookies
  Doughnuts, sweet rolls
  Pie
  Soft drinks (e.g., sodas, sweetened fruit drinks, punch, Kool-Aid)
Other Foods
  Chips
  Pork rinds
  Fruit leather

Appendix *D*

Resource Directory

THERE ARE HUNDREDS OF organizations providing direct and indirect services to people with disabilities, but only a partial selection is given here. The list of organizations assisting pregnant women is also partial. Many organizations provide more services than are mentioned. This directory emphasizes services that would be helpful for women who are pregnant or who are considering pregnancy.

If you cannot find the resource you need in this directory, it is likely that one of the other organizations listed can make an appropriate referral. Another excellent resource is the reference librarian at your public library. Librarians are trained to locate information; they are always eager to help; and they are usually able to answer questions by telephone.

If your local telephone directory does not list a local chapter of the organization you are looking for, the national headquarters may be able to give you a referral. The services offered by local chapters may vary. If your local chapter does not meet your needs, the national affiliate may be able to refer you to a chapter in a neighboring community, or to another organization. The State Department of Rehabilitation for each state usually offers many services, including referrals to the nearest independent living center.

RESOURCE CENTERS: United States

PREGNANCY, BIRTH, AND BREAST-FEEDING INFORMATION

American Academy of Husband-Coached Childbirth
P.O. Box 5224
Sherman Oaks, CA 91413 -5224
(818)768-6662/(800) 422-4784
www.bradleybirth.com

The American Academy of Husband-Coached Childbirth was founded by Robert A. Bradley, M.D. and Marjie and Jay Hathaway, AAHCC for the purpose of making childbirth education information more readily available.

ASPO/Lamaze International

2025 M Street NW # 800
Washington, D.C. 20036
(202) 367 1128
(800) 368-4404
www.lamaze.org

The American Society for Psychoprophylaxis in Obstetrics (ASPO) promotes the Lamaze Method, trains childbirth educators, and provides referrals to local teachers.

International Caesarean Awareness Network

1304 Kingsdale Avenue
Redondo Beach, CA 90278
(800) 686-ICAN
(310) 542-6400
Fax: (310) 542-5368
info@ican-online.org
www.ican-online.org

The International Caesarean Awareness Network, Inc. (ICAN) is a nonprofit organization founded by Esther Booth Zorn in 1982. ICAN's mission is to improve maternal-child health by preventing unnecessary caesareans through education, providing support for caesarean recovery, and promoting Vaginal Birth After Caesarean (VBAC).

International Childbirth Education Association (ICEA)

P.O. Box 20048
Minneapolis, MN 55420
(952) 854-8660
(800) 624-4934 (book center order line)
www.icea.org

Among other services, ICEA offers a wide variety of publications about pregnancy, childbirth, and breast-feeding. Also operates a mail-order bookstore. Call for information or catalogs.

La Leche League International: www.lalecheleague.org
The mission of La Leche is to help mothers worldwide to breast-feed, through mother-to-mother support, encouragement, information, and education, and to promote a better understanding of breast-feeding as an important element in the healthy development of the baby and mother. See the Web site for local phone contacts around the world.

Teratogenic Society (OTIS)
(866) 626-6847
www.otispregnancy.org
Checks medication and interaction with pregnancy and breast-feeding.

Planned Parenthood National Office
434 W. 33rd Street
New York, NY 10001
(800) 230-7526 (Routing number that will refer you to the closest chapter)
(800) 829-7732 (Planned Parenthood Federation of American)
www.plannedparenthood.org
Family planning and fertility information; referrals to local service providers.

Organizations Serving Individuals with Any Type of Disability

ABLEDATA
8630 Fenton Street, Suite 930
Silver Spring, MD 20910
(800) 227-0216
TTY: (301) 608-8912
Fax: (301) 608-8958
Assistive technology.

Disabled Right Advocate (DRA)
449 15th Street, Suite 303
Oakland, California 94612
(510) 451-8644
TTY: (510)-451-8716
Fax: (510) 451-8511
www.dralegal.org
Disability Rights Advocates is a national and international nonprofit organization dedicated to protecting and advancing the civil rights of people with disabilities. Operated by, and established for people with disabilities, DRA pursues its mission through research, education, and legal advocacy.

National Easter Seal Society
230 W. Monroe Street, Suite 1800
Chicago, IL 60606
(312) 726-6200
(800) 221-6827
www.easterseals.com

Distributes a wide variety of information on rehabilitation issues for children and adults. Referrals to local chapters throughout the country for information, rehabilitation, transportation, treatment, and other services.

ODPHP National Health Information Center
P.O. Box 1133
Washington, D.C. 20013
(301) 565-416
(800) 336-4797
Fax: (301) 984-4256
www.health.gov/nhic

Identifies health information resources and provides referrals to more than 1,000 health-related information organizations. Provides directories, bibliographies, and resource guides on health-related topics.

National Council on Independent Living
1916 Wilson Boulevard, Suite 209
Arlington, VA 22201
(703) 525-3406
(877) 525-3400
TTY: (703) 525-4153
Fax: (703) 525-3409
www.ncil.org

The National Council on Independent Living (NCIL) is a membership organization that advances the independent living philosophy, and advocates for the human rights of, and services for, people with disabilities, in order to further their full integration and participation in society. NCIL offers referrals to the local independent living centers.

National Library Service for the Blind and Physically Handicapped
Library of Congress
Washington, D.C. 20542
(202) 287-5100
(800) 424-9100
www.loc.gov/nls

A free national library program for individuals who cannot use standard printed materials. The national service also develops information packets, many of which are related to technology. The library may be able to refer you to a regional library near you that can provide disability-related information.

National Rehabilitation Information Center
4200 Forbes Boulevard, Suite 202
Lanham, MD 20706
(800) 346-2742
(301) 459-5900
TTY: (301) 459-5984
naricinfo@heitechservices.com

The National Rehabilitation Information Center (NARIC) is funded by the National Institute on Disability and Rehabilitation Research of the U.S. Department of Education (NIDRR). Its library facilitates access to NIDRR and Rehabilitation Services Administration (RSA) reports, and disseminates other rehabilitation-related information. NARIC's database, REHABDATA, lists over 19,000 documents including NIDRR and RSA reports, journal articles, and commercial publications. The database and library are available to the public, and information searches and referrals may be requested.

National Association of Protection and Advocacy Systems, Inc.
900 Second Street, NE, Suite 211
Washington, D.C. 20002
(202) 408-9514
Fax: 202-408-9520
www.NAPAS.org

The Protection and Advocacy Systems and Client Assistance Programs comprise the nationwide network of congressionally-mandated, legally-based disability rights agencies.

Parents with Disabilities On-line
www.disabledparent.com

Through the Looking Glass
2198 6th Street
Berkeley CA 94710
(510) 848-1112
(800) 644-2666
www.lookingglass.org

Through the Looking Glass is the first national resource center (NRC) for parents with disabilities in the United States. TLG provides direct and indirect services, as well as providing information on custody, adoption, pregnancy and birthing, and parenting adaptation and intervention. TLG also provides training and publications for all parents with disabilities and the professionals who work with them.

Organizations Serving Individuals with Specific Disabilities

Arthritis Foundation
Research Department
1330 West Peachtree Street, Suite 100
Atlanta, GA 30309

National Arthritis Foundation
P.O. Box 96280
Washington, D.C. 20077
(800) 933-0032
www.arthritis.org
Information and referral center.

Arthrogryposis Multiplex Congenita
Avenues, National Support Group for Arthrogryposis Multiplex Congenita
c/o Mary Ann Schmidt
P.O. Box 5192
Sonora, CA 95370
(209) 928-3688
www.sonnet.com/avenues

Information exchange for individuals with AMC, their families, and interested professionals. Newsletter, bibliography of research articles, and pamphlet available. Self-help orientation.

Epilepsy Foundation of America
4351 Garden City Drive
Landover, Maryland 20785
(301) 459-370
(800) EFA-1000
(800) 322-4050 (library service)
www.efa.org

Information for people with epilepsy, their families, and the general public.
Medical library service for health care professionals contains information on clinical and psychosocial aspects of epilepsy.

Hydrocephalus
http://members.aol.com/HydroWoman

International Polio Network
4207 Lindell Boulevard, Suite 110
St. Louis, Missouri 63108-2915
(341) 534-0475
gini_intl@msn.com

Lupus Foundation of America, Inc.
2000 L Street, N.W., Suite 710
Washington, D.C. 20036
(202) 349-1155
Fax: (202) 349-1156
www.lupus.org

Information and education about lupus, including a national newsletter and referrals to local chapters for support.

Muscular Dystrophy Association USA
3300 E. Sunrise Drive
Tucson, AZ 85718
(520) 529-2000
(650) 570-6166
(800) 572-1717
www.mdausa.org

Sponsors research on a number of disorders including dystrophies, myotonia, and Friedreich's ataxia. Referrals to local chapters, which may provide services including consultation, medical follow-up, and physical therapy.

Myasthenia Gravis Foundation of America
1821 University Ave. W., Suite S256
St. Paul, MN 55104
(651) 917-6256
(800) 541-5454
Fax: (651) 917-1835
www.myasthenia.org

Research and education; support for individuals and their families.

The National Multiple Sclerosis Society
150 Grand Avenue
Oakland, CA 94612
(800) Fight MS (800-344-4867)
www.nmss.org

National Spinal Cord Injury Association

6701 Democracy Boulevard, Suite 300-9
Bethesda, MD 20817
(800) 962-9629
(301) 214-4006
Fax: 301-881-9817
www.spinalcord.org/html/contact.php

"At NSCIA, we educate and empower survivors of spinal cord injury and disease to achieve and maintain the highest levels of independence, health, and personal fulfillment. We fulfill this mission by providing an innovative Peer Support Network, and by raising awareness about spinal cord injury and disease through education. Our education programs are developed to address information and issues important to our constituency, policymakers, the general public, and the media, including injury prevention, improvements in medical, rehabilitative and supportive services, research and public policy formulation."

Paralyzed Veterans of America

801 Eighteenth Street, NW
Washington, D.C. 20006-3517
PVA National Headquarters (800) 424-8200
PVA Health Care Hotline (800) 232-1782
www.pva.org

Osteogenesis Imperfecta Foundation

804 W. Diamond Avenue, Suite 210
Gaithersburg, MD 20878
(301) 947-0083
(800) 981-2663
Fax: (301) 947-0456
www.oif.org

Spina Bifida Association

4590 MacArthur Boulevard, NW, Suite 250
Washington, DC 20007-4226
(800) 621-3141
(202) 944-3285
Fax: (202) 944-3295
sbaa@sbaa.org
www.sbaa.org

Numerous programs include information and referral service; publishes newsletter and informational pamphlets.

National Scoliosis Foundation
(800) 673-6922
NSF@scoliosis.org
www.scoliosis.org/resources/medicalupdates/scoliosisandpregnancy.php

United Cerebral Palsy Associations
1660 L Street NW Suite 700
Washington, D.C. 20036
(800) 872-5827
www.ucp.org

National federation of state and local affiliates assisting individuals with CP and their families. The national organization can refer to local affiliates. Some of the local affiliates offer medical, therapeutic and social services, advocacy, and assistance with independent living.

RESOURCES: Worldwide

Centers for Independent Living and National Associations for Independent Living
www.independentliving.org/docs3/cils.html

DAWN Ontario: DisAbled Women's Network Ontario
Box 1138 North Bay
ON P1B 8K4
http://dawn.thot.net

DAWN Ontario is a progressive, volunteer-driven, feminist organization promoting social justice, gender equality, human rights, and the advancement of equality rights of disabled women through education, research, advocacy, coalition-building, resource development, and information and communication technology.

Disability, Pregnancy & Parenthood International (DPPI)
Unit F9, 89/93 Fonthill Road
London N4 3JH
Help line: 0800 018 4730
Text: 0800 018 9949
Admin: 020 7263 3088
Fax: 020 7263 6399
www.dppi.org.uk

This is a small, UK-based registered charity that is controlled by disabled parents. DPPI promotes better awareness and support for disabled people who are already parents and their families, those who wish to become parents and their families, and also for health and social work professionals, and other individuals and organizations concerned with disability and/or pregnancy and parenting. Provides information on pregnancy and babycare equipment.

Disabled Living Foundation and Disabled Living Foundation Equipment Centre (DLF)
380-384 Harrow Road
London W9 2HU
Equipment Centre (020) 7289-6111, ext.247
www.dlf.org.uk/about/contact.php

For over 30 years, the DLF has been working for freedom, empowerment, and choice for disabled and older people, and others who use equipment or assistive technologies to enhance their independence. They are the leading UK disability charity providing advice and information on equipment and assistive technologies for independent living.

PlanetAmber
www.planetamber.com/resources/189.html

"Planet Amber is a global information source for people with health impairments, their families, and for those who provide services and support. Our database includes links related to both specific health conditions, and resources covering universal health care issues. We offer a guide to communication connections and information related to care advice, services, and adaptive products. Explore the Resources section on our Web site to find the services and products that help make life easier, and allow accessible and independent living."

Assistive Equipment and Apparel

Accessible scales by Detecto: www.detectoscale.com
Offers products such as:
   Detecto Semi-Portable Wheelchair Scale; White.
   Capacity: 500 x .2 lb and 225 kg .1 kg
   Display: 7" high-contrast LCD
   Power source: 6 "C" size batteries
   Optional power supply available: Model# 728R90
   Platform: 30" L x 30" W x 2 1/2" H
   Dimensions: 30" L x 40" W x 4 1/2" H

   SECA 664 Digital Wheelchair Scale
   The 660-pound capacity of this wheelchair scale means that even heavy patients can be weighed with ease.

Welner Accessible Exam Table
Hausmann Industries Inc.
Contact Charles Cohen
130 Union Street
Northvale, NJ 07647
(201) 767-0255, ext.29
(888) 428-7626, ext.29
Fax: (877) 368-5081 or (651) 234-1209
charliec@hausmann.com

North Coast Medical Rehabilitation Catalog
(800) 821-9319

Fred Sammons Preston Rolyan Catalog
An Abilityone corporation
P.O. Box 5071
Bolingbrook, IL 60440
(800) 323-5547
Fax: (800) 547-4333
www.sammonsprestonrolyan.com

Leading Lady Companies
24050 Commerce Park
Beachwood, OH 44122
(216) 464-5490
(800) 321-4804
Fax: (216) 464-9365
Customer Service, Accounting, Fax: (216) 464-5456
www.leadinglady.com

This company manufactures an adaptive bra that closes with Velcro™ for women with arthritis, MS, TOS, and other dexterity problems.

Medela Inc
P.O. Box 660
McHenry, IL 60051
(800) 435-8316
(815) 363-1166 (USA)
(905) 795-0288 (Canada)
www.medela.com
Manufactures Breast Pumps Hands Free™

Whisper Wear Inc.
Marietta Georgia
(770) 984-0905
www.whisperwear.com

Medtronic Co.
(800) 328-0810
(763) 505-2634
www.medtronic.com
Manufactures Baclofen Pump

Neurocontrol
(216) 378-9106, ex 107
Fax: (216) 378-9116
txmina@ndimedical.com

Markets a device for assisting with bladder, bowel, and sexual function after spinal cord injury.

American Biosystem ABI Vest
1020 West County Road F
St. Paul, MN 55126
(800) 426-4224

Manufactures respiratory aid equipment.

Organizations That Adapt Baby Care Equipment

RESNA
http://www.resna.org/index.php; (703) 524-6686

RESNA is an interdisciplinary association of people with a common interest in technology and disability. Their purpose is to improve the potential of people with disabilities and help them to achieve their goals through the use of technology. They will connect you to a person in your area.

References

1. www.etenet.com/Apps/Library/Corporate.
2. www.mayoclinic.com.
3. Csuka ME. Disabling Rheumatologic Conditions Affecting Women. In: *Welner's Guide to the Care of Women with Disabilities.* Welner S, Haselstine F, Eds. Philadelphia: Lippincott Williams & Wilkins, 2004; p. 59–63.
4. www.peds.umn.edu/divisions/neonatology/hydro.html.
5. Silver R, Branch DW. Autoimmune disease in pregnancy, systemic lupus erythematosus and antiphospholipid syndrome. *Clinics in Perinatology* 1997; 24: 291–319.
6. www.wfubmc.edu/neuro/disease/neuromuscular.shtml.
7. www.chg.duke.edu/patients/lgmd.html.
8. www.oif.org/tier2/pregnancy.htm.
9. Robinson R. Spinal cord injury. Hendrick Health System. www.ehendrick.org/healthy/001281.htm. (October 2003).
10. Selmonosky C. TOS definition. Thoracic Outlet Syndrome. www.tos–syndrome.com/newpage2.htm#TOS percent20DEFINITION. (November 2002).
11. Pedersen S. Having a baby: how pregnancy affects women with limb loss. *InMotion* 2003; 13; 5:30–33.
12. What is arthrogryposis? *Avenues.* January 1992. www.sonnet.com/avenues/pamphlet.html.
13. Winch R, Bengtson L, McLaughlin J, et al. Women with cerebral palsy: obstetric experience and neonatal outcome. *Developmental Medicine in Child Neurology* 1993; 35:974–982.
14. Kappel B, Eriksen G, Hansen KB, et al. Short stature in Scandinavian women: an obstetrical risk factor. *Acta Obstetric Gynecology Scandinavian* 1987; 66:153–158.
15. Desai P, Hazra M, Trivedi LB. Pregnancy outcome in short–statured women. *Journal of the Indian Medical Association* 1989; 87:32–43.

16. Carstoniu J, Yee I, Halpern S. Clinical reports epidural anesthesia for caesarean section in an achondroplastic dwarf. *Canadian Journal of Anaesthesia* 1992; 39:708–111.

17. Bradley NK, Liakos AM, McAllister JP, et al. Maternal shunt dependency: implications for obstetrical care, neurosurgical, and pregnancy outcomes in a review of selected literature. *Neurosurgery* 1998; 43.

18. Farine D, Jackson U, Portale A, et al. Pregnancy complicated by maternal spina bifida: a report of two cases. *Journal of Reproductive Medicine* 1988; 33; 3:323–326.

19. Bradley NK. Hydrocephalus and pregnancy: the medical implications of maternal shunt dependency. Presented at the Annual Meeting of the Society for Research into Hydrocephalus and Spina Bifida, Manchester, UK, July 1–6, 1997.

20. Confavreux C, Hutchinson M, Hours M. Rate of pregnancy–related relapse in multiple sclerosis. *New England Journal of Medicine* 1998; 339:285–291.

21. Whitaker J. An editorial comment: Effects of pregnancy and delivery on disease activity in multiple sclerosis. *New England Journal of Medicine* 1998; 339–340.

22. Adelson R. The main event. *InsideMS*, April–June 2003; 21–28.

23. Batocchi AP, Majolini L, Evoli A, et al. Course and treatment of myasthenia gravis during pregnancy. *Journal of American Academy of Neurology* 1999; 52:447–452.

24. Byrne DL, Chappatte OA, Spencer GT, et al. Pregnancy complicated by Charcot Marie–Tooth disease requiring intermittent ventilation. *British Journal of Obstetrics & Gynaecology* 1992; 99:79–80.

25. King TE. Restrictive lung disease in pregnancy. *Clinical Chest Medicine* 1992; 13:607–622.

26. Gamzu R, Shenhav M, Fainaru O, et al. Impact of pregnancy on respiratory capacity in women with muscular dystrophy and kyphoscoliosis, a case study. *Journal of Reproductive Medicine* 2002; 47(1):53–56.

27. Schoneborn SR, Glauner B, Rohrig D, et al. Obstetric aspects in women with facioscapulohumeral muscular dystrophy, limb-girdle muscular dystrophy in congenital myopathies. *Archives of Neurology* 1997; 54:888–894.

28. Ayoubi JM, et al. Vaginal delivery in a woman with limb-girdle muscular dystrophy: a case study. *Journal of Reproductive Medicine* 2000; 45:498–500.

29. Carter G, Bonckat W. Successful pregnancy in the presence of spinal muscular atrophy: two case reports. *Arch Physical Medical Rehabilitation Journal* 1994; 75: 229–231.

30. Krakow D. *OI Issues: Pregnancy Considerations for Women with OI.* OI Osteogenesis Imperfecta Foundation. August 2003. www.oif.org/tier2/pregnancy.htm2004.

31. Gyermek. *Handbook on the Late Effects of Poliomyelitis for Physicians and Survivors,* Rev. Ed. Maynard FM, Headley JL, Eds. Saint Louis, MO: Gazette International Networking Institute (GINI) 1999; p. 91.

32. Selma H. Calmes, M.D., Chief Physician of Anesthesiology at Olive View/University of California Los Angeles Medical Center, Sylmar, California and Full Professor of Anesthesia at UCLA School of Medicine in Los Angeles.

33. Ostensen M. Pregnancy in patients with a history of juvenile rheumatoid arthritis. *Arthritis Rheumatology* 1991; 34:881–887.

34. Ostensen M, Ostensen H. Ankylosis spondylitis: the female aspect. *Rheumatoid* 1998; 25:120–124.

35. Blachek J. Scoliosis and pregnancy. March 24, 2004. www.scoliosis.org/resources/medicalupdates/scoliosisandpregnancy.php.

36. Jackson A. Pregnancy and Delivery. In *Women with Physical Disabilities: Achieving and Maintaining Health and Well-Being.* Krotoski D, Nosek M, Turk M, Eds. Baltimore: Paul H. Brooks Publishing, 1995; 92–94.

37. Petri M. Pregnancy in SLE. *Bailliere's Clinical Rheumatology.* Vol.12, No. 3 August 1998; 470–471.

38. Systemic lupus erythematosus (SLE) flares during pregnancy. *Accurate Diagnosis and Treatment of Rheumatic Diseases.* January 2002. www.accurheum.com/topics/pregsle-flare.htm.

39. Meng C, Lockshin M. Pregnancy in lupus. *Current Opinion in Rheumatology* 1999; 11:348–351.

40. Ostensen M, Ramsey-Goldman R. Treatments of inflammatory rheumatic disorders in pregnancy: what are the safest treatment options? *Drug Safety* 1998; 19 (5):389–410.

41. *Parade Magazine,* March 16, 2003; 11.

42. Pharmacy Direct USA. Ovulite saliva fertility ovulation tester. www.pharmacydirectusa.com/ovulation.htm (March 2003).

43. MMWR. Division of Reproductive Health, National Center for Chronic Disease Prevention and Health Promotion, et al. Contribution of assisted reproductive technology and ovulation-inducing drugs to triplet and higher-order multiple births—United States, 1980–1997. *MMWR* June 23, 2000; 49:535–538.

44. Toms BL, Kirshbaum M. *You May be Able to Adopt: A Guide to the Adoption Process for Prospective Mothers with Disabilities and Their Partners.* National Institute on Disability Rehabilitation and Research, U.S. Department of Education Grant #H133B30076. Berkeley, CA: Through the Looking Glass, 1997; 3.

45. Grose C. Chickenpox during pregnancy: still a feared complication. Virtual Hospital. August 2003. www.vh.org/adult/provider/obgyn/chickenpox.

46 About celiac disease. Celiac Disease Foundation. www.celiac.org.

47. pregnancy.about.com/library/weekly/aa120897.htm.

48. www.diagnosticultrasound.org.uk/nuchal_translucency.

49. Toms Barker L, Maralani V. *Challenges and Strategies of Disabled Parents: Findings from a National Survey of Parents with Disabilities: Final Report 1997.* Oakland, CA: Berkeley Planning Associates.

50. Eckhardt E, Waggoner NR. *Work Simplification in the Area of Child Care for Physically Handicapped Women.* OVR Special Project 37, Summary of Final Report June 15, 1955-December 31, 1960. Conducted by the School of Home Economics, University of Connecticut.

51. Bittle, JC. Mothers with Physical Limitations: Intimate Portraits of Fifteen Women and the Challenges They Face. Unpublished Masters Thesis, California State University, Sacramento.

52. Toms Barker L, Kirshbaum M. Teenagers and their parents. [National Institute on Disability Rehabilitation and Research, U.S. Department of Education Grant#H133G990130] Berkeley, CA Through the Looking Glass, 1997.

53. Olkin R, Abrams KY. Parents with Disabilities and Their Adolescent Children Final Report. Through the Looking Glass: Berkeley, CA. Supported by a grant from the National Institute of Disability and Rehabilitation Research, US Dept. of Ed; 2003. (H133G990130–00).

54. Fields A, Fields D. *Baby Bargains: Secrets to Saving 20 Percent to 50 Percent on Baby Furniture, Equipment, Clothes, Toys, Maternity Wear and Much, Much More!* Boulder, CO: Windsor Peak Press, 2001; 2–3.

55. From an interview with Sid Wolinski, Disability Rights Advocates, Oakland, CA. March, 2002.

56. Petri M. *Pregnancy and Rheumatic Disease.* Hopkins Lupus Pregnancy Center: 1987 to 1996. 1997; 23(1), 13.

57. Robin L. Goldfadden. *Through the Maze: A Guide to Health Care and Insurance Right and Resources for Californians with Disabilities.* Disabled Rights Advocates, Public Media.

58. Compiled by Janelle Durham. Sources: Food and Nutrition Board, National Academy of Sciences. *Family-Centered Maternity and Newborn Care* by Celeste Phillips. *Pregnancy, Childbirth, and the Newborn* by Simkin, Whalley, and Keppler. "Nutrition during Pregnancy" by Jo-Ann Heslin in *Childbirth Instructor*, Spring 1993. "Teaching Nutrition" by Jo-Ann Heslin in *Childbirth Instructor*, Spring 1995.

59. Noonan P, Stout F. Age of Discovery. *USA Weekend.* Jan. 17–19, 2003; 6–7.

60. Maynard FM, Headley JL. *Handbook on the Late Effects of Poliomyelitis for Physicians and Survivors* Rev. Ed. Saint Louis MO: Gazette International Networking Institute (GINI), 1999; 61.

61. Murray MT. *Encyclopedia of Nutritional Supplements* 1996; Rocklin, CA: Prima Publishing, 1996; 173.

62. Rothman JK, Lynn PH. Teratogenicity of high vitamin A intake. *New England Journal of Medicine* 1995; 21:1369–1373.

63. Rebar, Siega-Riz, et al. Vitamin C and the risk of preterm delivery. *American Journal of Obstetric Gynecology* 2003, Aug. 189:519–525; reprinted in *Journal Watch*, Vol. 01, 23, no. 20; 161.

64. Hill M. Development: anatomy.med.unsw. (October 2001).

65. Lipson J, Rogers J. Pregnancy, birth, and disability: women's health care experiences. *Health Care for Women International* 2000; 21:11–26.

66. Maynard FM, Headley JL. *Handbook on the Late Effects of Poliomyelitis for Physicians and Survivors* Rev. Ed. Saint Louis, MO: Gazette International Networking Institute (GINI), 1999; 8.

67. Personal Communications. March 1997. Sandra Welner, MD and author.

68. E-mail correspondence from Graham H. Creasey, MD, FRCSEd Consulting Physician Spinal Cord Injury Units VA and Metro Health Medical Centers Cleveland, Ohio.

69. www.cdc.gov/node.do/id/0900f3ec80010af9. www.embryology.med.unsw.edu.

70. Haddow J, Palomaki GE, Allan WC. Maternal thyroid deficiency during pregnancy and subsequent neuropsychological development of the child. *New England Journal of Medicine* Aug. 19, 1999, v. 341.

71. www.mtsinai.on.ca/pdmg/Tests/nuchal.htm.

72. www.youngliving.com.

73. www.dictionarybarn.com/ELECTROLYTE-IMBALANCE.php.

74. Damek DM, Shuster EA. Pregnancy and multiple sclerosis. *Mayo Clinic Proceedings* 1997; 72(10):977–989.

75. Welner S. Pregnancy in Women with Disabilities. In: *Cherry and Merkatz's Complication of Pregnancy* 5th edition. Philadelphia: Lippincott Williams & Wilkins, 2000; 829–838.

76. www.hmc.psu.edu/neurosurgery/aservices/baclofen.htm.

77. Nelson JL. Ostensin M. Pregnancy and rheumatoid arthritis. *Rheumatic Disease Clinics of North America* 1997; 23:195–212.

78. www.who.int/reproductive-health/.

79. Fausett M, Branch W. Autoimmunity and pregnancy loss. *Seminars in Reproductive Medicine* 2000; 18(4): 379–392.

80. Rosen I. Medical advances that can save your life. *Parade Magazine* Jan. 11, 2004; 4–6.

81. Golbus J, McCune WJ. Lupus nephritis: Classification, prognosis, immunopathogenesis and treatment. *Rheumatic Disease Clinics of North America* 1994; 20:213–242 (as cited Khamashta M, Ruiz-Irastorza G, Hughes G. *Systemic Lupus Erythematosus Flares During Pregnancy*) p. 25.

82. Douglas A. The top ten second trimester worries. *Parents Press* March 2002; 20.

83. www.books.md/C/dic/clonus.php.

84. Moser E, Ligon KM, Singer C, et al. Botulinum toxin: A Botox therapy during pregnancy. *Neurology* 1997 March; 48 (3 Suppl 2): A399.

85. Khamashta M, Guillermo RI, Hughes G. Systemic lupus erythematosus flares during pregnancy. *Rheumatic Disease Clinics of North America* 1994; 20:213–242.

86. *Williams Obstetrics*, 21st Ed. Cunningham G, Gant NF, Leveno KJ, et al., Eds. New York: McGraw-Hill Medical Publishing Division, 2001; 104.

87. www.niddk.nih.gov/health/digest/pubs/heartbrn/heartbrn.htm.

88. *Williams Obstetrics*, 21st Ed. Cunningham G, Gant NF, Leveno KJ, et al., Eds. New York: McGraw-Hill Medical Publishing Division, 2001; 1276.

89. From printed material of two presentations at two international forums in 1997 for the Consensus Conference on Complex Hydrocephalus and Complication of Hydrocephalus. http://members.aol.com/HydroWoman/.

90. Ledbetter S. *Preparing the Perineum for Delivery: Perineum Massage.* The Birth Institute and Birth & Bonding Family Center, 1126 Solano Ave., Albany, CA 94506.

91. *Williams Obstetrics*, 21st Ed. Cunningham G, Gant NF, Leveno KJ, et al., Eds. New York: McGraw-Hill Medical Publishing Division, 2001. Quoted from Eason and Feldman OB/Gyn 95:616 "much ado about a little cut"), p. 326.

92. Napoli M. Center for Medical Consumers in New York City. 2002 Gale Group Guide to Clinical Preventive Services, 2nd Ed. Prenatal Disorder. The draft of this

chapter was prepared for the U.S. Preventive Services Task Force by Steven H. Woolf, MD, MPH, and Douglas B. Kamerow, MD, MPH. http://cpmcnet.columbia.edu/texts/gcps/gcps0050.html.

93. *Williams Obstetrics, 21st Ed.* Cunningham G, Gant NF, Leveno KJ, et al., Eds. New York: McGraw-Hill Medical Publishing Division, 2001; 1417.

94. England P, Horowitz R. *Birthing from Within*. Partners Press.

95. Water Birth at Home. *Disability Pregnancy & Parenthood International* 1999; 25:1–99.

96. Ridgeway S. Reflections on multiple sclerosis, pregnancy and childbirth. *Disability Pregnancy & Parenthood International* July 1999; 27:5.

97. ACOG committee opinion. Delivery by vacuum extraction. American College of Obstetricians and Gynecologists. *International Journal of Gynecology and Obstetrics* 1999; 64(1):96. See also #209, 1998.

98. Personal Communications. March 2000. Dr. Richard Penn, a neurosurgeon with the University of Chicago. Dr. Penn has practiced neurosurgery in Chicago for 28 years. He is well known for his research and clinical work in drug delivery to the nervous system and for surgical treatments for movement disorders. He pioneered the use of implanted drug pumps to deliver medications directly to the spinal cord, implanting the first programmable pump for cancer pain and developing a new highly successful medicine for spasticity.

99. Dietz HP, Bennett MJ. The effect of childbirth on pelvic organ mobility. *Obstetrics and Gynecology* August 2003; 102:223–228. www.aafp.org/afp/20040301/tips/28.html.

100. *Vaginal Birth after Previous Caesarean Birth*, Clinical Practice Guidelines, Policy Statement. Society of Obstetricians and Gynecologists of Canada. Dec. 2001. www.calgary-healthregion.ca/hlthconn/items/vbac.htm (April 2004).

101. Mascola M, Repke J. Obstetric management of the high-risk lupus pregnancy. *Rheumatic Disease Clinic of North America* 1997; 23:129.

102. Zweiback M. Making sure baby gets enough milk. *Parents Press* May 1999; 13–16.

103. Curtis C. Fenugreek. Breast-feeding Online. www.breast-feedingonline.com/fenugreek.shtml (March 2004).

104. Nelson LM, Franklin GM, Jones MC. Risk of multiple sclerosis exacerbation during pregnancy and breast-feeding. *JAMA* 1988; 259 (23):3441–3443.

105. Barrett JH, Brennan P, Fiddler M. Breast-feeding and postpartum relapse in women with rheumatoid and inflammatory arthritis. (American College of Rheumatology) *Arthritis & Rheumatism* 2000; [43],5:1010–1015.

106. www.niams.nih.gov/hi/topics/lupus/lupusguide/luppdf/pregncy.pdf.

107. Noda B. Successful breastfeeding, a paraplegic mother's experience. *Disability Pregnancy & Parenthood International* January 1997, 17:6–8.

108. Neifert M. Breast-feeding after surgical procedure or breast cancer. *NAACOGS Clinical Issues Perinatal Women's Health Nurse* 1992; 3 (4): 673–682.

109. Vensand K, Rogers J, Tuleja C., et al. *Adaptive Baby Care Equipment: Guidelines, Prototypes & Resources.* National Institute on Disability, Rehabilitation, and Research, U.S. Depart-

ment of Education Grant #H133G10146. Berkeley, CA: Through the Looking Glass, 2000.

110. Brazelton, TB. *Infants and Mothers: Differences in Development.* New York, NY: Dell Publishing, 1983.

111. Meyer M. Beyond the baby blues. *Parade Magazine* Oct. 13, 2002; 11 (quoting Diane Dell Assistant Professor of Obstetrics-Gynecology at Duke University).

112. Ahokas A, Aito M, and Rimon R. Positive treatment of estradiol in postpartum psychosis: a pilot study. *Journal of Clinical Psychiatry* 2000; 61:166–169.

113. Darney P. Contraceptive Choices for Women with Disabilities. In: *Welner's Guide to the Care of Women with Disabilities.* Welner S, Haselstine F, Eds. Philadelphia: Lippincott Williams & Wilkins, 2004; 126–127.

114. Frederiksen M. Depot medroxyprogesterone acetate contraception in women with medical problems. *Journal of Reproductive Medicine* 1996; 41: 414–418.

115. www.plannedparenthood.org/BIRTH-CONTROL/depoforyou.htm.

116. Drey E, Darney P. Contraceptive Choices for Women with Disabilities. In: *Welner's Guide to the Care of Women with Disabilities.* Welner S, Haselstine F, Eds. Philadelphia: Lippincott Williams & Wilkins, 2004; 120.

117. *Contraceptive Technology*; New York: Ardent Media Inc., p. 518.

Recommended Reading

Eisenberg A, Murkoff H, and Hathaway S. *What to Expect When You Are Expecting.* New York, N.Y.: Workman Publishing, 1996.

Jacobson, DS. *The Question of David: A Disabled Mother's Journey Through Adoption, Family, and Life.* Berkeley, CA.: Creative Arts Book Company, 1999.

Neville H, Johnson D. *Temperament Tools: Working with Your Child's Inborn Traits.* Seattle, WA: Parenting Press 1998. www.TemperamentTools.com.

www.ctispregnancy.org

Index

A

Abdomen, postpartum changes in, 357
Abdominal muscle
   exercises, 139–145
   stretching, 183
Abortion, 33, 62, 110
Abruptio placentae, 316
Achondroplasia, 8
Active phase of labor, 265–268
Acupressure, 285–286
Advance planning, 112–113
Advanced Respirator, 161
Advocates, 113
AFP testing, 60
Afterpains, 352
Aging fears, 36
Alcohol intake, 128
Allergies, food, 127
Amenorrhoea, 156
American Academy of Husband-Coached
   Childbirth, 216
American Society for Psychoprophylaxis
   in Obstetrics, 216
Americans with Disabilities Act (ADA),
   86, 101
Amniocentesis, 25, 60, 61–62, 110,
   197–198, 225

Amniotic band syndrome, 4, 398
Amniotomy, 272, 273–274
Amputations, 4–5, 42–43, 399, 400,
   401, 474
Analgesics during labor, 294–295
Anemia, 123, 179, 351, 356
Anesthesia
   during caesarean sections, 319–322
   during labor
      general, 299
      local, 295
      regional, 295–299
   obstetric, 104–108
      consultation with anesthesiologist,
         104–105
      diagnostic tests and, 106
      drawbacks of, 105
      pain management options, 106
      past experiences with, 104
      questions to ask, 107
      recommendations regarding, 108
Anger, 64
Ankylosing spondylitis, 49
Anti-acetylcholine receptor antibody, 46
Antibiotics, for urinary tract infections,
   159
Anxiety during labor, 293

Apgar scores, 44, 299, 303
Appendicitis, 187
Appetite changes, 176–178
Aqua Socks, 289
Archives of Physical Medicine Rehabilitation, 91
Arthrogryposis, 5, 43, 402
Asexuality perceptions, 37
Aspirin, 163
Assistive devices, 206
Athetoid cerebral palsy, 6
Atresia, 60
Augmentation of labor, 274–277
Auscultation, 278
Autoimmune disorders, 13
Autonomic dysreflexia, 27
Avonox, 162

B

Baby Bargain Secrets, 77–78
Baby blues. *See* Mood changes
Back labor, 264–265, 291–292
Back pain
    in first trimester, 183
    during labor, 291–292
    in second trimester, 203–204
    in third trimester, 240–241
Baclofen Pump, 16, 183, 313
Barrier birth control methods, 384–388
Basal ganglia damage, 10
Basal temperature increase, as sign of
        pregnancy, 157
Bathing babies, 395
Baths during labor, 288–289
Bed rest, 251
Bed transfer, 244–245
Bending, 247
Betadine, 61
Betamethasone, 252
Betaseron, 162–163, 370
Biophysical profile, 226

Birth control methods
    barrier methods, 384–388
    birth control patch, 383–384
    birth control pills, 381–383
    breast feeding as, 379–380
    cervical caps, 387
    condoms, 384–385
    contraceptive foam, 387
    contraceptive hormones, 381–384
    contraceptive sponges, 387
    Depo-Provera, 383
    diaphragms, 385–386
    intrauterine devices, 387–388
    natural methods, 379–381
    Norplant hormonal implant, 383
    reliability of, 379
    rhythm method, 380
    sterilization, 388–389
    symptothermal method, 380–381
    tubal ligation, 388–389
    vasectomy, 388
Birth control patches, 383–384
Birth control pills, 381–383
Birth plans, 222–223
Birth weight, 117
Birthing chair, 305
Bladder control, 355
Bladder infections, 120, 182, 209
Bladder problems, 159–160
Bleeding, postpartum, 353, 357–358
Blood pressure, 165, 206–207, 268
Blood tests, 165–166, 171–172
    in ectopic pregnancies, 187
    in postpartum period, 348
    second trimester, 198
Blood thinners, 163
Blood volume
    in first trimester, 175
    in third trimester, 227
Bloody show, 260
Body image, 219
Body temperature, in first trimester, 175

Boppy, 393
Botox injections, 203
Bottle feeding, 371–373
Bradley method, 216–217
Braxton-Hicks contractions, 222, 229, 259, 260, 262, 264, 294
Breads, 484–485
Breast care, in postpartum period, 349
Breast changes
    in first trimester, 175
    postpartum, 356–357
    as sign of pregnancy, 157
    in third trimester, 228
Breast examinations, in postpartum period, 348
Breast feeding, 99–100, 328
    advantages of, 360–361
    art of, 362–365
    babies positioning, 364–365
    as birth control method, 379–380
    breast care and, 361–362
    combining with bottle feeding, 371–373
    comfortable brassieres, 363
    comfortable positioning, 363–364
    decision to breast feed, 359–360
    disability factors in, 366–370
    disadvantages of, 365–366
    fatigue and, 372–373
    helping baby during, 363
    infant problems with, 371
    medication and, 369–370
    mobility issues and, 370
    releasing baby from, 365
    using alternative breasts, 365
Breast pumps, 359
Breathing problems, 160–161, 210, 230–231
Breathing techniques, 283–284, 305–307
Breech presentations, 264, 277
Bright red spotting, 260
Budget management, 78

Burping technique, 373
Buttocks discomfort, 151

C
Caesarean section
    abruptio placentae, 316
    aftereffects of, 337–338
    anesthesia during, 319–322
    cord prolapse in early labor, 316
    disability indications for, 314–315
    emotional effects of, 333–337
    false assumptions, 312–314
    fetal distress, 317
    fetal position or presentation, 316
    fetopelvic disproportions, 315
    general herpes, 317–318
    home recovery, 331–333
    hospital stay, 326–331
    incisions, 323–324
    insufficient contractions, 316
    maternal illness, 318
    maternal immunization (Rh disease), 317
    obstetric indications for, 315–318
    placenta previa, 315
    postmature fetus, 317
    preeclampsia/eclampsia, 317
    preparation for, 318–319
    previous section and, 316
    pros and cons, 311–312
    recovery, 324–326
    special concerns, 311–312
    surgical process, 322–323
    vaginal birth after, 338–339
Calcium intake, 121–122
Calcium-rich foods, 482–483
Calcium supplements, 203
Calf stretches, 146–147
Calorie requirements, 118–119
Canadian crutches, 12

Candida infections, 232
Car transfer, 246
Careers and family, 80–81
Carpal tunnel syndrome, 4, 238
Carrying baby, 391–394
Catheterization, 169–170, 208, 239–240, 270
Celexa, 163
Celiac disease, 60
Central apnea, 9
Cephalopelvic disproportion, 277
Cerclage, 213
Cereals, 484–485
Cerebral palsy, 6–8, 43–44, 182, 403–410, 474
Cervical caps, 387
Cervical changes
 in first trimester, 175
 in second trimester, 213
 in third trimester, 228–230
Cervical examination, 222
Charcot-Marie-Tooth disease, 16–17, 46, 319, 321, 428–430
Chart on labor and deliveries, 474–475
Child care help, 69–70, 73, 78
Childbirth classes, 215–217
Childcare, physical consequences of, 56–57
Childhood experiences, 64
Childproofing home, 68–69
Chin tucks, 151
Chorea gravidarum, 186
Chorionic villus sampling, 60, 110, 174
Choroid plexus tumors, 12
Chronic childhood arthritis, 12
Chronic muscle pain syndrome, 10
Circulatory system, postpartum changes in, 356
Citrucel, 209
Cleft palate, 9
Clomid, 52, 95
Clonus, 203

Coaching during labor/delivery, 279–280
Codeine, 164, 184
Coffee intake, 128129
Colace, 184
Cold flashes, 292–293
Cold prolapse, caesarean sections and, 316
Communication importance, 111–112
Community relationships, 76–77
Complete blood count, 165
Complications of pregnancy
 first trimester
  chorea gravidarum, 186
  ectopic pregnancy, 186–187
  emotional concerns, 191–194
  fetal and placental development, 190–191
  miscarriage and threatened miscarriage, 187–189
  thrombophlebitis, 189–190
 second trimester
  cervical incompetence, 213
  intrauterine growth retardation, 214–215
  miscarriage or threatened miscarriage, 213–214
  placenta previa, 214
  placental abruption, 214
  preeclampsia, 211–213
 third trimester
  disability exacerbations, 249
  gestational diabetes, 247–248
  preeclampsia/eclampsia, 248–249
Conditioning exercises, 139
Condoms, 384–385
Congenital disabilities, 59–60
Congenital hip deformity, 11–12, 416
Congenital hip dislocation, 11
Congenital hip dysplasia, 9
Congenital hydrocephalus, 12, 417

Constipation, 183–184
    exercise to relieve, 152
    iron supplements and, 161–162
    in second trimester, 209
    in third trimester, 234–235
Contraception. *See* Birth control
Contraceptive foam, 387
Contraceptive hormones, 381–384
Contraceptive sponges, 387
Contraction chart, 262
Contractions, 258–264, 261–263, 266,
        277. *See also* Braxton-Hicks
        contractions
    in third trimester, 229
Contraindication for exercise, 136
Cool Touch cushion, 241
Corticosteroids, 163
Costochondritis, 183
Costs of birth, 101
Cradle transfers, 168–169
Cramping
    abdominal muscle, 183
    leg muscle, 183
    in second trimester, 202–203
Cravings, 127, 178
Crowning, 303
Curl-ups, 141–143
Cytomegalovirus infection, 59

                    D
Daily nutritional needs, 119
Dalkon Shield, 387
Decubitus ulcer (pressure sore), 5
Deep breathing, 144
Deep vein phlebitis, 189–190
Deep vein thrombosis, 48
Degenerative disk disease, 8, 410
Dehydration, 178
Delivery. *See* Labor and delivery
Demerol, 294
Depends, 209

Depo-Provera, 377, 383
Depression, 179. *See* Postpartum
        depression
Detecto, 172
Di-Tone, 177
Diabetes, gestational, 247–248
Diabetic neuropathy, 16
Diagnostic procedures, 106
    first trimester
        blood samples, 165–166, 171–172
        chorionic villus sampling, 174
        kidney malfunction tests, 170
        lung function tests, 171
        maternal alpha fetoprotein,
            170–171
        muscle strength tests, 171
        sonography, 173–174
        systemic lupus erythematosus, 171
        urine samples, 165, 172
    routine during labor/delivery
        cathetrization, 270
        internal examination, 268
        intravenous lines, 269–270
        pulse and blood pressure, 268
    second trimester
        amniocentesis, 197–198
        blood tests, 198
        fetal echocardiography, 197
        sonography, 196–197
        stress and non-stress tests, 198
    special during labor/delivery
        external monitoring, 270–272
        fetal scalp blood sampling, 273
        internal monitoring, 272
        ultrasound, 273
    third trimester, 225–227
Diapers, 394–395
Diaphragmatic hiatus, 233
Diaphragms, 385–386
Diastasis recti, 357
Diastrophic dysplasia, 9
Diet, in postpartum period, 348–349

Dietary changes, for morning sickness, 176–177

Digestive tract, postpartum changes in, 355–356

Dilation, 229

Diplegic cerebral palsy, 95

Disability health care specialists, 77

Disability indications for caesarean birth, 314–315

Disabled child, possibilities of having, 57–63

Discectomy, 8

Discharge, 222

Discomforts of pregnancy, 55–56, 463–473

  first trimester, 175–185
    abdominal muscle stretching/cramping, 183
    back pain, 183
    change in appetite, 176–178
    constipation, 183–184
    faintness, 180–181
    fatigue, 178–181
    headaches, 184
    leg muscle cramps, 183
    nausea, 176–178
    nosebleeds, 184
    urinary problems, 181–182
  second trimester, 201–211
    back pain, 203–204
    breathing problems, 210
    constipation, 209
    cramps, 202–203
    disability-specific complications, 211
    dizziness, 206–207
    edema, 210–211
    faintness, 206–207
    heartburn, 210
    mobility difficulties, 204–206
    muscle spasms, 203
    nasal congestion, 210
    urinary difficulties, 207–209

  third trimester
    back and leg pain, 240–241
    breathing difficulties, 230–231
    constipation, 234–235
    edema, 236–238
    headaches, 239
    heartburn, 232–234
    hemorrhoids, 235–236
    joints, 230
    mobility difficulties, 242–244
    painful or tingling hands, 238–239
    personal hygiene, 235
    sleeplessness, 241–242
    unusual problems, 230
    urinary problems, 239–240
    vaginitis, 231–232
    varicose veins, 236

Discrimination, 71, 84

Distal spinal muscular atrophy, 17

Ditropan, 182

Dizziness, in second trimester, 206–207

Doctors. *See also* Health care needs; Obstetrician; Office visits
  caesarian delivery by, 93
  on call, 95
  evaluation of, 86
  genetic counseling referrals, 93–94
  handling labor and delivery, 93
  handling unusual symptoms, 92–93
  interviewing, 87–89
  knowledge of disability, 90–91
  obstetrician and primary doctor relationship, 92
  office accommodations, 86–87
  questions for, 88, 89–94, 348–349
  unavailability and, 224
  when to call, 224

Doppler, 172–173

Doula, 279–280

Down's syndrome, 59, 61, 62, 174, 197

Doxycycline, 163
Dressing babies, 395
Dry mouth, 292
Dwarfism, 8–9, 44, 249, 320, 392,
    411–412, 474
Dysfunctional labor, 265
Dysreflexia, 170, 211, 258, 264,
    275–276
Dystocia, 265
Dystonia, 10, 413
Dystrophic dwarfism, 44

                    E
Early Care, 393
Early childhood, 73–74
Eating during labor, 281–282
Eclampsia, 248–249, 317. *See also*
    Preeclampsia
Ectopic pregnancy, 186–187
Edema, 210–211, 236–238
Effleurage, 286
Egg crate mattress, 291
Electrocardiograms, 106
Embolism, 236
Embrel, 162
Emotional aspects of parenting, 70
Emotional changes, postpartum,
    374–379
Emotional concerns
    first trimester, 191–194
    second trimester, 217–220
    third trimester, 254–256
Emotional effects of caesarean birth,
    333–337
Emotional reactions during delivery, 302
Emotional stress in postpartum period,
    350
Emotional support, 79–80
Empty calorie foods, 129
Endomyometritis, 347
Enemas, 282

Epidural anesthesia, 44, 106, 295–299,
    320–321
Epidural button, 298
Episiotomies, 250, 308, 354
Equinas valgus, 9
Equipment, baby, 390–391. *See also*
    Resource centers
Estrogen replacement therapy, 377
Exercises
    abdominal and lower back muscles,
        139–145
        curl-ups, 141–143
        deep breathing, 144
        leg lifts, 143
        pelvic tilts, 140–141
        pubococcygeal muscle
            strengthening, 144–145
    assisted, 133
    balanced program, 132–133
    conditions requiring restrictions of,
        137
    for constipation relief, 152
    contraindications for, 136
    general conditioning, 139
    importance of, 132
    informal, 137–138
    during labor, 282–283
    maximum heart rates during, 136
    negative experiences and, 134–135
    relaxation exercises, 150–152
        buttocks, 151
        feet, 151
        neck, 151–152
    safety guidelines, 133–135
    stretching, 145–150
        calf stretches, 146–147
        inner thigh stretches, 147–148
        low back stretches, 146
        seated trunk flexion, 146
        upper body stretches, 148–150
        upper limb stretches, 150

Exercises (*continued*)
   unassisted, 133
   wrist exercises, 150
   yoga, 138
Expectations, examining, 72

F

Facioscrapulohumeral muscular
   dystrophy, 46
Faintness, 180–181, 206–207
Falling fear, 35, 243
Familial spastic paresis, 6
Family planning. *See* Birth control
Father/partner attending birth, 100. *See
   also* Coaching
Fatigue, 42, 178–181, 350–352,
   372–373
Fears, 33, 37–38, 57–63, 256
Feeding schedules, 99
Feldenkreis method, 131
Fertility considerations, 51–52, 94–95
Fetal alcohol syndrome, 128
Fetal development
   in first trimester, 190–191
   in second trimester, 211
   in third trimester, 254
Fetal distress, 278–279, 317
Fetal echocardiography, in second
   trimester, 197
Fetal heart rate monitoring, 100,
   270–271, 272
Fetal movement, in second trimester,
   199–200
Fetal position, caesarean sections and,
   316
Fetal scalp blood sampling, 273
Fetopelvic disproportion, 93, 277, 315
Fever, 359
Fibromyalgia, 10, 186, 414
Fibrositis, 10
Financial considerations, 77–78

First trimester of pregnancy
   complications, 186–190
   disability issues, 159–162
   discomforts, 175–185
   emotional concerns, 191–194
   fetal and placental development,
      190–191
   initial signs and symptoms, 156–158
   medications, 162–165
   office visits, 158–159
   physical changes, 174–175
   physical examination, 165–170
   pregnancy and disability interaction,
      185–186
   special diagnostic tests, 170–174
Flashes, 292–293
Fluid intake, 120, 184, 234
Fluid leakage, 261
Foley catheter, 208, 270
Folic acid, 161
Food allergies, 127
Food guides, 479–490
Foot massage, 151
Forceps extraction, 277, 307
Forms, keeping copies of, 112
Freestanding birth centers, 101
Friedreich's ataxia, 17–18, 47, 430–431
Front packs, 391–394
Fruits and vegetables, 487–489
Furniture, baby, 390–391

G

General anesthesia
   in caesarean sections, 321–322
   during labor, 299
   recovery from, 325
Generic medications, 129
Genetic conditions, 59–60
Genetic counselors, 58, 59, 62, 93–94,
   109–111
Genetic testing, 60, 198

Genital herpes, 317–318
German measles, 165
Gestational diabetes, 201, 247–248
Glial scar formation, 14
Grains, 484–485
Grand mal seizures, 15

H
Hair changes, 184–185
Hairy nevus, 24
Hands, painful or tingling, 238–239
Head rolls, 151–152
Headaches, 184, 239, 264
Health care needs
  accommodations
    at doctor's office, 86–87
    at hospital, 97–98
  doctor evaluation, 86
  doctor's partners, 95–96
  fertility considerations, 94–95
  genetic counselors, 109–111
  home births, 101–104
  hospitals, 96–97
  interviewing doctors, 87–89
  mobility equipment, 114
  obstetric anesthesia, 104–108
  obstetrician selection, 83–86
  perinatologists, 108–109
  physical examinations, 94
  preauthorizations, 114
  questions about hospital services,
    98–101
  questions for doctors, 89–94
  support you need, 111–113
Health insurance, 77–78
Health Management Organizations
  (HMO), 85, 89
Heart rate during exercise, 136
Heart rate tests, 172
Heartburn, 210, 232–234
Hemorrhoids, 235–236, 356

Herbal tea, 128–129
Hernia, 233
High quadriplegia, 27
Hip dislocation, 11
Hip dysplasia, 11, 416
Hip dysplegia, 11, 415
Hitchhiker's thumb, 9
HIV-antibody tests, 165–166
Home births, 101–104
  convenience of, 103
  distance from hospital and, 103–104
  emergency equipment, 103
  midwives, 103
  reasons for, 102
  safety of, 102
Home pregnancy tests, 158
Home recovery, from caesarean section,
  331–333
Homework, 75
Hospitals
  birth-related services offered, 98
  breast feeding, 100
  care in postpartum period, 343–346
  costs, 101
  father's presence during birth, 100
  feeding schedules, 99
  fetal monitoring, 100
  intravenous needles, 100
  length of stay in, 98–99
  policies of, 96–97
  questions about services, 98–101
  reasonable accommodations at,
    97–98
  registered nurses, 98
  rooming-in, 99
  sibling visits, 100
  stay for caesarean sections, 326–331
Hot flashes, 292–293
Human chorionic gonadotropin, 157
Hydramnios, 214
Hydrocephalus, 44–45
Hydroxy-apatite, 122

Hydroxychloroquine, 51
Hyperemesis gravidarum, 177–178
Hyperreflexia, 27
Hypertension, pregnancy-induced, 51
Hypnosis, 287–288
Hypoxia, 214, 276

I

ICD 9 Codebook, 95
Ideal mother concept, 71–72
Idiopathic scoliosis, 49
Ileostomy, 61
Ileostomy bags, 208
Immunizations, 59
Incisions, caesarean, 323–324
Incontinence, 355
Induction of labor, 274–277
Infants, 72–73
Infections, postpartum, 358–359
Inner thigh stretches, 147–148
Insomnia, 376
Insufficient contractions, 277, 316
Intercostal muscles, 149
Intercostal stretches, 149
Internal examination during labor, 268
Intrauterine asphyxia, 44
Intrauterine birth control devices,
    387–388
Intrauterine growth retardation, 214–215
Intravenous immunoglobulin, 15
Intravenous lines, 269, 330
Intravenous needles, 100
Involution, 352
Iodine intake, 121
Iron intake, 122–123
Iron supplements, 234

J

Joint discomfort in third trimester, 230
Jump starting contractions, 275

Juvenile chronic polyarthritis, 12
Juvenile rheumatoid arthritis, 12–13, 49,
    418–421, 474

K

K-Y Jelly, 354
Kegel exercises, 144, 209
Kidney function in third trimester, 249
Kidney function tests, 170, 198
Kidney infections, 181, 208
Kidney problems, 159–160
Kidney stones, 182
Kyphoscoliosis, 46, 160

L

La Leche League, 337, 371
Labor and delivery
    active phase of labor, 265–268
    amniotomy in, 273–274
    anxiety about, 293
    apgar test, 303
    back labor, 264–265, 291–292
    backache, 291–292
    breathing techniques, 283–284,
        305–307
    breech presentation, 264
    comfortable position during delivery,
        304–305
    complications, 277–279
    coping with labor discomforts, 279
    delivery of baby, 299–303
    delivery of placenta, 308
    dry mouth or thirst, 292
    dysfunctional labor, 265
    early phase of labor, 259–265
    eating during labor, 281–282
    enemas, 282
    episiotomy, 308
    fetal distress, 278–279
    fetal scalp blood sampling, 273

fetopelvic or cephalopelvic disproportion, 277
forceps delivery, 307
hot and cold flashes, 292
induction and augmentation of labor, 274–277
insufficient contractions, 277
internal monitoring, 272
labor kit, 280
medication, 309
mild exercise and, 282–283
muscle cramps, 292
nausea, 292
nonpharmaceutical pain reduction, 299
pain relief, 294–299
perineum massage and, 250
phases of, 257
placenta previa, 278
post-term pregnancy, 253
postpartum stage, 309
precipitate labor, 265
preeclampsia, 277
premature placental separation, 278
preparing for, 249–250
preterm, 250–253
relaxation methods, 284–291
role of coach in, 279–281
routine diagnostic procedures, 268–270
signs and symptoms of, 258–259
sleepiness, 293
special diagnostic procedures, 270–273
transition phase of labor, 266–268
ultrasound during, 273
umbilical cord compression, 278
urge to push, 293–294
vacuum extraction, 307
Labor kit, 280
LaMaze method, 216–217
Laminectomy, 8
Laparoscopy, 37

Latent labor, 257
Leg lifts, 143
Leg pain, 240–241
Lightening, 229–230
Limb-girdle dystrophy, 18, 47, 432–434
Local anesthesia during labor, 295
Lofstram crutches, 12
Lomotil, 209
Long labors, 229
Lordosis (swayback), 5
Love relationships, 36. *See also* Marital relationships; Sexual relationships
Low back stretches, 146
Low blood pressure, 206–207
Lower back muscle exercises, 139–145
Lower limb amputation, 42–43
Lung function tests, 171
Lupus. *See* Systemic lupus erythematosus

M

Maalox, 233
Magnesium intake, 123
Magnetic resonance imaging (MRI), 106
Malignant tumors, 29
March of Dimes, 109
Marital relationships, 78–79. *See also* Love relationships
Massage, 250, 285–286
Maternal alpha fetoprotein tests, 170–171
Maternal illness, caesarean sections and, 318
Maternal immunization, caesarean sections and, 317
Maternal serum AFP, 60
Meconium in amniotic fluid, 278
Medical advice, doctor, 53–54
Medical issues in first trimester, 159–161
Medical procedures in third trimester
amniocentesis, 225–226
Rh antibody treatment, 225

Medical procedures in third trimester
(*continued*)
sonography, 226
stress and non-stress tests, 226–227
Medications
during breast feeding, 369–370
classifications, 42
for morning sickness, 177
in postpartum period, 349
in preterm labor, 252
Meningeal membrane, 24
Meningocele, 24
Meningomyocele, 24
Menstruation, 156
Midwives, 103
Migraines, 184
Milex Dilators, 314
Milk products, 482
Mineral intake
calcium and phosphorus, 121–122
iodine, 121
iron, 122–123
magnesium, 123
sodium, 121
zinc, 124
Mirrors in cathetrization, 208
Miscarriage
in first trimester, 187–189
accidents and, 187–188
disabilities and, 187–188
emotions and, 189
reasons for, 187
symptoms of, 188–189
threatened miscarriage, 188
in second trimester, 213–214
Mixed cerebral palsy, 6
Mobility difficulties, 39, 42
in second trimester, 204–206
in third trimester, 242–244
Mobility equipment, 42, 114
Mobility loss, 117
Monitoring rate of contractions, 271

Mood changes
postpartum, 374–377
sexual relationships and (*See* Sexual
relationship)
Morning sickness, 156, 176–178
Motrin, 164
Moving baby, 391–394
Mullerian anomaly, 6
Multifactorial conditions, 59–60
Multiple sclerosis, 14–16, 45, 179, 186,
312, 352, 367, 424–427, 474
Muscle cramps during labor, 292
Muscle spasms, 203, 302
Muscle strength tests, 171
Muscular dystrophy, 16, 18
Music during labor, 288
Myasthenia gravis, 16, 19, 46, 249, 251,
326, 352, 367, 434
Myopathic arthrogryposis, 5

N

Nasal congestion, 210
Natural births. *See* Homebirths
Nausea, 156–157, 176–178, 292
Neck and shoulder massage, 152
Neck exercises, 151–152
Neck side bending exercise, 152
Neck stretch, 152
Neonatal lupus, 51
Neural tube defects, 50
Neurogenic (spastic) bladder, 24
Neurologic disability, 107
Neuromuscular dysfunction, 46–51
Neurontin, 162
Newborns' and Mothers' Health
Protection Act, 97
Nipple soreness, 349
Nisentil, 295
Non-stress tests, 198, 226–227
Nondairy products, 483
Nonpharmaceutical pain reduction, 299

Nonprescription medications, 129
Norplant hormonal implants, 383
Nosebleeds, 184
Nuchal translucency, 62, 173–174
Nursing care, in postpartum period, 345–346
Nutrition
  allergies, 127
  calorie requirements, 118–119
  cravings, 127
  daily needs, 119
  finding right balance, 125
  fluids, 120
  minerals, 121–124
  in postpartum period, 351
  proteins, 120
  special concerns, 115–116
  vegetarian diets, 125–127
  vitamins and minerals, 118, 124–125
  weight gain, 116–118

O

Obstetricians
  finding, 85–86
  selecting, 83–84
Obstructive apnea, 9
Occupational therapy, 68–69, 116, 346
Office visits
  first trimester
    concluding, 173
    family medical history, 158
    gynecological history, 158
    medications, 162–165
    personal medical history, 158
    physical examination (*See* Physical examination)
    social history, 159
  postpartum period, 347–350
  second trimester, 195–196
  third trimester, 221–225
On-Q, 324

Ortho Evra, 383–384
Osteogenesis imperfecta, 20, 47, 59, 436–437, 475
Ovulite, 51
Oxycontin, 162
Oxytocin, 352–353, 358

P

Pack-N-Ride, 392
Pain management options, 106
Pain relief
  during labor/delivery
    analgesics and sedatives, 294–295
    anesthetics, 295–299
    nonpharmaceutical pain reduction, 299
  post-caesarean, 328–329
Paracervical block, 295
Parenthood
  arranging for help, 69–70
  attitudes towards, 6768
  combining career and family, 80–81
  community relationships, 76–77
  early childhood issues, 73–74
  emotional aspects of, 70
  emotional support during, 79–80
  financial considerations, 77–78
  ideal mother concept, 71–72
  infant issues, 72–73
  marital relationships and, 78–79
  occupational therapist role, 68–69
  personal qualities and, 72
  school-aged children issues, 74–75
  teenager issues, 75–76
Pediatrician selection, 225
Pelvic examination, 166–167
Pelvic tilts, 140–141
Perinatologists, 87, 108–109
Perineum examination, in postpartum period, 348
Perineum massage, 250

Perineum tears, 354
Peristalsis, 234
Personal hygiene, 235
Phenobarbital, 295
Phlebitis, 28
Phosphorous intake, 121–122
Physical changes
    in first trimester, 174–175
    in second trimester, 199–200
    in third trimester, 227–230
Physical examination
    first trimester
        blood tests, 165–166
        catheterization, 169–170
        diagnostic tests (See Diagnostic tests)
        dysreflexia during, 170
        finding comfortable position, 169
        heart rate, 172–173
        pelvic examination, 166–167
        routine, 165
        transferring issues, 167–169
        weight, 172
    postpartum period
        blood tests, 348
        breast examination, 348
        calves examination, 348
        perineum examination, 348
        rectal examination, 348
        routine checkup, 347–348
        vagina and uterus examination, 348
Physical stress, 57
Pitocin, 276
Pivot transfers, 168
Placenta, retained, 358
Placenta previa, 214, 278, 315
Placental abruption, 214
Placental delivery, 308–309
Placental development in first trimester,
    190–191
Planned Parenthood, 88
Plantar fasciitis, 8
Plasmapheresis, 199

PortaPak, 392
Positioning. See also Comfortable positioning
    during delivery, 303–305
    during labor, 289–291
Post-dural puncture headache, 321
Post-polio syndrome, 21–22, 48,
    438–440, 475
Post-term pregnancy, 253
Posterior presentations, 277
Postmature fetus, caesarean sections and,
    317
Postpartum depression, 375–377
Postpartum period
    abdominal changes in, 357
    bathing babies, 395
    birth control methods (See Birth
        control)
    bleeding in, 357–358
    breast changes in, 356–357
    breast feeding in (See Breast feeding)
    burping techniques, 373
    carrying and moving baby, 391–394
    changing diapers, 394–395
    circulatory changes in, 356
    combining breast and bottle feeding,
        371–373
    complications, 357–359
    digestive system changes in, 355–356
    disability related factors in, 366–370
    dressing babies, 395
    emotional changes, 373–374
    fatigue in, 350–352
    furniture and equipment, 390–391
    hospital care, 343–346
    infections in, 358–359
    leaving hospital, 347
    limitation issues, 370–371
    mood changes, 374–377
    office visits, 347–350
    sexual relationships in, 377–379
    urinary tract changes in, 355
    uterine contractions in, 352–353

vaginal changes in, 353–354
weight loss, 350
Preauthorization, insurance, 114
Prednisone, 164
Preeclampsia, 211–212, 238, 248–249,
    277, 317
Preferred Provider Organizations (PPO),
    85
Pregnancy
    best possible outcome, 3
    having more then one child, 64
    making primary concern, 2
    positive approach to, 1–2
    team approach to, 2–3
Pregnancy-induced hypertension, 51
Pregnancy tests, 157–158
Premature placental separation, 278
Presentation of fetus, 221–222
Pressure sores, 120, 161
Preterm labor, 250–253
Prilosec, 233
Primrose oil, 229
Prodromal labor, 257
Progressive relaxation, 285
Prolapsed uterus, 145
Prostaglandins to shorten labor, 229
Protein foods, 480–481
Protein requirements, 120
Proteinuria, 198, 211–212
Proximal focal femoral deficiency, 11
Prozac, 162
Pseudomonas infection, 209
Psychogenic rheumatism, 10
Pubococcygeal muscle exercises, 144–145
Pudendal block, 295
Pulse monitoring during labor, 268
Pyelonephritis, 181

Q

Quadriparesis, 28
Quadriplegia, 27, 39

R

Radicular pain, 25, 201–202
Rebelliousness in teenagers, 75
Recovery from caesarean sections,
    324–326
Rectal examination, in postpartum
    period, 348
Reflux, 232–234
Regional anesthesia
    in caesarean sections, 319–322
    during labor, 295–299
Registered nurses, 98
Reglan, 369
Rehabilitation, in postpartum period,
    349
Relaxation exercises, 150–152
Relaxation methods, 284–285
Relaxation techniques, 184
Remission of symptoms, 38
Resource centers
    any type of disability, 493–495
    assistive equipment and apparel,
        500–502
    baby care equipment, 502
    pregnancy, birth, and breast-feeding,
        491–493
    serving specific disabilities, 496–400
    worldwide, 499–500
Restrictions on exercise, 137
Retained placenta, 358
Rh antibody treatment, in third trimester,
    225
Rh disease, caesarean sections and, 317
Rh type, 165
Rheumatoid arthritis, 22–23, 49, 185,
    206, 440–442
Rhythm birth control method, 380
Rollator, 282, 305
Rolling boards, 291
Rooming-in, 99, 346
Rubella (German measles), 165
Ruptured membranes, 261

S

Sacral agenesis, 23–24, 442
Saddle block, 298–299
Safety guidelines for exercise, 135
Salt, 121
Sara's Ride, 393
School-aged children, 74–75
School issues with teenagers, 75
Sciatica, 241
Scoliosis, 49–50, 277, 298
Seabands, 177
Seated trunk flexion, 146
Seconal, 294
Second trimester of pregnancy
    childbirth classes, 215–217
    complications, 211–215
    diagnostic tests, 196–198
    discomforts, 201–211
    emotional concerns, 217–220
    fetal development, 211
    medical procedure, 199
    office visits, 195–196
    physical changes, 199–200
Sedatives during labor, 294–295
Self-esteem, 71
Self-examination of feelings, 35–36
Self-image, 36–37
Sexual activity, in third trimester, 224
Sexual relationship, 79, 254–255, 348,
        377–379. *See also* Birth control
        methods; Love relationships
Shower chairs, 289
Showers, 245
Shunt occlusion, 45
Shunts, 44–45
Sibling visitation in hospital, 100
Sickle cell anemia, 59
Sitting to standing, 244
Skin changes, 184–185, 228
Sleep loss, 57, 241–242, 250
Sleep position, 241–242

Smoking, 127–128
Social disapproval, 33
Sodium intake, 121
Sonography
    in ectopic pregnancies, 187
    in first trimester, 173–174
    in second trimester, 196–197
    in third trimester, 226
    in threatened miscarriages, 188
Spacing children, 65
Spastic cerebral palsy, 6
Spina bifida, 24–26, 50, 59–60, 443–447
Spinal anesthesia, in caesarean sections,
        320–321
Spinal cord dysfunction, 107, 229,
        263–264, 267, 475
Spinal cord injury, 26–29, 29–30, 50,
        251, 252–253, 267, 368,
        448–459
Spinal deformities, 298
Spinal muscular atrophy, 19–20, 47,
        435–436
Spinal tumor, 459–460
Spondyloepiphyseal dysplasia congenita,
        9, 413
Spotting, 224, 260
Sterilization, 95, 388–389
Still's disease, 12
Stopwatch, 281
Streptococcal infections, 221
Stress, 57
Stress incontinence, 209
Stress tests, 198, 226–227
Stretch marks, 228, 357
Stretching exercises, 145–150, 203
Strollers, 393–394
Suboccipital release, 152
Supplements, impact of pregnancy,
        176–177
Support, 111–113, 255
Supraclavicular tenderness, 30

Suprapubic catheter, 27
Surgery. *See* Caesarean sections
Sweets, 490
Swelling, 236–238
Symptothermal birth control method, 380–381
Systemic lupus erythematosis, 13–14, 50–51, 171, 188, 212, 251, 312, 314, 349, 352, 367–368, 377, 382, 421–423, 474

T

Tachycardias, 207
Tay Sachs disease, 59
Tea intake, 128–129
Teasing children, 74
Teenagers, 75–76
Temperature, 165
Tendonitis, 8
Tension myalgias, 10
Thirst during labor, 292
Thoracic outlet syndrome, 30–31, 461–462, 475
Threatened miscarriage, 187–189
Thromboembolism, 190
Thrombophlebitis, 189–190
Through the Maze, 96–97
Thyroid function tests, 166
Thyroxine, 121
Toco transducer, 271
Touch relaxation, 286
Transabdominal ultrasound, 62
Transcutaneous electrical nerve stimulation (TENS), 299
Transferring issues
  bed transfer, 244–245
  car transfer, 246
  cradle transfers, 168–169
  in physical examinations, 167–169
  pivot transfers, 168

points of discussion, 168
in second trimester, 205–206
shower or tub, 245
sitting to standing, 244
Transition stage of labor, 266–268
Transitional tasks, 391
Transvaginal ultrasound, 62
Trichomonas infections, 232
Tubal ectopic pregnancy, 187
Tubal ligation, 388–389
Tubs, 245
Tylenol, 164, 184

U

Ultrasound, 61, 62, 110, 173–174, 273
Ultrasound transducer, 271
Umbilical cord compression, 278
Unplanned pregnancies, 35
Unusual symptoms, 92–93
Upper body stretches, 148–150
Upper limb stretches, 150
Urge to push, 293–294
Urinary catheter, 329–330
Urinary difficulties, 181–182, 207–209, 239–240
Urinary tract, postpartum changes in, 355
Urinary tract infections, 159, 164, 181, 252
Urine tests, 165, 172
Urispas, 209
Urostomy, 26
Uterine bleeding, 357–358
Uterine contraction strength, 272
Uterine rupture, 301
Uterus
  changes in first trimester, 175
  changes in third trimester, 228–230
  examination in postpartum period, 348
  postpartum changes in, 352–353

V

Vacuum extraction, 277, 307
Vagina
   changes in first trimester, 175
   examination in postpartum period,
     348
   postpartum changes in, 353–354
Vaginal birth after caesarean section,
   338–341
Vaginitis, 231–232
Valium, 164
Valsalva maneuver, 305307
Variations in early labor, 264–265
Varicose veins, 236
Vasectomy, 388
Vegetarian diets, 125–127
Ventriculoatrial shunts, 44
Ventriculoperitoneal shunts, 44
Vertex presentation, 264
Visualization techniques, 286–287
Vital capacity measurement, 161
Vitamin A, 124
Vitamin B, 124–125
Vitamin C, 124
Vitamin C-rich foods, 486–487
Vitamin D, 125
Vitamin E, 124
Vomiting, 177–178

W

Warm showers during labor, 288–289
Water breaking, 260
Weight gain, 116–118, 165, 172, 201.
   See also Nutrition
Weight loss, in postpartum period, 350
Werdnig-Hoffman spinal muscular
   atrophy, 19
Wheelchairs, 42, 243–244, 393
Wrist exercises, 150
Wrist extension bilateral, 150
Wrist flexion, 150

X

X-rays, 106

Y

Yoga, 138

Z

Zinc intake, 124
Zofran, 177
Zoloft, 163